# Lu's Basic Toxicology

## Fundamentals, Target Organs, and Risk Assessment

Seventh Edition

# Lu's Basic Toxicology

## Fundamentals, Target Organs, and Risk Assessment

### Seventh Edition

Edited by

Byung-Mu Lee
Sam Kacew
Hyung Sik Kim

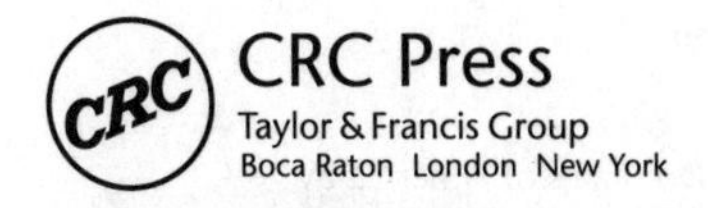


CRC Press is an imprint of the
Taylor & Francis Group, an **informa** business

CRC Press
Taylor & Francis Group
6000 Broken Sound Parkway NW, Suite 300
Boca Raton, FL 33487-2742



CRC Press is an imprint of Taylor & Francis Group, an Informa business



Printed on acid-free paper

International Standard Book Number-13: 978-1-138-03235-4 (Paperback); 978-1-138-08927-3 (Hardback)



**Library of Congress Cataloging-in-Publication Data**

Names: Byung-Mu Lee, author. | Kacew, Sam, author. | Kim, Hyung Sik, 1966- author. | Lu, Frank C. Basic toxicology.
Title: Lu's basic toxicology : fundamentals, target organs, and risk assessment / Byung-Mu Lee, Sam Kacew, Hyung Sik Kim.
Other titles: Basic toxicology
Description: Seventh edition. | Boca Raton : CRC Press, [2018] | Includes bibliographical references and index.
Identifiers: LCCN 2017010684| ISBN 9781138089273 (hardback : alk. paper) | ISBN 9781138032354 (paperback) | ISBN 9781315391700 (ebook) | ISBN 9781315391694 (ebook) | ISBN 9781315391687 (ebook) | ISBN 9781315391670 (ebook)
Subjects: LCSH: Toxicology.
Classification: LCC RA1211 .L8 2017 | DDC 615.9--dc23
LC record available at https://lccn.loc.gov/2017010684

**Visit the Taylor & Francis Web site at**
**http://www.taylorandfrancis.com**

**and the CRC Press Web site at**
**http://www.crcpress.com**

Printed and bound in the United States of America by
Edwards Brothers Malloy on sustainably sourced paper

# Contents

**Section II: Testing procedures for nontarget organ toxicities**



**Section III: Target organs and systems**

# Preface

Toxicology is an important life science. It is valuable in the protection of public health hazards associated with toxic substances in food, air, and water. It also provides a sound basis for formulating measures to protect the health of workers against toxicants in factories, farms, mines, and other occupational environments. Toxicology has played and will continue to play a significant role in the health and welfare of the world. Cognizant of the importance of toxicology, the World Health Organization (WHO) organized a toxicology training course in China in 1982, as part of the ongoing China–WHO collaborative program on medical sciences. The founding author (FCL) was invited to lectures on basic toxicology. The first edition of this book originated from those lecture notes.

Over the years, a number of important developments have occurred in toxicology. Furthermore, some readers of the book have suggested that discussions on a few groups of important chemicals and toxicants would not only provide some general knowledge of these substances, but also facilitate a deeper appreciation of the various aspects of toxicology. The book has received worldwide acceptance, as evidenced by its repeated editions and reprintings, and by the appearance of six foreign language versions (Chinese, French, Indonesian, Italian, Spanish, and Taiwan Chinese).

This new edition, prepared by invited scientists, has been further updated and expanded to include new chapters on clinical toxicology, chemicals and children, reproductive toxicology, and systems toxicology. There are chapters on lactation and occupational toxicology, as well as a chapter section describing the symptomatology of Gulf War syndrome and the probable toxicants implicated. The other chapters have been updated and expanded, notably those on the history of toxicology, carcinogenesis, mutagenesis, toxicology of organ systems—skin, liver, kidney, immune, and nanoparticle, endocrine, and safety/risk assessment. However, details of some toxicity tests have been abbreviated to keep the size of the book within bounds; the retained material is intended to portray more clearly the effects of toxicants.

It is hoped that these additions and updates will enhance the usefulness of the book. In making these changes, the authors have kept in mind the broad aim of the first edition, namely, a relatively comprehensive coverage of the subjects and brevity, thereby continuing to serve as an updated introductory text for toxicology students and for those involved in allied sciences who require a background in toxicology. Further, since toxicology is a vast and rapidly expanding subject, the book is likely to be useful to those who have become specialized in one or a few areas in toxicology, but wish to become more familiar in other areas. The extensive chemical index and subject index will facilitate the retrieval of specific topics.

**Byung-Mu Lee**
**Sam Kacew**
**Hyung Sik Kim**

# Editors

**Byung-Mu Lee, BS, MS, MSPH, Dr PH,** Division of Toxicology, College of Pharmacy, Sungkyunkwan University, South Korea, is associate editor of the *Journal of Toxicology and Environmental Health, Part A*; associate editor of *Food and Chemical Toxicology*; editorial board member of *Environmental Health Perspectives*; and advisory editor of *Archives of Toxicology*. He is currently the vice president of the International Association of Environmental Mutagenesis and Genomics Society (IAEMGS). He is the author of 230 papers and reviews, the *Encyclopedia of Environmental Health*, and 11 book chapters, as well as the coauthor of *Lu's Basic Toxicology*, Sixth Edition (Informa, 2013).

Prof. Lee has also been a research advisor of the Ministry of Food and Drug Safety, a committee advisor for the Ministry of Science, ICT, and Future Planning, the Ministry of Environment, and the Ministry of Human Health and Welfare in South Korea. He has been the president of the 13th International Congress of Toxicology (ICT XIII), the Korea Society of Toxicology (KSOT), and the Korea Environmental Mutagen Society (KEMS). He has been the vice president of the Asia Society of Toxicology (ASIATOX). He has organized eight workshops and three international symposia about toxicology, carcinogenesis, chemoprevention, endocrine disruption, and risk assessment. He has been a nominating committee member of the International Union of Toxicology (IUTOX) and deputy member of the Korean Pharmaceutical Society.

Prof. Lee has received numerous awards, including the Young Scientist Award, Brookhaven Symposium (U.S.); the Yun Ho Lee Award of Scientific Merit (International Aloe Science Council (U.S.); and the Merit Award from the Minister, Ministry of Food Drug Safety (Republic of Korea).

Prof. Lee's research areas include: carcinogenesis, chemoprevention, endocrine disruption, molecular epidemiology, biomarkers, systems toxicology, and risk assessment/management.

**Sam Kacew, PhD, ATS,** is an associate director of Toxicology, McLaughlin Centre for Population Health Risk Assessment at the University of Ottawa; professor of pharmacology, University of Ottawa; and scientist, Institute for Population Health, University of Ottawa.

Prof. Kacew is a visiting professor at the following institutions: the University of Guildford in Surrey, England; a Colgate-Palmolive visiting professor at the University of New Mexico; the Institute of Toxicology at National Taiwan University in Taipei, Taiwan; the Joszef Fodor National Center of Public Health in Budapest, Hungary; the Department of Occupational Health, Shanghai Medical University in Shanghai, China; the Zhehjiang University in Hangzhou, China; Nanjing Medical University, Nanjing, China; and the Division of Toxicology at Sungkyunkwan University in Suwon City, Korea.

Prof. Kacew is currently the editor-in-chief of the *Journal of Toxicology and Environmental Health, Part A, Current Issue*; editor-in-chief, *Journal of Toxicology and Environmental Health, Part B, Critical Reviews*; North American editor, *Toxicological and Environmental Chemistry*; associate editor of *Toxicology and Applied Pharmacology*; editor, *Encyclopedia of Environmental Health*; editor, *Lu's Basic Toxicology* (Fourth and Fifth editions); and guest editor of a special issue of *Toxicology and Applied Pharmacology* entitled "Toxicological Reviews in Fetal Childhood Development." He has edited several texts on pediatric toxicology and serves on several editorial boards. He has been a peer reviewer for the Environmental Protection Agency (EPA) on the Integrated Risk Information System (IRIS) documents, on the U.S. EPA Health Effects Assessment Summary Table (HEAST) chemicals, on the chemical-specific issue papers for the Superfund Technical Support Center (STSC) for the U.S. EPA, and has served on National Institutes of Health (NIH) grant study sections.

Prof. Kacew is a member of the Board on Environmental Studies and Toxicology (BEST) of the National Academy of Sciences (U.S.) and is a member of the Science Advisory Council (SAC) of the National American Flame Retardant Association (NAFRA).

Prof. Kacew has been a member of the board of trustees of Toxicology Excellence for Risk Assessment (TERA) and a member of the board of Review for Siloxane D5 appointed by the Minister of Environment of Canada. He has also been a member of the Committee on Toxicology of the National Academy of Sciences (NAS) of the United States and served as a chairman on the NAS Subcommittee on Iodotrifluoromethane; chairman on the NAS Subcommittee on Tetrachloroethylene; and a member of the NAS Subcommittees including Flame Retardants, Jet Propulsion Fuel-8, and Toxicologic and Radiologic Effects from Exposure to Depleted Uranium during and after Combat; and a member of the Advisory Expert Committee of the Canadian Network of Toxicology Centers. He served as a chairman of a U.S. EPA Panel on Peer Review Assessment of Toxicity

Values for Total Petroleum Hydrocarbons, member of the Panel on the Beryllium Lymphocyte Proliferation Screening Test, an expert panel member on the Breast Milk Monitoring for Environmental Chemicals in the United States, a core panel member of the Voluntary Children's Chemical Evaluation Program (VCCEP), part of a U.S. EPA initiative, expert panel member on the Pest Management Regulatory Agency of Health Canada on Citronella Science Review, expert panel member on drug-induced phospholipidosis to several pharmaceutical companies, expert panel member of the Council of Canadian Academies on Integrated Testing of Pesticides, and member of the Institute of Medicine (IOM) Committee on Blue Water Navy Vietnam Veterans and Agent Orange Exposure.

Prof. Kacew has received the Achievement Award of the Society of Toxicology of Canada in 1983, the Achievement Award of the Society of Toxicology in 1986, the ICI (Zeneca) Traveling Lectureship Award in 1991, the U.S.–China Foundation Award in 1995, the Colgate-Palmolive Visiting Professorship Award in 1997, and the Public Communications Award.

**Hyung Sik Kim, MS, PhD,** is a professor of the Division of Toxicology, College of Pharmacy, Sungkyunkwan University, South Korea.

Prof. Kim earned a PhD performing research on chemical carcinogenesis and chemoprevention at the College of Pharmacy, after which he joined the Korea Food and Drug Administration, serving as a senior researcher, where he was involved in reproductive and developmental toxicology and endocrine toxicology. He spent 2 years at the National Institutes of Health (NIH) in Bethesda, Maryland carrying out cancer and radiopharmaceutical research. Since 2003, he has been an assistant professor in the Division of Toxicology, College of Pharmacy at Pusan National University in South Korea.

He is a member of the American Association for Cancer Research (AACR), the Society of Toxicology (SOT), the International Congress of Toxicology (ICT), and the Korean Society of Toxicology (KSOT). He has published more than 210 papers and is the author of several book chapters included in the *Encyclopedia of Environmental Health, Reproductive and Developmental Toxicology,* and *Endocrine Disruptors,* among others. He is an editorial board member of the *Journal of Toxicology and Environmental Health, Part A,* an associate editor of the *Journal of Toxicological Sciences,* and an editorial board member of *Toxicological Research.*

Prof. Kim has served as an advisory committee member of government (National Food and Drug Safety, Ministry of Environment, Ministry of Health and Welfare) and has served as the vice chairman of the National Scientific Committee for the 13th International Congress of Toxicology (ICT) held in Seoul, Korea. He has also served as the vice chairman of the National Scientific Committee of the 8th International Congress of the Asian Society of Toxicology, held in Jeju, South Korea in 2015.

His primary research areas of interest are the identification of new cancer biomarkers, mechanisms of new anticancer agents, and cancer chemoprevention.

# Contributors

**Ok-Nam Bae, PhD**
**(Chapters 11, 16, 18, 19)**
College of Pharmacy
Hanyang University
Republic of Korea

**Kyung-Soo Chun, PhD**
**(Chapters 8, 9)**
College of Pharmacy
Keimyung University
Republic of Korea

**Ramesh C. Gupta, PhD**
**(Chapter 23)**
Murray State University
BVC Toxicology Department
Hopkinsville, Kentucky

**Gi-Wook Hwang, PhD**
**(Chapter 25)**
Graduate School of Pharmaceutical Sciences
Tohoku University
Sendai, Japan

**Tae Cheon Jeong, PhD**
**(Chapters 3, 14)**
College of Pharmacy
Yeungnam University
Gyeongsan, Republic of Korea

**Young-Suk Jung, PhD**
**(Chapters 12, 13)**
College of Pharmacy
Pusan National University
Busan, Republic of Korea

**Sam Kacew, PhD**
**(Chapters 17, 22, 26, 27, 28)**
McLaughlin Centre for Population Health Risk Assessment
University of Ottawa
Ontario, Canada

**Hyung Sik Kim, PhD**
**(Chapters 4, 5, 6, 8, 9, 13, 20, 21)**
Sunkyunkwan University
College of Pharmacy
Gyeonggi-do, Republic of Korea

**Kyu-Bong Kim, PhD**
**(Chapters 2, 7)**
College of Pharmacy
Dankook University
Chungnam, Republic of Korea

**Sang-Hyun Kim, PhD**
**(Chapter 24)**
Kyungpook National University
School of Medicine
Daegu, Republic of Korea

**Seok Kwon, PhD**
**(Chapter 30)**
Central Product Safety
Global Product Stewardship
Singapore Innovation Center
Procter & Gamble International Operations
Singapore

**Byung-Mu Lee, Dr PH**
**(Chapters 1, 8, 12, 22, 24, 26, 27, 29, 30)**
Sunkyunkwan University
College of Pharmacy
Gyeonggi-do, Republic of Korea

**Kyuhong Lee, PhD**
**(Chapter 15)**
Korea Institute of Toxicology
University of Science and Technology
Jeollabuk-do, Republic of Korea

**Semin Lee, PhD**
**(Chapter 7)**
School of Life Sciences
Ulsan National Institute of Science and Technology
Ulsan, Republic of Korea

**Pinpin Lin, PhD**
**(Chapter 4)**
National Health Research Institute
Taiwan

**Jung-Hwa Oh, PhD**
**(Chapter 7)**
Department of Predictive Toxicology
Korea Institute of Toxicology
Daejeon, Republic of Korea

**Helen E. Ritchie, PhD**
**(Chapter 10)**
Sydney Medical School
University of Sydney
Lidcombe, Australia

**William S. Webster, PhD**
**(Chapter 10)**
Department of Anatomy and Histology
University of Sydney
Sydney, Australia

*section one*

# *General principles of toxicology*

# chapter one

# History of toxicology

**Byung-Mu Lee**

Contents



## What is toxicology?

Toxicology (*toxicos*; poisonous + *logy*; science) also called *toxicological science* is the fusion of sciences based on biology, chemistry, physics, anatomy, physiology, pathology, psychology, zoology, pharmacology, genetics, biochemistry, statistics, and mathematics. Toxicology is traditionally defined as the science of poisons which are also termed as toxicants, toxic substances, toxins, xenobiotics, or stressors. A more descriptive definition of toxicology is the study of the nature and mechanisms underlying toxic effects exerted directly or indirectly by substances such as biological, chemical, physical, genetic, or psychological agents on living organisms and other biological systems. Toxicology also deals with quantitative or qualitative assessment of the adverse effects in relation to the concentration or dosage, duration, and frequency of exposure of the organisms.

The assessment of health hazards of industrial chemicals, environmental pollutants, and other substances represents an important element in the protection of the health of workers and members of communities.

In-depth studies of the nature and mechanism of the effects of toxicants are invaluable in the development of specific antidotes and other ameliorative measures. Along with other sciences, toxicology contributes to the development of safer chemicals used as drugs, food additives, and pesticides, as well as many useful industrial chemicals used for the fabrication of computers, cellular phones, televisions, and electronic equipment. Even the adverse effects per se are exploited in the pursuit of more effective insecticides, anthelmintics, antimicrobials, antivirals, and warfare agents. The purpose of toxicology is to protect humans or ecosystems from exposure to hazardous substances. Therefore, to ensure human safety, risk assessment which evaluates human safety based upon toxicological data and human exposure levels, in order to set human safe limits, may be considered one of the most important goals of toxicology (Song et al., 2013).

## *Mutiple fields of toxicology and applications*

Toxicology is a fusion science composed of multiple fields and has a broad scope. It deals with toxicity studies of substances used

1. In medicine for diagnostic, preventive, and therapeutic purposes.
2. In the food industry as direct and indirect additives.
3. In agriculture as pesticides, growth regulators, artificial pollinators, and animal feed additives.
4. In the chemical industry as solvents, components, and intermediates of plastics, components of electronic devices and many other types of chemicals. It is also concerned with the health effects of metals (as in mines and smelters), radiation, petroleum products, paper and pulp, flame retardants, toxic plants, and animal toxins. Overall, toxicology covers general safety issues in our lives and ecosystem.

Depending on the specific areas of toxicological application, toxicology can be subdivided into analytical toxicology, clinical toxicology, forensic toxicology, occupational toxicology, environmental toxicology, regulatory toxicology, and so forth. For example, a person may be exposed, accidentally or otherwise, to excessively large amounts of a toxicant and become severely intoxicated. If the identity of the toxicant is not known, *analytical toxicology* will be called upon to identify the toxicant through analysis of body fluids, stomach contents, suspected containers, and so forth. Those engaged in *clinical toxicology* administer antidotes, if available, to counter some specific toxicity, and take other measures to ameliorate the symptoms and signs and hasten the elimination of the toxicant from the body. There may also be legal implications, which is the task of *forensic toxicology*.

Intoxication may occur as a result of occupational exposure to toxicants. This may result in acute or chronic adverse effects. In either case, the problem is in the domain of *occupational toxicology*. The general public is exposed to a variety of toxicants, via air, water, and soil, or contact with skin as well as from food containing additives, pesticides, and contaminants, often at low levels that may be harmless acutely but may have long-term adverse effects. In pregnancy, the fetus is exposed via the maternal circulation while a lactating infant is exposed via breast milk. The sources of these substances, their transport, degradation, and bioconcentration in the environment, and their effects on humans are dealt with in *environmental toxicology*. *Regulatory toxicology* attempts to protect the public by setting laws, regulations, and standards to limit or suspend the use of toxic chemicals as well as defines use conditions for others. Some of the relevant laws in the United States are listed in Appendix 1.1.

To set meaningful regulations and standards, extensive profiles of the toxic effects are essential. Such profiles can only be established with a great variety of relevant and comprehensive toxicological data derived from *in vitro, in vivo,* and human studies, which form the foundation of regulatory toxicology.

The basic part of such studies is referred to as *conventional toxicology*. In addition, knowledge of the mechanism of action, provided by *mechanistic toxicology*, enhances the toxicological evaluation and provides a basis for other branches of toxicology. The knowledge gained is then utilized to assess the risk of adverse effects to the environment and humans and is termed a risk assessment. A health risk assessment constitutes a written document based upon all pertinent scientific information regarding toxicology, human experiences, environmental fate, and exposure scenario. These data are subject to critique and interpretation. The aim of a risk assessment is to estimate the potential of an adverse effect in humans and wildlife ecological systems caused by exposure to a specific amount of toxic substances. Risk assessments include several elements such as

1. Description of the potential adverse health effects based on an evaluation of results of epidemiological, clinical, preclinical, and environmental research.
2. Extrapolation from these results to predict the type and estimate the extent of adverse health effects in humans under given conditions of exposure.
3. Assessments as to the number and characteristics of individuals exposed at various intensities and durations.
4. Summary judgments on the existence and overall magnitude of the public health problem given the information of (1), (2), and (3) (Paustenbach, 2002). Risk characterization represents the final and

the most critical step in the risk assessment process whereby data on the dose–response relationship of a chemical are integrated with estimates of the degree of exposure in a population to estimate the likelihood and severity of human health risk (Williams and Paustenbach, 2002; Song et al., 2013).

## *History of toxicology in early stage*

In ancient times, human poisonings occurred after exposure to a numerous unknown or known poisons from different sources such as animals, plants, soil, air, and water. Some plants and heavy metals used for poisons in the world are listed in Table 1.1.

Ebers Papyrus is probably the oldest document that provides human toxicological information on poisons in BC 1500. It attests to awareness of the toxic effects of a number of substances—such as snake venom, poisonous plants like hemlock and aconite, and the toxic heavy metals arsenic, lead, and antimony. Some of these were actually used (intentionally for their adverse effects) for hunting, warfare, suicide, or homicide. For centuries, homicides with toxic substances were common in Europe, thus stimulating continual efforts toward the discovery and development of preventive and antidotal measures. The following are some famous examples of ancient poisonings in humans.

Socrates (BC 470–399), a Greek philosopher, died of hemlock poisoning (according to Plato). Hemlock (*Conium maculatum*) contains coniine, one of the active toxic ingredients and other toxic alkaloids (cicutoxin, oenanthotoxin, virol A, virol C, C17–polyacetylenes) that cause nausea, vomiting, diarrhea, tachycardia, cardiac dysrhythmias, mydriasis, renal failure, coma, respiratory impairment, and death (Schep et al., 2009). Cleopatra (BC 69–30), was made Cleopatra VII and became Queen of Egypt when her father Ptolemy XII died. Although her death is still a mystery, three possible scenarios for her death were suggested (Wexler, 2014): (a) committed suicide on August 12, BC 30, by means of an Egyptian serpent, referred to as her asp (Espinoza, 2001); (b) committed suicide by poison (possibly hidden somewhere in her mausoleum); (c) poisoned by Octavian and/or his men (Orland et al., 1990). Nero (AD 37–68) became Roman Emperor after the death of his adopted father, the Emperor Claudius in AD 54 (possibly by being poisoned with a mushroom). Nero was known as one of the most infamous men who used poisons to murder his rivals as well as his brother-in-law.

Mithridates VI (131–63 BC), the King Mithridates VI of Pontus, was known to expose himself and his prisoners to test poisons and antidotes. He would take small amounts of poison, not exceeding the toxic dosage, and gradually increase the doses until successfully acquiring immunity or tolerance. For this reason, the term "mithridatic" was coined meaning

*Table 1.1* List of poisonous plants in the world

| Plants | Ingredients | Toxic effect | Country | Year | Ref. |
|---|---|---|---|---|---|
| Aconite (*Aconitum napellus*) | Aconitine, yunaconitin, mesaconitine, hypaconitine | Cardiotoxicity, neurotoxicity | Europe, North America | – | Chan, 2009 |
| Chinese tallowtree (*Sapium sebiferum*) | Toxalbumin, saponin | Diarrhea, listlessness, weakness, dehydration | China | 1700s | Everest et al., 2005; NCSU, 2011 |
| Colchicum (*Colchicum autumnale*) | Alkaloid colchicine | Arrhythmias, liver failure, pancreatitis, alopecia | Europe | – | Jaeger and Flesch, 1990; Brvar et al., 2004 |
| Deadly nightshade (*Atropa belladonna*) | Atropine, hyoscyamine, scopolamine | Dryness of mouth, ileus, tachycardia | Europe, Asia | Roman times | Rajput, 2013 |
| Hellebore (*Helleborus niger*) | Cardiac glycosides, helleborin, hellebrin, | Dermatitis, convulsions, respiratory failure | Europe | 1400 BC | Schep et al., 2009; Cornell University, 2015 |
| Hemlock (*Conium maculatum*) | Cicutoxin, virol A, virol C, oenanthotoxin, C17-polyacetylenes | Tachycardia, mydriasis, renal failure, coma | North America, UK | – | |
| Henbane (*Hyoscyamus nigar*) | Atropine, hyoscyamine, scopolamine | Dry mouth, delirium, hallucinations, blurred vision, tachycardia | Europe, Africa | 681 AD | Alizadeh et al., 2014 |

*(Continued)*

***Table 1.1 (Continued)*** List of poisonous plants in the world

| Plants | Ingredients | Toxic effect | Country | Year | Ref. |
|---|---|---|---|---|---|
| Mandrake (*Atropa mandragora*) | Solanum alkaloids, tropane alkaloids | Mydriasis, blurred vision, headache, vomiting | Europe | – | Tsiligianni et al., 2009 |
| Mushrooms (*Amonita muscaria*) | Ibotenic acid, muscinol | Confusion, mydriasis, drowsiness | Italy | – | Michelot & Melendez-Howell, 2003 |
| Opium (*Papaver somniferum*) | Codeine, heroin, morphine, urushiol | Stupor, coma, death, liver and kidney toxicity | Eurasia, Korea | 1500 BC | Park et al., 2000; NSM, 2016 |
| Thorn apple (*Datura stramonium*) | Atropine, scopolamine, hyosciamine | Mydriasis, tachycardia, hallucinations | U.S., Asia | – | Thabet et al., 1999 |
| Yew (*Taxus accato*) | Taxine, paclitaxel, cephalomannine | Cardiac arrest, respiratory paralysis, ataxia, death | Canada | – | Cope, 2005; Perju-Dumbrava et al., 2013 |

"immunized or tolerable to a poison." Mithridate (originating from mithridatium), a combination of small doses of poisons invented by Mithridates VI, refers to an antidote or detoxifying agent against poison.

Hippocrates (BC 460–370) was a Greek physician—usually called the father of medicine—he is considered one of the important contributors for the development of clinical toxicology. Maimonides (1135–1204) published his famous medical work *Poisons and Their Antidotes* in 1198. Paracelsus (1493–1541) stated: "No substance is a poison by itself. It is the dose (the amount of the exposure) that makes a substance a poison" and "the right dose differentiates a poison from a remedy." These statements laid the foundation for the concept of the "dose–response relation" and the "therapeutic index" (TI) developed later. In addition, Paracelsus described in his book *Bergsucht* (1533–1534) the clinical manifestations of chronic arsenic and mercury poisoning as well as miner's disease. He might be considered the forefather of occupational toxicology. Orfila (1787–1853), a Spain-born French toxicologist and chemist, wrote an important treatise (1814–1815) describing a systematic correlation between the chemical and biological information on certain poisons. He also devised methods for detecting poisons and pointed to the necessity of chemical analysis for legal proof of lethal intoxication. The introduction of this approach ushered in a specialty area of modern toxicology: forensic toxicology. Ralph Waldo Emerson (1803–1882), American poet, essayist, philosopher, and journalist, had this ironic comment about poison: "Tobacco, coffee, alcohol, hashish, prussic acid, strychnine, are weak dilutions: the surest poison is time." —*Old Age*

## History of toxicology in modern stage

Due to the growing concern of human safety in modern society, people tend to demand improvements in health and living conditions, including nutrition, clothing, dwelling, and transportation. To meet this goal, a great variety of chemicals need to be manufactured and used in a way not to exceed human safety limits. It has been estimated that tens of thousands of different chemicals are used in commercial production in industrialized countries. In one way or another, these chemicals come in contact with various segments of the population, that is, individuals engaged in manufacturing, handling, usage (e.g., painters, applicators of pesticides), consumption (e.g., drugs, food additives, natural food products, or nutraceuticals), or misusage (e.g., suicide, accidental poisoning, and environmental disasters). Further, individuals may be exposed to more persistent chemicals via various environmental media and be affected more insidiously. To illustrate the devastating effects of toxicants, some examples of massive acute and long-term human poisonings are listed in

Appendix 1.2. In some of these episodes, a considerable amount of sophisticated toxicological investigation was conducted before the etiology was ascertained. These and other tragic outbreaks of massive chemical poisonings resulted in intensified testing programs, which revealed the great diversity of the nature and site of toxic effects. This revelation, in turn, has called for more studies using a greater number of animals, a greater number of indicators of toxicity, biomonitoring of chemicals, and so forth. There is, therefore, a need to render the task of toxicologically assessing the vast number of chemicals (by using increasingly more complex testing procedures) more manageable. To pursue this goal, criteria have been proposed and adopted for the selection of chemicals to be tested according to their priority. In addition, the "tier systems" allow decisions to be made at different stages of toxicological testing, thus avoiding unnecessary studies. If a chemical is found to be exceedingly toxic using a simplified "tier 1" screen such as loss of renal creatinine excretion and histopathology damage, then the compound is removed from the market does not require more sophisticated "tier 2" or "tier 3" testing. This procedure is particularly remarkable because the current testing system for carcinogenicity, mutagenicity, immunotoxicity, and reproductive capacity is quite expensive and involves a multitude of tests.

Because the number of individuals exposed to these chemicals is large, society cannot defer appropriate control until serious injuries have appeared. The modern toxicologist, therefore, needs to attempt to identify, where possible, indicators of exposure, and early reversible signs of adverse health effects. These will permit the formulation of decisions at the appropriate step to safeguard the health of individuals, either as occupational workers or in exposed communities. Achievements in these areas have assisted responsible personnel in instituting appropriate medical surveillance of occupational workers and other exposed populations. Notable examples are the use of cholinesterase inhibition as an indicator of exposure to organophosphorus pesticides as well as various biochemical parameters to monitor exposure to lead. Such "biological markers" or "biomarkers" are intended to measure exposure to toxicants or their effects as well as to detect susceptible population groups (NRC, 1987); they are used for clinical diagnosis, monitoring of occupational workers, and facilitating safety/risk assessment (WHO, 1993).

An important function of toxicology is to determine safe levels of exposure to natural and synthetic chemicals, thereby preventing the adverse effects of exposures to toxicants. The U.S. Food and Drug Administration (FDA) took one of the earliest official actions in this field. It stipulated that a 100-fold margin was required for the permission to use a food additive. In other words, a chemical additive should not occur in the total human diet in a quantity greater than one-hundredth of the amount that is the maximum safe dosage in long-term animal experiments (Lehman and Fitzhugh, 1954). While evaluating a number of food additives in 1961, the World Health Organization (WHO) coined the term "acceptable daily intake (ADI)" (WHO, 1962). Using the ADI procedure, WHO has since convened annual meetings of experts in the field of food additives, contaminants, residues of veterinary drugs, and pesticides. Assessment of these chemicals resulted, where appropriate, in the assignment of ADIs. Since then, the term "ADI" and the WHO evaluations have been adopted by regulatory agencies in many nations. The inception, evolution, and application of ADI have been outlined by Lu (1988). For toxicants in the occupational settings, quantitative assessments are provided in terms of "threshold limit values" (TLVs) (Federal Register, 1971).

These determinations involve comprehensive studies of the toxic properties, demonstration of dosages that produce no observable adverse effects, establishment of dose–effect and dose–response relationships, and toxicokinetic and biotransformation studies. The greatly increased scope and the multiplicity of subdisciplines as outlined above provide a vivid view of recent progress in toxicology.

## *Human poisonings and progress in toxicology*

Rehn (1895), a German surgeon, reported tumors in the urinary bladders of three men who had worked in an aniline factory. The role of aniline and aniline dyes as etiological agents was confirmed only some 40 years later after carrying out much experimental investigations in animals (Hueper et al., 1938), and extensive epidemiological studies (Case et al., 1954). This discovery led to improved occupational standards and more stringent controls of food colors derived from coal tar.

In the late 1950s, thalidomide was widely used as a sedative. It has a very low acute toxicity and readily met the toxicity-testing protocol prevailing at that time. However, a rare form of congenital malformation, phocomelia (the virtual absence of extremities), was observed among some offspring of mothers who had taken this drug during the first trimester (Lenz and Knapp, 1962). This tragedy led to the explosive development of teratology (developmental toxicology), an important specialty area of toxicology. The importance of modifying factors has been dramatized by the tragic effect of cobalt among heavy beer drinkers.

The once prevalent lead poisoning in certain areas of industrialized countries has now largely disappeared. This great accomplishment in the field of public health has resulted from the implementation of control measures devised on the basis of the knowledge gained from the numerous toxicological studies of lead. However, this has now raised new concerns. Lead has been replaced by the gasoline additive methylcyclopentadienyl manganese tricarbonyl (MMT). Combustion of MMT-containing gasoline generates tailpipe emissions of manganese (Mn) and studies demonstrated that Mn produces central nervous system disturbances (Gwiadza et al., 2007). Thus, it should be kept in mind that the removal and replacement of one chemical with another does not necessarily reduce the risk for the development of adverse effects.

Many cases of serious illness (that culminated in permanent paralysis and death) were reported in Minamata and Niigata in Japan in the 1950s and 1960s, respectively (Study Group of Minamata Disease, 1968; Tsubaki and Irukayama, 1977). The cause of the illness was eventually traced to methylmercury found in fish caught locally. The fish were contaminated with this chemical, either discharged untreated into the water by a factory, or from elemental mercury discharged by the factory and methylated through microorganisms in the mud. As a result, measures to rehabilitate the surviving patients and to establish legal controls over the factories were instituted.

On the other hand, the cause of another mysterious illness in Japan, known as "itai-itai" disease, remains unsolved, although cadmium apparently played a role. The patients had resided for many years in the vicinity of mines and where the cadmium levels in rice and water were excessive.

A more solid foundation in the assessment of risks of chemical carcinogens resulted from recent advances in epidemiology, long-term animal studies, short-term mutagenesis/carcinogenesis tests, and mechanistic investigations; as well as the realization that carcinogens differ in their potency, latency, and mode of action depending on species, strains, and gender.

## *Toxicity versus other considerations*

Human exposure to toxic substances should be avoided, but the human exposure level needs to be determined considering cost (the severity of the effects, reduction cost) and benefit (health protection, benefit from life convenience). Some substances produce mild, transient, or reversible effects, whereas those of others may be irreversible, serious, and even fatal. Exposure to the former type of substances might thus be acceptable, but, as a rule, not the latter. There are exceptions, such as methylmercury which is extremely toxic and is present in many species of fish. Because of the nutritional value of fish, permissible levels of methylmercury are established to minimize the risk, and yet not deny this valuable source of nutrients. Another is aflatoxin $B_1$, which is one of the most potent carcinogens present in a variety of foods. However, food in which it appears is not banned as long as the toxin does not exceed the permissible levels.

The complex nature of assessing the toxicity of a substance in light of its benefits is also exemplified by the toxicology seen in lactation and over-the-counter (OTC) products. The former involves weighing the benefits of breastfeeding versus the toxicity of certain potential contaminants. OTC products, when improperly used, present toxicological problems. However, the value of these products in general cannot be ignored. There is a growing debate about natural food products (nutraceuticals), where some accept the benefits, yet these products have not been assessed toxicologically and there are reports of adverse effects. Therefore, the therapeutic value of these products is subject to debate and needs extensive study as the number of consumers is in the millions and the toxicity remains unknown.

The perception of risk and benefits to society are crucial. It is clearly documented that the introduction of chemicals to control infectious diseases and the reduction of occupational exposure (through the use of protective gear) has increased human life expectancy. However, to completely eliminate all risks requires excessively high costs. Hence, it may not be beneficial if society demands that all risks be removed no matter what the costs are. In essence, by completely removing all chemicals and potential risks, the life expectancy will decrease and mortality will rise. The concept of an acceptable risk to benefit ratio needs to be kept in mind. The dilemmas involved in these topics are further described and discussed in other chapters.

## *Toxicology in the future*

The need of new substances will undoubtedly continue as some of them will treat or prevent a variety of diseases, which are currently untreatable or unpreventable. Others will render food more plentiful, tastier, and hopefully healthier. Still others will improve living conditions in various ways. At the same time, people are more conscious of subtle adverse effects on health and expect the new substances to be "absolutely safe." Further, the disposal of these substances and their byproducts is expected to produce no environmental hazards, adversely affecting humans and the ecosystem.

To satisfy these seemingly irreconcilable societal demands, a toxicologist needs to conduct a series of studies on each new substance:

1. Is it readily absorbed, distributed to specific organs, stored, and/or readily excreted?
2. Is it detoxicated or bioactivated?
3. What kind of adverse effects does it induce and what are the host and environmental factors (termed confounding factors), which can alter these effects?
4. How does it produce the effect on a cellular and molecular level?

5. What type of "general toxicity" does it produce?
6. What organs are its targets?
7. What is its predominant mechanism of action? How or can it be eliminated from the organism?

Answers to these and other questions will provide a scientific basis for assessing its safety and risk for the intended use. It is evident that the multitude of studies involved will place increasing demands on the limited facilities for toxicological testing and on the short supply of qualified personnel. It is of utmost importance, therefore, that toxicity data generated anywhere be accepted internationally. However, to ensure general acceptance, data need to meet certain standards. All countries involved in toxicological testing should adopt the "Good Laboratory Practice" (GLP) promulgated by the U.S. Food and Drug Administration (FDA, 1980) and the Organization of Economic Cooperation and Development (OECD, 1982).

To streamline the long and costly testing of each chemical separately, there have been schemes that test a representative chemical extensively and verify the results on other members of the group with minimal testing. This practice has been adopted successfully when the substances included in a group are essentially similar. A proposal to ban all chlorine compounds, however, appears to have gone too far in ignoring the great diversity of the toxic nature and potency of such a large group of substances (Karol, 1995). Similar calls for the ban of substances containing bromine, especially flame retardants present in furniture, computers, and televisions—which are crucial for protection against fire damage, have been instituted by a segment of the population based on the adverse effects of these chemicals. It will be a major challenge to determine how a variety of chemicals can be rationally grouped for toxicological testing and assessment purposes.

## *Development and validation of a toxicity test system*

There have been recent trends designed to simplify and hasten the testing systems which include a reduction in the use of lab animals and supplement (or supplant) them with *in vitro* studies. This is done partly in response to a societal call for the abolishment of animal testing on humane grounds.

Isolated organs, cultured tissues and cells, and lower forms of life will be increasingly used. Further, such test systems will likely be faster and less expensive and will augment the variety of studies, especially those related to the mechanism of toxicity. An understanding of the mechanism of action of a chemical is often valuable in providing a sounder basis for the assessment of its safety and risk. Other types of improvements of the testing procedure with respect to simplicity and reliability will continue to be made. Currently, there is a major movement termed "Toxicity Testing in the Twenty-First Century" using computational models developed to predict the toxicity of chemicals based upon *in vitro* data (Rhomberg, 2010; Roggen, 2011). Although this will go a long way in reducing animal testing, the computational model cannot always predict effects *in vivo* in animals and humans. One must bear in mind that this is only a model and can have a useful function as a "tier 1" screen; therefore, *in vivo* testing will still be required.

Recently, systems toxicology (i.e., toxicogenomics, toxicoproteomics, and toxicometabolomics) has been considered a promising approach to develop new biomarkers comprehensively for predicting stage-dependent toxicity of substances and risk assessment (McHale et al., 2010; Yang et al., 2010; Kim et al., 2015) (see Chapter 7).

Advances made in biochemical and toxicokinetic studies as well as those in genetic toxicology, immunotoxicology, reproductive toxicology, morphological studies on a subcellular level, and biochemical studies on a molecular and genetic level have all contributed to a better understanding of the nature, site, and mechanisms of action of toxicants. For example, technological breakthroughs enabled *in vitro* studies to demonstrate whether hepatocytes or nonparenchymal cells affected by a chemical carcinogen are related to differences in their ability to repair the DNA damage induced by the chemical. Studies using isolated nephrons have provided insight into the site and mode of action of nephrotoxicants. Various other types of *in vitro* studies demonstrated the possibility of their use in screening toxicants for specific effects such as mutagenicity and dermal irritancy. Numerous studies showed that responses to toxicants are better correlated with the effective dose, that is, the concentration of the toxicant at the target site of action, rather than the administered dose. Further, it is important that one knows whether the effects observed result mainly or entirely from an active metabolite, or from the concentration of the metabolite formed rather than that of the parent chemical.

## *Adverse outcome pathways*

To manifest adverse effects in target organs of organisms, alterations of critical biochemical or molecular molecules are involved in important physiological and pathological pathways. For these reasons, OECD proposed adverse outcome pathways (AOPs) and a guideline was also suggested to study a sequential chain of causally linked events at different levels of biological organization that led to an adverse health or ecotoxicological effect (OECD, 2013). In 2014, OECD launched its knowledge base upon AOP in collaboration with the U.S. Environmental Protection Agency (EPA) and the European Commission Joint Research Centre (JRC). Further, AOP-Wiki platform was developed and the latest version of all AOPs (version 2.0 of the AOP-Wiki, December 4, 2016) is available at: https://aopwiki.org/. This wiki is based upon the Chemical Mode of Action developed by the EPA under the auspices of the WHO International Programme on Chemical Safety (IPCS) Mode of Action Steering Group and is jointly led by the OECD and the JRC (AOPWiki, 2016). Another AOP Knowledge Base (AOP KB) module, a web-based platform, is Effectopedia (The Online Encyclopedia of AOPs, available at: http://effectopedia.org/), especially adapted for development of quantitative AOPs.

An AOP is a conceptual framework which integrates all known toxicological and molecular information, and is the sequential progression of events from molecular initiating event (MIE) to *in vivo* outcome of interest. It includes a broader set of pathways in which (1) chemical interacts with a biological target (e.g., DNA, protein, lipids, etc.); (2) sequential series of biological activities (e.g., gene activation, altered tissue development, etc.); (3) sinal adverse effect relevance to human or ecological risk assessors (e.g., mortality, disrupted reproduction, cancer, or extinction, etc.) (OECD, 2011).

This AOP approach may contribute to elucidation of mechanisms of toxicity, development of alternative toxicity testing, detoxification agents, and diagnosis of toxicities or diseases, which might be related to new drug development by modifying the molecular pathways. Application of AOP will be discussed in more detail in Chapter 16.

## *About the book*

As noted earlier, to provide a basis for proper assessment of the safety or risk of a chemical and for a variety of other purposes, toxicology is increasingly becoming a multifaceted science. To facilitate the acquisition of a broad knowledge of toxicology, this book covers four major areas.

Section I: Describes general topics related to absorption, distribution, and excretion of toxicants, their transformation in the body, the various types of toxic effects they exert, and the host and environmental factors that modify these effects.

Section II: Deals with procedures used in determining the general and specific toxic effects.

Section III: Describes the organ/system-specific toxicants and the procedures most commonly used to detect their effects.

Section IV: Discusses several major groups of toxicants such as food additives and contaminants, pesticides, metals, various environmental pollutants, toxicants in the workplace, clinical toxicology dealing with OTC preparations, and risk assessment. The last chapter outlines the widely adopted approaches to the assessment of safety and risk of noncarcinogenic and carcinogenic substances. In addition, two indices are appended listing chemicals and subjects, respectively, to assist the reader in retrieving relevant parts of the text.

## *Appendix 1.1 U.S. laws that have a basis in toxicology*

| Responsible agency | Law (year enacted) |
|---|---|
| Food and Drug Administration (FDA) | Federal Food and Drugs Act (FFDA) (1906) |
| | Federal Food, Drug, and Cosmetic Act (FD&C) (1938) |
| Environmental Protection Agency (EPA) | Federal Insecticide, Fungicide, and Rodenticide Act (FIFRA) (1947) |
| | Clean Air Act (CAA) (1963) |
| | Safe Drinking Water Act (SDWA) (1974) |
| | Toxic Substances Control Act (TSCA) (1976) |
| Consumer Product Safety Commission (CPSC) | Consumer Product Safety Act (CPSA) (1972) |
| | Federal Hazardous Substances Act (FHSA) (1960) |
| Occupational Safety and Health Administration (OSHA) | Occupational Safety and Health Act (OSHA) (1970) |

# *Appendix 1.2 Examples of outbreaks of mass poisoning in humans*

| Location and year | Toxicant | Adverse effect | Number affected |
|---|---|---|---|
| Detroit, MI, 1930 | Tri-*o*-cresyl phosphate in "ginger jake" | Delayed neurotoxicity | 16,000 |
| London, UK, 1952 | $SO_2$ and suspended PM in air | Deaths | 3000 |
| Toyama, Japan, 1950s | Cadmium in rice | *Itai-itai* disease | 200[a] |
| Minamata, Japan, 1950s | Methylmercury in fish | Minamata disease | 200[a,b] |
| Southeast Turkey, 1956 | Hexachlorobenzene in wheat | Porphyria, neurological diseases | 4000 |
| Morocco, 1959 | Tri-*o*-cresyl phosphate in adulterated oil | Delayed neurotoxicity | 10,000 |
| Western Europe, late 1950s–1960s | Thalidomide | Phocomelia | 10,000 |
| Fukuoka, Japan, 1968 | PCBs | Skin disease, weakness | 1700 |
| Iraq, 1972 | Methylmercury in wheat | Deaths | 500 |
| | | Nonfatal cases | 50,000 |
| Madrid, Spain, 1981 | Toxic oil in food | Deaths | 340 |
| | | Nonfatal cases | 20,000 |
| Bhopal, India, 1984 | Methyl isocyanate released into air | Deaths | 6000 |
| | | Nonfatal cases | 200,000 |
| Chernobyl, USSR, 1986 | Radioactivity release | Deaths | 31 |
| | | Cancer death estimate | 8000 |
| China, 2008 | Melamine in milk | Deaths | 6 |
| | | Infant illness, kidney | 300,000 |
| Fukushima, Japan, 2011 | Radioactivity release | Deaths | 1700 |
| | | Cancer death estimate | 1000 |

[a] Many more cases with mild or moderate symptoms and signs of intoxication.
[b] Hundreds of cases occurred in Niigata, Japan, in the 1960s from the same source, fish.

## References

Alizadeh A, Moshiri M, Alizadeh J, Balali-Mood M (2014). Black henbane and its toxicity—A descriptive review. *Avicenna J Phytomed*. 4(5), 297–311.

AOPWiki (Adverse Outcome Pathway Wiki). (2016). Available at: https://aopwiki.org/.

Brvar M, Kozelj G, Mozina M, Bune M (2004). Acute poisoning with autumn crocus (*Colchicum autumnale* L.). *Wien Klin Wochenschr*. 116(5–6), 205–8.

Case RAM, Hosker ME, McDonald DB et al. (1954). Tumours of the urinary bladder in workmen engaged in the manufacture and use of certain dyestuff intermediates in the British chemical industry. *Br J Ind Med*. 11, 75–104.

Chan TY (2009). Aconite poisoning. *Clin Toxicol (Phila)*. 47(4), 279–85.

Cope RB (2005). The dangers of yew ingestion. *Toxicology Brief*. College of Veterinary Medicine. 646–50.

Cornell University. (2015). *Helleborus niger*—Christmas Rose. College of Agriculture and Life Science. Available at: http://poisonousplants.ansci.cornell.edu/christmasrose/christmasrose.html.

Espinoza R (2001). In relation to Cleopatra and snake bites. *Rev Med Chil*. 129,1222–6.

Everest JW, Powe Jr. TA, and Freeman JD (2005). Poisonous Plants of the Southeastern United States. Alabama Cooperative Extension System. Available at: http://www.aces.edu/pubs/docs/A/ANR-0975/ANR-0975.pdf.

FDA. (1980). Code of Federal Regulations, Title 21, Food and Drugs. Part 58. Washington, DC U.S. Government Printing Office.

Federal Register. (1971). Threshold Limit Values Adopted by the American Conference of Governmental Industrial Hygienists. 36(105), May 29, 1968. Washington, DC U.S. Government Printing Office.

Gwiadza R, Lucchini R, Smith D (2007). Adequacy and consistency of animal studies to evaluate the neurotoxicity of chronic low-level manganese exposure in humans. *J Toxicol Environ Health A*. 70, 594–605.

Hueper WC, Wiley FH, Wolfe HD (1938). Experimental production of bladder tumors in dogs by administration of beta-naphthylamine. *J Ind Hyg Toxicol*. 20, 46–84.

Jaeger A, Flesch F (1990). *Colchicum autumnale* L. INCHEM. Available at: http://www.inchem.org/documents/pims/plant/pim142.htm.

Karol MH (1995). Toxicologic principles do not support the banning of chlorine: A society of toxicology position paper. *Fundam Appl Toxicol*. 24, 1–2.

Kim DH, Kwack SJ, Yoon KS, Choi JS, Lee BM (2015). 4-Hydroxynonenal: A superior oxidative biomarker compared to malondialdehyde and carbonyl content induced by carbon tetrachloride in rats. *J Toxicol Environ Health. A*, 78(16), 1051–62.

Lehman AJ, Fitzhugh OG (1954). 100-fold margin of safety. *Q Bull Assoc Food Drug Officials U.S.* 18, 33–5.

Lenz W, Knapp K (1962). Thalidomide embryopathy. *Arch Environ Health*. 5, 100–5.

Lu FC (1988). Acceptable daily intakes: Inception, evolution and application. *Regul Toxicol Pharmacol*. 8, 45–60.

McHale CM, Zhang L, Hubbard AE et al. (2010). Toxicogenomic profiling of chemically exposed humans in risk assessment. *Mutat Res*. 705, 172–83.

Michelot D, Melendez-Howell LM (2003). *Amanita muscaria*: Chemistry, biology, toxicology, and ethnomycology. *Mycol Res*. 107(2), 131–46.

NCSU (NC State University). (2011). Invasive, Exotic Plants of the Southeast: Chinese Tallow Tree. 2011. Going Native. Available at: https://www.ncsu.edu/goingnative/howto/mapping/invexse/chineset.html.

NRC (National Research Council). (1987). Committee on Biological Markers. Biological markers in environmental health research. *Environ Health Perspect.* 74, 3–9.

NSM (Nova Scotia Museum-Poison Plant Patch). (2016). Poppy (*Papavar* species). Available at: https://novascotia.ca/museum/poison/default.asp?section=species&id=102.

OECD. (1982). Good Laboratory Practice in the Testing of Chemicals. Paris, France. Organization of Economic Cooperation and Development.

OECD. (2011). Report of the Workshop on Using Mechanistic Information in Forming Chemical Categories. OECD Environment, Health and Safety Publications Series on Testing and Assessment No. 138. ENV/JM/MONO(2011)8. Available at: http://www.oecd.org/chemicalsafety/adverse-outcome-pathways-molecular-screening-and-toxicogenomics.htm.

OECD. (2013). Guidance Document on Developing and Assessing Adverse Outcome Pathways. Series on Testing and Assessment No. 184. JT03338300. ENV/JM/ENV/JM/MONO(2013)6.

Orland RM, Orland FJ, Orland PT (1990). Psychiatric assessment of Cleopatra: A challenging evaluation. *Psychopathology.* 23, 169–75.

Park SD, Lee SW, Chun JH, Cha SH (2000). Clinical features of 31 patients with systemic contact dermatitis due to the ingestion of Rhus (lacquer). *Br J Dermatol.* 142(5), 937–42.

Paustenbach DJ (2002). *Human and Ecological Risk Assessment. Theory and Practice.* New York: John Wiley & Sons.

Perju-Dumbrava D, Morar S, Chiroban O, Lechintan E, Cioca A (2013). Suicidal poisoning by ingestion of Taxus Baccata leaves. Case report and literature review. *Rom J Leg Med.* 21, 115–8.

Rajput H (2013). Effects of *Atropa belladonna* as an anti-cholinergic. Rajput. *Nat Prod Chem Res.* 1, 1.

Rehn L (1895). Blasengeschwulste bei fuchsin-arbeiten. *Arch Klin Chir.* 50, 588.

Rhomberg LR (2010). Toxicity testing in the 21st century: How will it affect risk assessment? *J Toxicol Environ Health B Crit Rev.* 13, 361–75.

Roggen EL (2011). In vitro toxicity testing in the twenty-first century. *Front Pharmacol.* 2, 1–3.

Schep LJ, Slaughter RJ, Becket G, Beasley DM (2009). Poisoning due to water hemlock. *Clin Toxicol (Phila).* 47(4), 270–8.

Song JB, Ahn IY, Cho KT, Kim YJ, Kim HS, Lee BM (2013). Development and application of risk management system in Korea for consumer products to comply with global harmonization. *J Toxicol Environ Health Part B.* 16(1), 1–16.

Study Group of Minamata Disease. (1968). *Minamata Disease.* Minamata, Japan: Minamata University.

Thabet H, Brahmi N, Amamou M, Ben Salah N, Hedhili A, Yacoub M (1999). *Datura stramonium* poisonings in humans. *Vet Human Toxicol.* 41(5), 320–1.

Tsiligianni IG, Vasilopoulos TK, Papadokostakis PK, Arseni GK, Eleni A, Lionis CD (2009). A two cases clinical report of mandragora poisoning in primary care in Crete, Greece: Two case report. *Cases J.* 2, 9331.

Tsubaki T, Irukayama K (1977). *Minamata Disease: Methyl Mercury Poisoning in Minamata and Niigata, Japan*. New York: Elsevier Scientific.
Wexler P (2014). The death of Cleopatra: Suicide by snakebite or poisoned by her enemies? In *History of Toxicology and Environmental Health*. Toxicology in Antiquity, Vol. I. London: Academic Press. p. 16.
WHO. (1962). Sixth Report of the Joint FAD/WHO Expert Committee on Food Additives. Geneva, Switzerland: World Health Organization.
WHO. (1993). Biomarkers and risk assessment: Concepts and principles. *Environ Health Criteria*. 155.
Williams PRD, Paustenbach DJ (2002). Risk characterization: Principles and practice. *J Toxicol Environ Health B*. 5, 337–406.
Yang B, Wang Q, Lei R et al. (2010). Systems toxicology used in nanotoxicology: Mechanistic insights into the hepatotoxicity of nano-copper particles from toxicogenomics. *J Nanosci Nanotechnol*. 10, 8527–37.

# *chapter two*

# *Toxicokinetics of xenobiotics*

***Kyu-Bong Kim***

*Contents*



## *Introduction*

Xenobiotics exert adverse effects through toxicokinetics (TK) and toxicodynamics (TD). Toxicokinetics or pharmacokinetics is a science that indicates the quantitative fate of a xenobiotic in the body whereas toxicodynamics is a process of interaction between active forms of xenobiotics and biomolecules such as DNA, protein, and lipids. Physiological and biochemical processes in the body undergo absorption, distribution, metabolism, and excretion (ADME) of toxicants, which may explain how to predict potential biological

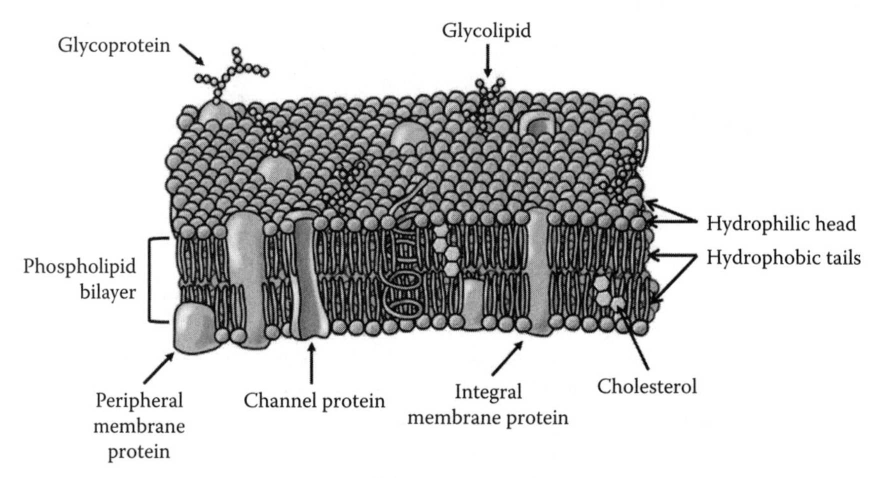


***Figure 2.1*** Schematic diagram of a biological membrane. Spheres represent head groups (phosphatidylcholine) and lines indicate tail ends of lipids. Black, white, and stippled spheres indicate different kinds of lipids. Large bodies represent proteins; some are located on the surface, others within the membrane. Glycoproteins or glycolipids are attached to proteins and lipids on the surface of cell membrane. (Adapted from Singer SJ, Nicolson GC, *Science*, 175, 720–31, 1972.)

activities. Absorption, the first step of TK, can be defined as systematical entry of xenobiotics into the body via the bloodstream. Metabolism (biotransformation) will be discussed separately in Chapter 3. A xenobiotic needs to pass through various membranes to be absorbed, distributed, and excreted. A cell membrane generally consists of a biomolecular layer of lipid molecules with proteins scattered throughout the membrane (Figure 2.1).

There are four mechanisms by which a toxicant may pass through a cell membrane; the most important of them is passive diffusion through the membrane. The others are filtration through the membrane pores, carrier-mediated transport, and engulfing by the cell. The last two mechanisms are different in that the cell takes an active part in the transfer of a toxicant across its membranes.

## *Transport system of xenobiotics*

### *Passive diffusion*

Simple passive diffusion is defined as the movement of toxicants from areas of higher concentration to areas of lower concentration, which does not require energy. On the other hand, when molecules travel from a region of low concentration to a region of high concentration, it is called active transport and requires energy. Most toxicants cross cell membranes by simple and passive diffusion. The rate of passage is related directly to the concentration gradient across the membrane and to the lipid solubility. For example, mannitol is hardly absorbed (<2%), acetylsalicylic acid is fairly well absorbed (21%), and thiopental is even more readily absorbed (67%). It is noteworthy that the chloroform:water partition of the nonionized forms of these chemicals is, respectively, <0.002, 2, and 100. For references to this and other examples, see Hogben et al. (1958).

Many toxicants are ionizable. The ionized form is often unable to penetrate the cell membrane because of its low lipid solubility. On the other hand, the nonionized form is likely sufficiently lipid-soluble, and its rate of penetration depends upon the lipid solubility. The extent of ionization of weak organic acids and bases depends upon the pH of the medium. Thus, for the former, such as benzoic acid, diffusion is facilitated in an acidic environment, where this chemical exists mainly in the nonionized form; for the latter, such as aniline, diffusion is facilitated in a basic environment (Figures 2.2 and 2.3).

## *Filtration*

The membranes of the capillaries and glomeruli have relatively large pores (about 70 nm) and allow molecules smaller than albumin (molecular

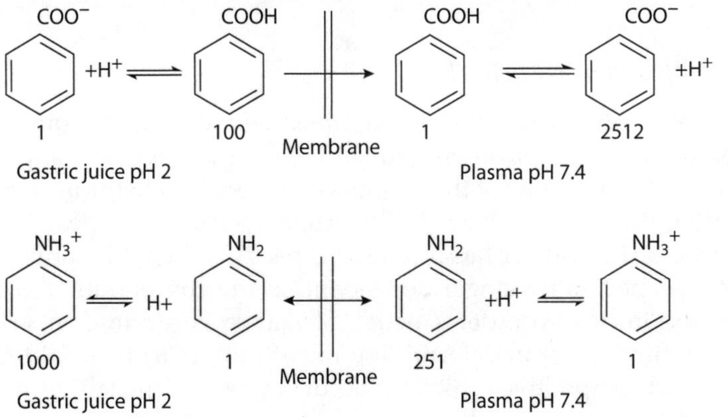

***Figure 2.2*** Disposition of benzoic acid and aniline ingastric juice and plasma. Figures immediately below the structural formulas represent proportions of ionized and nonionized forms. (From Timbrell JA, *Principles of Biochemical Toxicology*, London, UK: Taylor & Francis, 1991.)

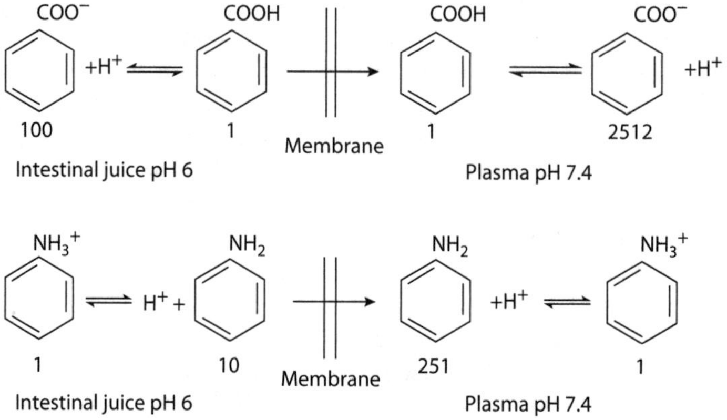

*Figure 2.3* Disposition of benzoic acid and aniline in intestinal juice and plasma. (From Timbrell JA, *Principles of Biochemical Toxicology*, London, UK: Taylor & Francis, 1991.)

weight 60,000 Da) to pass through. Bulk flow of water through these pores results from hydrostatic and/or osmotic pressure and act as a carrier of toxicants. The pores in most cells, however, are relatively small (about 4 nm) and allow chemicals only up to a molecular weight of 100–200 Da to pass through. Chemicals of larger molecules, therefore, filter into and out of the capillaries. They can, therefore, establish equilibrium between the concentrations in plasma and in the extracellular fluid, but cannot do so by filtration between the extracellular and intracellular fluids.

## *Carrier-mediated transport*

This involves the formation of a complex between the chemical and a macromolecular carrier on one side of the membrane. The complex then diffuses to the other side of the membrane, where the chemical is released. Thereafter, the carrier returns to the original surface to repeat the transport process. The carrier has a limited capacity. When it is saturated, the rate of transport is no longer dependent on the concentration of chemical and assumes zero order kinetics. Structure, conformation, size, and charge are important in determining the affinity of a chemical for a carrier site, and competitive inhibition occurs among chemicals with similar characteristics.

*Active transport* involves a carrier that moves molecules across a membrane against a concentration gradient, or, if the molecule is an ion, against an electrochemical gradient. It is selective for specific structural features of chemicals. It requires the expenditure of metabolic energy by hydrolysis of adenosine triphosphate and can be inhibited by poisons that interfere with cell metabolism.

*Facilitated diffusion* is similar to active transport but does not move molecules against concentration or electrochemical gradient. Further, it is not energy-dependent, and metabolic poisons do not inhibit this process. Therefore, facilitated diffusion is classified as a passive transport system. Glucose, sodium ions, and chloride ions are examples of substances using facilitated diffusion to efficiently cross plasma membranes.

### *Engulfing by the cell (endocytosis)*

Particles may be engulfed by cells. When the particles are solid, the process is called phagocytosis and when they are liquid, it is called pinocytosis. This process is also called active transport and requires energy. Such special transport systems are important for the removal of particulate matter from the alveoli and of certain toxic substances from the blood by the reticuloendothelial system. Carrageenans (molecular weight about 10,000–40,000 Da) are also absorbed from the gut by this process.

## *Absorption pathways*

The main routes by which toxicants are absorbed are the GI tract, lungs, and skin. However, in toxicologic studies, special routes such as intravenous, intraperitoneal, intradermal, intramuscular, and subcutaneous injections are also used. Other minor routes include intracardiac and intra-articular injection, and intraosseous infusion.

### *Gastrointestinal tract*

Many toxicants enter the GI tract along with food and water, or alone as drugs or other types of chemicals. With the exception of those that are caustic or irritating to the mucosa, most toxicants do not exert any toxic effect unless they are absorbed. Absorption takes place along the entire GI tract. For example, certain drugs are administered as sublingual tablets and suppositories to be absorbed in the mouth and rectum, respectively. However, the mouth and rectum are, in general, insignificant sites of absorption of environmental chemicals.

The stomach is a significant site of absorption, especially for weak acids, which exist in the diffusible, nonionized, and lipid-soluble form. On the other hand, weak bases are highly ionized in the acidic gastric juice (pH about 2) and therefore not readily absorbable. The difference in absorption is further amplified by the circulating plasma. Weak acids exist mainly in ionized form in plasma and are carried away, whereas weak bases exist in nonionized form and diffuse back to the stomach. The influence of these factors, using benzoic acid and aniline as examples, is shown in Figure 2.2.

In the intestine, weak acids will exist mainly in the ionized form and hence are less readily absorbable. However, upon entering the blood, they become ionized and thus will not readily diffuse back. On the other hand, weak bases will exist mainly in the nonionized form; hence more readily absorbable, as shown in Figure 2.3. However, the Henderson–Hasselbach equation is not the only determination of GI absorption. It should be noted that intestinal absorption is further enhanced by long contact time, the large surface area provided by the villi and microvilli, and blood flow rate.

In the intestine, there are special carrier-mediated transport systems that are responsible for absorption of nutrients, such as monosaccharides, amino acids, and elements such as iron, calcium, and sodium. However, a few toxicants, such as 5-fluorouracil (5-FU), thallium, and lead, are known to be absorbable from the intestine by active transport systems. Those toxicants have shown potential competition with nutrients because of transportation using the same specialized transporter: 5-FU for the pyridium transport system; thallium for the iron transport system; lead for the calcium transporter. In addition, particulate matters such as those of the azo dyes and polystyrene latex enter the intestinal cell by pinocytosis.

## *Respiratory tract*

The main site of absorption in the respiratory tract is the alveoli in the lungs. This is especially true for gases such as carbon monoxide, nitrogen oxides, and sulfur dioxide, and for vapors of volatile liquids such as benzene and carbon tetrachloride. Their ready absorption is related to the large alveolar area, high blood flow, and proximity of the blood to the alveolar air.

The rate of absorption is dependent upon the solubility of the gas in the blood—the more soluble it is, the faster the absorption. However, equilibrium between the air and blood is reached more slowly for more soluble chemicals, such as chloroform, compared with less soluble chemicals, such as ethylene. This is because the more soluble a chemical, the more of it can be dissolved in the blood. As the alveolar air carries only a limited amount of the chemical, greater respiratory rates and a longer time are required to attain equilibrium. This takes even longer if the chemical is also deposited in fat tissue.

In addition to gases and vapors, liquid aerosols and airborne particles may also be absorbed. The inhalational absorption of gases and vapors is influenced by the partitioning of the substance between blood and gas phase according to its solubility and tissue affinity. In contrast, the inhalational absorption of aerosols and particles is determined by aerosol or particle size, and the water solubility of any substance contained in the aerosol or particle. In general, large particles (>10 μm) do not enter the respiratory tract; when they do, they are deposited in the nose and disposed of by wiping, blowing, and sneezing. Very small particles (<0.01 μm) are likely to be exhaled. Those in the range of 0.01–10 μm are deposited in various parts of the respiratory tract (Oberdorster et al., 2005). The larger ones are likely to be deposited in the nasopharynx and absorbed either through the epithelium of this region or through the GI tract epithelium after they are swallowed along with the mucus. Smaller particles are deposited in the trachea, bronchi, and bronchioli, and are then either aspirated onto the mucociliary escalator or engulfed by phagocytes. The particles carried up by the escalator will be coughed up or swallowed. The phagocytes with engulfed particles are absorbed into the lymphatics. Some free particles also migrate into the lymphatics. Soluble particles may be absorbed through the epithelium into the blood.

The Task Group on Lung Dynamics (1966) provides a detailed examination of how particles of various sizes are deposited, in different parts of the respiratory tract. However, as a rough estimate, 25% of inhaled particles are exhaled, 50% are deposited in the upper respiratory tract, and 25% are deposited in the lower respiratory tract (Morrow et al., 1966).

## *Skin*

In general, the skin is the largest organ and relatively impermeable, and therefore it constitutes a good barrier, separating the organism from its environment. However, some chemicals are absorbed through the skin in sufficient quantities to produce systemic effects.

A chemical may be absorbed via the hair follicles or through the cells of the sweat glands or sebaceous glands. These are, however, minor routes for absorption because they constitute only a small surface area of the skin. Therefore, percutaneous absorption of a chemical is essentially through the skin proper, which consists of the epidermis and dermis (Figure 16.1 of Chapter 16).

The first phase of percutaneous absorption is diffusion of the toxicant through the epidermis, the most important barrier, and especially its stratum corneum. The stratum corneum consists of several layers of thin, cohesive, dead cells that contain a chemically resistant material (protein filament). Small amounts of polar substances appear to diffuse through the outer surface of the protein filaments of the hydrated stratum corneum; nonpolar substances dissolve in and diffuse through the lipid matrix between the protein filaments. All toxicants pass through the stratum corneum by passive diffusion and this process is the rate-limiting step in skin absorption.

In the human stratum corneum, there are significant differences in structure and chemistry from one region of the body to another, which are reflected in the permeability to chemicals. For example, toxicants cross the scrotum readily, cross the abdominal skin less readily, and cross the sole and palm with great difficulty (Zbinden, 1976).

The second phase of percutaneous absorption is diffusion of the toxicant through the dermis, which contains a porous, nonselective, aqueous diffusion medium. Therefore, it is less effective as a barrier than the stratum corneum. As a consequence, abrasion or removal of the latter causes a marked increase in the percutaneous absorption. Acids, alkalis, and mustard gases also increase absorption by injuring this barrier. Some solvents, notably dimethyl sulfoxide, also enhance dermal permeability.

## *Distribution in organs*

After a chemical enters the blood, it is distributed rapidly throughout the body. The rate of distribution to each organ is related to the speed and amount of blood that flows through the organ, the ease with which the chemical crosses the local capillary wall and the cell membrane, and affinity of components of the organ for the chemical.

### *Barriers*

The *blood–brain barrier* (BBB) is located at the brain capillary wall. The capillary endothelial cells are tightly joined, leaving few or no pores between these cells (Bradbury, 1984). Thus, the toxicant has to pass through the capillary endothelium itself. A lack of vesicles in these cells further reduces their transport ability. Finally, the protein concentration of the interstitial fluid in the brain is low, in contrast to that in other organs; protein binding therefore does not serve as a mechanism for the transfer of toxicants from blood to the brain. For these reasons, the penetration of toxicants into the brain depends upon their lipid solubility. An example is the toxicant methylmercury, which enters the brain readily and whose main target is the central nervous system. In contrast, inorganic mercury compounds are not lipid soluble, do not enter the brain readily, and exert their main adverse effects not on the brain but on the kidney. Glucose is transported across the brain capillary wall by the glucose transporter 2 (GLUT2). Active transport systems also play a major role in limiting the distribution of xenobiotics in the brain. The BBB is composed of various members of the ATP-binding cassette transporter (ABC) and solute carrier transporter (SLC) families, adenosine triphosphate (ATP)-dependent transporters. Efflux transporters (MDR1, BCRP, MRP1, 2, 4, and 5) are located on the apical plasma membrane and act to pump xenobiotics absorbed into the capillary endothelial cells out into the blood. The BBB is not completely developed in newborns, and therefore some xenobiotics are more toxic to newborns than adults. For instance, morphine is more toxic to immature rats than adult ones because of the higher disposition to morphine of the brain of newborns; deltamethrin, a synthetic pyrethroid insecticide, is more toxic to younger rats than adult ones because the brain disposition is higher in younger animals (Kim et al., 2010).

The *placental barrier* differs anatomically among various animal species. There are six layers of cells between fetal and maternal blood in some species, whereas in others there is only one layer. Further, the number of layers may change as gestation progresses. Although the relationship of the number of layers of the placenta to its permeability needs quantitative determination, the placental barrier does impede transfer of toxicants to the fetus, which is therefore protected to some extent. However, the concentration of a toxicant such as methylmercury may be higher in certain fetal organs, such as the brain, because of the less-effective fetal blood–brain barrier. On the other hand, the fetal concentration of the food coloring amaranth is only 0.03–0.06% of that of the mother (Munro and Willes, 1978).

Other barriers are also present in organs such as the eyes and testes. In addition, the erythrocyte plays an interesting role in the distribution of certain toxicants. For example, its membrane acts as a barrier against the penetration of inorganic mercury compounds but not that of alkyl mercury. Further, there is affinity of the erythrocyte cytoplasm for alkyl mercury compounds. Because of these factors, the concentration of inorganic mercury compounds in the erythrocytes is only about half that in the plasma, whereas that of methylmercury in the erythrocyte is about 10 times higher than that in the plasma (WHO, 1976).

## Binding and storage

As noted above, binding of a chemical in a tissue results in a higher concentration in that tissue. There are two major types of binding. The covalent type of binding is irreversible and is, in general, associated with significant toxic effects. The noncovalent binding usually accounts for a major portion of the dose and is reversible. Therefore, this process plays an important role in the distribution of toxicants in various organs and tissues. There are several types of noncovalent binding as outlined by Guthrie (1980). In general, storage of toxicants in nontarget organs may be considered as the first step to protect our body, but their chronic release from nontarget organs into the body may produce chronic intoxication later.

*Plasma proteins* bind normal physiological constituents in the body as well as many foreign compounds. Most of the latter are bound to the albumin and are therefore not immediately available for distribution to the extravascular space. However, since binding is reversible, it permits the bound chemical to dissociate from the protein, thereby replenishing the level of unbound chemical, which may then cross the capillary endothelium. The toxicologic significance of the binding can be illustrated by the possible induction of coma by the administration of sulfonamide drugs to patients who are taking antidiabetic drugs. The antidiabetic drugs are bound to the plasma proteins but may be replaced by the sulfonamide drugs, which have a greater affinity for the plasma protein. The anti-diabetic drugs thus released may precipitate a hypoglycemic coma. This is an example of drug–drug interaction through plasma protein binding that has toxicological significance. Other types of plasma proteins for storage are lipoproteins (for vitamins, cholesterol, steroid, lipid soluble agents, and basic drugs), gamma globulins for antigens, transferrin for iron, and ceruloplasmin for copper.

The *liver* and *kidney* have a higher capacity for binding chemicals. This characteristic may be related to their metabolic and excretory function. Certain proteins have been identified in these organs for their specific binding property, such as metallothionein (MT), which is important for the binding of cadmium in liver and kidney, and possibly also for transfer of the metal from liver to kidney. Binding of a substance increases its concentration in an organ rapidly. For example, 30 minutes after a single administration of lead, its concentration in the liver is 50 times higher than in plasma. MTs might also be upregulated in various organs/tissues by inflammatory stimuli, suggesting the possible target of MTs in inflammatory diseases (Inoue et al., 2009). MTs (e.g., MT-I, MT-II, MT-III, and MT-IV, and other isoforms) exert various biological effects on heavy metal homeostasis, cancer, circulation, diabetes, the immune system, and antioxidative defense (Thirumoorthy et al., 2011).

*Adipose tissue* is an important storage depot for lipid-soluble substances such as dichlorodiphenyltrichloroethane (DDT), dieldrin, and polychlorinated biphenyls (PCBs). These chemicals appear to be stored in the adipose tissue by simple dissolution in the neutral fats. There exists the potential that the plasma concentration of the substances stored in the fat may increase sharply as a result of rapid mobilization of fat following starvation. Conjugation of fatty acid to toxicants, such as DDT, may also be a mechanism by which these chemicals are retained in the lipid-containing tissues and cells of the body (Leighty et al., 1980).

*Bone* is a major site for storage of such toxicants as fluoride, lead, and strontium. The storage takes place by an exchange adsorption reaction between the toxicants in the interstitial fluid and the hydroxyapatite crystals of bone mineral. By virtue of similarities in size and charge, $F^-$ may readily replace $OH^-$, and calcium may be replaced by lead or strontium. These stored substances are released by ionic exchange and by dissolution of bone crystals through osteoclastic activity.

## *Excretion pathways*

After absorption and distribution in the organism, toxicants are excreted, rapidly or slowly. A generally accepted indicator of the rate of elimination of a toxicant is its "half-life" ($t_{1/2}$), which is the time required to remove 50% of it from the bloodstream.

The toxicants are excreted as the parent chemicals, as their metabolites, and/or as conjugates of them. The principal routes of excretion are the urine and feces, but the liver and lungs are also important excretory organs for certain types of chemicals such as bilirubin and diethyl ether. In addition, there are a number of other minor routes for excretion, including sweat, saliva, and milk.

### *Urinary excretion*

The kidney is an important organ for the elimination of xenobiotics because most chemicals are excreted from blood by urine rather than any other pathway. The kidney receives about 25% of cardiac output, and about one-fifth of the blood in the kidney is filtered at the glomeruli. Overall, the kidney removes toxicants from the body by the same mechanisms as those used in the removal of end products of normal metabolism, namely, glomerular filtration, tubular diffusion, and tubular secretion.

The glomerular capillaries have large pores (70 nm); therefore, most toxicants will be filtered at the glomerulus, except those that are very large (greater than 60,000 Da) or those that are tightly bound to plasma protein. Once a toxicant enters the glomerular filtrate, it will either be passively reabsorbed across the tubular cells if it has a high lipid/water partition coefficient or remains in the tubular lumen and be excreted if it is a polar compound.

A toxicant can also be excreted through the tubules into the urine by passive diffusion. As urine is normally acidic, this process plays a role in the excretion of organic bases. On the other hand, organic acids are unlikely to be excreted by passive diffusion through the tubular cells. However, weak acids are often metabolized to stronger acids, thereby increasing the percentage of the ionic forms that are not reabsorbed through the tubular cells and are thus excreted.

Certain toxicants might be secreted by the cells of the proximal tubules into the urine. There are two distinct secretory mechanisms, one for organic acids (e.g., glucuronide and sulfate conjugates) and the other for organic bases. Protein-bound toxicants are also secreted, provided binding is reversible. Further, chemicals of similar characteristics compete for the same transport system. For example, probenecid increases the serum levels of penicillin and prolongs its activity by blocking its tubular excretion (Nierenberg, 1987).

### *Biliary excretion*

The liver is also an important organ for excretion of toxicants, especially for compounds with high polarity (anionic and cationic), conjugates of compounds bound to plasma proteins, and compounds with molecular weights greater than 300 Da. The factors determining whether a xenobiotic is excreted via bile or urine are not fully understood. However, it is generally recognized that a xenobiotic or its conjugate with molecular weight over 300 Da may be easily excreted via bile, whereas low-molecular-weight compounds are poorly eliminated via bile. In general, once these compounds are in the bile, they are not reabsorbed into the blood and are excreted via the feces. However, there are exceptions, such as the glucuronide conjugates, which are hydrolyzed by intestinal flora, enabling the reabsorption of free toxicants.

The importance of the biliary route of excretion for some chemicals has been demonstrated in experiments that showed a several-fold increase of the acute toxicity in animals with ligated bile ducts. Such chemicals include digoxin, indocyanine green, ouabain, and, most dramatically, diethylstilbestrol (DES) (Klaassen, 1973; Harrison and Gibaldi, 1976). The toxicity of DES is increased 130-fold in rats with ligated bile ducts rather than in sham-operated rats (Klaassen, 1973).

### *Lungs*

Substances that exist in the gaseous phase at body temperature are excreted mainly by the lungs. Volatile liquids are also readily excreted via the expired air. Highly soluble liquids such as chloroform and halothane are excreted slowly because of their storage in adipose tissue and the limited ventilation volume. Excretion of toxicants from the lung is accomplished by simple diffusion through cell membranes. The breakdown of compounds to constituents such as carbon dioxide results in excretion of this gas via the lungs.

### *Other routes*

The *gastrointestinal tract* is not a major route of excretion of toxicants. However, because the human stomach and intestine secretes each about

3 L of fluid per day, some toxicants are excreted along with the fluid. The excretion is mainly by diffusion, and thus the rate depends on the $pK_a$ of the toxicant and the pH of the stomach and intestine.

The excretion of toxicants in mother's *milk* is not important as far as the host organism is concerned. However, the presence of toxic substances in milk may be toxicologically significant because these chemicals are transferred through the milk from mother to nursing child and from cows to humans. The excretion is also via simple diffusion. As milk is slightly acidic, basic compounds reach a higher level in milk than in plasma, while the opposite is true with acidic compounds. Lipophilic compounds such as aldrin, chlordane, DDT, and PCBs also reach a higher level in milk because of its higher fat content (Van den Berg et al., 1987; Li et al., 1995).

*Sweat* and *saliva* are also minor routes of excretion of toxicants. The excretion also occurs by diffusion; thus it is confined to the nonionized, lipid-soluble forms of the toxicants. Substances excreted in the saliva are usually swallowed and then become available for reabsorption in the GI tract.

## Physiologically based pharmacokinetic modeling

Physiologically based pharmacokinetic (PBPK) models represent the body as a set of functional compartments, for example blood, brain, liver, kidneys, muscle, skin, and the remainder of the body. A schematic PBPK model for deltamethrin, a pesticide, is illustrated in Figure 2.4. All compartments need not necessarily be involved, as shown in Figure 2.5, as a PBPK model for methylene chloride, where brain, as opposed to deltamethrin, is not a significant target. Table 2.1 shows various parameters used in the mouse, rat, and human PBPK model structure of Figure 2.5 to simulate pharmacokinetics (PK) of methylene chloride. PBPK facilitates simulation of PK profiles of chemicals on the basis of available information on relevant physiological, physicochemical, and biochemical factors (Thompson et al., 2008). These models utilize biological information to predict the disposition of chemicals for which limited human data are available. It is essential to understand that the chemical is present at low or pharmacological levels and the responses are linear. PBPK models are becoming increasingly important in chemical health risk assessment. In order to construct PBPK models to predict the disposition of chemicals, it is important to take into account genetic makeup, life stage, and health status, because these are confounding factors that may affect the disposition and subsequently the risk assessment. The PBPK model for an infant is markedly different from that of an adult and thus the risk for a child, in general, is greater than that for an adult (Price et al., 2003). Governmental agencies have come to rely in recent years on PBPK modeling as an essential tool in the overall assessment of a chemical hazard for humans.

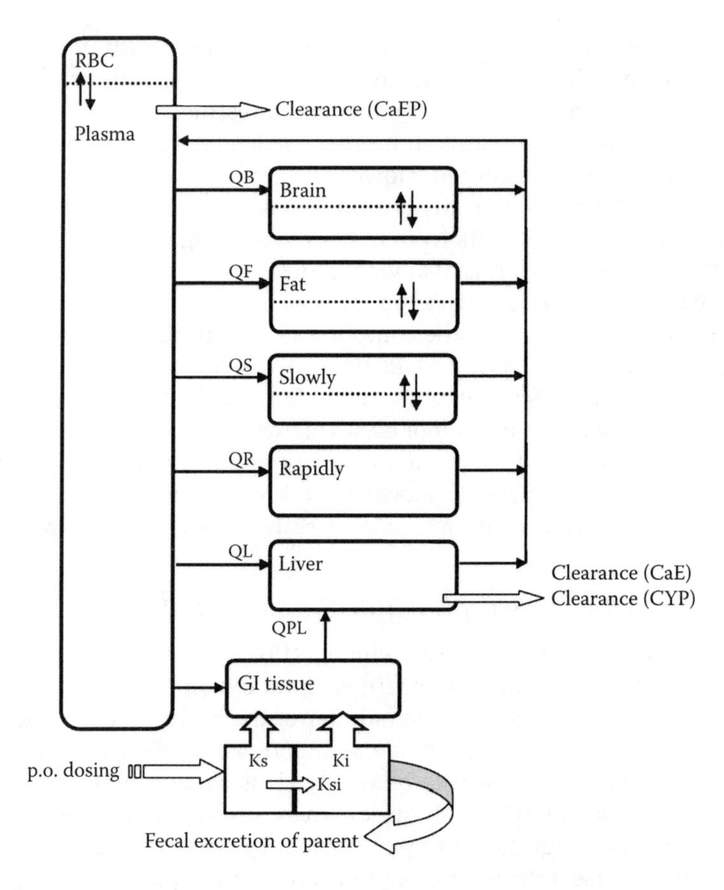


***Figure 2.4*** Schematic diagram of physiologically based pharmacokinetic model for assessing doses of deltamethrin, a pyrethroid pesticide. (Adapted from Tornero-Velez R, Mirfazaelian A, Kim KB et al., *Toxicol. Appl. Pharmacol.*, 244, 208–17, 2010.)

The advantages of PBPK models over classic PK models are that (1) PBPK models describe the time course of deposition of xenobiotics to any organ or tissue including blood; (2) the same PBPK models predict the toxicokinetics (TK) of xenobiotics across species by allometric scaling, or different exposure routes; (3) PBPK models estimate the effects of changing physiological parameters on xenobiotic concentrations in tissue; (4) nonlinear PK or saturable processes, such as metabolism and binding, are readily accommodated (Andersen et al., 2005).

A further step is the use of physiologically based toxicokinetic (PBTK) models where the chemical is present in excessive or toxic levels and where the responses do not follow a linear pattern (Dixit et al.,

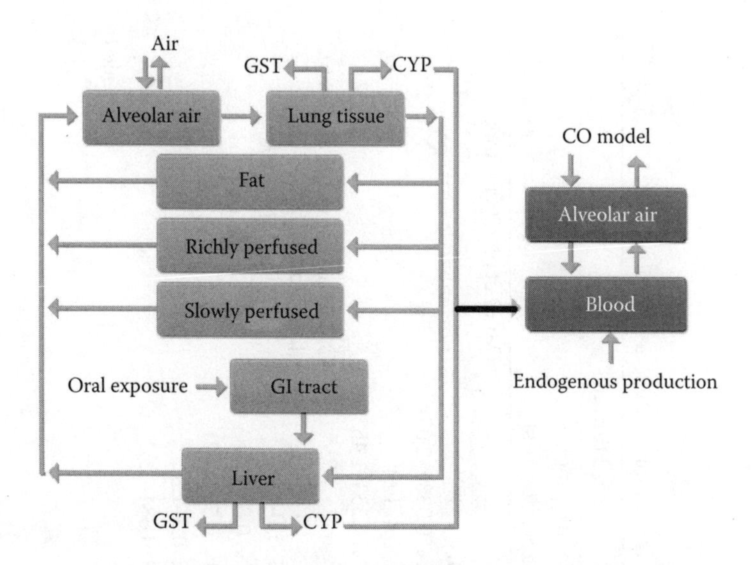


***Figure 2.5*** Schematic diagram of physiologically based pharmacokinetic model for methylene chloride. Methylene chloride can be absorbed through oral or inhalation route and then is eliminated by hepatic metabolism or activated through cytochrome P-450. (Adapted from David RM, Clewell HJ, Gentry PR et al., *Regul. Toxicol. Pharmacol.*, 45, 55–65, 2006.)

2003). Toxicokinetic models are often defined based upon the nature of the rate processes such as absorption across the GI tract, hepatic metabolism, or elimination by the kidney. A conceptual representation of a PBTK model for volatile organic chemicals is illustrated in Figure 2.6. At toxic concentrations, the solubility of chemicals is altered leading to different absorption patterns, excess bioavailability and accumulation, and predictability of chemical disposition becomes less reliable. A TK model is only a tool to estimate chemical concentrations, generating parameters that are useful for further analysis and quantification of the biological processes under study. Toxicokinetics serves as a bridge for extrapolating chemical concentrations across different species, from *in vitro* to *in vivo* studies, from chemical exposure to systemic dose in risk assessment, or as a link between physiology or genetics and chemical disposition in populations of animals and humans.

## *Levels of toxicants in the body*

The nature and intensity of the effects of a chemical depend upon its concentration at the site of action, namely, the effective dose rather than the administered dose. The level in the target organ is, in general, a function

***Table 2.1*** Parameters for the mouse, rat, and human PBPK model for methylene chloride

| | | | Human | | |
|---|---|---|---|---|---|
| Parameter | Mouse mean | Rat value | Mean | CV/GSD (shape, bounds) | Sources |
| **Fractional flow rates (fraction of cardiac output)** | | | | | David et al. (2006); then normalized; $Qi = \frac{QC \cdot QiC}{\sum QjC}$ |
| QFC (Fat) | 0.05 | 0.09 | 0.05 | 0.3 (N, 0.1–1.9) | |
| QLC (Liver) | 0.24 | 0.20 | 0.26 | 0.35 (N, 0.0385–2.05) | |
| QRC (Rapidly perfused tissues) | 0.52 | 0.56 | 0.50 | 0.2 (N, 0.4–1.6) | |
| QSC (Slowly perfused tissues) | 0.19 | 0.15 | 0.19 | 0.15 (N, 0.553–1.453) | |
| **Fractional tissue volumes (fraction of BW)** | | | | | Otherwise David et al. (2006); then normalized; $Vi = \frac{0.9215 \cdot BW \cdot ViC}{\sum VjC}$ |
| VFC (Fat) | 0.04 | 0.07 | f (age, gender) | 0.3 (N, 0.1–1.9) | |
| VLC (Liver) | 0.04 | 0.04 | f (age) | 0.05 (N, 0.85–1.15 | |
| VluC (Lung) | 0.0115 | 0.0115 | 0.0115 | 0.14 (N, 0.58–1.42) | |
| VRC (Rapidly perfused tissues) | 0.05 | 0.05 | 0.064 | 0.1 (N, 0.7–1.3) | |
| VSC (Slowly perfused tissues) | 0.78 | 0.75 | 0.63 | 0.3 (N, 0.684–1.32 | |

(*Continued*)

*Table 2.1 (Continued)* Parameters for the mouse, rat, and human PBPK model for methylene chloride

| Parameter | Mouse mean | Rat value | Human: Mean | Human: CV/GSD (shape, bounds) | Human: Sources |
|---|---|---|---|---|---|
| **Partition coefficients** | | | | | GM and GSD/GM values Converted from arithmetic mean & SDs of David et al. (2006) |
| PB (Blood/air) | 23.0 | 19.4 | 9.7 | 1.1 (LN, 0.738–1.34) | |
| PF (Fat/blood) | 5.1 | 6.19 | 11.9 | 1.34 (LN, 0.413–2.41) | |
| PL (Liver/blood) | 1.6 | 0.73 | 1.43 | 1.22 (N, 0.552–1.81) | |
| PLu (Lung/blood) | 0.46 | 0.46 | 1.43 | . | |
| PR (Rapidly perfused/blood) | 0.52 | 0.73 | 1.43 | . | |
| PS (Slowly perfused/blood) | 0.44 | 0.41 | 0.80 | 1.22 (LN, 0.555–1.83) | |
| **Flow rates** | | | | | QCC; vprv = VPR/$VPR_{mean}$ |
| QCC (Cardiac output (L/hr/$kg^{0.74}$)) | 24.2 | 14.99 | $QCC_{mean}$ = f (QAlvC) | QCC = $QCC_{mean}$/prv | |

*Source:* Adapted from David RM, Clewell HJ, Gentry PR et al. *Regul. Toxicol. Pharmacol.*, 45, 55–65, 2006.

*Abbreviations:* CV, coefficient of variation; GM, geometric mean; GSD, geometric standard deviation; QCC, cardiac output; SD, standard deviation.

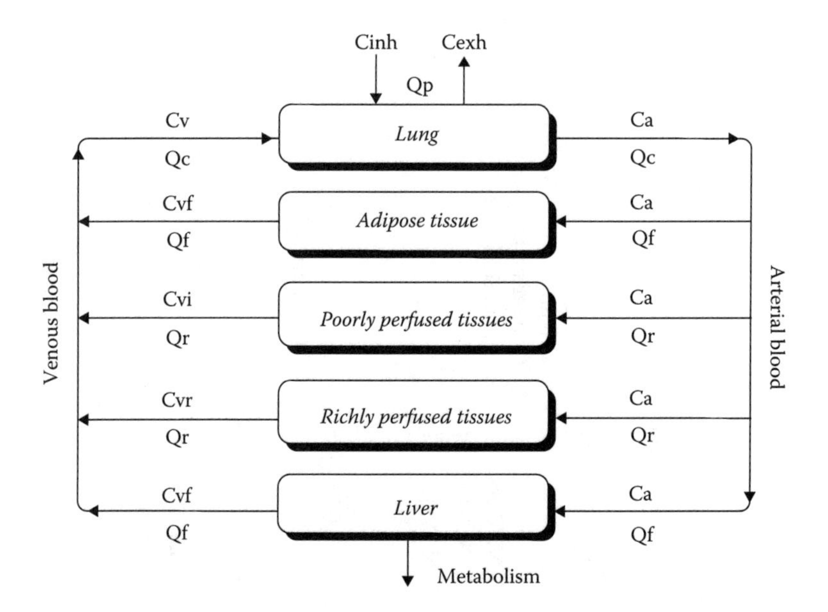


***Figure 2.6*** Conceptual representation of PBTK model for volatile organic chemicals. Qp and Qc refer to alveolar ventilation rate and cardiac output. Cinh, Cexh, Cv, and Ca refer to chemical concentration in inhaled air, exhaled air, venous blood, and arterial blood, respectively. Cvf and Qf refer to venous blood concentrations leaving tissue compartments and blood flow to tissues (i.e., f, adipose tissue; s, slowly perfused tissues; r, richly perfused tissues; and l, liver). (From Haddad S, Charest-Tardif G, Krishnan K, *J. Toxicol. Environ. Health.*, A 61, 209–23, 2000.)

of the blood level. However, binding of a toxicant in a tissue increases its level, whereas tissue barriers tend to reduce the level. As the blood level is more readily determined, especially over a time period, it is the parameter often used in TK studies.

While the toxicant is being absorbed, its blood level rises. In the meantime, the rates of its excretion, biotransformation (Chapter 3), and distribution to other organs and tissues also increase. The curve depicting the blood level against time and the area under that curve (AUC) are useful tools in TK. In a series of experimental studies, Smyth and Hottendorf (1980) demonstrated that the AUC for a solution of a chemical is, in general, greater than that for its suspension, and it is greater for acidic than for basic chemicals. They also illustrated the effects of the route of administration, dose level, and dosing vehicle on the AUC.

The influence of the rate of excretion on the blood level is shown in Figure 2.7. Saccharin is rapidly excreted; hence its blood level drops rapidly,

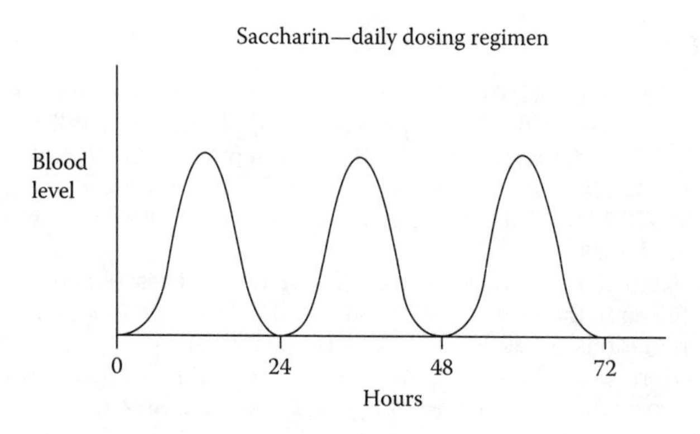


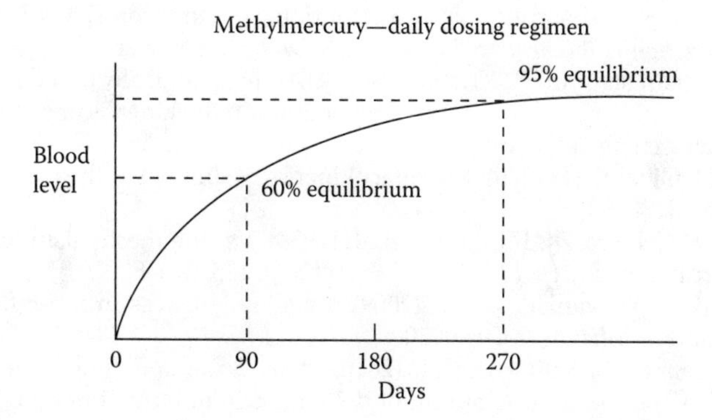


***Figure 2.7*** Comparative chemobiokinetics of saccharin and methylmercury chloride. (From Munro IO, Willes AF, *Chemical Toxicology of Food*, Amsterdam, The Netherlands Elsevier/North Holland, 1978.)

even after repeated administration. On the other hand, methylmercury is excreted slowly; its gradual accumulation culminates in a near plateau only after 270 days (Munro and Willes, 1978). It should be noted that the blood level of a chemical does not necessarily correlate with toxicity. In the case of blood lead levels, the concentration found was high but did not appear to correlate with any adverse effects, especially in children. The blood chemical concentration is simply a marker of exposure and not necessarily toxicity.

Methods for determining the rate and extent of absorption, distribution, binding, storage, and excretion at various organs and tissues are found in the literature. A summary of some of them is given in a WHO publication and OECD guideline (WHO, 1986; OECD, 2009).

## *References*

Andersen ME, Yang RSH, Clewell HJ, Reddy MB (2005). Introduction: A historical perspective of the development and applications of PBPK models. In: Reddy MB, Yang RSH, Clewell HJ, Andersen ME, eds. *Physiologically Based Pharmacokinetic Modeling*. Hoboken, NJ: John Wiley & Sons.

Bradbury MWB (1984). The structure and function of the blood–brain barrier. *Fed Proc*. 43, 186–90.

David RM, Clewell HJ, Gentry PR et al. (2006). Revised assessment of cancer risk to dichloromethane II. Application of probabilistic methods to cancer risk determinations. *Regul Toxicol Pharmacol*. 45, 55–65.

Dixit R, Riviere J, Krishnan K et al. (2003). Toxicokinetics and physiologically based toxicokinetics in toxicology and risk assessment. *J Toxicol Environ Health B*. 6, 1–40.

Guthrie FE (1980). Absorption and distribution. In: Hodgson E, Guthrie FE, eds. *Introduction to Biochemical Toxicology*. New York: Elsevier.

Haddad S, Charest-Tardif G, Krishnan K (2000). Physiologically based modeling of the maximal effect of metabolic interactions on the kinetics of components of complex chemical mixtures. *J Toxicol Environ Health*. A 61, 209–23.

Harrison LI, Gibaldi M (1976). Pharmacokinetics of digoxin in the rat. *Drug Metab Dispos*. 4, 88–93.

Hogben CAM, Tocco DJ, Brodie BB et al. (1958). On the mechanism of intestinal absorption of drugs. *J Pharmacol Exp Therap*. 125, 275–82.

Inoue K, Takano H, Shimada A et al. (2009). Metallothionein as an anti-inflammatory mediator. *Mediators Inflamm*. 2009, 7.

Kim KB, Anand SS, Kim HJ et al. (2010). Age, dose, and time-dependency of plasma and tissue distribution of deltamethrin in immature rats. *Toxicol Sci*. 115, 354–68.

Klaassen CD (1973). Comparison of the toxicity of chemicals in newborn rats to bile duct-ligated and sham-operated rats and mice. *Toxicol Appl Pharmacol*. 24, 37–44.

Leighty EG, Fentiman AF Jr, Thompson RM (1980). Conjugation of fatty acids to DDT in the rat: Possible mechanism for retention. *Toxicology*. 15, 77–82.

Li X, Weber LWD, Rozman KK (1995). Toxicokinetics of 2,3,7,8-tetrachlorodibenzo-p-dioxin (TCDD) in female Sprague-Dawley rats including placental and lactational transfer to fetuses and neonates. *Fudnam Appl Toxicol*. 27, 70–6.

Morrow PE, Hodge HC, Newman WF et al. (1966). Deposition and retention models for internal dosimetry of the human respiratory tract. *Health Phys*. 12, 173–207.

Munro IO, Willes AF (1978). Reproductive toxicity and the problems of in vitro exposure. In: Galli A, Paoletti R, Veterazzi G, eds. *Chemical Toxicology of Food*. Amsterdam, The Netherlands Elsevier/North Holland.

Nierenberg DW (1987). Drug inhibition of penicillin tubular secretion: Concordance between in vitro and clinical findings. *J Pharmacol Exp Ther*. 240, 713–6.

Oberdorster G, Oberdorster E, Oberdorster J (2005). Nanotoxicology: An emerging discipline evolving from studies of ultrafine particles. *Environ Health Perspect*. 113, 823–39.

OECD. (2009). OECD guideline for the testing of chemicals draft proposal for a revised TG: 417 Toxicokinetics. Available from: http://www.oecd.org/dataoecd/26/32/44216274.pdf.

Price K, Haddad S, Krishnan K (2003). Physiological modeling of age-specific changes in the pharmacokinetics of organic chemicals in children. *J Toxicol Environ Health*. A 66, 417–33.

Singer SJ, Nicolson GC (1972). The fluid mosaic model of the structure of cell membranes. *Science*. 175, 720–31.

Smyth AD, Hottendorf GH (1980). Application of pharmacokinetics and biopharmaceutics in the design of toxicological studies. *Toxicol Appl Pharmacol*. 53, 179–95.

Task Group on Lung Dynamics. (1966). Deposition and retention models for internal dosimetry of the human respiratory tract. *Health Phys*. 12, 173–207.

Thirumoorthy N, Shyam Sunder A, Manisenthil Kumar K et al. (2011). A review of Metallothionein isoforms and their role in pathophysiology. *World J Surg Oncol*. 20, 9–54.

Thompson CM, Sonawane B, Barton HA et al. (2008). Approaches for applications of physiologically based pharmacokinetic models in risk assessment. *J Toxicol Environ Health B*. 11, 519–47.

Timbrell JA (1991). *Principles of Biochemical Toxicology*. London: Taylor & Francis.

Tornero-Velez R, Mirfazaelian A, Kim KB et al. (2010). Evaluation of deltamethrin kinetics and dosimetry in the maturing rat using a PBPK model. *Toxicol Appl Pharmacol*. 244, 208–17.

Van den Berg M, Heeremans C, Veerhoven E, Olie K (1987). Transfer of polychlorinated dibenzo-*p*-dioxins and dibenzofurans to fatal and neonatal rats. *Fundam Appl Toxicol*. 9, 635–44.

WHO. (1976). Mercury: Environmental Health Criteria 1. Geneva, Switzerland: World Health Organization, p. 70.

WHO. (1986). Principles of Toxicokinetic Studies. Environmental Health Criteria 57. Geneva, Switzerland: World Health Organization.

Zbinden G (1976). Percutaneous drug permeation. In: *Progress in Toxicology, vol. 2*. New York: Springer-Verlag.

# *chapter three*

# *Biotransformation of toxicants*

***Tae Cheon Jeong***

*Contents*

## *General considerations*

Once a toxicant is absorbed into an organism through various routes, such as the mouth, blood, lung, skin, eye, or nasal mucosa, it is distributed to various parts of the body, including the excretory organs. Many chemicals are known to undergo biotransformation (metabolic transformation or metabolism), which is catalyzed by enzymes present in the blood and tissues. Although the most important site of such reactions is the liver, other organs also contribute in some extent. Examples are the lungs, stomach, intestine, skin, and kidneys. During the process of biotransformation, "xenobiotics" (foreign substances to an organism or toxic substances) can be either activated to toxic form(s) or inactivated to nontoxic form(s) to become reactive or nonreactive with biomolecules such as DNA, RNA, proteins, and lipids.

There are two types of biotransformation:

1. Phase I, involving oxidation, reduction, and hydrolysis may be considered degradation reactions.
2. Phase II, involving the production of a compound (a conjugate) that is biosynthesized from the toxicant, or its metabolite, plus an endogenous substrate may be considered conjugation reactions.

Biotransformation is, therefore, a process that, in general, converts the parent compounds into metabolites and then forms conjugates, but it may involve only one of these reactions. In other words, it is defined as a converting process of lipophilicity to hydrophilicity, or a process of an absorbable to an excretal form. For example, benzene undergoes oxidation, a phase I reaction, to form phenol, which conjugates with sulfate, a phase II reaction. However, when the administered chemical is phenol, it will be conjugated with sulfate without a phase I reaction. The metabolites and conjugates are usually more water-soluble and more polar, hence more readily excretable. Biotransformation mediated by phase I and II metabolizing enzymes can, therefore, be considered a mechanism of detoxication or bioinactivation in general by the host organism.

However, it must be noted that in certain cases metabolites are more toxic than parent compounds. Such reactions are known as "bioactivation." This is frequently noted with chemicals that induce cancer where the metabolite and not the parent compound is the culprit. In fact, most of carcinogens require metabolic activation by certain enzymes for inducing cancer. Aflatoxin $B_1$ and benzo(a)pyrene are such examples.

The rate of biotransformation and the type of biotransformation of a toxicant often differ from one species of animal to another and even from one strain to another, a fact that often accounts for differences in toxicity in these animals (see Chapter 5). The age and gender of the animal and its exposures to other chemicals may also alter biotransformation. Genetic polymorphisms in xenobiotic-metabolizing enzymes and transporter have been considered a critical factor for individual susceptibility or variation in toxic responses (Ginsberg et al., 2009; Johansson and Ingelman-Sundberg, 2011). Knowledge of such factors is important in the design of toxicological studies and in the interpretation of health hazards attributed to human toxicants.

## *Phase I (degradation) reactions*

The three types of phase I reactions, namely, oxidation, reduction, and hydrolysis, are briefly described. Although many exceptions exist, as a general rule the enzymes show broad substrate specificities because a limited number of enzymes metabolize a great number of substrates.

### *Oxidation*

The biotransformation of a great variety of chemicals involves oxidative processes. The most important enzyme systems catalyzing these processes include cytochrome P450 (CYP) and NADPH CYP reductase. In these reactions, one atom of molecular oxygen is reduced to water and the other is incorporated into the substrate as follows: $SH + O_2 + NADPH + H^+ \rightarrow SOH + H_2O + NADP^+$, where S is the substrate.

Cytochrome-linked monooxygenases (oxidases) are located in the endoplasmic reticulum. When a cell is homogenized, the endoplasmic reticulum breaks down to small vesicles known as microsomes. Because of the location of these enzymes and the wide variety of chemicals that they catalyze, they are also known as microsomal mixed-function oxidases (MFOs). The human CYP MFO system consists of more than 60 isozymes in humans, which metabolize a great variety of chemicals as shown in this chapter. In addition, oxidation of a number of toxicants is catalyzed by non-microsomal oxidoreductases that are located in the mitochondrial fraction in the 100,000 *g* supernatant of tissue homogenates.

Oxidation may take place in a variety of reactions, and often more than one metabolite is formed. The following are some examples.

#### *Microsomal oxidation*

1. Aliphatic oxidation involves oxidation of the aliphatic side chains of aromatic chemicals: for example, *n*-propylbenzene → 3-phenylpropan-1-ol, 3-phenylpropan-2-ol, and 3-phenylpropan-3-ol, as well as aliphatic compounds such as *n*-hexane.

2. Aromatic hydroxylation generally proceeds through an epoxide intermediate: for example, naphthalene → naphthalene-1, 2-epoxide → 1-naphthol + 2-naphthol.
3. Epoxidation: for example, aldrin → dieldrin.
4. Oxidative deamination: for example, amphetamine → phenylacetone.
5. *N*-Dealkylation: for example, *N,N*-dimethyl-*p*-nitrophenyl carbamate → *N*-methyl-*p*-nitrophenyl carbamate.
6. *O*-Dealkylation: for example, *p*-nitroanisole → *p*-nitrophenol.
7. *S*-Dealkylation: for example, 6-methylmercaptopurine → 6-mercaptopurine.
8. *N*-Oxidation: for example, trimethylamine → trimethylamine oxide.
9. *N*-Hydroxylation: for example, aniline → phenylhydroxylamine.
10. *P*-Oxidation: for example, diphenylmethylphosphine → diphenylmethylphosphine oxide.
11. Sulfoxidation: for example, methiocarb → methiocarb sulfone.
12. Desulfuration involves the replacement of S by O: for example, parathion → paraoxon.

#### *Non-microsomal oxidations catalyzed by enzymes in mitochondria, cytosol, and nuclei*

1. Amine oxidation: Monoamine oxidase is located in mitochondria and diamine oxidase is a cytosolic enzyme. Both are involved in the oxidation of the primary, secondary, and tertiary amines, such as 5-hydroxytryptamine and putrescine into their corresponding aldehydes.
2. Alcohol and aldehyde dehydrogenations are catalyzed, respectively, by alcohol dehydrogenase and aldehyde dehydrogenase: for example, ethanol → acetaldehyde → acetic acid.

### *Reduction*

Toxicants may undergo reductions through the function of reductases. These reactions are less active in mammalian tissues but more so in intestinal bacteria, because the distant part of the intestine, where reduction is more favorable than oxidation, lacks oxygen. A notable example is reduction of prontosil to sulfanilamide, converting an inactive chemical to an effective antibacterial drug.

#### *Microsomal reduction*

1. Nitro reduction: for example, nitrobenzene → nitrosobenzene → phenyl hydroxylamine → aniline.
2. Azo reduction: for example, azobenzene → aniline.

Non-microsomal reductions occur via the reverse reaction of alcohol dehydrogenases (see the section, "Non-Microsomal Oxidations Catalyzed by Enzymes in Mitochondria, Cytosol, and Nuclei").

### *Hydrolysis*

Many toxicants contain ester-type bonds and are subject to hydrolysis. These are essentially esters, amides, and compounds of phosphate. Mammalian tissues, including the plasma, contain a large number of nonspecific esterases and amidases, which are involved in hydrolysis. The esterases, usually located in the soluble fraction of the cell, may be broadly categorized into four classes:

1. Arylesterases, which hydrolyze aromatic esters
2. Carboxyl esterases, which hydrolyze aliphatic esters
3. Cholinesterases, which hydrolyze esters in which the alcohol moiety is choline
4. Acetyl esterases, which hydrolyze esters in which the acid moiety is acetic acid

In contrast to esterases, amidases cannot be classified according to substrate specificity. Of equal importance, enzymatic hydrolysis of amides proceeds more slowly than that of esters, probably a result of the lack of substrate specificity. An example is procaineamide, a drug used for arrhythmia, which is metabolized slowly. On the other hand, structurally similar procaine, a local anesthetic containing a carboxyl ester, cannot be used for systemic purposes because it is metabolized too quickly.

## *Phase II (conjugation) reactions*

Phase II reactions involve several types of endogenous metabolites that, as noted above, may form conjugates with toxicants per se or their metabolites. These conjugates are generally more water soluble and more readily excretable. This is because the physiological transport mechanisms for endogenous metabolites also recognize the conjugates and hence facilitate their excretion.

### *Glucuronide formation*

This is the most common and important type of conjugation. The enzymes catalyzing this reaction are uridine diphosphate-glucuronosyl transferases (UGTs) and the coenzyme is uridine-5′-diphospho-α-D-glucuronic acid (UDP-GA). This enzyme is located in the endoplasmic reticulum.

There are four classes of chemical compounds that are capable of forming conjugates with glucuronic acid: (1) aliphatic or aromatic alcohols; (2) carboxylic acids; (3) sulfhydryl compounds; and (4) amines. Bilirubin, the product from heme metabolism, is solely glucuronidated for excretion. An individual who lacks certain UGTs exhibits hyperbilirubinemia (i.e., Crigler-Najjar syndrome) due to the absence of bilirubin glucuronidation.

### *Sulfate conjugation*

This reaction is catalyzed by sulfotransferases. These enzymes are found primarily in the cytosolic fraction of the liver, kidneys, and intestines. The coenzyme is 3-phosphoadenosine-5′-phosphosulfate. The functional groups of the foreign compounds for sulfate transfer are phenols and aliphatic alcohols as well as aromatic amines.

### *Methylation*

This reaction is catalyzed by methyl transferases. The coenzyme is *S*-adenosylmethionine. Methylation is not a major route of biotransformation of toxicants. Further, it does not always increase the water solubility of the methylated products. The enzymes are located in both the mitochondrial and cytosolic fractions.

### *Acetylation*

Acetylation involves transfer of acetyl groups to primary aromatic amines, hydrazines, hydrazides, sulfonamides, and certain primary aliphatic amines. The enzyme and coenzyme involved are, respectively, *N*-acetyl transferases (NATs) and acetyl coenzyme A. In certain cases, such as isoniazid, acetylation results in a decrease not only in water solubility of an amine but also in toxicity. NATs show genetic polymorphism. Fast acetylators acetylate isoniazid to its diacetylated metabolite compared to slow acetylators. For this reason, slow acetylators are more sensitive to isoniazid-induced toxicity compared to fast acetylators.

### *Amino acid conjugation*

This conjugation is catalyzed by amino acid conjugates and coenzyme A. Aromatic carboxylic acids, arylacetic acids, and aryl-substituted acrylic acids form conjugates with not only α-amino acids, mainly glycine, but also with glutamine in humans (and certain monkeys) and ornithine in birds. Taurine, an example of β-amino acid, forms a conjugate with cholic acid.

## *Glutathione conjugation*

This important reaction is affected by glutathione *S*-transferases and the cofactor glutathione (GSH, a tripeptide; γ-glu-cys-gly). GSH conjugates subsequently undergo enzymatic cleavage and acetylation, forming *N*-acetylcysteine (mercapturic acid) derivatives of the toxicants, which are readily excreted. Examples of chemicals such as epoxides and aromatic halogens that conjugate with GSH are shown in Figure 3.1. In addition, GSH might conjugate unsaturated aliphatic compounds and displace the nitro groups in chemicals.

In the process of biotransformation of toxicants, a number of highly reactive electrophilic metabolites are formed. In particular, the generation of reactive oxygen species (ROS) is believed to be responsible for the cancer produced by diesel exhaust particles. Some of these metabolites react with cellular constituents and produce cell death, induce tumor formation, or affect immune function. The role of GSH is to react with the electrophilic metabolites such as ROS and thus prevent their harmful effects on the cells. However, exposure to excessive amounts of such reactive substances might deplete GSH, thereby resulting in marked toxic effects. An example of the decreased levels of GSH by acetaminophen and concomitant increase in covalent binding to macromolecules is shown in Figure 3.2. Similarly, 3-methylindole is bioactivated mainly in lungs and, after diminishing GSH concentrations, produces lung damage (Adams et al., 1988). Further, certain GSH conjugates may become toxic

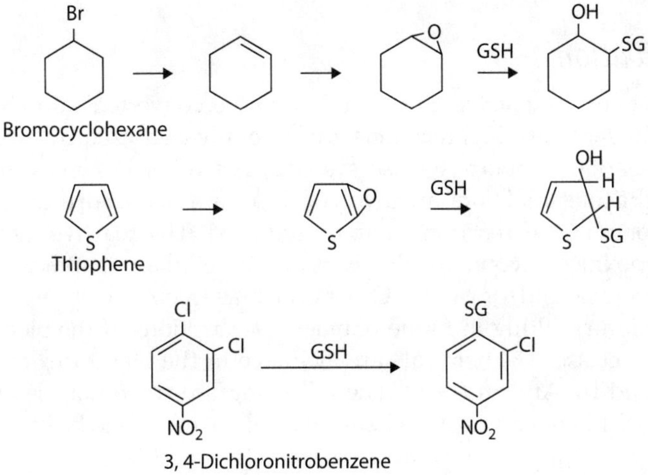

***Figure 3.1*** Conjugation of epoxide and dehalogenation catalyzed by glutathione (GSH) transferase. (From Timbrell JA, *Principles of Biochemical Toxicology*, London, UK: Taylor & Francis, 1991.)

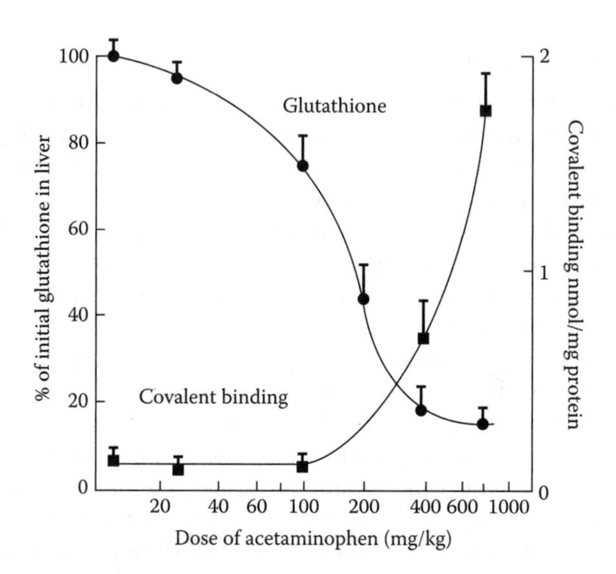


***Figure 3.2*** Protective effect of glutathione against covalent binding of acetaminophen to liver proteins. (From Wills ED, *Testing for Toxicity*, London, UK: Taylor & Francis, 1981.)

(Anders et al., 1988). For additional information on the biological functions of GSH in the conjugation of electrophiles and as antioxidants, see DeLeve and Kaplowitz (1991) and Commandeur et al. (1995).

## *Bioactivation*

Certain chemically stable compounds may be converted into chemically reactive metabolites. The reactions are generally catalyzed by cytochrome P450-dependent monooxygenase systems, but other enzymes, including those of the intestinal flora, are involved in certain cases. Further, additional phase I or phase II reactions may be required. The reactive metabolites, such as epoxides, become covalently bound to cellular macromolecules and induce necrosis and/or cancer. Others, such as free radicals, produce lipid peroxidation resulting in tissue damage. Descriptions of the bioactivation of various classes of chemicals are available in the literature, such as the book edited by Anders (1985). The following are some notable examples. Appendix 3.1 lists a number of chemicals that are known to be bioactivated.

### *Epoxide formation*

Many aromatic compounds are converted to epoxides by microsomal mixed-function oxidase systems. The biotransformation of bromobenzene

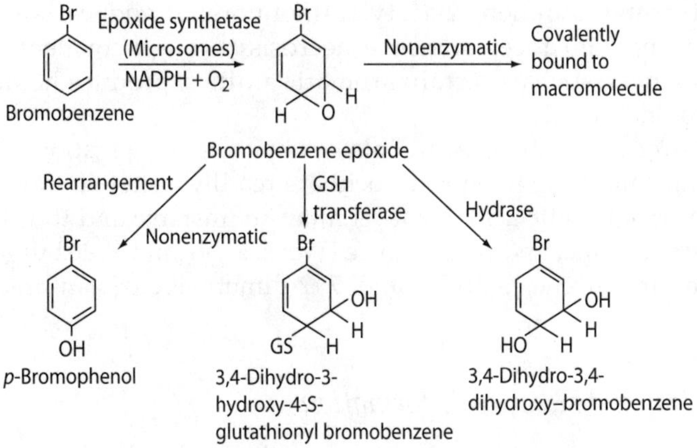

Br Epoxide synthetase (Microsomes) NADPH + $O_2$ Br
Bromobenzene
H O H
Nonenzymatic
Covalently bound to macromolecule
Bromobenzene epoxide
Rearrangement Nonenzymatic
GSH transferase
Hydrase
Br OH
p-Bromophenol
Br OH H GS H
3,4-Dihydro-3-hydroxy-4-S-glutathionyl bromobenzene
Br OH H HO H
3,4-Dihydro-3,4-dihydroxy–bromobenzene

***Figure 3.3*** The bromobenzene epoxide formed from the parent chemical may covalently bind to macromolecules, but such binding may be minimal when the other metabolic routes are predominant. (From Gillette JR, Mitchell JR, *Handbook of Experimental Pharmacology*, New York, Springer-Verlag, 359–82, 1975.)

to its epoxide and subsequent reactions serves as an interesting example of bioactivation and its consequences. These are depicted in Figure 3.3.

Although bromobenzene epoxide may become covalently bound to tissue macromolecules and produce injury, the alternative routes of metabolism may prevent or reduce the injury. The most important of these routes is conjugation with GSH. This reaction is important in that it serves as a protective mechanism. Only after hepatic levels of reduced GSH have been greatly depleted will the bromobenzene epoxide significantly bind to macromolecules and result in hepatic necrosis. Depletion of GSH occurs when an excessive dose of bromobenzene is present or when there has been an induction of microsomal enzymes; both conditions increase the amount of bromobenzene epoxide. Other reactions include a nonenzymatic arrangement to form *p*-bromophenol and the formation of 3,4-dihydro-3,4-dihydroxy-bromobenzene catalyzed by hydrolyzing enzymes.

Other chemicals that undergo epoxidation include aflatoxin $B_1$, benzene, benzo(a)pyrene, furosemide, olefins, polychlorinated, and polybrominated biphenyls, trichloroethylene, and vinyl chloride. Bioactivation takes place mainly in the liver, and the resulting reactive metabolites induce toxicity through covalent binding with macromolecules in the tissue, resulting in necrosis or cancer formation.

## N-*hydroxylation*

Microsomal enzymes from many tissues might *N*-hydroxylate a variety of chemicals. Some of the *N*-hydroxy metabolites, such as those of acetaminophen, 2-acetylaminofluorene, and certain aminoazo dyes, induce cancer or tissue necrosis through covalent binding, whereas others, such as certain aromatic amines, produce hemolysis or methemoglobinemia.

*N*-hydroxy metabolites are also subject to conjugation reactions. Their conjugates with glucuronic acid are readily excreted; those formed with sulfuric or acetic acid, however, may be unstable and thus be mutagenic, carcinogenic, and highly toxic (Weisburger and Weisburger, 1973). 2-Acetylaminoflurene, safrole, and 7,12-dimethylbenz[a]anthracene are examples.

### *Free radical and superoxide formation*

Free radicals are unstable and highly reactive molecules that are capable of existing independently, contain one or more unpaired electrons, have an extremely short half-life, and seek to gain additional electrons to have complete pairs or to bind to other molecules to increase their stability. Certain halogen-containing compounds undergo metabolism to form free radicals. For example, carbon tetrachloride forms a trichloromethyl radical, which initiates peroxidation of polyunsaturated lipid as well as covalently binds to protein and unsaturated lipid. These initial reactions are followed by disturbances of various cellular components, as described in Chapter 12. Halothane and bromotrichloromethane are other examples of chemicals that may form free radicals. The herbicide paraquat is known to produce superoxide radicals which produce pulmonary toxicity (Halliwell et al., 1992).

It should be noted that during the metabolic process some chemicals produce not only their reactive metabolites, but generate free radicals such as ROS (radical forms: superoxide anion, hydroxyl radical, peroxyl and alkoxyl radical; non-radical forms: $O_3$, $H_2O_2$, hypochlorous acid, and singlet oxygen) or chemical radicals. For example, benzo(a)pyrene (BaP) produces an ultimate metabolite [e.g., benzo(a)pyrene 7,8-diol 9,10-epoxide (BPDE)], ROS, and BaP radical cation (Jiang et al., 2007). Free radicals such as ROS, reactive nitrogen species (radical forms: nitric oxide and nitrogen dioxide; non-radical forms: peroxynitrite, nitroxyl anion, nitrosyl cation, nitronium anion, nitrous acid, etc.), and organic radicals activate nonreactive toxicants to form biologically reactive intermediates or reactive toxicants without metabolizing enzymes. Free radicals play a central role in toxicological sciences and are involved in various types of toxic manifestations and common mechanisms of toxic actions (Choi and Lee, 2004). Therefore, toxic effects may be ameliorated or prevented by scavenging free radicals with antioxidants, such as antioxidant vitamins, curcumin, isoflavonoids, resveratrol, and plant polysaccharides.

### *Other pathways*

Ethanol can be oxidized by a dehydrogenase to acetaldehyde, which has been implicated in some of the manifestations of alcohol toxicity. Pyrrolizidine alkaloids are dehydrogenated to reactive pyrrole derivatives, which are carcinogenic. There is evidence confirming that the acute toxicity of aliphatic nitriles is attributable to the cyanide released through hepatic microsomal enzyme activities (Willhite and Smith, 1981).

### *Activation in the GI tract*

Nitrites and certain amines react in the acidic environment of the stomach to form nitrosamines, many of which have been shown to be potent carcinogens, and nitrates, which, under certain conditions, are converted to nitrites that may induce methemoglobinemia. The artificial sweetener cyclamate is converted by intestinal bacteria to cyclohexylamine, which induces testicular atrophy. Cycasin is converted by intestinal microbiota to its aglycone, methylazoxymethanol, which is hepatotoxic and produces tumors. The role of intestinal microbiota in metabolic activation of certain drugs and toxicants are now evident. Intestinal microbiota increase the toxicity of chemicals by producing toxic or carcinogenic metabolites which sometimes would not be formed in tissues (Jeong et al., 2013; Kang et al., 2013).

## *Complex nature of biotransformation*

Toxicants generally undergo several types of biotransformation, resulting in a variety of metabolites and conjugates. Some of the various metabolites and conjugates of bromobenzene are shown in Figure 3.3. Organophosphorus insecticides, such as fenitrothion, chlorofenvinphos, and omethoate, may be metabolized through dealkylation, oxidation, desulfuration, or hydrolysis, yielding 10 or more different metabolites.

Parathion, an organophosphorus pesticide, is bioactivated in the liver to paraoxon, which is a more potent cholinesterase inhibitor. Infusion of parathion by way of the vena cava, bypassing the liver, therefore produced little cholinesterase inhibition, but a moderate effect was induced following infusion by way of the portal vein. On the other hand, infusion of paraoxon via the vena cava nearly completely blocked cholinesterase activity, whereas it exerts negligible effect after an infusion via the portal vein, since it is detoxicated in the liver (Westermann, 1961).

A reactive metabolite formed in a phase I reaction may be further metabolized, such as carbon tetrachloride and halothane. Such a metabolite may also be followed by a phase II reaction to produce another reactive metabolite. For example, 2-acetylaminofluorene after *N*-hydroxylation undergoes acetylation or forms sulfate or GSH conjugates, all of which are highly reactive.

The relative importance of various types of biotransformation of a toxicant depends upon many host, environmental, and chemical factors as well as toxicant dose. Since the metabolites resulting from different types of biotransformation are often markedly different in their effects, the toxicity of a chemical can be greatly altered by these factors, as discussed in Chapter 5.

Some of the metabolic reactions take place in sequence; hence interference with the normal metabolic pathway may exert considerable influence on toxic effects. For example, ethanol is normally metabolized through the intermediary product acetaldehyde. In normal humans the acetaldehyde formed is rapidly further metabolized to acetate, which in turn is converted to carbon dioxide and water. However, if the aldehyde dehydrogenase is inhibited, such as after the administration of disulfiram, the level of acetaldehyde rises and results in distress symptoms such as nausea, vomiting, headache, and palpitations.

A toxicant may be transformed in one organ to a stable proximate metabolite, which is transported to another organ and metabolizes to the ultimate toxic metabolite (Cohen, 1986).

Reeves (1981) provided a number of examples of biotransformation of "typical" chemicals, as well as a limited generalization of the typical routes of foreign compound metabolism in humans (Figure 3.4).

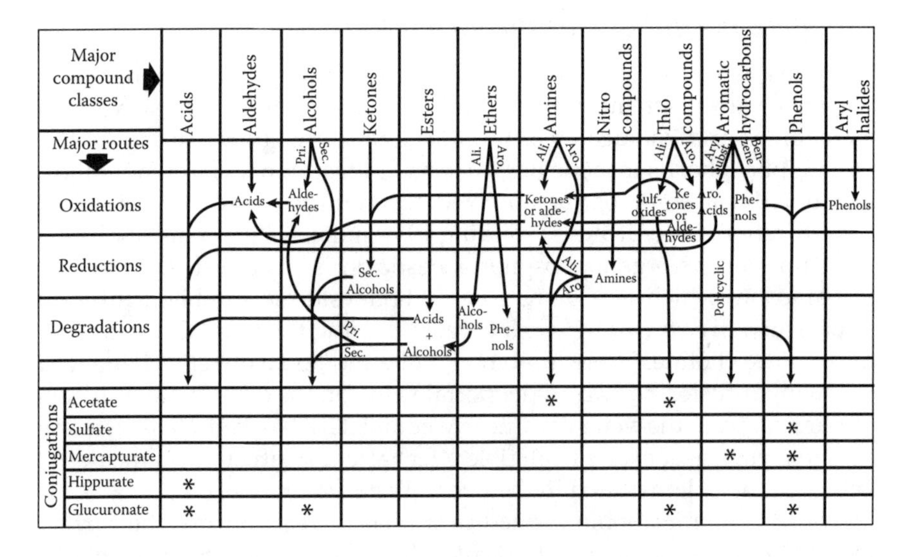


*Figure 3.4* Typical routes of foreign compound metabolism in humans. (From Reeves AL, *Toxicology: Principles and Practices, Vol. 1,* New York: John Wiley, 1981.)

## Developmental and childhood considerations

The ability to handle chemicals in the fetus, infant, and child varies distinctly from that in the adult. Makri et al. (2004) described the metabolic characteristics of neonates to the adolescent, which would ultimately affect the susceptibility of the subject to various chemicals. In general, a neonate, infant, or child is more susceptible to chemical exposure. The age categories are as follows: neonate is 0–1 month, infant from 1 month to 2 years, preschool from 2 to 6 years, the child from 6 to 12 years, and adolescent from 12 to 16 years. Cytochrome P450 is low from 0 to 1 year, which indicates that a chemical half-life is longer and elimination is prolonged. In essence, this manifests itself as a higher susceptibility to chemical effects. Alcohol dehydrogenase is barely detectable in the infant and present at 5 years of age, indicating an inability to handle alcohol and thus toxic consequences to the infant. Glucuronidation pathways and acetylation capacity are not available until 3 years of age, again indicating an enhanced susceptibility. Although sulfate conjugation is higher from 0 to 3 years, the capacity falls at the adult level 3 to 10 years. The difficulty here is that sulfation is not a predominant route for elimination of various compounds and thus results in enhanced chemical susceptibility.

The U.S. Environmental Protection Agency cancer risk assessment guidance recommends a default assumption that children are inherently up to 10 times more sensitive than adults to carcinogen exposures. However, as pointed out by Pyatt et al. (2007), there is no evidence that children are at an increased risk for chemically induced acute myelogenous leukemia development. In fact, it would appear that the risk for drug-induced leukemia development is actually lower in younger children. These findings clearly demonstrate that generalized observations in toxicology can result in miscalculations of risk and unnecessary concerns. The need for extensive data in making decisions, especially as it pertains to sensitive subpopulations, is warranted.

## Elderly

It is also important to bear in mind that the metabolic pathways are age-dependent and less reliable in the elderly, which is also manifested as an increased susceptibility to toxicity in the elderly. Generally, the elderly are a population that is exposed to multidrug therapy, resulting in drug interactions and a reduced capacity of the liver to handle these agents. With concurrent environmental chemical exposure and multidrug administration in a subject with a compromised ability to eliminate chemicals, the occurrence of toxicity attributed to environmental chemicals can be additive or synergistic.

## *Appendix 3.1 Examples of bioactivation*[a]

| Parent compound | Toxic metabolite | Mechanism of toxicity | Toxic effect |
|---|---|---|---|
| Acetaminophen | *N*-acetyl-*p*-benzoquinone imine | Covalent binding | Hepatic necrosis, GI bleeding, nephrotoxicity |
| 2-Acetylaminofluorene (AAF) | *N*-hydroxy-AAF, sulfate ester | Covalent binding | Cancers (liver, kidney, bladder) |
| Aflatoxin $B_1$ | Aflatoxin-8,9-epoxide | Covalent binding | Hepatic cancer |
| Allyl formate | Acrolein | Covalent binding | Hepatic necrosis, lung toxicity |
| Amiodarone | Des ethyl amiodarone | Ethylation | Pulmonary fibrosis, thyroid abnormalities, ophthalmological effects, neurological changes |
| Amygdalin | Mandelo nitrile, hydrogen cyanide | Cyanide formation | Cytotoxic hypoxia, toxicity of nervous, cardiovascular, and respiratory systems |
| *N*-arylsuccinimide | 3,5-Dichlorophenyl-2-hydroxysuccinimide | Oxidation and hydrolysis | Nephrotoxicity |
| Benzene | Benzene epoxide → hydroquinone, 1,2,4-trihydroxybenzene | Covalent binding | Bone marrow depression, leukemia |
| Benzo(a)pyrene (BaP) | BaP-7,8-epoxide → (+)BaP-7,8-diol-9,10-epoxide [(+)BPDE-I] | Covalent binding | Cancers (lung, stomach, cervix, skin) |
| Bromobenzene | 2-Bromoquinone, 4-bromoquinone, bromobenzene epoxides | Covalent binding | Hepatic, renal, bronchiolar toxicity |
| 1,3-Butadiene | 3,4-Epoxy-1-butene (EB) 1,2:3,4-diepoxybutane (DEB), 3,4-epoxy-1,2-butanediol (EB diol) | Covalent binding | Cancer (stomach, blood, lymphatic system), hepatic necrosis, narcosis, reproductive toxicity |

(*Continued*)

| Parent compound | Toxic metabolite | Mechanism of toxicity | Toxic effect |
|---|---|---|---|
| 2-Butoxyethanol | 2-Butoxyacetic acid | Oxidation | Hemolytic disorders |
| Carbon tetrachloride | Trichloro methane free radical | Covalent binding | Hepatic necrosis, hepatic cancer, neurotoxicity |
| Carcinogenic alkyl nitrosamines | α-Hydroxylation | Alkylation | Cancer (liver, esophagus, many organs) |
| Carcinogenic aminoazo dyes | *N*-hydroxy derivatives | Covalent binding | Hepatic cancer, bladder cancer |
| Carcinogenic polycyclic aromatic hydrocarbons (PAHs) | PAH-diolepoxide | Covalent binding | Cancers (lung, skin, stomach) |
| Chloroform | Phosgen | Covalent binding | Hepatic, renal necrosis |
| Cycasin | Methylazoxymethanol, gut flora | Alkylation | Cancers (liver, kidney, intestine), hepatic necrosis |
| Cyclophosphamide | Phosphoramide mustard | Alkylation | Cytotoxic, nephrotoxicity |
| Formaldehyde | | Covalent binding | Nasal cancer, leukemia? |
| Fluoroacetate | Fluoro citrate | Enzyme inhibition | General toxicity |
| Furosemide | Epoxide? | Covalent binding | Hepatic, renal necrosis |
| Halothane | Free radical | Covalent binding | Hepatic necrosis |
| Isoniazid | *N*-hydroxy acetyl hydranize | Covalent binding | Hepatic necrosis |
| Metam sodium | (Metabolite of) methyl isothiocyanate | Reduction | Immunosuppression, spontaneous abortion with increased frequency, asthma |

(*Continued*)

| Parent compound | Toxic metabolite | Mechanism of toxicity | Toxic effect |
|---|---|---|---|
| Methemoglobin-producing aromatic amines and nitro compounds | *N*-hydroxy metabolites | Cyclic oxidoreduction | Methemoglobinemia |
| Methoxyflurane | Inorganic fluoride | Enzyme inhibition | Renal failure |
| Monocrotaline | Monocrotaline pyrrole | Electrophile monocrotaline pyrrole → formation of free radical | Lung and liver damage |
| Naphthylamine | *N*-hydroxy naphthylamine | Covalent binding | Bladder cancer |
| Nitrates | Nitrites | Hemoglobin oxidation | Methemoglobinemia |
| Nitrites plus secondary or tertiary amines | Nitrosamines | Alkylation | Hepatic, pulmonary cancers |

(*Continued*)

| Parent compound | Toxic metabolite | Mechanism of toxicity | Toxic effect |
|---|---|---|---|
| Parathion | Paraoxon | Covalent binding to cholinesterase | Neuromuscular paralysis |
| Purine and pyrimidine base analogues | Mononucleotides, nucleotide triphosphates | Lethal synthesis, lethal incorporation | Cytotoxicity |
| Safrole (also known as shikimol) | 1′-Hydroxy safrole | Covalent binding | Cancers |
| Styrene | Styrene oxide | Covalent binding | Lung tumors |
| Urethane (ethyl carbamate) | *N*-hydroxy urethane, vinyl carbamate epoxide | Alkylation | Cancers (liver, lung), cytotoxicity |
| Vinyl chloride | Chloroethylene epoxide | Covalent binding | Liver cancer |

[a] The site of bioactivation is the liver, except as otherwise noted. Covalent binding refers to DNA, protein, or lipid adduct formation with reactive metabolites of chemicals or reactive chemicals themselves.

## References

Adams JD Jr, Laegreid WW, Huijzer JC et al. (1988). Pathology and glutathione status in 3-methylindole-treated rodents. *Res Commun Chem Pathol Pharmacol.* 60, 323–36.

Anders MW (1985). *Bioactivation of Foreign Compounds.* New York: Academic Press.

Anders MW, Lash L, Dekant W et al. (1988). Biosynthesis and biotransformation of glutathione S-conjugates to toxic metabolites. *CRC Crit Rev Toxicol.* 18, 311.

Choi SM, Lee BM (2004). An alternative mode of action of endocrine-disrupting chemicals and chemoprevention. *J Toxicol Environ Health B Crit Rev.* 7, 451–63.

Cohen GM (1986). Basic principles of target organ toxicity. In: Cohen GM, ed. *Target Organ Toxicity.* Boca Raton, FL: CRC Press.

Commandeur JNML, Stijntjes GJ, Vermeulen NPE (1995). Enzymes and transport systems involved in the formation and disposition of glutathione S-conjugates. *Pharmacol Revs.* 47, 271–330.

DeLeve LD, Kaplowitz N (1991). Glutathione metabolism and its role in hepatotoxicity. *Pharmacol Ther.* 52, 287–305.

Gillette JR, Mitchell JR (1975). Drug actions and interactions: Theoretical considerations. In: Eichler O, Farah A, Herken H, Welch AD, eds. *Handbook of Experimental Pharmacology. New Series, vol. 28.* New York: Springer-Verlag, 359–82.

Ginsberg G, Smolenski S, Hattis D et al. (2009). Genetic polymorphism in glutathione transferases (GST): Population distribution of GSTM1, T1, and P1 conjugating activity. *J Toxicol Environ Health B Crit Rev.* 12, 389–439.

Halliwell B, Gutteridge JMC, Cross CE (1992). Free radicals, antioxidants and human diseases—Where are we now? *J Lab Clin Med.* 119, 598–620.

Jeong HG, Kang MJ, Kim HG et al. (2013). Role of intestinal microflora in xenobiotic-induced toxicity. *Mol Nutr Food Res.* 57, 84–99.

Jiang H, Gelhaus SL, Mangal D et al. (2007). Metabolism of benzo(a)pyrene in human bronchoalveolar H358 cells using liquid chromatography-mass spectrometry. *Chem Res Toxicol.* 20, 1331–41.

Johansson I, Ingelman-Sundberg M (2011). Genetic polymorphism and toxicology—with emphasis on cytochrome p450. *Toxicol Sci.* 120, 1–13.

Kang MJ, Kim HG, Kim JS et al. (2013). The effect of gut microbiota on drug metabolism. *Expert Opin Drug Metab Toxicol.* 9, 1295–308.

Makri A, Goveia M, Balbus J et al. (2004). Children's susceptibility to chemicals: A review by developmental stage. *J Toxicol Environ Health B.* 7, 417–35.

Pyatt DW, Aylward LL, Hays SM (2007). Is age an independent risk factor for chemically induced acute myelogenous leukemia in children? *J Toxicol Environ Health B.* 10, 379–400.

Reeves AL (1981). The metabolism of foreign compounds. In: Reeves AL, ed. *Toxicology: Principles and Practices, Vol 1.* New York: John Wiley.

Timbrell JA (1991). *Principles of Biochemical Toxicology.* London, UK: Taylor & Francis.

Weisburger JH, Weisburger EK (1973). Biochemical formation and pharmacological, toxicological and pathological properties of hydroxylamines and hydroxyamic acids. *Pharmacol Rev.* 25, 166.

Westermann EO (1961). Bioactivation of parathion. Proceedings of International Pharmacology Meeting 6: 205. In: Ariens EJ, Simmonis AM, Offermeier J, eds. *Introduction to General Toxicology*. New York: Academic Press, 147.

Willhite CC, Smith RP (1981). The role of cyanide liberation in the acute toxicity of aliphatic nitriles. *Toxicol Appl Pharmacol*. 59, 589–602.

Wills ED (1981). The role of glutathione in drug metabolism and the protection of the liver against toxic metabolites. In: Gorrod JW, ed. *Testing for Toxicity*. London, UK: Taylor & Francis.

# *chapter four*

# *Mechanisms of toxic effects*

***Hyung Sik Kim and Pinpin Lin***

*Contents*

## *Introduction*

As a function of dose and exposure duration, xenobiotics (also termed stressors) produce adverse responses in biomolecules (DNA, protein, lipids), cells, tissues, organs, and the body. Toxic effects vary in nature, potency, target organ, and mechanism of action (MOA). A better understanding of their characteristics can improve the assessment of the associated health hazards and facilitate development of rational, preventive, and therapeutic measures.

All adverse effects result from biochemical interactions between toxicants (and/or their metabolites) and certain structures of the organism. The structure may be nonspecific, such as any tissue in direct contact with corrosive chemicals. More often it is specific, involving a particular subcellular structure. A variety of structures may be affected.

The nature of effects may also vary from organ to organ. The organ-specific effects will be discussed in some detail in the chapters found in Section III of this book. In some cases, the reason for a particular organ being affected is known. This knowledge is useful in many ways and a few examples are described in this chapter.

## *Spectrum of toxic effects*

The great variety of toxic effects can be grouped according to target organ, MOA, or other characteristics such as those discussed below.

### *Local and systemic effects*

Certain chemicals produce injuries at the site of first contact with an organism. These local effects are induced by caustic substances acting on the gastrointestinal tract, by corrosive materials on the eyes or skin, and by irritant gases and vapors on the respiratory tract. Electrophilic or nucleophilic groups that could haptenize protein act through covalent modification, for example: aldehydes, ketone, codicils, quinones, other conjugated unsaturated functional groups, or epoxy groups.

Systemic effects result only after the toxicant has been absorbed and distributed to other parts of the body. Most toxicants exert their main

***Table 4.1*** Chemicals that cause systemic effects

| Mode of toxicity | Chemicals groups |
|---|---|
| Toxicity caused by electrophiles | Acyl halides<br>Aryl halides<br>Azides and S-mustards<br>Epoxides<br>Nitroso groups conjugated double bonds<br>Aromatic nitro, azo, or amine groups |
| Free radical formation | Aminophenols<br>Catechols, quinines, hydroquinones<br>Metal complexes (iron and chromium), polycyclic aromatics |
| Receptor-mediated mechanisms | Environmental estrogens<br>Fibrates, phthalates<br>Polychlorinated aromatics (Ah receptor ligands)<br>Retinoids (retinoic acid receptor ligands) |

*Source:* Cooke MW, Ferner RE, *Arch Emerg Med*, 10, 368–371. 1993.

effects on one or a few organs. These organs are referred to as the "target organs" of these toxicants. A target organ does not necessarily have the highest concentration of the toxicants in the organism. For example, the target organ of dichlorodiphenyltrichloroethane (DDT) is the central nervous system, but it is concentrated in adipose tissues.

Systemic toxicity is frequently mediated by the presence of reactive functional groups (whether present in the parent compound or introduced via biotransformation). Reactive compounds or metabolites may exert adverse effects by modification of cellular macromolecules (proteins, RNA, DNA). This results in destruction or dysfunction of the target molecules. In addition, covalent modification of target molecules, which are covalently modified, may render them "foreign" or antigenic (immune response). DNA-reactive chemicals have genotoxic potential (DNA adducts formation), free radical formation, and receptor-mediated mechanisms (see Table 4.1).

## *Reversible and irreversible effects*

Reversible effects of toxicants are those that disappear following cessation of exposure to them and thereafter toxicants are detoxified and eliminated. Irreversible effects, in contrast, persist or even progress after exposure is discontinued. Certain effects, which are irreversible, include carcinomas, teratogenesis, damage to neurons, and liver cirrhosis. In toxicology, irreversible effects are more important than reversible effects because the former are chronic and difficult to treat. Certain effects are considered irreversible even though they disappear sometime after cessation of exposure. For example, the "irreversible" cholinesterase-inhibiting insecticides inhibit the activity of this enzyme for a period of time that approximates the time required for the synthesis and replacement of the enzyme. Injury to the nervous system is usually irreversible since neuronal cells cannot divide and be replaced.

The effect produced by a toxicant may be reversible if the organism is exposed at a low concentration and/or for a short duration, whereas irreversible effects may be produced at higher concentrations and/or for longer periods of exposure.

### *Immediate and delayed effects*

Many toxicants produce immediate adverse effects, which develop shortly after a single exposure, a notable example being cyanide poisoning. However, lethal doses of 2,3,7,8-tetrachlorodibenzodioxan (TCDD) result in death of experimental animals after more than 2 weeks (Alarie, 1981; Chanter and Heywood, 1982). To characterize the acute toxicity of different chemicals, $LD_{50}$ values are frequently used as a basis for comparison. The $LD_{50}$ values for number of chemicals administered to rats are given in Table 4.2. However, animal-welfare groups have campaigned against $LD_{50}$ testing using experimental animals. Several countries, including the United Kingdom, have taken steps to ban the oral $LD_{50}$, and the Organization for Economic Cooperation and Development (OECD) abolished the requirement for the oral test in 2001.

***Table 4.2*** Chemicals and their $LD_{50}$ values

| Compounds | $LD_{50}$ value (mg/kg) |
|---|---|
| Ethanol | 7060 (rat, oral) |
| Sodium bicarbonate | 4200 (rat, oral) |
| Sodium chloride | 3000 (rat, oral) |
| Vitamin A | 2000 (rat, oral) |
| Aspirin | 200 (rat, oral) |
| Phenobarbital sodium | 350 (rat, oral) |
| Paraquat | 120 (rat, oral) |
| Aldrin | 46 (rat, oral) |
| Tetrodotoxin | 0.1 (rat, oral) |
| 2,3,7,8-tetrachlorodibenzodioxan (TCDD) | 0.001 (rat, oral) |
| Botulinum toxin | 0.00001 (rat, oral) |

Delayed effects occur after a lapse of some time. Carcinogenic effects generally become manifest 10–20 years after the initial exposure in humans; even in rodents, a lapse of many months is required. In some cases, for example, diethylstilbestrol (DES) was taken by pregnant mothers to prevent miscarriages (Roy et al., 1997; Dean, 1998). However, vaginal adenocarcinomas occurred in the daughters of mothers taking DES. This effect took 15–20 years to develop not in the target subject but was found in the offspring. In addition, in men there was evidence of reproductive dysfunction and increased occurrence of prostatic and testicular cancers. To determine these and other delayed effects of toxicants, chronic studies are essential not only in the directly exposed individual but also in the fetus or offspring.

## *Morphological, functional, and biochemical effects*

Morphological effects refer to gross and microscopic changes in the morphology of the tissues. Many of these effects, such as necrosis and neoplasia, are irreversible and serious often resulting in mortality. Functional effects usually represent reversible changes in the function of target organs. The function of the liver and kidney (e.g., rate of excretion of dyes) are commonly tested in toxicological studies.

Functional effects are in general reversible, whereas morphological effects are not, and functional changes are generally detected earlier or in animals exposed to lower doses than those with morphological changes. In addition, functional tests are valuable in following the progress of effects on target organs in long-term studies in animals and humans. It is worthwhile noting that functional tests can be positive for an adverse effect, yet there is no morphological evidence. An example is the presence of depleted uranium producing proteinuria, indicative of a renal functional alteration, but there are no apparent morphological changes (NAS, 2008). The role of concentration of depleted uranium at the target site may be important as lower amounts of this metal may produce the effect seen, but in concentrations not sufficient to induce morphological alterations. This is of particular concern for veterans of the Gulf War and for the assessment of hazard characterization. However, the results are often more variable.

Although all adverse effects are associated with biochemical alterations, in routine toxicity testing, "biochemical effects" usually refer to those without apparent morphological changes. An example of such effects is the cholinesterase inhibition following exposure to organophosphate and carbamate insecticides. Another example is δ-aminolevulinic acid dehydratase inhibition in lead poisoning (see Chapter 25).

## *Allergic and idiosyncratic reactions*

Allergic reaction (also known as hypersensitivity and sensitization reaction) to a toxicant results from previous sensitization to that toxicant or a chemically similar one. The chemical acts as a hapten and combines with an endogenous protein to form an antigen, which in turn elicits the formation of antibodies. A subsequent exposure to the chemical results in an antigen–antibody interaction, which provokes the typical manifestations of allergy. Thus, this reaction is different from the usual toxic effects, first because a previous exposure is required, and second because a typical sigmoid dose–response curve is usually not demonstrable with allergic reactions. Nevertheless, threshold doses were demonstrable for the induction as well as the challenge in dermal sensitization (Koschier et al., 1983). In addition to the immune response described above, humans also generate self- or autoantigens, constituents of the body's own tissues in response to a specific humoral or cell-mediated immune response termed as autoimmunity. An example of an autoimmune disease is systemic lupus erythematosus (SLE), and a chemical implicated in SLE occurrence is trichloroethene (Wang et al., 2007).

Generally an idiosyncratic reaction is a genetically determined abnormal reactivity to a chemical. Some patients exhibit prolonged muscular reaction and apnea following a standard dose of succinylcholine. These patients have a deficiency of serum cholinesterase, which normally degrades the muscle relaxant rapidly. Similarly, individuals with a deficiency of NADH methemoglobinemia reductase are abnormally sensitive to nitrites and other chemicals that produce methemoglobinemia. Several studies demonstrated that susceptibility to arsenic-induced cancer development was dependent on genetic polymorphism. Arsenic metabolism is dependent on methylene tetrafolate reductase and glutathione S-transferases. Polymorphisms in these enzymes result in differences in arsenic metabolism and thus differences in susceptibility to cancer induction (Steinmaus et al., 2007).

## *Graded and quantal responses*

Effects on body weight, food consumption, and enzyme inhibition are examples of graded responses. On the other hand, mortality and tumor formation are examples of quantal (all-or-none) responses. Both types of responses may be analyzed statistically, as illustrated in Chapter 6.

The relationship between dose and response usually follows an S-shaped curve. Figure 4.1a and b is a schematic representation of most chemicals and that of certain essential nutrients, respectively. The latter is exemplified by thiamine and ascorbic acid. Insufficient intake of these

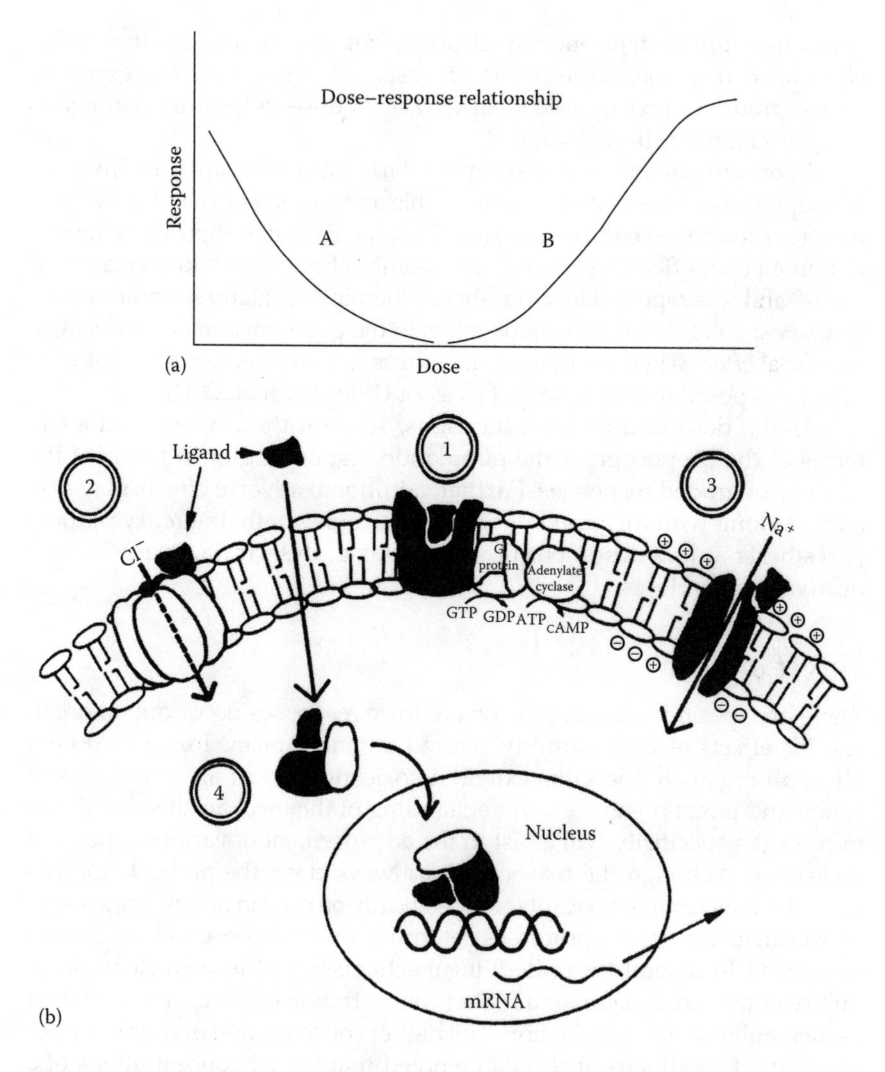


***Figure 4.1*** (a) Schematic representation of dose–response relationship. *Curve A*: certain essential nutrients, with which the response (deficiency syndrome) increases along with decreased intake. *Curve B*: most chemicals with which the response (toxic effects) increases along with increased intake. Certain substances, for example, selenium, exhibit both types of responses. (b) Schematic representation of the four classes of receptors. 1. G-protein coupled receptor, 2. ligand-gated ion channel, 3. voltage-gated ion channel, and 4. intracellular receptor. (From Mailman RB, Lawler CP, *Introduction to Biochemical Toxicology*, Appleton & Lange, Norwalk, CT, 1994.)

vitamins induces deficiency syndromes, but higher intakes are readily eliminated in urine. Selenium is an essential element but an excessive intake produces toxicity (see Chapter 21); its dose–response relationship is represented by curves A and B.

Another type of dose–response relationship (J-shaped or inverted U-shaped) consists of an effect observable at doses lower than the NOAEL (no-observed adverse-effect level) (see Chapter 25) and is opposite to the predominant toxic effect (e.g., stimulation vs. inhibition). This is known as "hormesis" and was reported for a number of chemicals (Calabrese and Baldwin, 2001). Post-conditioning hormesis refers to the phenomenon of producing a beneficial effect when applying a mild stress to cells or organisms that were initially exposed to a high dose of stressor (Wiegant et al., 2011).

As the dose of a toxicant increases, so does the response, either in terms of the proportion of the population responding or in terms of the severity of graded responses. Further, additional adverse effects may also appear along with increased doses. For example, methylmercury induces paresthesia at low doses, but produces ataxia, dysarthria, deafness, and death at higher doses.

## *Target organs*

There are specific target organs where toxic responses occur due to organ specific effects or organ affinity, termed organotropism. Toxicants do not affect all organs to the same extent. A toxicant may act at several sites of action and target organs. An understanding of the mechanisms that determine organ specificity will assist in the advancement of various aspects of toxicology. Although the reason is not always clear, the probable mechanisms by which many toxicants act specifically on certain organs are known. However, toxicokinetics processes determine toxicant concentrations in target organs. In general, the underlying mechanism is either a greater susceptibility of the target organ or a higher concentration of the chemical and/or its metabolite at the site of action. The higher concentration may arise under a variety of conditions. It should be noted that higher concentrations of a compound may be present, for example, in adipose tissue for DDT, yet the effect produced is in the brain at lower amounts. The concentration at the target tissue and receptor need to be sufficient for a period of time to produce an effect but this amount may not be the highest in the body. Further, the route of exposure might also be responsible for a specific target toxicity.

### *Sensitivity of the organ*

Neurons and myocardium depend primarily on adenosine triphosphate (ATP) generated by mitochondrial oxidation with little capacity for anaerobic metabolism, and there are rapid ionic shifts through the cell membrane. Neurons and myocardium are, therefore, especially sensitive to lack of oxygen resulting from disorders of the vascular system or of hemoglobin (e.g., carbon monoxide poisoning). Rapidly dividing cells, such as those in the bone marrow and intestinal mucosa, are more susceptible to mitotic poisons (e.g., methotrexate).

### *Distribution*

The respiratory tract and skin are target organs of industrial and environmental toxicants because these are the sites of absorption. An example is provided by bis(chloromethyl) ether, which produces skin tumors in humans when applied topically, but induces tumors in the respiratory tract after exposure by inhalation.

On a unit weight basis, the liver and kidney have a higher volume of blood flow, and thus are in general exposed to toxicants to a greater extent. In addition, these organs have greater metabolic and excretory functions, which also render them more susceptible to toxicants. Being lipophilic, methylmercury crosses the blood–brain barrier and exerts its toxic effects on the nervous system. Inorganic mercury compounds, in contrast, are not able to cross the blood–brain barrier and are not neurotoxic.

Radiation may oxidatively damage DNA by free radical generation and induce tumors. Ultraviolet light has little penetrating power and therefore only produces skin tumors, whereas ionizing radiation may penetrate tissues and induce leukemia and other types of cancer.

### *Selective uptake*

Certain cells have a high affinity for selected chemicals. For example, in the respiratory tract, the type I and type II alveolar epithelial cells, which have an active uptake system for endogenous polyamines, take up paraquat, a structurally similar chemical. This process results in damage of the local tissue even when paraquat is administered orally.

Melanin is present in the eyes, inner ear, and so forth. Drugs such as chloroquine and kanamycin that have an affinity for melanin may accumulate, after prolonged administration, in these organs and produce damage. Strontium-90 (Sr-90) with a half-life of 28 years is selectively deposited in the bone and induces tumors of the bone.

### *Biotransformation*

As a result of *bioactivation*, reactive metabolites are formed. The liver, being a major site of biotransformation, is susceptible to the action of many toxicants. However, there are exceptions. For example, certain metabolites are sufficiently stable; they may affect other organs after being transported there. Thus bromobenzene, though bioactivated in the liver, affects the kidney.

With some toxicants, bioactivation at certain sites is predominately responsible for observable effects. For example, the organophosphorothioate insecticides, such as parathion, are mainly bioactivated in the liver, but the abundance of detoxifying enzymes and of reactive but noncritical binding sites there prevent any overt signs of toxicity. On the other hand, nervous tissue contains less bioactivating enzymes, but because bioactivation takes place near critical target sites, that is, the synapses, the main toxic manifestations of this group of toxicants arise from the nervous system.

The bioactivating enzymes are not necessarily evenly distributed in an organ or tissue. For example, Clara cells (nonciliated bronchiolar epithelial cells) constitute only 1% of cells in the lung, yet they contain a major portion of the pulmonary cytochrome P-450. The lung is therefore more susceptible to damage by such toxicants as 4-ipomeanol and carbon tetrachloride ($CCl_4$). Recently, Clara cells were found to metabolize styrene to styrene oxide that ultimately results in lung carcinoma. A similar situation exists in the kidney. The proximal tubules, especially the S3 cells, located in the pars recta portion of these tubules have the highest concentrations of this enzyme system; hence the most susceptible parts of the kidney are the proximal tubules, especially its pars recta portion. The nephrotoxicity of haloalkenes is attributed to renal metabolites generated in the kidney.

## *Repair and adaptation*

Many toxicants alter macromolecules, which eventually induce cellular dysfunctions. Progression of toxicity can be intercepted by repair mechanisms. Repair mechanisms include repair of protein, lipid and DNA at the molecular levels. For example, protein disulfides are reduced by thioredox and glutaredoxin pathways. Once protein is oxidized, the catalytic thiol groups in these proteins are recycled by reduction with NADPH. Further, damaged proteins can be refolded with the action of chaperone protein or degraded following ubiquitination in proteasomes. Peroxidized lipids may be reduced by the glutathione-peroxidase or peroxiredoxin pathways. DNA modifications can be repaired by direct repair ($O^6$-alkylguanine-DNA-alkyltransferase), excision repair (AP endonuclease, nucleotide-excision repair, or PARP), or recombinational repair (Kleihues and Cooper, 1976).

Adaptation is defined as a hazard-induced capability of the organism to defend against the hazard and increase tolerance to it. Many of these adaptations regain or preserve biological homeostasis by (1) decreasing delivery to the target; (2) diminishing target density or responsiveness; (3) increasing repair; (4) compensating dysfunction and (5) epigenetic modifications. Epigenetic modifications include DNA methylation, covalent modifications of histone proteins, and regulation by noncoding RNAs, among others, which play a significant role in normal development and genome stability and constitute a mechanism of genome adaptation to external stimuli.

## *Mechanisms of action*

Although the mechanisms of action (MOA) of all toxicants are not fully understood, a number of biochemical reactions are likely involved. The underlying processes/subcellular sites are listed, along with some exemplary toxicants, in Table 4.3.

The table clearly shows the diverse nature of the mechanisms as well as the multiple processes/sites that are involved in the action of a number of toxicants. For many of the toxicants listed in Table 4.3, the mechanisms will be described, along with their toxic manifestations, in the relevant chapters.

### *Calcium homeostasis*

Of the various MOA, disturbance of calcium homeostasis merits special mention because of its importance and complexity. The extracellular level of $Ca2^+$ is more than 10 times higher than in cytosol. The ionic differential is maintained by a variety of mechanisms, including the $Ca2^+$ transporting ATPase at the plasma membrane, the storage in the endoplasmic reticulum, mitochondria, and nucleus as well as the binding with intracellular calmodulin. Increase in cytosolic $Ca2^+$ may be produced via different mechanisms. For example, $CCl_4$ and bromobenzene act through inhibition of $Ca2^+$ ATPase, acetaminophen, and $CCl_4$ through damage of plasma membrane, and cadmium by release of $Ca2^+$ from mitochondria. The rise in cytosolic $Ca2^+$ may affect the cytoskeleton thereby damaging cellular integrity either directly or through $Ca2^+$-activated proteases. Oxidant stress produces injury in lungs through an increase in $Ca2^+$ in alveolar macrophages by a Ca-mediated signaling (Hoyal et al., 1998). In addition, 2,3,7,8-tetrachlorodibenzo-*p*-dioxin (TCDD) may promote "apoptosis" (programmed cell death) by combining with Ah receptors, increasing intracellular $Ca2^+$ thus activating endonuclease and inducing DNA breakdown (Timbrell, 1991; Halliwell and Cross, 1994).

Most of the reactions take place at various subcellular sites. Table 12.1 in Chapter 12 lists a number of hepatotoxicants along with the organelles affected.

*Table 4.3* Some mechanisms of toxic action[a]

| Mechanism of action | Process/subcellular site | Examples of toxicants |
|---|---|---|
| Perturbation of cellular activity | Neurotransmitters | Botulinum toxin, organophosphate pesticides |
| Perturbation of cellular activity | Receptors | Amitrole, DES, retinoic acid, TCDD |
| | Enzymes | Fluoroacetate, cyanide, organophosphate pesticides |
| | Transport proteins | CO, nitrites |
| Interference with membrane function | Excitable membrane: Ion influx | DDT, saxitoxin, tetrodotoxin |
| | Membrane: Fluidity | Organic solvents (e.g., $CCl_4$, chloroform), ethanol |
| | Lysosomal membranes | $CCl_4$, phosphorus, phalloidin |
| | Mitochondrial membranes | $CCl_4$, organotins, phosphorus |
| Interference with cellular energy production | Hemoglobin | CO, nitrites |
| | Oxidative phosphorylation: Uncoupling | Dinitrophenol, organotins |
| | Electron transport: Inhibition | Cyanide, rotenone |
| | Carbohydrate metabolism: Inhibition | Fluoroacetate |
| Covalent binding to biomolecules | Lipids: Peroxidation | $CCl_4$, ozone, paraquat, phenytoin, free radicals |
| | Glutathione: Depletion | Acetaminophen |
| | Protein thiols: Oxidation | Acetaminophen, phenytoin |
| | Nucleic acids | Reactive carcinogens, mutagens, teratogens |
| Perturbation of calcium homeostasis | Cytoskeleton, etc. | Arsenic, cobalt, doxorubicin, microcystin, paraquat, phalloidin |
| | Apoptosis | TCDD |
| Perturbation of redox homeostasis | Mitochondria | Paraquat, doxorubicin |
| Dysregulation of gene expression | Transcription | DES, TCDD, DDT |
| | Signal transduction | Arsenic, Fumonisin B |

*Abbreviations:* TCDD, (2,3,7,8-tetrachlorodibenzo-*p*-dioxin), DDT, dichlorodiphenyl trichloroethane, DES, diethylstilbestrol.

[a] The toxic effects of a number of the toxicants are described in other sections. For the relevant page, refer to the Chemical Index.

## *Reactive oxygen species*

Reactive oxygen species (ROS) play an important role in adverse effects in health such as chronic inflammation, autoimmune diseases (diabetes, rheumatoid arthritis, lupus), cardiovascular diseases (atherosclerosis, hypertension, ischemia/reperfusion injury), fibrotic disease (pulmonary and liver fibrosis, diabetic nephropathy), neurological disorders (Parkinson's, Alzheimer's, schizophrenia), infectious diseases (septic shock, influenza, hepatitis, HIV), and cancer (Halliwell, 1997; Thomas and Kalyanaraman, 1997; Poyton et al., 2009). In contrast, ROS also plays a key role in several physiologic processes such as normal vascular cell functioning and maintaining vascular diameter regulation by immune response, signaling molecules, or regulating glucose uptake. Further, ROS participate in the regulation of differentiation, proliferation, growth, apoptosis, and cytoskeletal regulation (Görlach et al., 2015).

Most types of ROS including hydroxyl or peroxyl radicals, hydrogen peroxide and superoxide radical anion, have long been implicated in oxidative damage inflicted on fatty acids, DNA, and proteins as well as other cellular components (Figure 4.2). ROS can be produced from pollutants, tobacco, smoke, drugs, xenobiotics, or radiation (x-rays, $\gamma$-rays, UV light). Environmental pollutants produce ROS during metabolic activation (e.g., benzo(a)pyrene) and chemicals that promote superoxide formation such as quinones, nitroaromatics, bipyrimidiulium herbicides, chemicals that are metabolized to radicals (Fu et al., 2012), or chemicals that release iron and copper that promote the formation of hydroxyl radicals (Park et al., 2005).

Benzo(a)pyrene (B[a]P) acts as an inducer of CYP1A1 enzyme activity which converts the chemical into more polar, oxygenated products, facilitating their elimination from the cell. The metabolism of B(a)P via CYP1A1 generates ROS, which disrupts the intracellular oxidant/antioxidant balance (Mangal et al., 2009). In the process of B(a)P metabolism, major primary and secondary metabolites of B(a)P are formed (epoxides or hydroxyl metabolites), and then further oxidation results in the formation of quinines, diols, and diol epoxides. These predominant quinines affect the redox cycle between hydroquinone and semiquinone intermediates to generate ROS such as superoxide anion, $H_2O_2$, and hydroxyl radicals by Fenton chemistry. For example, formation of the B(a)P-1,6-quinone and B(a)P-3,6-quinone occurred in sera 3 hours after B(a)P treatment. Further, the time-dependent pattern of serum lipid peroxidation and level of erythrocyte antioxidant enzymes were found to be related to concentrations of the BaP-quinone metabolites. These results suggest that BaP-quinine metabolites generated ROS result through oxidative alteration of lipids and antioxidant enzymes in the blood, and might be

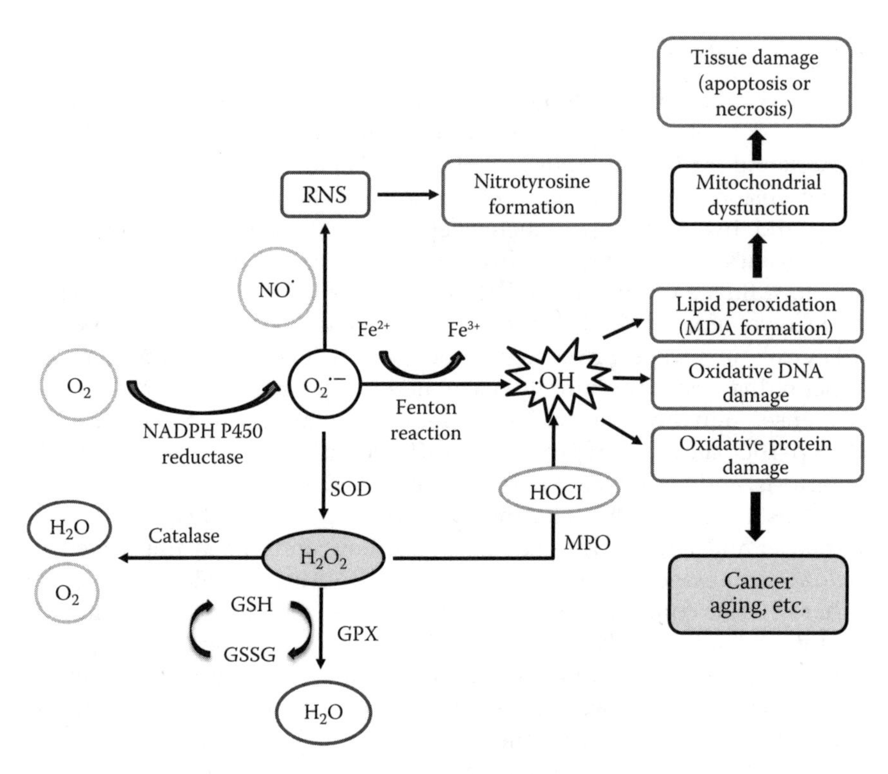


***Figure 4.2*** Pathways illustrating the sources of reactive oxygen species and its physiological roles in the development of cancer and diseases. (From Mailman RB, Lawler CP, *Introduction to Biochemical Toxicology*, Appleton & Lange, Norwalk, CT, 1994.)

associated with B[a]P-related vascular toxicity including carcinogenesis (Kim et al., 2000).

Chemotherapeutic drugs exert cytotoxicity through generation of ROS to cancer cells. For example, cisplatin and adriamycin appear to produce ROS at excessive levels, resulting in DNA damage and cell death (Pogrebniak et al., 1991). Although acetaminophen is safe at low doses, APAP overdose mediated hepatic injury due to its metabolism to hepatotoxic *N*-acetyl-*p*-benzoquinone imine (NAPQI), catalyzed by CYP2E1, and via the direct activation of JNK-dependent cell death pathway (Figure 4.3). In contrast, ROS are produced as a normal product of cellular metabolism. In particular, one major contributor to oxidative damage is hydrogen peroxide ($H_2O_2$), which is converted from superoxide that leaks from the mitochondria. Catalase and superoxide dismutase (SOD) ameliorate the damaging effects of hydrogen peroxide and superoxide, respectively, by

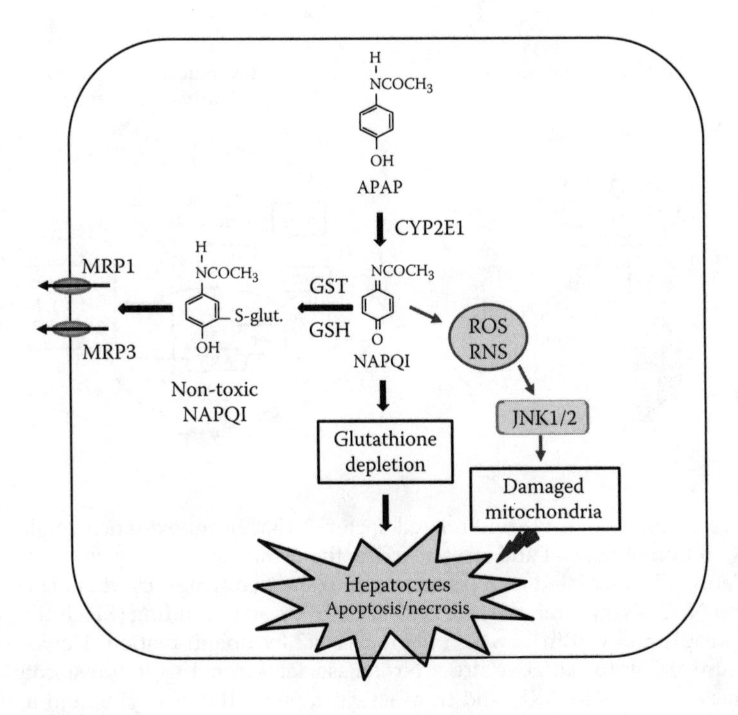


***Figure 4.3*** Schematic representation on the role of acetaminophen-induced hepatotoxicity.

converting these compounds into oxygen and hydrogen peroxide (which is later converted to water), resulting in production of benign molecules.

ROS as second messengers are important for the expression of several transcription factors and other signal transduction molecules such as heat shock-inducing factors and nuclear factors (Finkel, 2011). For example, nuclear factor (erythroid-derived 2) factor 2 (Nrf2) is increasingly recognized as a crucial transcription factor, which mediates protection against electrophiles and oxidants, and enhances cell survival in many tissues (Ma, 2013). Nrf2 binds to antioxidant response elements (AREs), specific sequences present in the promoter regions of its target genes, as a heterodimer with a small Maf protein, and stimulates transcription of antioxidant proteins including heme oxygenase-1 (HO-1), gluthatione S-transferases (GSTs), NAD(P)H: quinone oxidoreductase 1 (NQO1), thioredoxin, thioredoxin reductase, as well as proteins involved in scavenging ROS and glutathione (GSH) biosynthesis and regeneration (Figure 4.4).

In this role, Nrf2 functions as a xenobiotic-activated receptor (XAR) to regulate the adaptive response to oxidants and electrophiles. Disruption of the Nrf2-antioxidant axis leads to increased oxidative stress and DNA

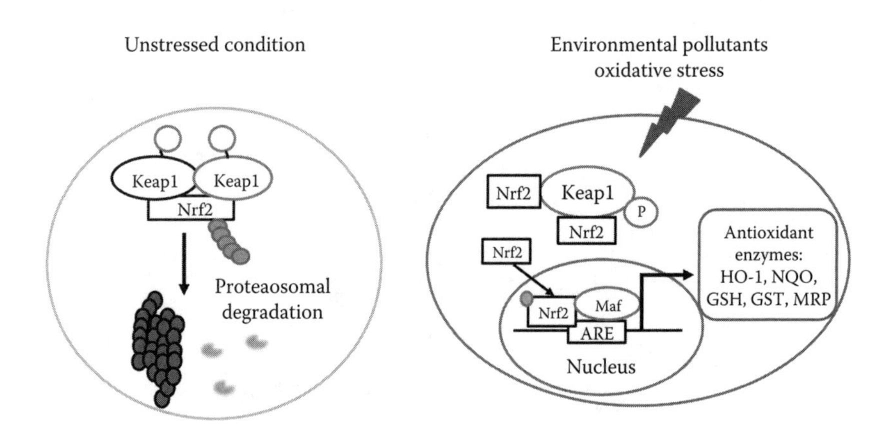


***Figure 4.4*** Nuclear erythroid-related factor 2 (Nrf2) antioxidant signaling on the condition of normal and stress. Nrf2 is the principal transcription factor that regulates ARE-mediated expression of antioxidant enzymes. Under normal conditions, Nrf2 is sequestered in the cytoplasm by an actin-binding (Kelch-like) protein (Keap1) and Cullin 3, which degrade Nrf2 by ubiquitination. However, on exposure of cells to oxidative stress, Nrf2 dissociates from Keap1, translocates into the nucleus, binds to ARE, and transactivates phase II detoxifying and antioxidant genes such as catalase, superoxide dismutase (SOD), glutathione reductase, and glutathione peroxidase.

damage in the initiation of cellular transformation in the prostate gland (Kensler et al., 2007; Frohlich et al., 2008; Ma, 2013).

# *Molecular targets: Chemical nature*

## *Proteins*

### *Receptors*

Receptors are located across plasma membranes, or in cytosol, or in the nucleus, and serve to transmit physical or chemical signals to the cell. There are many types of receptors that serve a variety of functions. Toxicants are known to affect some of them (see the section "Receptors" at the end of this chapter).

### *Enzymes*

Enzymes are common targets of toxicants. The enzyme effects may be specific, such as the inhibition of acetylcholinesterase (AChE). They may be reversible, such as the case with a number of carbamate insecticides on AChE. Irreversible enzyme inhibition is exemplified by di-isopropyl fluorophosphate, which covalently bind with the enzymes.

The effects may be nonspecific. For example, lead and mercury are inhibitors of a great variety of enzymes. However, some enzymes are more susceptible: for example, δ-aminolevulinic acid dehydrase is especially sensitive to lead, and its activity in erythrocytes is used as an early indicator of lead poisoning.

The last step of the oxidation of many chemicals is catalyzed by the cytochrome oxidase chain. Hydrocyanic acid binds with iron in these enzymes and blocks their redox function. The aerobic respiration of cells is then arrested and biochemical asphyxia ensues.

An enzyme can also be inhibited by a chemical derived by synthesis from the toxicant such as fluoroacetic acid and its derivatives. The process is known as *lethal synthesis*. Fluoroacetic acid is metabolized as acetic acid in the citric acid cycle and fluorocitric acid is synthesized, instead of citric acid. Since fluorocitric acid is an inhibitor of aconitase, further metabolism, and consequently the energy production, is blocked. In a somewhat similar manner, amino acid antagonists (e.g., azaserine and fluorophenylalanine) interfere with utilization of specific amino acids in the synthesis of proteins. The energy that is liberated by biochemical oxidation is normally stored in the form of high-energy phosphates. *Uncoupling agents* such as dinitrophenol interfere with the synthesis of energy-rich phosphates, and thus the energy is liberated as heat instead of being stored.

### *Carriers*

Carriers such as hemoglobin can be affected by a toxicant through preferential binding. For example, carbon monoxide binds hemoglobin at the site where oxygen is normally bound. Because of its greater affinity for hemoglobin, it inactivates hemoglobin and generates manifestations of oxygen deficiency in tissues.

Oxygen transport can also be impaired by an accumulation of methemoglobin, which is an oxidation product of hemoglobin with no oxygen binding ability. In normal individuals, the trace amount of methemoglobin present is readily reduced to hemoglobin. Certain toxicants, such as nitrites and aromatic amines, enhance formation of methemoglobin and overwhelm the normal process of its reduction to hemoglobin. Subjects with glucose-6-phosphatase dehydrogenase deficiency have a lower capacity to regenerate hemoglobin from methemoglobin and are thus prone to develop methemoglobinemia.

P-glycoprotein is a transmembrane protein expressed by the small intestine, kidneys, liver, placenta, and the blood–brain barrier (Abu-Qare et al., 2003). The function of P-glycoprotein is to bind to a chemical and then transport the agent from the cell; in essence, it serves as a carrier of xenobiotic from the cell. Compounds such as ivermectin, chlorpyrifos, and endosulfan showed decreased effectiveness due to increased expression of P-glycoprotein, which acts as a protective transporter.

### Structural proteins

Extracellular structural proteins such as collagen are unlikely to be affected by toxicants. However, toxicants such as ozone and asbestos may produce an increase in fibroblasts and deposition of collagen in the lungs (Chapter 12). Intracellular structural proteins, such as cytoskeleton, may be damaged by toxicants such as arsenic (Li and Chou, 1992) paraquat (Li et al., 1987), benzene (Ross, 2000), styrene (Cohen et al., 2002), and deoxynivalenol (Pestka and Smolinski, 2005).

### Coenzymes

Coenzymes are essential for the normal function of enzymes. Their levels in the body can be diminished by toxicants that inhibit their synthesis. For example, pyrithiamine inhibits thiamine kinase, which is responsible for the formation of the coenzyme thiamine pyrophosphate. NADPH is destroyed in the presence of free radicals, which can be produced by such toxicants as carbon tetrachloride. Metal-dependent enzymes are blocked by chelating agents (e.g., cyanides and dithiocarbamates) through removal of metal coenzymes such as copper and zinc.

### Lipids

*Peroxidation* of polyenoic fatty acids has been suggested as a mechanism of the necrotizing action of a number of toxicants, such as carbon tetrachloride, ozone, and estrogen (Roy et al., 2007). The culprit is believed to be ROS that are generated by the transformation of the chemical with subsequent ROS interaction with membrane lipid. The resulting outcome is cellular death or necrosis. Covalent binding of benzo(a)pyrene diolepoxide to triglyceride may be associated with the epigenetic mechanism of benzo(a)pyrene carcinogenesis (Kwack and Lee, 2000; Park et al., 2002).

*Cell membrane* derangement may result after exposure to various types of toxicants. The general anesthetics, ether and halothane, as well as many other lipophilic substances accumulate in cell membranes and thereby interfere with transport of oxygen and glucose into the cell resulting in narcosis. The cells of the central nervous system are especially susceptible to a lowering of oxygen tension and glucose levels and are therefore among the first to be deleteriously affected by these substances. Membrane dissolution follows contact with organic solvents and amphoteric detergents.

The ions of mercury and cadmium form complexes with phospholipid bases and expand the surface area of the membrane, thereby altering its function. Lead ion increases the fragility of erythrocytes and results in hemolysis. The oxygen-carrying function of hemoglobin is lost after it escapes from hemolyzed erythrocytes.

### Nucleic acids

*Covalent binding* between a toxicant (such as alkylating agents) and replicating DNA and RNA induces cancer, mutations, and teratogenesis. Such toxicants may also exert immunosuppressive effects.

*Antimetabolites* such as aminopterin and methotrexate may be incorporated into DNA and RNA and then interfere with their replication.

### Others

*Hypersensitivity reactions* result from repeated exposure to a particular substance or to its chemically related substances. The latter phenomenon is referred to as cross sensitization. The substance, if it is a large polypeptide, acts as an antigen and stimulates the body to form antibodies. Otherwise, the substance acts as a hapten and combines with proteins in the body to form antigens. The reaction between an antigen from a subsequent exposure and the corresponding antibodies results in release of histamine, bradykinin, and other constituents. The reaction has a typical pattern irrespective of the nature of the antigen. Photosensitization reaction is somewhat similar except sunlight is also required for its induction (see Chapters 11, 12, and 15).

*Corrosive agents* such as strong acids and bases destroy local tissues by precipitating cellular proteins. Irritation of the underlying tissues occurs as a consequence.

*Blockade* of renal and biliary tubules may follow precipitation of relatively insoluble toxicants or their metabolites. For example, acetyl sulfapyridine, a metabolite of sulfapyridine, may block renal tubules; harmol glucuronide from harmol may produce cholestasis.

## Receptors

### Historical notes

It has long been observed that a number of poisons and toxins exert certain specific biological effects. John N. Langley proposed in 1905 the concept of a "receptive substance." That the receptors are protein in nature was first suggested by Welsh and Taub (1951). To demonstrate the protein nature of acetylcholine receptors, Lu (1952) showed that the stimulant effect of acetylcholine on isolated rabbit ileum was lost after the ileum was treated with the proteolytic enzyme trypsin (10 mg/100 ml, for 30 min). That the effect was on the receptor rather than the muscle was demonstrated by the fact that the treated ileum still responded to barium chloride, a direct-acting muscle stimulant. In 1971, Cuatrecasas observed that trypsin, at the same concentration as that used by Lu, eliminated the activity of insulin receptors (Cuatrecasas, 1971).

In the 1970s, cholinergic receptors (ChR) were solubilized, isolated, and characterized by several groups of investigators. The amino acid composition of ChR was reported by Heilbronn et al. (1975). They also found that ChR contained about 6% carbohydrates. Although it has been generally agreed that the ligand–receptor complex would initiate responses in the cells, it was Rodbell et al. (1971) who proposed that a "transducer" was required to act between the receptor and the effector. This "transducer" was later confirmed as the G-proteins (Gilman, 1987).

## *Definition*

Receptors refer to macromolecules that bind small molecules (commonly termed ligands, e.g., xenobiotics) with high affinity and specificity that initiates a characteristic biochemical effect, and subsequently changes physiological functions (e.g., toxicity). The ligand that binds with the receptor may be an "agonist" or an "antagonist." An agonist induces the "physiological" function of the receptor, whereas an antagonist blocks its functions. For example, methacholine is an agonist interacting with certain cholinergic receptors, mimicking the effects of acetylcholine, whereas atropine, an antagonist, blocks these effects. Both types exert adverse health effects. In addition, an agonist may cause a toxic effect by failing to dissociate from the receptor readily enough, thereby preventing further action of the endogenous messenger, and an antagonist competes with the messenger for the site on the receptor and blocks the action of the latter. In addition, a toxicant may induce tolerance to its toxicity by reducing the number of receptors, as shown by Costa et al. (1981) thru the chronic treatment with an organophosphate AChE inhibitor.

## *Receptor families*

Agonists that bind to receptors may elicit physiological functions by a direct intracellular effect or by releasing another intracellular regulatory molecule, known as a second messenger. Some receptors may interact with closely associated cellular proteins to generate its effects. Receptors are divided into four families, based on the effector mechanisms:

(i) G-protein coupled receptors; (ii) ion channels; (iii) membrane-bound receptors with integral enzyme activity; and (iv) intracellular receptors. With the G-protein coupled receptors (Figure 4.2), binding with a ligand results in the activation of the G-protein, converting guanosine triphosphate to guanosine diphosphate, which stimulates or inhibits a specific enzyme (adenylate cyclase or phospholipase C), followed by the formation of a "second messenger," for example, cAMP (from ATP), diacylglycerol, or phosphoinositol. The second messenger then initiates the cellular response—the biological effect. Many neurotransmitter receptors are G-protein coupled receptors, such as dopamine, adrenergic, and muscarinic cholinergic receptors. Their ligands include analogs of these neurotransmitters, such as ephedrine and diphtheria toxin.

Some membrane-bound receptors contain transmembrane segments and a cytosolic domain with intrinsic enzyme activity or a direct association with cytoplasmic enzymes. Ligand binding to the extracellular domain induces enzyme activity on the intracellular side. Ligands of these receptors include growth factors and cytokine receptors. Enzymes-linked receptors include receptor tyrosine kinase, serine/threonine-specific protein kinase, and guanylate cyclase.

Intracellular receptors are located in the cytosol or nucleus (Figure 4.2). The main endogenous ligands are estrogens, androgens, progestins, glucocorticoids, and mineralocorticoids. A representative toxicant that binds with this type of receptor is TCDD. It binds with the Ah receptor in the cytosol, but translocates to the nucleus after binding. For additional details see Mitchell (1992) and Mailman and Lawler (1994). The molecular mechanisms of polybrominated biphenyl ether (PBDE) toxicities have been carried out through the hormone receptor pathways, including TR, ER, AR, PR, and AhR. These stages include receptor binding, receptor conformation change, co-activator or co-repressor recruitment, HRE binding, and gene expression. This review focuses on the toxicology of endocrine-disrupting chemicals (see Chapter 21).

The ion channels are transmembrane proteins with ion channels. These receptors can be activated by ligand binding or by voltage change, termed ligand-gated or voltage-gated ion channels. Upon binding with a ligand, the ligand-gated ion channels undergo conformational changes resulting in the opening of the channel. This process allows changes of $Na^+$, $K^+$, $Cl^-$, or $Ca2^+$ concentrations across the plasma membrane. Nicotinic cholinergic and $GABA_A$ receptors belong to this class. In addition, glutamate and chemicals such as kainate, diazepam, barbiturates, and picrotoxin also act on this type of ion-channel receptors. The voltage-gated in channels are located across plasma membranes of excitable cells such as neurons and their axons. At present, no endogenous ligands are known. However, the neurotoxins, namely tetrodotoxin and saxitoxin (see Chapter 18), bind to a site near the extracellular opening of the $Na^+$ channel and block entry of $Na^+$ through the channel, thereby interfering with the conduction of nerve impulse.

## *Receptors in toxicology*

The receptor concept has been valuable in advancing our understanding of certain biochemical, physiological, and pharmacological effects, as well as facilitating the development of drugs. Its role in toxicology is evidenced by an increasing number of receptors being recognized as mediators of the effects of toxicants.

Poland and Knutson (1982) reviewed the extensive literature on TCDD and related halogenated aromatic hydrocarbons with respect to their toxicity, their ability to induce aryl hydrocarbon hydroxylase, and their affinity for a cytosol receptor. It was suggested that TCDD binds with the Ah (aromatic hydrocarbon) receptor. The TCDD–receptor complex translocates to the nucleus and there interacts with specific genomic recognition sites. This initiates transcription and translation of the specific genes that code for aryl hydrocarbon hydroxylase. A preponderance of evidence suggests that most of the TCDD toxicities are receptor mediated. It was also noted that the concentration of this cytosol receptor is higher in the liver of C57 BL/6 mice than that of DBA/2 mice, and that the former strain of mouse was more susceptible than the latter with respect to TCDD-induced thymus involution, teratogenesis, and hepatic porphyria. Further, genetic evidence indicated that the *Ah* locus in mice was the structural gene for the cytosol receptor (see also Whitlock, 1990; Okey et al., 1994).

Many neurotoxicants act through receptors on the central, peripheral, and autonomic nervous systems. For example, certain organophosphorus compounds act not only through acetylcholine but also on muscarinic receptors (Huff et al., 1994). The receptors for 12,0-tetradecanoyl phorbol 13-acetate (TPA) and retinoic acid are worth noting. TPA, a tumor promoter, binds with a receptor that initiates a chain of events leading to selected replication of initiated cells (Blumberg et al., 1983). Retinoic acid, similar to TCDD, acts on an estrogen receptor to exert teratogenic and other effects (Lu et al., 1994). A few examples of toxicants that act through receptors are mentioned in the previous section. Peroxisome proliferators such as the hypolipidemic drug clofibrate and the plasticizers phthalate esters are active on the peroxisome proliferator-activated receptors (PPARα, PPARβ/δ, and PPARγ) that are involved in the metabolism of polyunsaturated fatty acids and anti-inflammatories (Varga et al., 2011). Further, many immunotoxicants act through specific receptors on T cell, B cell, cytokine, polymorphonuclear cells, and monocytes (Lad et al., 1995).

Aberrant expression and regulation of insulin-like growth factor binding protein 3 regulates normal and malignant cell growth (Zou et al., 1998).

## *References*

Abu-Qare AW, Elmasry E, Abou-Donia MB (2003). A role for P-glycoprotein in environmental toxicology. *J Toxicol Environ Health B.* 6, 279–288.

Alarie Y (1981). Dose–response analysis in animal studies: Prediction of human responses. *Environ Health Perspect.* 42, 9–13.

Blumberg PM, Delcos BK, Dunn JA et al. (1983). Phorbol ester receptors and the in vitro effects of tumor promoters. *Ann N Y Acad Sci.* 407, 303–315.

Calabrese EJ, Baldwin LA (2001). The frequency of U-shaped dose responses in the toxicological literature. *Toxicol Sci.* 62, 330–338.

Chanter DO, Heywood R (1982). The LD50 test: Some considerations of precision. *Toxicol Lett.* 10, 303–307.

Cohen JT, Carlson G, Charnley G et al. (2002). A comprehensive evaluation of the potential health risks associated with occupational and environmental exposure to styrene. *J Toxicol Environ Health B.* 5, 1–263.

Cooke MW, Ferner RE (1993). Chemical burns causing systemic toxicity. *Arch Emerg Med.* 10, 368–371.

Costa LG, Schwab BW, Hand H et al. (1981). Reduced [H3] quinuclidinyl benzilate binding to muscarinic receptors in disulfoton-tolerant mice. *Toxicol Appl Pharmacol.* 60, 441–450.

Cuatrecasas P (1971). Perturbation of the insulin receptor of isolated fat cells with proteolytic enzymes. *J Biol Chem.* 246, 6522–6531.

Dean BS (1998). Diethylstilbesterol. In: Wexler P, ed. *Encyclopedia of Toxicology.* New York: Academic Press, 477–478.

Finkel T (2011). Signal transduction by reactive oxygen species. *J Cell Biol.* 194, 7–15.

Frohlich DA, McCabe MT, Arnold RS, Day ML (2008). The role of Nrf2 in increased reactive oxygen species and DNA damage in prostate tumorigenesis. *Oncogene.* 27, 4353–4362.

Fu PP, Xia Q, Sun X, Yu H (2012). Phototoxicity and environmental transformation of polycyclic aromatic hydrocarbons (PAHs)-light-induced reactive oxygen species, lipid peroxidation, and DNA damage. *J Environ Sci Health C Environ Carcinog Ecotoxicol Rev.* 30, 1–41.

Gilman AG (1987). G-proteins: Transducers of receptor-generated signals. *Ann Rev Biochem.* 56, 615–649.

Görlach A, Dimova EY, Petry A et al. (2015). Reactive oxygen species, nutrition, hypoxia and diseases: Problems solved? *Redox Biol.* 6, 372–385.

Halliwell B (1997). *Oxygen Radicals and Disease Process.* Thomas CE, Kalyanaraman B, eds. Hardwood Academic Publishers, The Netherlands, 1–14.

Halliwell B, Cross CE (1994). Oxygen-derived species: Their relation to human disease and environmental stress. *Environ Health Persp.* 102(Suppl 10), 5–12.

Heilbronn E, Mattsson C, Elfman L (1975). Biochemical and physical properties of the nicotinic ACh receptor from *Torpedo marmorata.* In: Wollemann M, ed. *Properties of Purified Cholinergic and Adrenergic Receptors, Vol. 37.* New York: Elsevier.

Hoyal CR, Giron-Calle J, Forman HJ (1998). The alveolar macrophage as a model of calcium signaling in oxidative stress. *J Toxicol Environ Health B.* 1, 117–134.

Huff RA, Corcoran JJ, Anderson JK et al. (1994). Chloropyrifos oxon binds directly to muscarinic receptors and inhibits cAMP accumulation in rat striatum. *J Pharmacol Exp Therap.* 269, 329–335.

Kensler TW, Wakabayashi N, Biswal S (2007). Cell survival responses to environmental stresses via the Keap1-Nrf2-ARE pathway. *Annu Rev Pharmacol Toxicol.* 47, 89–116.

Kim HS, Kwack SJ, Lee BM (2000). Lipid peroxidation, antioxidant enzymes, and benzo(a)pyrene-quinones in the blood of rats treated with benzo(a)pyrene. *Chem Biol Interact.* 127, 139–150.

Kleihues P, Cooper HK (1976). Repair excision of alkylated bases from DNA in vivo. *Oncology.* 33, 86–88.

Koschier FJ, Burden EJ, Brunkhorst CS et al. (1983). Concentration-dependent elicitation of dermal sensitization in guinea pigs treated with 2,4-toluene diisocyanate. *Toxicol Appl Pharmacol.* 67, 401–407.

Kwack SJ, Lee BM (2000). Correlation between DNA or protein adducts and benzo(a) pyrene diol epoxide I-triglyceride adduct detected in vitro and in vivo. *Carcinogenesis.* 21, 629–632.

Lad PM, Kapstein JS, Lin CE, eds. (1995). *Signal Transduction in Leukocytes. G-Protein-Related and Other Pathways.* Boca Raton, FL: CRC Press.

Li W, Chou IN (1992). Effects of sodium arsenite on the cytoskeleton and cellular glutathione levels in cultured cells. *Toxicol Appl Pharmacol.* 114, 132–139.

Li W, Zhao Y, Chou IN (1987). Paraquat-induced cytoskeletal injury in cultured cells. *Toxicol Appl Pharmacol.* 91, 96–106.

Lu FC (1952). The effects of proteolytic enzymes on the isolated rabbit intestine. *Br J Pharmacol* 7, 624–640.

Lu Y, Wang X, Safe S (1994). Interaction of 2,3,7,8-tetrachlorodibenzo-*p*-dioxin and retinoic acid in MCF-7 human breast cancer cells. *Toxicol Appl Pharmacol.* 127, 1–8.

Ma Q (2013). Role of Nrf2 in Oxidative Stress and Toxicity. *Annu Rev Pharmacol Toxicol.* 53, 401–426.

Mailman RB, Lawler CP (1994). Toxicant-receptor interactions: Fundamental principles. In: Hodgson E, Levi PE, eds. *Introduction to Biochemical Toxicology.* Norwalk, CT: Appleton & Lange.

Mangal D, Vudathala D, Park JH et al. (2009). Analysis of 7,8-dihydro-8-oxo-2′-deoxyguanosine in cellular DNA during oxidative stress. *Chem Res Toxicol* 22, 788–797.

Mitchell RH (1992). Inositol lipids in cellular signalling mechanisms. *Trends Biochem Sci.* 17, 274–276.

NAS (National Academy of Sciences). (2008). *Review of the Toxicologic and Radiologic Risks to Military Personnel from Exposure to Depleted Uranium During and After Combat.* Washington, DC: National Academies Press.

Okey AB, Riddick DS, Harper PA (1994). The Ah receptor: Mediator of the toxicity of 2,3,7,8-tetrachlorodibenzo-*p*-dioxin (TCDD) and related compounds. *Toxicol Lett.* 70, 1–22.

Park HS, Park YA, Lee BM (2002). Effects of pH and temperature on benzo[a] pyrene-DNA, -protein, and -lipid adducts in primary rat hepatocytes. *J Toxicol Environ Health A.* 65, 205–214.

Park JH, Gopishetty S, Szewczuk LM et al. (2005). Troxel AB, Harvey RG, Penning TM. Formation of 8-oxo-7,8-dihydro-2′-deoxyguanosine (8-oxo-dGuo) by PAH *o*-quinones: Involvement of reactive oxygen species and copper(II)/copper(I) redox cycling. *Chem Res Toxicol.* 18, 1026–1037.

Pestka JJ, Smolinski AT (2005). Deoxynivalenol: Toxicology and potential effects on humans. *J Toxicol Environ Health B.* 8, 39–69.

Pogrebniak HW, Matthews W, Pass HI (1991). Chemotherapy amplifies production of tumor necrosis factor. *Surgery.* 110, 231–237.

Poland A, Knutson JC (1982). 2,3,7,8-Tetrachlorodibenzo-*p*-dioxin and related halogenated aromatic hydrocarbons: Examination of the mechanism of toxicity. *Annu Rev Pharmacol Toxicol.* 22, 517–554.

Poyton RO, Ball KA, Castello PR (2009). Mitochondrial generation of free radicals and hypoxic signaling. *Trends Endocrinol Metab.* 20, 332–340.

Rodbell M, Birnbaumer L, Pohl SL et al. (1971). The glucagon sensitive adenyl cyclase system in plasma membranes of rat liver. V. An obligatory role of guanyl nucleotides in glucagon action. *J Biol Chem.* 246, 1877–1887.

Ross D (2000). The role of metabolism and specific metabolites in benzene-induced toxicity: Evidence and issues. *J Toxicol Environ Health A.* 61, 357–372.

Roy D, Cai Q, Felty Q et al. (2007). Estrogen-induced generation of reactive oxygen and nitrogen species, gene damage and estrogen-dependent cancers. *J Toxicol Environ Health B.* 10, 235–257.

Roy D, Palangat M, Chen C-W et al. (1997). Biochemical and molecular changes at the cellular level in response to exposure to environmental estrogen-like chemicals. *J Toxicol Environ Health.* 50, 1–29.

Steinmaus C, Moore LE, Shipp M et al. (2007). Genetic polymorphisms in MTHFR 677 and 1298, GSTM1 and T1 and metabolism of arsenic. *J Toxicol Environ Health A.* 70, 159–170.

Thomas CE and Kalyanaraman B eds. (1997). *Oxygen Radicals and the Disease Process.* The Netherlands: Hardwood Academic Publishers.

Timbrell JA (1991). *Principles of Biochemical Toxicology.* London: Taylor & Francis.

Varga T, Czimmerer Z, Nagy L (2011). PPARs are a unique set of fatty acid regulated transcription factors controlling both lipid metabolism and inflammation. *Biochim Biophys Acta.* 1812, 1007–1022.

Wang G, Ansari GAS, Khan MF (2007). Involvement of lipid peroxidation-derived aldehyde–protein adduct in autoimmunity mediated by trichloroethene. *J Toxicol Environ Health A.* 70, 1977–1985.

Welsh JH, Taub R (1951). The significance of the carbonyl group and ether oxygen in the reaction of acetylcholine with receptor substance. *J Pharmacol Exp Ther.* 103, 62–73.

Whitlock JP Jr. (1990). Genetic and molecular aspects of 2,3,7,8-tetrachlorodibenzo-*p*-dioxin action. *Ann Rev Pharmacol Toxicol.* 30, 251–277.

Wiegant FA, Prins HA, Van Wijk R (2011). Postconditioning hormesis put in perspective: An overview of experimental and clinical studies. *Dose Response.* 9, 209–224.

Zou T, Fleisher AS, Kong D et al. (1998). Sequence alterations of insulin-like growth factor binding protein 3 in neoplastic and normal gastrointestinal tissues. *Cancer Res.* 58, 4802–4804.

# *chapter five*

# *Modifying factors of toxic effects*

***Hyung Sik Kim***

*Contents*



## *General considerations*

Toxicity is an inherent property of a toxic substance; however, the nature and extent of the toxic manifestations in an organism that is exposed to the substance depends upon a variety of factors. The obvious ones are dose of the substance and duration of exposure. However, factors also include less obvious host factors such as the species and strain of an animal, gender and age, nutritional and hormonal status as well as presence of medical conditions such as hypertension or compromised function as in AIDS. Various environmental factors (physical and social factors, housing, and temperature) also play a part. In addition, the toxic effect of a chemical may be influenced by simultaneous, concurrent, or prior exposure to other compounds.

The adverse effects may be modified in a number of ways: alterations in absorption, distribution, and excretion of a chemical; an increase or a decrease of its biotransformation; and changes of the sensitivity of the receptor at the target organ. An example is the combination of *N,N*-diethyl-*m*-toluamide (DEET), an insect repellent; pyridostigmine (PB), an anti-nerve agent; and permethrin, an insecticide used in the Gulf War. PB by itself did not produce any adverse effects but when combined with DEET, the veterans complained of neurotoxicity. Studies showed that DEET application to skin changed dermal properties such that PB was absorbed to a greater extent and thus toxicity occurred.

A clear understanding of the existence of these factors and of their mode of action is important in designing the protocols of toxicological investigation. It is equally important in evaluating the significance of the toxicological data and in assessing the safety/risk to humans under specified conditions of exposure. Some of these are discussed in this chapter.

The most common mechanism underlying various modifying factors is differences in the rate of detoxication. However, differences in bioactivation, and toxicokinetic, toxicodynamic, physiological, psychological, and anatomic characteristics are responsible for a number of modifying factors. Examples are listed in Table 5.1.

## Host factors

### Species, strain, and individual

In general, different species of animals respond similarly to most toxicants. However, differences in toxic effects from one species to another have long been recognized. This is clearly demonstrated for the most toxic chemical known, dioxin: the $LD_{50}$ is 2 μg/kg for a guinea pig; 50 μg/kg for a rabbit; 200 μg/kg for a mouse, and 2000 μg/kg for a hamster. Knowledge in this field has been used to develop, for example, pesticides, which are more toxic to pests than to humans and other mammals. Among the various species of mammals, most effects of toxicants are somewhat more similar. This fact forms the basis of predicting the toxicity to humans based on results obtained in toxicological studies conducted in other mammals, such as rat, mouse, dog, rabbit, and monkey. There are, however, notable differences in toxicity even among mammals (Williams, 1974).

Some of these differences may be attributed to variations in detoxication mechanisms. Differences in response to hexobarbital, although less marked, also exist among various strains of mice (Jay, 1955). For example, the sleeping time induced in several species of lab animals by hexobarbital shows marked differences, which are attributable to the activity of the detoxication enzyme as shown in Table 5.2.

***Table 5.1*** Mechanisms[a] underlying certain modifying factors

| Toxicant | Responsible mechanism | Toxic response |
|---|---|---|
| | **Bioactivation differences** | |
| 2-Naphthylamine | 2-Naphthyl hydroxylamine | Bladder tumor in dog, human, but not in rat, mouse |
| Acetylaminofluorene | *N*-hydroxy metabolite | Carcinogenic in rat, mouse, and hamster, but not in guinea pigs |
| | **Toxicokinetic characteristics** | |
| Lead, cadmium | Greater absorption in the young | Greater toxic effects |
| Penicillin, tetracycline | Slower excretion in the young | Longer half-life |
| Morphine | Blood–brain barrier inefficient in the young | Greater CNS effect |
| Sulfur dioxide | Higher breathing rate in the young | Greater lung damage |
| | **Toxicodynamic characteristics** | |
| DDT | Susceptibility of receptor | Less susceptible in the young |
| | **Anatomic characteristics** | |
| Butylated hydroxyanisole, butylated hydroxytoluene | Presence of forestomach in rat | Hyperplasia of forestomach |
| *Physiological characteristics* | | |
| Squill | Vomiting reflex | Absence in rat leading to toxic effect |

[a] Other than detoxication.

Other examples include ethylene glycol and aniline. Ethylene glycol is metabolized to oxalic acid, which is responsible for the toxicity, or to carbon dioxide. The magnitude of the toxicity of ethylene glycol in animals is in the following order: cat > rat > rabbit and this is the same for the extent of oxalic acid production. Aniline is metabolized in the cat and dog mainly to *o*-aminophenol, which is more toxic, but it is metabolized mainly to *p*-aminophenol in the rat and hamster, which are less susceptible to aniline (Timbrell, 1991).

***Table 5.2*** Species differences in the duration of action and metabolism of hexobarbital[a]

| Species | Duration of action (min) | Plasma half-life (min) | Relative enzyme activity (μg/g/hr) | Plasma level on awakening (μg/mL) |
|---|---|---|---|---|
| Mouse | 12 | 19 | 598 | 89 |
| Rabbit | 49 | 60 | 196 | 57 |
| Rat | 90 | 140 | 135 | 64 |
| Dog | 315 | 260 | 36 | 19 |

*Source:* Quinn GP et al. *Biochem. Pharmacol.* 1, 152–159, 1958.

[a] Dose of barbiturate 50 mg/kg in dogs and 100 mg/kg in the other animals.

Differences in bioactivation also account for many dissimilarities of toxicity. A notable example is 2-naphthylamine, which produces bladder tumors in the dog and human but not in the rat, rabbit, or guinea pig. Dogs and humans, but not the other species, excrete the carcinogenic metabolite 2-naphthyl hydroxylamine (Miller et al., 1964). Acetylaminofluorene (AAF) is carcinogenic to many species of animals but not to guinea pig. However, the *N*-hydroxy metabolite of AAF is carcinogenic to all animals including guinea pigs, demonstrating that differences between guinea pigs and the other animals is not in their response to the toxicant but in bioactivation (Weisburger and Weisburger, 1973).

Although differences in biotransformation, including bioactivation, account for species variation in susceptibility to a great majority of chemicals, other factors such as absorption, distribution, and excretion also play a part. In addition, variations in physiological functions are important in toxic manifestations in response to such toxicants as squill. This toxic chemical is a good rodenticide because rats cannot vomit, whereas humans and many other mammals can eliminate this poison by vomiting (Doull, 1980). Anatomic differences may also be responsible, such as with butylated hydroxyanisole.

Target organ is the primary or most sensitive organ affected by exposure to toxic substances. The same chemical entering the body with different routes of exposure, dosages, gender, and species may affect the sensitivity to target organ toxicity. Aflatoxin $B_1$ ($AFB_1$) is a well-known hepatocarcinogen in all animal species. A wide variation in $LD_{50}$ values has been obtained in animals treated with single doses of $AFB_1$. $LD_{50}$ values of $AFB_1$ range from 0.5 to 10 mg/kg body weight as described in Table 5.3. Species differences were demonstrated in their susceptibility for acute and chronic exposure to aflatoxins. The enhanced sensitivity to $AFB_1$-induced

***Table 5.3*** Acute aflatoxin $B_1$ LD50 (mg/kg, p.o.) in various animal species

| Species | LD 50 (mg/kg, oral) |
|---|---|
| Rabbit | 0.3 |
| Cat | 0.55 |
| Dog | 0.55–1.0 |
| Pig | 0.6 |
| Rat | 6.0–7.0 |
| Mouse | 9.0 |
| Hamster | 10.2 |

hepatocarcinogenicity in newborn and adult mice after liver injury is closely related to a lower level of glutathione S-transferase (GST) activity in liver, as compared to hepatic activity in normal adult mice (Sell, 2003). Further, humans are highly susceptible to the toxic and carcinogenic effects of $AFB_1$ due to relatively low expression of mGSTA3 activity for aflatoxin-8,9-epoxide. However, mice are resistant to $AFB_1$ because of a high expression of mGSTA3 in their liver (Hayes et al., 1992; van Ness et al., 1998).

With the diversity in the number of rat strains available, it should not be surprising that there are differences in chemical-induced sensitivities. In general, each chemical induces a change in all rat strains, but the degree of the effect varies among strains (Table 5.4). However, there may be no response in humans. Clearly, there are hormonal differences between males and females, but the precise role of these hormones in strain-associated chemical-induced outcomes still remains to be established. It should be noted that the reproductive cycle in female F344 rats is dramatically different from that of Sprague–Dawley rats (Kacew et al., 1995) (Table 5.4). Consequently, the incidence of spontaneous and chemical-induced mammary tumorigenicity is markedly higher in Sprague–Dawley rats, as this stock possesses greater estrogen levels. The human does not resemble the Sprague–Dawley strain and thus findings cannot be applied to humans. In comparing both males and females of the same strain, in general, chemicals including nitrosamines, decalin, hydroquinone, or chloroform induce markedly greater responses in the male (Kacew and Festing, 1995). It is of interest that in studies where males and females of different strains are compared, the males of certain strains are far more susceptible to adverse effects. Less dramatic, but more consistently greater susceptibility to many drugs has been reported to exist among Indonesians, and perhaps also other Asians (Darmansjah and Muchtar, 1992).

***Table 5.4*** Strain-related differences in drug-induced responses

| | | Strain/stock | |
|---|---|---|---|
| **Parameter** | **Tissue** | **Resistant**[a] | **Susceptible** |
| Ciprofibrate-induced peroxisomal proliferation | Liver | Sprague–Dawley | Long-Evans |
| Acetaminophen-induced necrosis | Kidney | Sprague–Dawley | F344 |
| Streptozotocin-induced autoimmune reactivity | Popliteal lymph node | F344 | Sprague–Dawley or Wistar |
| Amiodarone-induced phospholipidosis | Lung | Sprague–Dawley | F344 |
| Diethyl stilbesterol-induced carcinoma | Mammary tissue | COP | F344 |
| Saccharin-induced histopathological changes | Urinary bladder | Sprague–Dawley | Wistar |
| Mepirizole-induced ulceration | Duodenum | DONYRU | Sprague–Dawley or F344 |
| Azaserine-induced carcinoma | Pancreas | F344 | Wistar |
| β-adrenoceptor suppression of lipolysis | Adipocyte | Wistar | Sprague–Dawley |
| Diethyl stilbesterol-induced prolactin secretion | Pituitary | Sprague–Dawley | F344 |

[a] Resistant does not imply a lack of effect but a significantly lower responsiveness than susceptible.

## *Gender, hormonal status, and pregnancy*

Male and female animals of the same strain and species usually react to toxicants similarly. There are, however, notable quantitative differences in their susceptibility, especially in rats. For example, many barbiturates induce more prolonged sleep in female rats than in male ones. The shorter duration of action of hexobarbital in male rats is related to their higher activity of liver microsomal enzymes to hydroxylate this chemical. This higher activity can be reduced by castration or pretreatment with estrogen. Similarly, male rats demethylate aminopyrine and acetylate sulfanilamide faster than females, thus males are less susceptible.

Female rats are also more susceptible than males to organophosphorus insecticides such as azinphos-methyl and parathion. Castration and hormone treatment reverse this difference. Further, weaning rats of both genders are equally susceptible to these toxicants. However, unlike hexobarbital, parathion is metabolized more rapidly in the female than in the male rat. This faster metabolism of parathion results in a higher concentration of its metabolite, paraoxon, which is more toxic than the parent compound. This higher toxicity resulting from greater bioactivation in female rats, compared with males, is also true with aldrin and heptachlor, which undergo epoxidation. Female rats are also more susceptible to warfarin and strychnine. On the other hand, male rats are more susceptible than females to ergot and lead.

Differences in susceptibility between genders are also seen with other chemicals. For example, chloroform is acutely nephrotoxic in the male mouse but not in the female. Castration or the administration of estrogens reduces this effect in males, and treatment with androgens enhances susceptibility to chloroform in females. The greater susceptibility of male mice was explained on the basis of a higher concentration of cytochrome P-450 (Smith et al., 1983). Strain and gender also play an important role in hyaline droplet nephropathy. Administration of decalin to male F-344, Sprague–Dawley, Buffalo, or BN rats increased $\alpha 2_{\mu}$-globulin content associated with hyaline droplet formation. In contrast, female F-344, SD, Buffalo, and BN rats showed no evidence of hyaline droplet formation or accumulation of $\alpha 2_{\mu}$-globulin. It is of interest that both male and female NCI-Black Reiter (NBR) rats resembled female responsiveness, as there was no hyaline droplet nephropathy. Clearly, the decalin-induced hyaline droplet nephropathy is strain related, but the role of male hormones is difficult to decipher due to the lack of response noted in NBR male rats. However, there are marked differences in endogenous circulating testosterone levels among strains and this may account for the differences between NBR and other strains. It is also conceivable that NBR male rats, unlike Sprague–Dawley or F-344, lack the gene necessary to synthesize $\alpha 2_{\mu}$-globulin. Nicotine is also more toxic to the male mouse, and digoxin is more toxic to the male dog. However, the female cat is more susceptible to dinitrophenol and the female rabbit is more so to benzene.

Imbalances of non-sex hormones also alter susceptibility of animals to toxicants. Hyperthyroidism, hyperinsulinism, adrenalectomy, and stimulation of the pituitary–adrenal axis have all been shown to be capable of modifying the effects of certain toxicants (Doull, 1980; Hodgson, 1987).

## *Age*

Toxicants exert greater effects in young animals than in adults because of a less developed detoxication capability. In general, it has long been recognized that neonates and very young animals are more susceptible to toxicants such as morphine. For a great majority of toxicants, the young are 1.5–10 times more susceptible than adults (Goldenthal, 1971). In the case of DDT, the $LD_{50}$ for a newborn is greater than 4000 mg/kg and falls to 730 mg/kg at 10 days; 190 mg/kg at 4 months, and is 220 mg/kg in the adult. This clearly shows that the neonate is less susceptible than the adult to DDT-mediated lethality. Hence, it is important to emphasize that there are exceptions to the general rules that the young are always more sensitive than adults to chemical exposure.

The available information indicates that the greater susceptibility of the young animals to many toxicants might be attributed to deficiencies of various detoxication enzyme systems (Makri et al., 2004). Both phase I and phase II reactions may be responsible. For example, hexobarbital at a dose of 10 mg/kg induced a sleeping time of longer than 360 minutes in 1-day-old mice compared with 27 min in the 21-day-old mice. The proportion of hexobarbital metabolized by oxidation in 3 hours in these animals was 0% and 21–33%, respectively (Jondorf et al., 1959). On the other hand, chloramphenicol is excreted mainly as a glucuronide conjugate. When a dose of 50 mg/kg was given to 1- or 2-day-old infants, the blood levels were 15 μg/mL or higher over a period of 48 hours. In contrast, children aged 1–11 years maintained such blood levels for only 12 hours (Weiss et al., 1960). Further, the route of exposure plays a significant role in the susceptibility of infants to air pollutants. The lung epithelium is not fully developed until the age of 4 (Foos et al., 2008). Children have a larger lung surface area per kilogram than adults and breathe a greater volume of air per kilogram. Hence, air pollution may exert persistent effects on respiratory health, especially in the young. It should be kept in mind that the immune system is immature during this period and it has been postulated that the rise in asthma frequency is attributable to the greater inhalation exposure to pollutants in association with immune function immaturity.

However, not all chemicals are more toxic to the young. Certain substances, notably CNS stimulants, are less toxic to neonates. Lu et al. (1965) reported that the effect of $LD_{50}$ of DDT was more than 20 times greater in newborn rats than in adults, in sharp contrast to the effect of malathion on age (Table 5.5). This insensitivity to the toxicity of DDT may be reassuring in assessing the potential risk of this pesticide, because of the larger intake in young babies via breast feeding and cow's milk, especially on the unit body weight basis.

The effect of age on the susceptibility to other CNS stimulants including other organochlorine insecticides (dieldrin) appears less marked (generally in the range of 2- to 10-fold). Most organophosphorus pesticides such as malathion are more toxic to the young; schradan (octamethyl pyrophosphoramide) and phenyl-thiourea are notable exceptions (Brodeur and DuBois, 1963).

Apart from differences in biotransformation, other factors also play a role. For example, a lower susceptibility at the receptor has been found to

***Table 5.5*** Effect of age on acute toxicity of Malathion, DDT, and Dieldrin in rats

| Pesticide | Age | $LD_{50}$ (mg/kg) with 95% CI Limits | |
|---|---|---|---|
| Malathion | Newborn | 134.4 | (94.0–190.8) |
| | Pre-weaning | 925.5 | (679.01–261.0) |
| | Adult | 3697.0 | (3179.0–4251.0) |
| DDT | Newborn | >4000.0 | |
| | Pre-weaning | 437.8 | (346.3–553.9) |
| | Adult | 194.5 | (158.7–238.3) |
| Dieldrin | Newborn | 167.8 | (140.8–200.0) |
| | Pre-weaning | 24.9 | (19.7–31.5) |
| | Adult | 37.0 | (27.4–50.1) |

*Source:* Lu FC, Jessup DC, Lavellee A, *Food Cosmet. Toxicol.*, 3, 591–596,1965.

be the reason for the relative insensitivity of young rats to DDT (Henderson and Woolley, 1969).

Certain toxicants are absorbed to a greater extent by the young than by adults. For example, young children absorb 4–5 times more lead than adults (McCabe, 1979) and 20 times more cadmium (Sasser and Jarbor, 1977). The greater susceptibility of the young to morphine is attributable to a less efficient blood–brain barrier, as is vividly illustrated in Figure 5.1 (Kupferberg and Way, 1963). Penicillin and tetracycline are excreted more slowly and hence are more toxic in the young (Lu, 1970). Ouabain is about 40 times more toxic in newborn rats than in adults because the adult rat liver is more efficient in removing this cardiac glycoside from the plasma. The higher incidence of methemoglobinemia in young infants has been explained on the basis that their lower gastric acidity allows upward migration of intestinal microbial flora and reduction of nitrates to a greater extent. Further, young infants have a higher proportion of fetal hemoglobin, which is more readily oxidized to methemoglobin (WHO, 1977).

There is evidence that the newborn is more susceptible to such carcinogens as $AFB_1$. $AFB_1$ is seven times more toxic in newborn (1-day-old) rats than adults because of an undeveloped blood–brain barrier. Adult mice tolerate high doses of $AFB_1$ (up to 60 mg/kg) without manifesting toxic or carcinogenic effects (Wogan, 1969; Vesselinovitch et al., 1972). However, mice are prone to $AFB_1$-induced toxicity if the toxin is administered during the first week after birth, with males being significantly more sensitive than females (Ueno et al., 1991). In addition, the susceptibility to $AFB_1$ increases in adult mice if hepatocyte proliferation is stimulated following partial hepatectomy or $CCl_4$-induced injury (Arora, 1981), or during chronic regenerative hyperplasia (Sell et al., 1991). The enhanced sensitivity to $AFB_1$ hepatocarcinogenicity in newborn and adult mice after liver

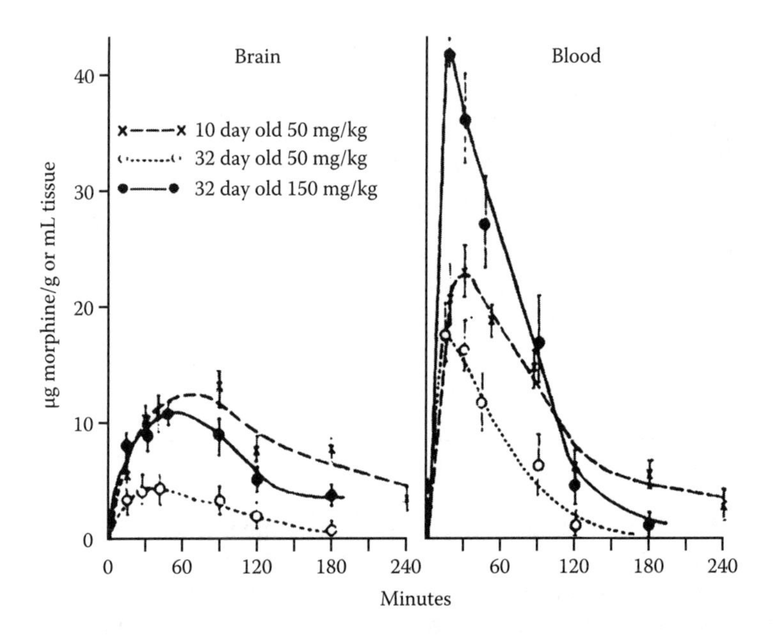


*Figure 5.1* Brain and blood levels of free morphine at specific time intervals following intraperitoneal injections of morphine. Bracketed vertical lines show the standard error observed, using four animals per point. (From Kupferberg HJ, Way EL, *J. Pharmacol. Exp. Ther.*, 141, 105–112, 1963.)

injury is closely related to a lower level of GST activity in the liver, as compared to the hepatic activity in normal adult mice (Sell, 2003). The resistance of adult mice to $AFB_1$ has been suggested to be due to constitutive expression in mouse liver of mGSTA3, which exhibits high catalytic activity toward $AFB_1$ (Degen and Neumann, 1981; Ilic et al., 2010).

Further, fetuses, but not embryos of rodents are more susceptible. For example, there was a 50-fold increase in the potency of ethylnitrosourea. This is also true with nonhuman primates, except the maximal effects that occur during the first third of gestation. If this is true with human fetuses, then they may be exposed to carcinogens before mothers are aware of their pregnancies (Rice, 1979).

Old animals and humans are also more susceptible to certain chemicals. This problem has not been studied as extensively as in the young. However, the available evidence indicates that aged patients are generally more sensitive to many drugs. The possible mechanisms include reduced detoxication and an impaired renal excretion (Goldstein, 1990). In addition, the distribution of chemicals in the body may also be altered because of increased body fat and decreased body water (Jarvik et al., 1981). A number of drugs were found to be likely to induce more severe signs of toxicity. These include most CNS depressants, certain antibiotics, cardiac glycosides, and hypotensive agents (WHO, 1981; Rochon et al., 1999).

## *Nutritional status*

The principal biotransformation of toxicants, as noted in Chapter 3, is catalyzed by the microsomal mixed-function oxidases (MFO). A deficiency of essential fatty acids generally depresses MFO activities. This is also true with protein deficiency. The decreased MFO has different effects on the toxicity of chemicals. For example, hexobarbital and aminopyrine are detoxicated by these enzymes and are thus more toxic to rats and mice with these nutrient deficiencies. On the other hand, the toxicities of aflatoxin A, carbon tetrachloride, and heptachlor are lower in such animals because of their depressed bioactivation of these toxicants. Rats fed low-protein diets were 2–26 times more sensitive to a variety of pesticides (Boyd, 1972). MFO activities decrease in animals fed high levels of carbohydrates.

A number of carcinogenesis studies demonstrated that restriction of food intake decreases tumor yield. Deficiency of protein generally lowers the tumorigenicity of carcinogens, such as aflatoxin $B_1$ and dimethyl nitrosamine (DMN). The importance of diet on carcinogenesis is further demonstrated by the fact that rats and mice fed diets rich in fats have higher tumor incidences compared with those that are given a restricted diet.

Vitamin A deficiency depresses the MFO. In general, this is also true with deficiencies of vitamins C and E. But thiamine deficiency has the opposite effect. Vitamin A deficiency, in addition, increases the susceptibility of the respiratory tract to carcinogens (Nettesheim et al., 1979). Some foods contain appreciable amounts of chemicals that are potent inducers of MFO, such as safrole, flavones, xanthines, and indoles. In addition, potent inducers such as DDT and polychlorinated biphenyls are present as contaminants in many foods.

## *Diseases*

The liver is the main organ wherein biotransformation of chemicals takes place. Diseases like acute and chronic hepatitis, cirrhosis of the liver and hepatic necrosis often decrease the process of biotransformation. The microsomal and non-microsomal enzyme systems as well as the phase II reactions may be affected.

Renal diseases may also affect the toxic manifestations of chemicals. This effect stems from disturbances of the excretory and metabolic functions of the kidney. Endocrine disorders such as diabetes mellitus compromise the immune system and thus the ability of individuals to cope with stress induced by chemicals. Heart diseases, when severe, increase toxicity of chemicals by impairing hepatic and renal circulation, thus affecting the metabolic and excretory functions of these organs. Respiratory tract disorders such as asthma render subjects more susceptible to air pollutants such as $SO_2$.

### *Genetic factors*

Apart from differences in susceptibility that exist from one species to another and from one strain to another, there are also variables among individuals of the same species and same strain. The metabolism of toxic chemical may be modified by inherited and induced variation in CYPs, acetyltransferase (NAT), and GST genes. For example, some individuals may not respond to acetaminophen medication while others fall into a deep sleep at a similar dose. In general, the genetic polymorphisms may affect the level of expression, the catalytic activity of metabolic, or detoxify enzymes, thereby influencing the toxicity susceptibility of toxicants (Miller et al., 2001). Among them, CYP polymorphisms provide important genetic information that helps to understand the adverse effects of chemicals on humans. For drug metabolism, the most important CYP polymorphisms are those of genes coding for CYP2C9, CYP2C19, CYP2D6, or CYP3A4/5, which result in therapeutic failure or severe adverse reactions (Zanger et al., 2001; Ingelman-Sundberg and Sim, 2010; Preissner et al., 2013). Genes coding for CYP1A1, CYP1A2, CYP1B1, or CYP2E1 are among the most responsible for biotransformation of chemicals, especially for metabolic activation of pre-carcinogens. There is evidence of association between gene polymorphism and cancer susceptibility (Bartsch et al., 2000).

Other genetic polymorphisms have been widely studied in humans. For example, there are "slow inactivators," who are deficient in NAT. Such individuals acetylate isoniazid only slowly and are thus likely to suffer from peripheral neuropathy resulting from an accumulation of isoniazid (Cohen et al., 1974). On the other hand, people with more efficient NAT require larger doses of isoniazid to obtain its therapeutic effect and are thus more likely to suffer from hepatic damage. It is estimated that 45% of Caucasians lack a functional GSTM1 allele, while 20% of Caucasians lack a functional GSTT1 allele. One of the consequences of inheriting a nonfunctional GSTM1 allele appears to be an increased risk for cancer, particularly of the bladder and lung (Bell et al., 1993a,b; Brockmoller et al., 1996).

Glucose-6-phosphate dehydrogenase (G6PD) deficiency indirectly affects xenobiotic toxicity. G6PD is an enzyme in the hexose monophosphate shunt, a principal source of NADPH, which restores oxidized glutathione,

GS-SG, to its reduced form (GSH) in red blood cells and many tissues (Beutler and Duparc, 2007; Nkhoma et al., 2009). Numerous drugs and electrophilic metabolites affect GSH levels, leading to GSH deficiency, especially in G6PD-deficient patients with a low GSH reserve. GSH deficiency in red blood cells results in membrane fragility and hemolysis; hence, hemolytic anemia often ensues. G6PD and altered stability of reduced glutathione are responsible for hemolytic anemia in subjects exposed to primaquine, anti-pyrine, and similar agents (Carson et al., 1956; Calabrese et al., 1979; Cappellini and Fiorelli, 2008; Rochforda et al., 2013).

Variants of base excision and nucleotide excision repair genes (XRCC1 and XPD) appear to modify exposure-induced damage from cigarette smoke and radiation. Investigations are underway to discover genetic variation in environmental response genes and determine if this variation exerts any effect on gene function or if it is associated with disease risk. These and other results are discussed in the context of evaluating inherited or acquired susceptibility risk factors for environmentally associated diseases.

## *Environmental factors*

### *Physical factors*

Changes in temperature may alter toxicity. For example, colchicine and digitalis are more toxic to rat than frog, but toxicity to the frog can be increased by raising the environmental temperature. The duration of the response, however, is shorter when the temperature is higher. The effect of environmental temperature on the magnitude and duration of the response is apparently related to the temperature-dependent biochemical reactions responsible for the effect and biotransformation of the chemical.

Researchers' interest in the effect of barometric pressure on the toxicity of chemicals stems from human exposure to these substances in space and in saturation diving vehicles. At high altitudes, the toxicity of digitalis and strychnine is decreased, whereas that of amphetamine is increased. The influence of changes in barometric pressure on the toxicity of chemicals seems attributable mainly, if not entirely, to altered oxygen tension rather than to a direct pressure effect.

Whole-body irradiation increases the toxicity of CNS stimulants but decreases that of CNS depressants. However, it has no marked effect on analgesics such as morphine. More details and literature citations have been provided by Doull (1980).

The effects of toxicants often show a diurnal pattern that is mainly related to the light cycle. In the rat and the mouse, the activities of cytochrome P-450 are greatest at the beginning of the dark phase.

### Social factors

It is well known that animal husbandry and a variety of social factors modify the toxicities of chemicals: the handling of animals, housing (singly or in groups), types of cage, supplier, and bedding materials are all important factors. Some examples of the influence of environmental factors on toxicity are given in Chapter 6.

## Chemical interactions

### Types of interaction

The toxicity of a chemical in an organism may be increased or decreased by a simultaneous or consecutive exposure to another chemical (Table 6.1 of Chapter 6). If the combined effect is equal to the sum of the effect of each substance given alone, the interaction is considered to be *additive*; for example, combinations of most organophosphorus pesticides on cholinesterase activity. If the combined effect is greater than the sum, the interaction is considered to be *synergistic*; for example, carbon tetrachloride and ethanol on the liver, and asbestos exposure and cigarette smoking on the lungs. In the latter example, Selikoff et al. (1968) reported that there was a 5-fold increase in lung cancer incidence among asbestos workers, an 11-fold rise among cigarette smokers, and a 55-fold increase among asbestos workers who were cigarette smokers. The term *potentiation* is used to describe the situation in which the toxicity of a substance on an organ is markedly increased by another substance that by itself exerts no significant toxic effect on that organ. For example, isopropanol exerts no marked effect on the liver, but it significantly increases the hepatotoxicity of carbon tetrachloride. Similarly, trichloroethylene (TCE), which exerts little effect on the liver, enhances the hepatotoxicity of carbon tetrachloride, as measured by the release of liver enzymes ALT, SDH, and AST (Borzelleca et al., 1990).

The exposure of an organism to one chemical may reduce the toxicity of another. *Chemical antagonism* denotes the situation wherein a reaction between the two chemicals produces a less toxic product, for example, chelation of heavy metals by dimercaprol. *Functional antagonism* exists when two chemicals produce opposite effects on the same physiological parameters, such as the counteraction between CNS stimulants and depressants. *Competitive antagonism* exists when the agonist and antagonist act on the same receptor, such as the blockade of the effects of nicotine on ganglia by ganglionic blocking agents. *Noncompetitive antagonism* exists when the toxic effect of one chemical is blocked by another not acting on the same receptor. For example, atropine reduces the toxicity of acetyl-cholinesterase (AChE) inhibitors not by blocking the receptors on the AChE, but by blocking the receptors for the accumulated acetylcholine.

## *Mechanisms of action*

Chemical interactions are achieved through a variety of mechanisms. For instance, nitrites and certain amines react in the stomach to form nitrosamines, the majority of which are potent carcinogens, and thus greatly increase toxicity. On the other hand, the action of many antidotes is based upon their interaction with toxicants; for example, thiosulfate is used in cases of cyanide poisoning. Further, a chemical may displace another from its binding site on plasma protein and thereby increase its effective concentration. A chemical may modify the renal excretion of weak acids and weak bases by altering the pH of urine. Competition for the same renal transport system by one chemical might hinder the excretion of another. A notable example is administration of probenecid along with penicillin to reduce renal excretion of the antibiotic, thereby prolonging its duration of action.

One important type of interaction involves the binding of chemicals with their specific receptors. An antagonist blocks the action of an agonist, such as a neurotransmitter or a hormone, by preventing the binding of the agonist to the receptor.

Another important type of interaction results from alterations in biotransformation of one chemical by another. Some chemicals are *inducers* of xenobiotic metabolizing enzymes. These compounds augment activities of these enzymes, perhaps mainly by de novo synthesis. The common inducers include phenobarbital, 3-methylcholanthrene (3-MC), polychlorinated biphenyl, DDT, and BaP. The inducers may lower the toxicity of other chemicals by accelerating their detoxication; for example, pretreatment with phenobarbital shortens the sleeping time induced by hexobarbital and the paralysis induced by zoxazolamine. Such pretreatment also reduces the plasma level of aflatoxins (Wong et al., 1981). In addition, 3-MC pretreatment greatly reduces the liver necrosis produced by bromobenzene, probably by enhancing the activity of the epoxide hydrase (see Figure 3.3 of Chapter 3). On the other hand, pretreatment with phenobarbital augments the toxicity of acetaminophen and bromobenzene, apparently by increasing the number of toxic metabolites formed. Repeated administration of a chemical may induce its metabolizing enzymes, as shown with vinyl chloride.

Piperonyl butoxide, isoniazid, SKF 525 A, and related chemicals are inhibitors of various xenobiotic-metabolizing enzymes. For instance, piperonyl butoxide enhances toxicity of pyrethrum in insects by inhibiting their MFO that detoxifies this insecticide. Isoniazid, when taken along with diphenylhydantoin, lengthens the plasma half-life of the antiepileptic drug and increases its toxicity. Iproniazid inhibits monoamine oxidase and augments the cardiovascular effects of tyramine, which is found in cheese and is normally readily metabolized by the oxidase.

### Characteristics of enzyme induction

Because of the importance of the effect of enzyme induction, numerous studies were conducted on certain inducers, notably phenobarbital and polycyclic aromatic hydrocarbons (PAHs). These two types of inducers differ in several aspects. For example, phenobarbital markedly increases the liver weight and the smooth endoplasmic reticulum, but PAHs such as 3-MC and BaP exert little effect on these parameters. Phenobarbital augments mainly the amounts of cytochrome P-450 and NADPH cytochrome *c* reductase. PAHs produce little effect on these enzymes, but raise the amounts of cytochrome P-448, which is also known as $P_1$-450, and aryl hydrocarbon hydroxylase (AHH). These isozymes exhibit different substrate specificity and hence alter the effects of toxicants differently (Sipes and Gandolfi, 1993).

### Interactions as toxicological tools

Studies on chemical interaction are conducted not only to determine the effects of combinations of chemicals, but the data thereof are also useful in assessing health hazards associated with exposures to such combinations. These studies are also conducted to elucidate the nature and the mode of action of the toxicity of one chemical by the administration of another, as well as to bring out the weak or latent effects of chemicals.

It needs to be made abundantly clear that in reality exposure may not be strictly to one compound but to a mixture of chemicals. Agency for Toxic Substances and Disease Registry (ATSDR) has deemed that exposure to chemical mixtures is one of the priority areas of concern and has significant health implications (DeRosa et al., 2004). Data in this scientific field is sorely lacking and one cannot assume or presume that the compounds will act synergistically or antagonistically. However, it is known that exposure to a mixture of low levels of benzene, ethyl benzene, toluene, and xylene (BTEX) has severe neurotoxicity consequences.

## References

Arora RG (1981). Enhanced susceptibility to aflatoxin $B_1$ toxicity in weanling mice pretreated with carbon tetrachloride. *Acta Pathol Microbiol Scand.* A 89, 303–8.

Bartsch H, Nair U, Risch A, Rojas M, Wikman H, Alexandrov K (2000). Genetic polymorphism of CYP genes, alone or in combination, as a risk modifier of tobacco-related cancers. *Cancer Epidemiol Biomarkers Prev.* 9, 3–28.

Beutler E, Duparc S (2007). G6PD Deficiency Working Group Glucose-6-phosphate dehydrogenase deficiency and antimalarial drug development. *Am J Trop Med Hyg.* 77, 779–89.

Bell JA, Taylor JA, Butler MA et al. (1993a). Genotype/phenotype discordance for human arylamine *N*-acetyltransferase (NAT2) reveals a new slow-acetylator allele common in African-Americans. *Carcinogenesis.* 14, 1689–92.
Bell DA, Taylor JA, Paulson DF et al. (1993b). Genetic risk and carcinogen exposure: A common inherited defect of the carcinogen-metabolism gene glutathione *S*-transferase M1 (GSTM1) that increases susceptibility to bladder cancer. *J Natl Cancer Inst.* 85, 1159–64.
Borzelleca JF, O'Hara TM, Gennings C et al. (1990). Interactions of water contaminants. *Fundam Appl Toxicol.* 14, 477–90.
Boyd EM (1972). *Protein Deficiency and Pesticide Toxicity.* Springfield, IL: Charles C Thomas.
Brockmoller J, Cascorbi I, Kerb R, Roots I (1996). Combined analysis of inherited polymorphisms in arylamine *N*-acetyltransferase 2, glutathione *S*-transferases M1 and T1, microsomal epoxide hydrolase, and cytochrome P450 enzymes as modulators of bladder cancer risk. *Cancer Res.* 56, 3915–25.
Brodeur J, DuBois KP (1963). Comparison of acute toxicity of anticholinesterase insecticides to weanling and adult male rats. *Proc Soc Exp Biol Med.* 114, 509–11.
Calabrese EJ, Moore G, Brown R (1979). Effects of environmental oxidant stressors on individuals with a G-6-PD deficiency with particular reference to an animal model. *Environ Health Persp.* 29, 49–55.
Cappellini MD, Fiorelli G (2008). Glucose-6-phosphate dehydrogenase deficiency. *Lancet.* 371, 64–74.
Carson PE, Alving AS, Flanagan CL, Ickes CE (1956). Enzymatic deficiency in primaquine-sensitive erythrocytes. *Science.* 124, 484–5.
Cohen LK, George W, Smith R (1974). Isoniazid-induced acne and pellagra. Occurrence in slow inactivators of isoniazid. *Arch Dermatol.* 109, 377–81.
Darmansjah I, Muchtar A (1992). Dose–response variation among different populations. *Clin Pharmacol Therap.* 52, 449–52.
Degen GH, Neumann HG (1981). Differences in aflatoxin $B_1$ susceptibility of rat and mouse are correlated with the capability in vitro to inactivate aflatoxin $B_1$ epoxide. *Carcinogenesis.* 2, 229–306.
DeRosa CT, El-Masri HA, Pohl H et al. (2004). Implications of chemical mixtures in public health practice. *J Toxicol Environ Health B.* 7, 339–50.
Doull J (1980). Factors influencing toxicology. In: Doull J, Klaassen CD, Amdur MO, eds. *Casarett and Doull's Toxicology.* New York: Macmillan.
Foos B, Marty M, Schwartz J et al. (2008). Focusing on children's inhalation dosimetry and health effects for risk assessment: An introduction. *J Toxicol Environ Health A.* 71, 149–65.
Goldenthal EI (1971). A compilation of LD50 values in newborn and adult animals. *Toxicol Appl Pharmacol.* 18, 185–207.
Goldstein RS (1990). Drug-induced nephrotoxicity in middle-aged and senescent rats. In: *Proceedings of the V International Congress of Toxicology.* London, UK: Taylor & Francis.
Hayes JD, Judah DJ, Neal GE, Nguyen T (1992). Molecular cloning and heterologous expression of a cDNA encoding a mouse glutathione S transferase Yc subunit possessing high catalytic activity for aflatoxin $B_1$-8,9-epoxide. *Biochem J.* 285, 173–80.

Henderson GL, Woolley DA (1969). Studies on the relative insensitivity of the immature rat to the neurotoxic effects of DDT. *J Pharmacol Exp Ther.* 170, 173–80.

Hodgson E (1987). Modification of metabolism. In: Hodgson E, Levi PE, eds. *Modern Toxicology.* New York: Elsevier.

Ilic Z, Crawford D, Egner PA, Sell S (2010). Glutathione-S-transferase A3 knockout mice are sensitive to acute cytotoxic and genotoxic effects of aflatoxin $B_1$. *Toxicol Appl Pharmacol.* 242, 241–6.

Ingelman-Sundberg M, Sim SC (2010). Pharmacogenetic biomarkers as tools for improved drug therapy; emphasis on the cytochrome P450 system. *Biochem Biophy Res Commun.* 396, 90–4.

Jarvik LF, Greenblatt DJ, Harman D (1981). *Clinical Pharmacology and the Aged Patient.* New York: Raven Press.

Jay GE Jr (1955). Variation in response of various mouse strains to hexobarbital (Evipal). *Proc Soc Exp Biol Med.* 90, 378–80.

Jondorf WR, Maickel RP, Brodie BB (1959). Inability of newborn mice and guinea pigs to metabolize drugs. *Biochem Pharmacol.* 1, 352–4.

Kacew S, Festing MFW (1995). Role of rat strain in the differential sensitivity to pharmaceutical agents and naturally occurring substances. *J Toxicol Environ Health.* 47, 1–30.

Kacew S, Ruben Z, McConnell RF (1995). Strain as a determinant factor in the differential responsiveness of rats to chemicals. *Toxicol Pathol.* 23, 701–14.

Kupferberg HJ, Way EL (1963). Pharmacologic basis for the increased sensitivity of the newborn rat to morphine. *J Pharmacol Exp Ther.* 141, 105–12.

Lu FC (1970). Significance of age of test animals in food additive evaluation. In: Roe FJC, ed. *Metabolic Aspects of Food Safety.* Oxford, UK: Blackwell Scientific.

Lu FC, Jessup DC, Lavellee A (1965). Toxicity of pesticides in young versus adult rats. *Food Cosmet Toxicol.* 3, 591–6.

Makri A, Goveia M, Balbus J et al. (2004). Children's susceptibility to chemicals: A review by developmental stage. *J Toxicol Environ Health B.* 7, 417–35.

McCabe EB (1979). Age and sensitivity to lead toxicity: A review. *Environ Health Persp.* 29, 29–33.

Miller EC, Miller JH, Enomotor M (1964). The comparative carcinogenetics of 2-acetylaminofluorene and its *N*-hydroxy metabolite in mice, hamsters and guinea pigs. *Cancer Res.* 24, 2018–32.

Miller MC, Mohrenweiser HW, Bell DA (2001). Genetic variability in susceptibility and response to toxicants. *Toxicol Lett.* 120: 269–80.

Nettesheim P, Snyder C, Kim JCS (1979). Vitamin A and the susceptibility of respiratory tract tissues to carcinogenic insult. *Environ Health Persp.* 29, 89–93.

Nkhoma ET, Poole C, Vannappagari V, Hall SA, Beutler E (2009). The global prevalence of glucose-6-phosphate dehydrogenase deficiency: A systematic review and metaanalysis. *Blood Cells Mol Dis.* 42, 267–78.

Preissner SC, Hoffmann MF, Preissner R et al. (2013). Polymorphic cytochrome P450 enzymes (CYPs) and their role in personalized therapy. *PLOS One.* 8, e82562.

Quinn GP, Axelrod J, Brodie BB (1958). Species, strain and sex differences in metabolism of hexobarbitone, amidopyrine, antipyrine and aniline. *Biochem Pharmacol.* 1, 152–9.

Rice JM (1979). Perinatal period and pregnancy: Intervals of high risk for chemical carcinogens. *Environ Health Persp.* 29, 23–7.

Rochforda R, Ohrtb C, Paul C et al. (2013). Humanized mouse model of glucose 6-phosphate dehydrogenase deficiency for in vivo assessment of hemolytic toxicity. *PNAS*. 110, 17486–91.
Rochon PA, Anderson GM, Tu JV et al. (1999). Age and gender-related use of low dose drug therapy. *J Am Geriatr Soc*. 47, 954–9.
Sasser LB, Jarbor GE (1977). Intestinal absorption and retention of cadmium in neonatal rat. *Toxicol Appl Pharmacol*. 41, 423–31.
Selikoff IJ, Hammond EC, Churg J (1968). Asbestos exposure, smoking, and neoplasia. *J Am Med Assoc*. 204, 106–12.
Sell S (2003). Mouse models to study the interaction of risk factors for human liver cancer. *Cancer Res*. 63, 7553–62.
Sell S, Hunt JM, Dunsford HA, Chisari FV (1991). Synergy between hepatitis B virus expression and chemical hepatocarcinogens in transgenic mice. *Cancer Res*. 51, 1278–85.
Sipes IG, Gandolfi AJ (1993). Biotransformation of toxicants. In: Amdur MO, Doull J, Klaassen CD, eds. *Casarett and Doull's Toxicology*. New York: McGraw-Hill.
Smith JH, Maita K, Adler V et al. (1983). Effect of sex hormone status on chloroform nephrotoxicity and renal drug metabolizing enzymes. *Toxicol Lett*. 28(Suppl 1), 23.
Timbrell JA (1991). *Principles of Biochemical Toxicology*. London, UK: Taylor & Francis.
Ueno Y, Kobayashi T, Yamamura H et al. (1991). Effects of long term feeding of nivalenol on aflatoxin $B_1$ initiated hepatocarcinogenesis in mice. *IARC Sci Publ*. 105, 420–3.
van Ness KP, McHugh TE, Bammler TK, Eaton DE (1998). Identification of amino acid residues essential for high aflatoxin $B_1$-8,9-epoxide conjugation activity in alpha class glutathione S-transferases through site-directed mutagenesis. *Toxicol Appl Pharmacol*. 152, 166–74.
Vesselinovitch SD, Mihailovich N, Wogan GN et al. (1972). Aflatoxin $B_1$, a hepatocarcinogen in the infant mouse. *Cancer Res*. 32, 2289–91.
Weisburger JH, Weisburger EK (1973). Biochemical formation and pharmacological, toxicological and pathological properties of hydroxylamines and hydroxamic acids. *Pharmacol Rev*. 25, 166.
Weiss CG, Glazko AJ, Weston A (1960). Chloramphenicol in the newborn in-fant. a physicologic explanation of its toxicity when given in excessive doses. *N Engl J Med*. 262, 787–94.
WHO. (1977). Nitrates, nitrites and *N*-nitroso compounds. Environmental Health Criteria 5. Geneva: World Health Organization.
WHO. (1981). Health care in the elderly: Report of the technical group on use of medicaments by the elderly. *Drugs*. 22, 279–94.
Williams RT (1974). Inter-species variations in the metabolism of xenobiotics. *Biochem Soc Trans*. 2, 359–77.
Wogan GN (1969). Metabolism and biochemical effects of aflatoxins. Goldblatt LA ed. *Aflatoxin—Scientific Background Control and Implications*. New York: Academic Press, 151–86.
Wong ZA, Wei Ching I, Rice DW et al. (1981). Effects of phenobarbital pretreatment on the metabolism and toxicokinetics of aflatoxin $B_1$ in the rhesus monkey. *Toxicol Appl Pharmacol*. 60, 387–97.
Zanger UM, Fischer J, Raimundo S et al. (2001). Comprehensive analysis of the genetic factors determining expression and function of hepatic CYP2D6. *Pharmacogenetics*. 11, 573–85.

# chapter six

# Conventional toxicity studies

*Hyung Sik Kim*

*Contents*

# *Introduction*

## *Usefulness*

The purpose of classical toxicology is to investigate poisonings of toxic substances and mechanisms of action. Recently, toxicology has been paying attention to the study of the interaction between chemical agents and biological systems. Although the subject of toxicology is quite complex, it is necessary to understand the characteristics of xenobiotics, physicochemical properties, routes of exposure, duration, gender, exposure scenarios, and susceptibilities that affect adverse outcomes of toxic substances. As noted in prior chapters, toxicants vary greatly in their potency, target organs, and modes of action. To provide the proper orientation for additional in-depth targeted studies, conventional toxicity studies are generally carried out first. These studies are designed to provide indications of the appropriate dosage ranges, the probable adverse effects, the target organs (e.g., liver) or systems (e.g., respiratory), and the special toxicities (e.g., carcinogenicity). In this chapter, we describe the purpose and principal methods of conventional toxicity studies.

In addition to providing preliminary information for proper orientation of additional investigations, the conventional toxicity studies per se yield data that can be used to assess the nature of the adverse effects and the "no-observed adverse effect level" (NOAEL) of the toxicant, which are required in the safety assessment described in Chapter 27. For example, approximately half of the pesticides evaluated by the WHO Expert Committee on Pesticide Residues in the past 30 years have been based on conventional toxicity studies, despite the extensive database that is also available (Lu, 1995).

## *Categories*

In order to examine the different effects associated with various lengths of exposure, the conventional studies are generally divided into four categories:

1. *Acute* toxicity studies involve either a single administration of the chemical under test or several administrations within a 24-hour period. In this study, the lethal dose 50% ($LD_{50}$) and acute toxicities are determined within 14 days of treatment.

2. *Short-term* (also known as subacute and subchronic) toxicity studies involve repeated administrations, usually on a daily or five times per week basis, over a period of about 10% of the life span, namely, 3 months in rats and 1 or 2 years in dogs. However, shorter durations such as 14- and 28-day treatments have also been used by some investigators.
3. *Long-term* (also known as chronic) toxicity studies involve repeated administrations over the entire life span of the test animals or at least a major fraction of it, for example, 18 months in mice, 24 months in rats, and 7–10 years in dogs and monkeys. These types of studies are essential for assessment of the carcinogenic potential of chemicals.
4. *Multigenerational* studies involve the administration of compounds to the parent or first generation, and subsequently compounds are given to the offspring for a second generation. These types of studies are crucial for assessment of reproductive capability as well as for determination of developmental functions.

## *Importance of selection of animal strains*

In the search for compounds to enhance our living standards, there is a necessity for understanding normal human functions and mechanisms which underlie dysfunction in these processes. Utilization of a suitable animal model, which simulates humans, is necessary to develop new pharmaceutical agents to alleviate diseases or chemicals to enhance our lifestyle. It is incumbent upon investigators to choose a species in which pharmacokinetic principles are established and resemble those of humans. The choice of rodents has specific advantages because of similarities in toxicokinetic and toxicodynamic parameters. Other advantages include usability, low cost, ease of breeding, and an extensive literature database to compare to present research. Factors that need to be recognized as playing an important role in chemical-induced outcomes include strain, supplier, gender, and dietary intake. This is especially critical in the risk-assessment process.

In an effort to establish animal models to extrapolate to human responses, one must be apprised that choosing the rat strain can affect the responses observed under normal or chemically altered conditions. Even by limiting genetic variability by simply using the same strain, factors such as supplier and dietary intake can bring about differences in the responsiveness of one strain as well as between strains. In addition, the target receptor should be present in the test species. Furthermore, the rodent may be susceptible while the human is nonresponsive.

## *Acute toxicity studies*

Acute toxicity testing may be used in risk assessments of toxicants for humans or environmental organisms. These studies are designed either to determine the median lethal dose ($LD_{50}$) of the toxicant, or a rough estimate of it. The $LD_{50}$ has been defined as "a statistically derived expression of a single dose of a material that can be expected to kill 50% of the animals, after administration of a single dose in a period not exceeding 24 hours, up to a limit of 2 g/kg." In addition, such studies may also indicate the probable target organ of the chemical and its specific toxic effect as well as provide guidance on the doses to be used in the more prolonged studies. Therefore, the main goals of acute toxicity testing are to:

1. Identify adverse outcomes due to acute high dosing of a substance
2. Provide information needed for the dose selection in prolonged toxicity studies
3. Generate data for potential adverse effects of a substance on animals, humans, and the environment
4. Provide the basis for which other testing programs may be designed

In certain cases, especially those with low acute toxicities, it may not be necessary to determine the precise $LD_{50}$s. Simple lethality data can serve useful purposes. For example, synergistic and antagonistic effects can be demonstrated using some animals as shown by the data presented in Table 6.1. Furthermore, even the information that a sufficiently large dose produces few or no deaths may suffice. This *limit test* has been applied. For example, a number of food colors were given to rats at a dose of 2 g/kg. Since none of the rats died, it was considered sufficient to rule out any serious

***Table 6.1*** Using lethality in demonstrating chemical interaction

| Lethality (number of deaths/number on test) | | | |
|---|---|---|---|
| $KBrO_3$ (mg/kg) | Control (saline) | Cysteine[a] (400 mg/kg) | Diethyl maleate[b] (0.7 mL/kg) |
| 169 | 5/5 | 0/5 | |
| 130 | 5/5 | 0/5 | |
| 49 | 0/5 | | 4/5 |
| 29 | 0/5 | | 4/5 |

*Source:* Kurakawa Y, Takamura N et al., *J. Am. Coll. Toxicol.*, 6, 487–501, 1987.
*Note:* With five animals per dose group, the interactions between $KBrO_3$ and the "antagonist" (cysteine) and a "synergist" (diethyl maleate) are evident.

[a] Antagonistic.
[b] Synergistic.

acute toxicity and no $LD_{50}$ was determined (Lu and Lavallée, 1965). This view was accepted by the Joint FAO/WHO Expert Committee on Food Additives (WHO, 1966). The EPA (1994) recommends the use of 5 g/kg.

When the route of exposure is inhalation, the endpoint is either the median lethal concentration ($LC_{50}$) with a given duration of exposure or the median lethal time ($LT_{50}$) with a given concentration of the chemical in the air.

## Experimental design

### Selection of species of animal

The species selection should be made using a combination of ethical, scientific, and practical considerations to obtain the best possible prediction of human response. In general, the rat, and sometimes the mouse, is selected for use in determining the $LD_{50}$. The preference stems from the fact that they are economical, readily available, and easy to handle. Further, there are more toxicological data on these species of animals, a fact that facilitates comparisons of toxicities to other chemicals.

Sometimes a nonrodent species is desirable. This is true, especially when the $LD_{50}$ values in rats and mice are markedly different or when the pattern or rate of biotransformation in humans is known to be significantly different from rats and mice.

The $LD_{50}$ determination is preferably done in animals of both genders, and also in adult and young animals, because of their differences in susceptibility. In recent years, the use of an $LD_{50}$ has been supplanted due to the unnecessary overuse of too many animals, and the data generated are not essential for determination of risk for humans. The beneficial value of $LD_{50}$ data does not outweigh the cost of animal welfare.

## Route of administration

Generally, the toxicant is administered by the route by which humans will be exposed. The oral route is most commonly used. The dermal and inhalation routes are used increasingly, not only for chemicals that are intended for human use by such routes but also for chemicals whose health hazards to personnel handling these chemicals are to be assessed (see Chapters 12 and 15). Parenteral routes are mainly used in assessing the acute toxicity of parenteral drugs. In addition, immediate or very prompt and complete, or nearly complete absorption generally follow intravenous and intraperitoneal injection. The intravenous route is advantageous in the determination of the distribution of a compound in the organic system and given in a radioactive form.

## *Dosage and number of animals*

To properly ascertain an $LD_{50}$, it is necessary to try to select a dose that will kill about half of the animals, another that will kill more than half (preferably less than 90%), and a third dose that will kill less than half (preferably more than 10%) of the animals. OECD (1992), among others, recommends a "Sighting" study to aid in the selection of the doses, which can be accomplished with no more than five animals. Dosing of the animals is done sequentially, with at least a 24-hour interval to allow adjustment of the dose that the next animal is to receive. Such tests use at least 30 animals per test chemical and require the death of animals as an endpoint, regardless of the suffering caused. In 2001, the OECD agreed that the $LD_{50}$ test for acute oral toxicity should be abolished and deleted from the OECD manual of internationally accepted test guidelines by the end of 2002 (OECD, 2002).

For most chemicals, however, approximate $LD_{50}$s are adequate. These doses can be estimated using six to nine animals (Bruce, 1985). As indicated previously, this type of study is outdated and not necessary in light of the cost to animals in order to gain data of limited value.

Several alternative methods have been developed which use fewer animals, and in some cases replace death as the endpoint with signs of significant toxicity instead. Information on similar chemicals is used to guide the selection of initial dose levels and the tests are designed to avoid or minimize lethality or severe toxicity. These methods have replaced the $LD_{50}$ test for acute oral toxicity, but several acute tests such as those involving inhalation, dermal, and eye exposure have yet to be modified. This modification to the classical $LD_{50}$ test includes the fixed-dose procedure, OECD TG 420, the acute-toxic-class method, OECD TG 423, and the up-and-down procedure, OECD TG 425.

There are also some limitations for $LD_{50}$ studies such as: the $LD_{50}$ gives a measure of the immediate or acute toxicity; results may vary greatly. $LD_{50}$ is not tested on humans; all relation to humans are only a guess. The $LD_{50}$ test is neither reliable nor useful because the human lethal dose can't be predicted from animal studies. Several countries, including the United Kingdom and the OECD, have taken steps to ban the oral $LD_{50}$ (OECD, 2002).

## *Observations and examinations*

After administering the toxicant to the animals, they should be examined for the number and time of death in order to estimate the $LD_{50}$. More importantly, their signs of toxicity should be recorded. Table 6.2 provides a list of body organs and systems that might be affected, along with the

***Table 6.2*** Relationship between toxic signs and body organs or systems

| System | Toxic signs |
|---|---|
| Autonomic | Relaxed nictitating membrane, exophthalmos, nasal discharge, salivation, diarrhea, urination, piloerection |
| Behavioral | Sedation, restlessness, sitting position—head up, staring straight ahead, drooping head, severe depression, excessive preening, gnawing paws, panting, irritability, aggressive and defensive hostility, fear, confusion, bizarre activity |
| Sensory | Sensitivity to pain, righting, corneal, labyrinth, placing, and hindlimb reflex; sensitivity to sound and touch; nystagmus, phonation |
| Neuromuscular | Decreased and increased activity, fasciculation, tremors, convulsions, ataxia, prostration, straub tail, hindlimb weakness, pain and hindlimb reflexes (absent or diminished), opisthotonos, muscle tone, death |
| Cardiovascular | Increased and decreased heart rate, cyanosis, vasoconstriction, vasodilation, hemorrhage |
| Respiratory | Hypopnea, dyspnea, gasping, apnea |
| Ocular | Mydriasis, miosis, lacrimation, ptosis, nystagmus, cycloplegia, pupillary light reflex |
| Gastrointestinal, gastrourinary | Salivation, retching, diarrhea, bloody stool and urine, constipation, rhinorrhea, emesis, involuntary urination and defecation |
| Cutaneous | Piloerection, wet dog shakes, erythema, edema, necrosis, swelling |

*Source:* McNamara BP, *New Concepts in Safety Evaluation*, Hemisphere, Washington, DC., 1976.

specific signs of toxicity. The observation period should be sufficiently long so that delayed effects, including death, would not be missed. The period is usually 7–14 days but may be much longer.

Gross autopsies should be performed on all animals that have died, as well as on at least some of the survivors, especially those that are morbid at the termination of the experiment. Autopsy can provide useful information on the target organ, especially when death does not occur shortly after the dosing. Histopathological examination of selected organs and tissues may also be indicated.

## *Multiple endpoint evaluation*

To derive additional information concerning the chemical on test, the toxic signs, such as those listed in Table 6.2, should be critically observed and recorded for evaluating nonlethal endpoints. These endpoints may assist in characterizing the nature of the toxicant.

## *Evaluation of the data*

### *Dose–response relationship*

The dose–response relationship is a fundamental concept in toxicology and the basis for measurement of the relative harmfulness of a chemical. A dose–response relationship is defined as a consistent mathematical and biologically plausible correlation between the number of individuals responding and a given dose over an exposure period. When the mortality, or the frequency of other effects expressed in percentages, is plotted against the dose on a logarithmic scale, an S-shaped curve is obtained (Figure 6.1, Curve B). The central portion of the curve (between 16% and 84% response) is sufficiently straight for estimating the $LD_{50}$ or $ED_{50.}$ However, a much wider range of the curve can be straightened by converting the percentages to probit units. This procedure is especially useful in estimating, for example, the $LD_{01}$ or $LD_{99,}$ when the extreme ends of this curve have to be used.

The probit units correspond to normal equivalent deviations around the mean, for example, +1, +2, +3… and –1, –2, –3… deviations, whereas the mean value itself has a zero deviation. However, to avoid negative numbers, the probit units are obtained by adding five to these deviations. The corresponding figures in these systems are as follows:

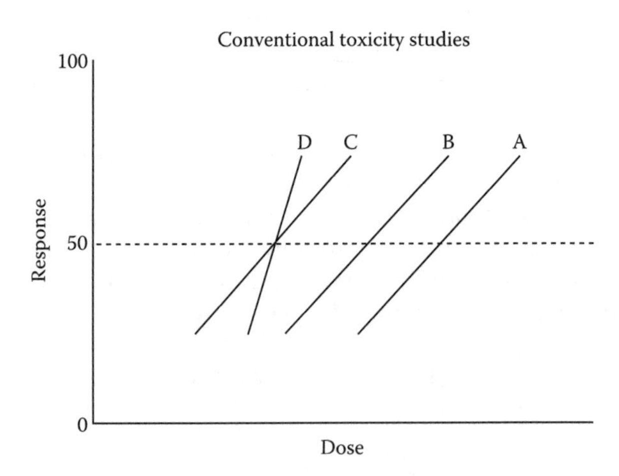


*Figure 6.1* Median lethal doses and slopes of the dose–response (death) relationships of four chemicals. Chemical A is less toxic than the others. Chemical C is as toxic as D at the median lethal dose level but is more toxic at lower dose levels. Chemical B is less toxic than D at the median lethal dose level, but it may be more or less so at lower doses.

Detailed methods for estimating the $LD_{50}$ and its standard errors are given in many papers and books on statistics, including those of Bliss (1957), Finney (1971), and Weil (1952).

| Deviations | Probit | % Response |
|---|---|---|
| –3 | 2 | 0.1 |
| –2 | 3 | 2.3 |
| –1 | 4 | 15.9 |
| 0 | 5 | 50 |
| 1 | 6 | 84.1 |
| 2 | 7 | 97.7 |
| 3 | 8 | 99.9 |

### *Relative potency*

The potency of toxicants varies significantly. Table 6.3 illustrates the range of $LD_{50}$ values. To render $LD_{50}$ values more meaningful, it is advisable to also determine their standard errors (or the confidence limits) and the slopes of the dose–response curves. The importance of the slope can be readily appreciated when comparing two substances with similar $LD_{50}$s. The one with a flatter slope will likely produce more deaths than the other

***Table 6.3*** Acute $LD_{50}$ values for a variety of chemical agents

| Agent | Species | $LD_{50}$ (mg/kg body weight) |
|---|---|---|
| Ethanol | Mouse | 10,000 |
| Sodium chloride | Mouse | 4000 |
| Ferrous sulfate | Rat | 1500 |
| Morphine sulfate | Rat | 900 |
| Phenobarbital, sodium | Rat | 150 |
| DDT | Rat | 100 |
| Picrotoxin | Rat | 5 |
| Strychnine sulfate | Rat | 2 |
| Nicotine | Rat | 1 |
| *d*-Tubocurarine | Rat | 0.5 |
| Hemicholinium-3 | Rat | 0.2 |
| Tetrodotoxin | Rat | 0.1 |
| Dioxin (TCDD) | Guinea pig | 0.001 |
| Botulinum toxin | Rat | 0.00001 |

*Source:* Loomis T, *Essentials of Toxicology*, 3rd ed., Lea and Febiger, Philadelphia, PA, 1978.

*Table 6.4* Dose–response relationships[a]

| Aflatoxin $B_1$[b] | | | | Botulinum toxin[c] | |
|---|---|---|---|---|---|
| Dose (ppb) | Response (tumor) | Dose (pg) | Response (death) | Dose (pg) | Response (death) |
| 0 | 0/18 | 1 | 0/10 | 34 | 11/30 |
| 1 | 2/22 | 5 | 0/10 | 37 | 10/30 |
| 5 | 1/22 | 10 | 0/30 | 40 | 16/30 |
| 15 | 4/21 | 15 | 0/30 | 45 | 26/30 |
| 50 | 20/25 | 20 | 0/30 | 50 | 26/30 |
| 100 | 28/28 | 24 | 0/30 | 55 | 17/30 |
| | | 27 | 0/30 | 60 | 22/30 |
| | | 30 | 4/30 | 65 | 20/30 |

[a] Note relatively shallow dose–response relationship with aflatoxin $B_1$ wherein a 100-fold increase existed between the minimal and maximal effective doses, in contrast to the steep slope of botulinum toxin where there was a mere 50% increase.
[b] From Food Safety Council, *Food. Cosmet. Toxicol.*, 16, 1–136, 1978.
[c] Data supplied by E.J. Schantz (Food Research Institute, University of Wisconsin, Madison, Wisconsin, USA). Part of the data also appears in: Food Safety Council, *Food. Cosmet. Toxicol.*, 16, 1–136, 1978.

at doses smaller than the $LD_{50}$s (Figure 6.1, chemicals C and D). The examples in Table 6.4 illustrate the marked differences in slopes.

## *Use of $LD_{50}$ values and signs of toxicity*

These values are useful in a number of ways.

1. Classification of chemicals according to relative toxicity. A common classification is shown in Table 6.5.
2. Other uses include evaluation of the hazard from accidental overdosage; planning subacute and chronic toxicity studies in animals; providing information about (a) variations in response among

*Table 6.5* Acute oral toxicity categories

| Category | $LD_{50}$ |
|---|---|
| Supertoxic (mg/kg) | 5 or less |
| Extremely toxic (mg/kg) | 5–50 |
| Highly toxic (mg/kg) | 50–500 |
| Moderately toxic (g/kg) | 0.5–5 |
| Slightly toxic (g/kg) | 5–15 |
| Practically nontoxic (g/kg) | >15 |

*Source:* Data quoted from Food Safety Council, *Food Cosmet Toxicol.* 16, 1–136, 1978.

*Table 6.6* Comparison of different methods

| Contents | Method Karber | Method of Miller and Tainter | Method of Lorke |
|---|---|---|---|
| No. of rodents used | More than necessary | More than necessary | Appropriate |
| Expenditure | High | High | Average |
| Accuracy of results | Inaccurate | Inaccurate | Doubtful |

*Source:* Paramveer D, Chanchal MK, Paresh M et al., *J. Chem. Pharm. Res.*, 6, 450–453, 2010.

different animal species and strains; (b) the susceptibility of a particular animal population; and (c) quality control of chemical products to detect toxic impurities, etc.

For toxicants with important health implications (e.g., TCDD), $LD_{50}$s are determined in several species of animals. The extent of variation of these values indicates the range of differences in the toxicokinetics and/or toxicodynamics among these species. Guidelines for acute oral, dermal, and inhalation toxicity studies have been published by various national and international agencies (e.g., EPA, 1994). However, the prevailing advice is to estimate approximate $LD_{50}$s unless otherwise indicated.

The deletion of the $LD_{50}$ test from the OECD guidelines was due to three alternative methods being adopted, which all involve more humane treatment of the animals and use fewer animals than the $LD_{50}$ test. They record toxicity signs in place of death (Table 6.6).

## *Short-term and long-term toxicity studies*

Humans are more often exposed to chemicals at levels much lower than those that are acutely fatal, but they are exposed over longer periods of time. To assess the nature of the toxic effects under these more realistic situations, short-term and long-term toxicity studies are conducted. These studies are also known as subacute (or subchronic) and chronic toxicity studies. The procedures involved in these two types are similar except their duration. These studies are conducted to determine the organs affected by different dose levels and to assess the nature of chemicals under more realistic situations than the acute toxicity studies. Three dose levels are normally used. Dosages are generally selected on the basis of information obtained in acute toxicity studies using both $LD_{50}$ and the slope of the dose–response curve. Chronic toxicity studies are basically carried out to determine the organs affected and to check whether the drug is potentially carcinogenic or not. These test extends over a long period of time and involve large groups of laboratory animals.

## *Experimental design*

### *Species and number*

Generally, two or more species of animals are used. Ideally, the animals chosen should biotransform the chemical in a manner essentially identical to humans. Since this is often unattainable, rats and dogs are usually selected. This preference is based on their appropriate size, ready availability, and the great preponderance of toxicological information on chemicals for these animals. As noted in Chapter 5, different strains of rats may respond markedly differently to toxicants.

Equal numbers of male and female animals should be used. Generally, 10–50 rats are used in each dose group, as well as in the control group. As a rule, this procedure should provide data that are statistically analyzable. Smaller numbers of rats (10 animals/group/gender; thus a total of 50 animals for four groups plus control) are used because of the greater number of examinations that can be made on each animal and because of their size and the expense involved.

### *Route of administration*

The chemical should be administered according to the route of the intended use or exposure in humans. For most chemicals, the common route is oral. The preferred procedure is to incorporate the chemical in the diet, therefore drinking water is sometimes used as the vessel. The latter method is advisable when the chemical might react with a component in the diet. The chemical, especially if it is reactive, volatile, or unpalatable, is often administered by gavage or in gelatin capsules, a procedure more often used in dogs. The daily dose of the chemical may also be incorporated in a bolus of canned dog food.

Dermal application, exposure by inhalation, and parenteral routes are used for special purposes, such as industrial and agricultural products, and drugs.

### *Dosage and duration*

As the aims of these studies are to determine the nature and site of the toxic effects, as well as the NOAEL, it is advisable to select three doses: (i) a dose that is high enough to elicit definite signs of toxicity but not high enough to kill many of the animals; (ii) a low dose that is expected to induce no toxic effect; and (iii) an intermediate dose. Sometimes, one or more additional doses are included to ensure that the above objectives are achieved. As noted earlier, a control group must be included. These animals will not receive the chemical under test but must be given the vehicle used in the study.

The doses are generally selected on the basis of the information obtained in the acute toxicity studies, using both the $LD_{50}$ and the slope of the dose–response curve. Any information on related chemicals and on their metabolism, especially the presence or absence of bioaccumulation, is also taken into account. Sometimes, a range-finding or dose range-finding study is performed. It consists of dosing 5 rats of each gender at each of the 3 or 4 dose levels for 7 days. The criteria for assessing toxic effects are mortality, body weight gain, relative liver and kidney weight, and food consumption. The results from 7-day tests are generally better than the $LD_{50}$ values in predicting the dose levels for the longer-term toxicity study.

In studies in rats, the dose levels may be constant concentrations and expressed in mg/kg diet (ppm) or constant dosage and expressed in mg/kg of body weight of the animals. As the animal grows, there are changes in the body weight as well as in the food consumption. For a constant dose regimen, the concentration of the chemical must therefore be adjusted periodically to maintain a relatively constant dose in mg/kg body weight. This is usually done at weekly intervals during the period of rapid growth and biweekly thereafter.

In the short-term studies, the duration in rats is generally 90 days. In dogs, the duration is often extended to 6 months or even 1 year. The duration of long-term studies in rats is generally 24 months, and 7 or more years in dogs.

## *Observations and examinations*

### *Body weight and food consumption*

Body weight and food consumption should be determined weekly. Decreased body weight gain is a simple, yet sensitive, index of adverse effects. Food consumption is also a useful indicator. In addition, a marked decrease in food consumption can induce effects that mimic or aggravate the toxic manifestations of the chemical. In such cases, *paired feeding* or parenteral feeding may have to be instituted. When the animals receiving the toxicant are affected more than those maintained on a reduced feed alone, then the toxicant, apart from the undernutrition, is responsible for the effect.

### *General observations*

These should include appearance, behavior, and any abnormality. Dead and moribund animals should be removed from the cages for gross and possibly microscopic examination. Frequent observation is necessary to minimize cannibalism.

## *Laboratory tests*

*Hematological* examinations usually include hematocrit, hemoglobin, erythrocyte count, total leukocyte count, and differential leukocyte count. All dogs should be sampled before the initiation of treatment and at 1 week, 1 month, and at the end. Tests at other intervals may be warranted. Because of the small blood volume of rats, only half of them are sampled at various intervals, while the others are sampled only at the end. Special tests such as reticulocyte count, platelet count, methemoglobin, and glucose-6-phosphate dehydrogenase (G-6-PD) may be indicated.

*Clinical laboratory* tests usually include fasting blood glucose, serum aspartate aminotransferase (AST or SGOT), alanine aminotransferase (ALT or SGPT), alkaline phosphatase (AP), creatine kinase (CK), lactate dehydrogenase (LDH), total protein, albumin, globulin, blood urea nitrogen (BUN), triglycerides, cholesterol, creatinine, and such elements as sodium, potassium, calcium, and chloride. Other tests may be done where indicated. For example, cholinesterase activity is assessed when testing organophosphorus and carbamate pesticides.

*Urinalysis* usually includes color, specific gravity, pH, protein, glucose, creatinine, ketones, formed elements (red blood cells, etc.), and crystalline and amorphous materials.

## *Postmortem examination*

Whenever possible, all animals that are found dead or dying should be subjected to a gross pathological examination. If the state of the tissue permits, histological examinations should also be done. In addition, the weight of a number of organs, either in absolute values or in terms of the body weight, should be determined as they serve as useful indicators of toxicity.

The organs that are usually weighed are the liver, kidneys, adrenals, heart, brain, thyroid, and testes or ovaries. Those that are histologically examined are the following: all gross lesions, the brain (three levels), spinal cord, eye and optic nerve, a major salivary gland, the thymus, thyroid, heart, aorta, lung with a bronchus, stomach, small intestine (three levels), large intestine (two levels), adrenal glands, pancreas, liver, gallbladder (if present), spleen, kidneys, urinary bladder, skeletal muscle, and bone and its marrow.

A list indicating the correlation between general observations, clinical laboratory tests, and postmortem examinations is produced as Appendix 6.1.

WHO (1978, 1990) and the U.S. Environmental Protection Agency (EPA, 1994), among others, have published guidelines for short-term and long-term studies.

## *Evaluation*

Comprehensive short-term and long-term toxicity studies, using the various parameters of observations and examinations described earlier, usually yield information on the toxicity of the chemical under test, with respect to the target organs, the effects on these organs, and the dose–effect and dose–response relationships. Such information often provides indications on the additional specific types of studies that should be conducted. The quantitative data from the short-term and other studies have been suggested for use in the determination of the NOAEL. This suggestion, however, has not been widely accepted because it is considered more prudent to use the data from long-term studies. This is especially true for chemicals (e.g., food additives, pesticides, and environmental pollutants) which humans may be exposed to for a lifetime. On the other hand, short-term studies may suffice in testing chemicals present in pharmaceuticals as they are used for short durations. However, in the case of occupational exposure, one needs to be cognizant that chemicals may cause delayed effects long after exposure as in the case of asbestos workers. It should also be kept in mind that confounding factors such as cigarette smoking or diet also exert effects on the responses to chemical exposures.

The NOAEL from the long-term studies, along with data on their acute toxicity and metabolism as well as information from genetic, reproductive, and any other studies, are used in determining their "acceptable daily intakes" for humans. For further discussion on the procedure used for this purpose, see Chapter 27.

## *Good laboratory practice*

In 1975 and 1976, the U.S. Food and Drug Administration (FDA) raised questions about the integrity of toxicological data received from certain laboratories. On inspecting these facilities, FDA discovered a number of unacceptable laboratory practices, such as selective reporting, underreporting, lack of adherence to a specified protocol, poor animal care procedures, poor record-keeping, and inadequate supervision of personnel. In an attempt to improve the validity of the data, FDA proposed a set of regulations for good laboratory practice in 1978. These were later included in the Regulation for the Enforcement of the Federal Food, Drug, and Cosmetic Act.

These regulations (FDA, 1987) contain detailed guidance on provisions for the following:

1. Personnel, stipulating the responsibilities of the study director, testing facility management, and quality assurance unit
2. Facilities for animal care, animal supply, and handling test and control chemicals

3. Equipment, regarding its design, maintenance, and calibration
4. Testing facilities operation, including standard operating procedures, reagents and solutions, and animal care
5. Test and control chemicals, such as their characterization and handling
6. The protocol and conduct of a laboratory study
7. Records, their storage, retrieval, and retention, as well as the preparation and contents of reports
8. Disqualifications of testing facilities

The U.S. Environmental Protection Agency also proposed a set of good laboratory practice standards. They contain provisions similar to those of the FDA regulation regarding testing of health effects. Furthermore, EPA standards also contain provisions for environmental effects testing. At an international level, OECD (1982) has also produced a set of similar guidelines. Good Manufacturing Practice and Good Clinical Practice are also needed to implement quality standards in drug research and development in pharmaceutical companies.

### *Prospect of new test methods*

Toxicity testing plays a crucial role in ascertaining the toxic effect and characterization of a test substance. Toxicity obtained in animal studies occurs with similar incidence and severity in humans. An *in vitro* toxicity study using high-throughput screening (HTS) for toxicological risk assessment is currently being performed by the EPA ToxCast program (Dix et al., 2007). This program aims to develop a cost- and time-efficient approach to predict the potential toxicological risks of environmental chemicals for human health. However, the use of animals in toxicity testing is most likely to continue for the foreseeable future because of the benefits they offer in examining whole functioning organisms. Recently, integration of new techniques into existing protocols such as genomics, proteomics, and metabonomics will become a growing practice in the future (see Chapter 8). The introduction of systems toxicity studies provide greater understanding of chemical toxicity in conventional laboratory models and will be an important factor in the future of toxicity testing. New toxicity models under development include transgenic animals, the long-term exposure of hepatocyte cultures and tissue slices, and further development of methods for testing mechanisms of carcinogenicity. Stem cells remain the great hope of toxicity testing (van Vliet, 2011).

## Appendix 6.1 General observations, clinical laboratory tests, and pathology examinations that may be used in short- and long-term toxicity studies

| Organ or organ system | General observations | Clinical laboratory tests on blood | Pathology examination[a] |
|---|---|---|---|
| Liver | Discoloration of mucus membranes, edema, ascites | ALT (SGPT), AP, AST (SGOT), LDH cholesterol, total protein, albumin, globulin | Liver |
| Urinary system | Urine volume, consistency, color | BUN, total protein, albumin, globulin, glucose | |
| Gastrointestinal (GI) system | Diarrhea, vomit, stool, appetite | Total protein, albumin, globulin, sodium, potassium | Stomach, GI tract, gallbladder (if present), salivary gland, pancreas |
| Nervous system | Posture, movements, responses, behavior | | Brain, spinal cord, and sciatic nerve |
| Eye | Appearance, discharge, ophthalmological examination | | Eye and optic nerves |
| Respiratory system | Rate, coughing, nasal discharge | Total protein, albumin, globulin | One lung with a major bronchus |
| Hematopoietic system | Discoloration of mucus membranes, lethargy, weakness | Packed red cell volume, hemoglobin, erythrocyte count, total and differential leukocyte count, platelet count, prothrombin time, activated partial thromboplastin time | Spleen, thymus, mesenteric lymph nodes, bone marrow smear and section |

(Continued)

| Organ or organ system | General observations | Clinical laboratory tests on blood | Pathology examination[a] |
|---|---|---|---|
| Reproductive system | Appearance and palpation of external reproductive organs | FSH, LH, estrogen, testosterone | Testes and epididymis or ovaries. Uterus or prostate and seminal vesicles[b] |
| Endocrine system | Skin, hair coat, body weight, urine, and stool characteristics | Glucose, Na, K, AP (dog), cholesterol | Thyroid, adrenal, pancreas |
| Skeletal system | Growth, deformation, lameness | Calcium, phosphorus, AP | Bone and breakage strength |
| Cardiovascular system | Rate and characteristic of pulse, rhythm, edema, ascites | Creatine kinase, LDH | Heart, aorta, small arteries in other tissues |
| Skin | Color, appearance, odor, hair coat | Total protein, albumin, globulin | Only in dermal studies |
| Muscle | Size, weakness, wasting, decreased activity | AST creatine, phosphokinase | Only if indicated by observations, clinical chemistry, or gross lesion |
| Bone | Deformity, weakness | Calcium, phosphorus, uric acid, AP | Spongy appearance |

*Source:* Workshop on Subchronic Toxicity Testing, Proceedings of the Workshop, Springfield, VA: National Technical Information Service,1980.

[a] All animals should undergo a thorough gross examination; organs or tissues listed should be examined microscopically.

[b] These organs should also be weighed.

## Further reading

Ecobichon DJ (1992). *The Basis of Toxicity Testing*. Boca Raton, FL: CRC Press.

## References

Bliss CL (1957). Some principles of bioassay. *Am Sci.* 45, 449–66.

Bruce RD (1985). An up-and-down procedure for acute toxicity testing. *Fundam Appl Toxicol.* 5, 151–7.

Dix DJ, Houck KA, Martin MT et al. (2007). The ToxCast program for prioritizing toxicity testing of environmental chemicals. *Toxicol Sci.* 95, 5–12.

EPA. (1994). Health Effects Test Guidelines. Hazard Evaluation. Code of Federal Regulations, Title 40, Parts 792, 798.

FDA. (1987). Good laboratory practice regulations; Final rule. Fed Reg 52, 33768–82.

Finney DJ (1971). *Probit Analysis*. Cambridge, MA: Cambridge University Press.

Food Safety Council. (1978). Proposed system for food safety assessment. *Food Cosmet Toxicol.* 16, 1–136.

Kurakawa Y, Takamura N et al. (1987). Comparative studies on lipid peroxidation in the kidney of rats, mice and hamsters and the effect of cysteine, glutathione and diethyl maleate treatment on mortality and nephrotoxicity after administration of potassium bromate. *J Am Coll Toxicol.* 6, 487–501.

Loomis T (1978). *Essentials of Toxicology*, 3rd ed. Philadelphia, PA: Lea and Febiger.

Lu FC (1995). A review of the acceptable daily intakes of pesticides assessed by WHO. *Regul Toxicol Pharmacol.* 21, 352–64.

Lu FC, Lavallée A (1965). The acute toxicity of some synthetic colors used in drugs and foods. *Can Pharm J* 97, 30.

McNamara BP (1976). Concepts in health evaluation of commercial and industrial chemicals. In: Mehlman MA, Shapiro RE, Blumenthal H, eds. *New Concepts in Safety Evaluation*. Washington, DC: Hemisphere.

OECD. (1982). Good Laboratory Practice in the Testing of Chemicals. Organization of Economic Cooperation and Development. France.

OECD. (1992). OECD Guidelines for Testing Chemicals. Acute Oral Toxicity. Organization of Economic Cooperation and Development. France.

OECD. (2002). Guidance Document on Acute Oral Toxicity. Environmental Health and Safety Monograph Series on Testing and Assessment. France.

Paramveer D, Chanchal MK, Paresh M et al. (2010). Effective alternative methods of $LD_{50}$ help to save number of experimental animals. *J Chem Pharm Res.* 6, 450–3.

van Vliet E (2011). Current standing and future prospects for the technologies proposed to transform toxicity testing in the 21st century. *ALTEX*. 28, 17–44.

Weil CS (1952). Tables for convenient calculation of median effective dose ($LD_{50}$ or $ED_{50}$) and instructions for their use. *Biometrics.* 8, 249–63.

WHO. (1966). Specifications for Identity and Purity and Toxicological Evaluation of Food Colors, WHO/Food Add./66.25. Geneva, Switzerland: World Health Organization.

WHO. (1978). Principles and Methods for Evaluating the Toxicity of Chemicals. Part I, Environmental Health Criteria 6. Geneva, Switzerland: World Health Organization.

WHO. (1990). Principles for Toxicological Assessment of Pesticide Residues in Food. Environ Health Criteria 104. Geneva, Switzerland: World Health Organization.

Workshop on Subchronic Toxicity Testing. (1980). In: Page N, Sawbney D, Ryon MG, eds. Proceedings of the Workshop EPA–560/11–80–028. Springfield, VA: National Technical Information Service.

# chapter seven

# Systems toxicology

***Kyu-Bong Kim, Semin Lee, and Jung-Hwa Oh***

*Contents*

## *Introduction*

Traditional toxicological studies use lab animals to identify chemical safety for humans, but often require a great deal of time and money. Traditional toxicological studies also rarely determine the mechanism of toxic action. Recently established high-end technologies have been used to explore toxicology since the completion of the human genome project. The term *toxicogenomics* is a combination of toxicology and genomics (mainly transcriptomics; a gene expression profile). In early 2000, the United States (U.S.) government adopted this tool and the National Institute of Environmental Health Sciences (NIEHS) created the National Center for Toxicogenomics (NCT). Tennant (2002) stated that "The Center's mission is to promote the evolution and coordinated use of gene expression technologies and to apply them to the assessment of toxicologic effects in humans. The primary goal is to provide a worldwide reference system of genome-wide gene expression data and to develop a knowledge base of chemical effects in biological systems." Waters and Fostel (2004) also emphasized "that toxicology is gradually evolving into a systems toxicology that will eventually allow us to describe all the toxicological interactions within a living system under stress and to predict the modes of action." Currently, multi-omics methods were developed for biological research. These approaches may help to understand mechanism of toxic action, the adverse outcome pathway (AOP) in toxicological research (Joyce and Palsson, 2006). The integration of multi-omics data derived from toxicants have represented well the AOP by combinations from genes to organs (Figure 7.1). Considering the spatial and temporal bounds, the systems toxicology elucidates the complex and unique AOP at system level.

Systems toxicology is the integrative analysis of multi-omics to determine multiple levels of biological adverse effects by a toxicant (Table 7.1). These toxicity profiles produced by multi-omics such as genome, proteome, and metabolome provide biomarkers of adverse effects. It is generally recognized that biological response to a toxicant initiates gene expression, through protein alterations to change of metabolites. The advent of functional genomics and systems toxicology has opened the door to understanding the complex interactions among genome, transcriptome, proteome, and metabolome on a cell, tissue, and biofluid, as well as on a holistic level (Table 7.1). Figure 7.1 illustrates multi-omics technologies involved in systems toxicology and Figure 7.2 shows the generalized process of multi-omics analysis for systems toxicology. In this chapter, new multi-omics technologies and their toxicological applications are discussed.

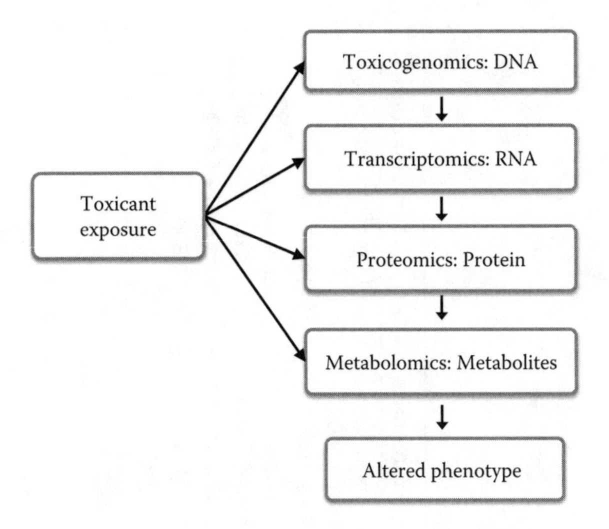


***Figure 7.1*** Multi-omics technologies employed in systems toxicology. The integration of -omics sciences may lead to a better comprehensive understanding of toxicological science or systems toxicology. (From Kim KB, Lee BM, *Toxicol. Res.*, 25, 59–69, 2009b.)

## Toxicogenomics

Cunningham and Lehman-McKeeman (2005) suggested a role for toxicogenomics in mechanistic and predictive toxicology. Initially, microarray technology used a two color fluorescent dye for competitive target binding (Schena et al., 1995). Many individual labs installed a DNA chip fabrication system for the production of in-house DNA chips while many commercial DNA chips also appeared on the market. Over the past two decades, the microarray has been the core technology employed for gene expression profiling in drug screening and toxicology research. Although microarray technology has been the most widely accepted methodology for gene expression profiling, some limitations remain. Mortazavi et al. (2008) raised several areas of concern regarding microarrays including the detection of RNA splice patterns and coverage of all possible genes. The use of RNA sequencing (RNA-Seq) to map and quantify transcriptomes was proposed to overcome these limitations. Recent consortium projects such as SEQC/MAQCIII compared RNA-Seq and microarray data. Wang et al. (2009) concluded that there was concordance in differentially expressed genes and enriched pathways between different platforms, but that this concordance was affected by gene abundance and by mechanistic complexity. Further, Wang et al. (2009) showed that gene expression patterns from RNA-Seq are

***Table 7.1*** Comparison of multi-omic methods

| | Toxicogenomics | Transcriptomics | Proteomics | Metabolomics |
|---|---|---|---|---|
| Target material | Gene, chromosome (genetic code) | mRNA (genetic code) | Protein (function of the protein) | Low molecular weight metabolites |
| Molecular weight (Da) | 100,000–120,000 | 100,000–120,000 | 5,000–20,000 | 100–5,000 |
| Characteristics | Context independent | Context dependent | Separation, characterization | Separation, characterization |
| Analytical methods | DNA sequencer | Hybridization | 2D gel, MALDI TOF | NMR, MS, GC, LC |
| Numbers in humans | 30,000 genome | | $>10^9$ | ~2,500 |

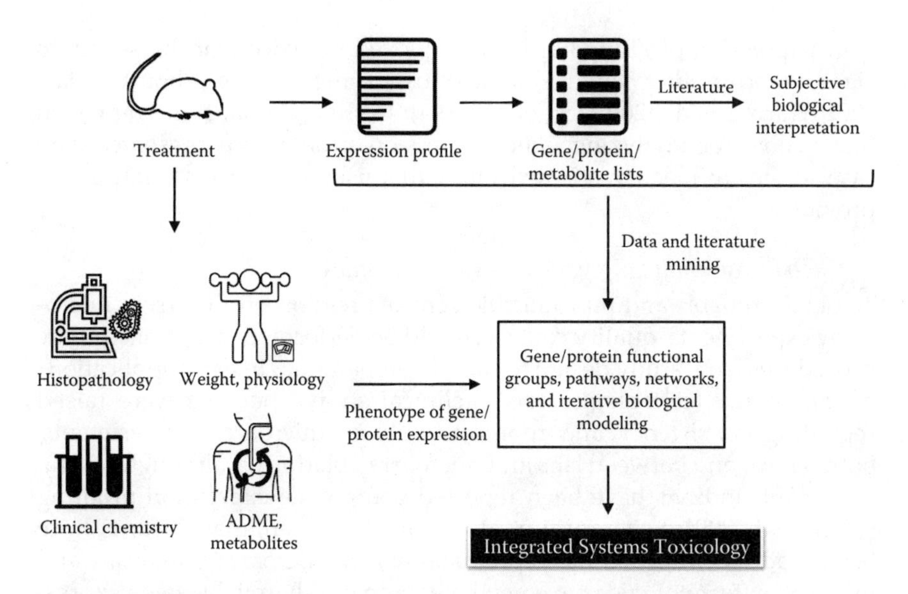


***Figure 7.2*** The process of multi-omic analysis for systems toxicology. This figure shows the path from initial observation (animal, upper left) to an integrated genomic, proteomic, and metabolomic analysis and then to systems toxicology. The -omics data stream is represented by the right path leading from the animal to the knowledge base; the traditional toxicological approach is represented by the downward path. The middle path involves information on gene/protein functional groups, pathways, networks, and iterative biological modeling and leads to a better understanding of systems toxicology. ADME: absorption, distribution, metabolism, and excretion.

consistent with the results of quantitative real-time polymerase chain reaction (qRT-PCR) in comparison with microarray data, due to the accuracy of identifying rarely expressed genes on the RNA-Seq platform. Previous investigations indicated that biological complexity, including all of the possible genes, would be valuable for prediction of the mechanistic toxicity; thus, genomic applications may play a key role in clinical and regulatory decision making. The toxicological evaluation process requires an interdisciplinary approach using experimental data; therefore, the application of numerous tools is necessary. The use of advanced technologies to assess chemical and drug safety is thus needed. In this chapter, we describe new technologies involving genomics data and their toxicological applications.

## *Gene expression profiling using microarray analysis*

Microarray technology has been widely used in preclinical studies to examine various cellular responses associated with toxicity. Comprehensive gene expression profiling has been employed in toxicological research to classify and predict chemical toxicity using microarrays (Thomas et al., 2001; Waring et al., 2001; Oh et al., 2014). In this section, some representative tools for analyzing gene expression profiles are presented and case studies in mechanistic toxicology that used microarray analysis are provided.

#### *Tools for analyzing gene expression profiles*

To obtain reliable and reproducible gene expression profiles from microarray experiments, quality control should be performed at all stages of the procedures from study design to sample preparation. In early applications of microarray technologies for preclinical study, concerns were raised regarding consistency and reproducibility of microarray experiments, both within and between labs and microarray platforms, although several important findings have been reported using gene expression profiling (Mah et al., 2004; Severgnini et al., 2006). Since then, many efforts have been made to improve the reproducibility of microarray analysis, and microarray technologies have generated apparently reliable gene expression data based on standardized procedures using commercial microarray platforms (Burgoon, 2006; Guo et al., 2006).

The term *gene expression profiling* is generally defined as analysis of the expression level of a gene transcript that is translated into proteins as well as of noncoding RNAs such as microRNA (miRNA). This section focuses on the widely employed method of miRNA profiling. The general strategy for analyzing gene expression profiling begins with selecting differentially expressed genes. These are genes that exhibit upregulation or downregulation and are identified by comparison among experimental groups; this procedure is briefly described here. After the final step of the scanning process in the microarray experiment, the raw signal intensity is preprocessed for data acquisition, background correction, and normalization using methods such as RMA, PLIER, and MAS 5.0. Normalization algorithms are selected according to the study design and experimental conditions of the microarray. Differentially expressed genes are identified based on relative fold changes and statistical testing among experimental groups. The *t*-test and analysis of variance (ANOVA) are used for comparisons of two or several experimental groups, respectively. When differentially expressed genes are identified using multiple comparisons, a false discovery correction needs to be applied. In gene expression analysis, Bonferroni or Benjamini and Hochberg corrections are often used to determine the *P* value. Bonferroni is a more conservative method, while Benjamini and Hochberg correction is more often used to determine the false discovery rate (FDR) (Reiner et al., 2003; Lesack and Naugler, 2011).

Gene sets of interest with similar expression patterns may be further classified using clustering analysis. Principal component analysis (PCA) can be used to group the samples by plotting the samples in multiple dimensions according to dominant expression patterns and variation (Ringner, 2008). PCA is an easy method to visualize similarities and differences among experimental samples by exploring the variation in gene expression without directly analyzing the gene expression patterns. Hierarchical clustering, *k*-means clustering, and self-organizing map (SOM) methods are popular for clustering closely related genes or samples with similar expression patterns (D'Haeseleer, 2005). The goal of these clustering methods is to subdivide the gene sets into smaller clusters exhibiting similar gene expression patterns. Hierarchical clustering can be used to visualize gene expression as a heat map as well as a dendrogram based on correlation distance algorithms. The *k*-means clustering method subdivides the most closely related genes into a defined number (*k*) of clusters. SOM is a method to cluster gene expression patterns based on hypothetical neural structure connecting neighboring clusters with similar expression patterns. Although one can refine gene sets with similar gene expression patterns using these methods, more functional analysis is needed to understand the molecular mechanism underlying the toxic responses.

To understand the biological functions of differentially expressed genes, further statistical analysis of pathways, gene enrichment, and networking are needed. Genes related to the same biological functions are ranked and annotated using statistical methods such as Fisher's exact test or Gene Set Enrichment Analysis (GSEA) (Bayerlova et al., 2015). Network analysis of differentially expressed genes also provides information regarding the genes' biological functions including molecular function and disease or pathological endpoints. Based on pathway and networking analyses, the key molecules related to biological functions are visualized to illustrate gene–gene and gene–protein interactions (Figure 7.3).

For gene expression analysis, useful open source and commercial tools are available. Among freely available programs, Bioconductor based on the R platform and ArrayTrack developed by the U.S. Food and Drug Administration (FDA) can be used to identify differentially expressed genes and analyze gene clustering using various algorithms (Xu et al., 2010). Commercially available software such as GeneSpring GX (Agilent Technologies, Santa Clara, California), GeneXplain (GeneXplain, Germany), and Array Suite (OmicSoft, Cary, North Carolina) are also available for easy analysis on most microarray platforms. To analyze the pathways and networks of significantly upregulated or downregulated genes, there are numerous free and commercial resources available, as shown in Table 7.2. Network analysis comprehensively examines

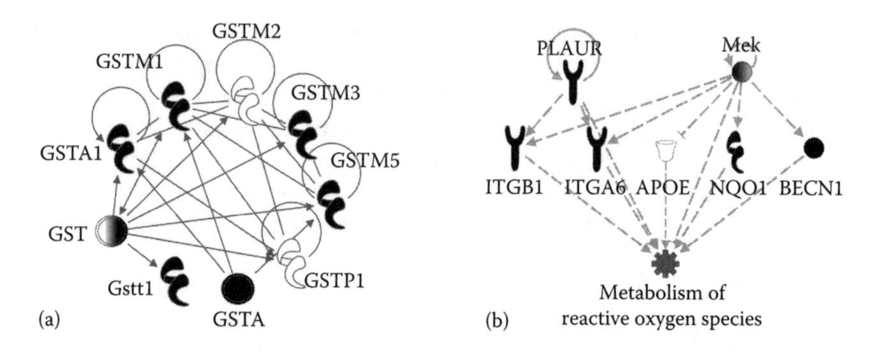


***Figure 7.3*** Network and regulatory effect analyses of differentially expressed genes in the acetaminophen (APAP) treated group based on Ingenuity Pathway Analysis software. The black and white colors represent overexpression and downregulation compared to controls, respectively. (a) Networking analysis indicates that GST (glutathione S-transferase) is a core regulator among the genes significantly affected by APAP treatment. GSTA1, GST alpha1; GSTM1, GST mu 1; GSTM2, GST mu 2; GSTM3, GST mu 3; GSTM5, GST mu 5; GSTP1, GST pi 1; Gstt1, GST theta 1; MGST2, microsomal GST 2. (b) Regulatory effects of differentially expressed genes are predicted based on Ingenuity Systems Knowledge Base. The results indicate several upstream regulators including PLAUR (plasminogen activator, urokinase receptor) and Mek (mitogen-activated protein kinase) regulate gene expression changes in the downstream region and may lead to the metabolism of reactive oxidative stress in the APAP treated group. ITGB1, integrin subunit beta 1; ITGA6, integrin subunit alpha 6; APOE, apolipoprotein E; NQO1, NAD(P)H quinone dehydrogenase 1; BECN1, beclin 1.

molecular interactions including gene–gene, protein–protein, gene–protein, drug–protein, or other chemical–protein interactions (Wu et al., 2012; Zhao et al., 2012; Glaab and Schneider, 2015). As described in this section, the various analysis tools available for gene expression profiling provide insights into the mode of toxic action (Enayetallah et al., 2013; Hoeng et al., 2014). Through further experimental validation of gene function, novel targets of toxicity or regulatory factors that trigger toxic responses may be revealed using comprehensive analysis of gene expression profiles.

*Case studies about mechanistic toxicology using microarray analysis* Recently, many mechanistic analyses of toxicological outcomes have been reported based on gene expression analysis, and case studies of idiosyncratic liver injury and cellular toxic mechanisms are discussed in this section. Idiosyncratic drug-induced liver injury (IDILI) is a major cause of the withdrawal or warning labeling of drugs on the market, and has become a major obstacle to the development of new drugs as it is not apparent in the preclinical and clinical stages (Roth and Ganey, 2011; Hussaini and

***Table 7.2*** Publicly and commercially available resources for pathway or networking analysis of differentially expressed genes

| Resource | Website | References |
|---|---|---|
| | **Publicly available** | |
| KEGG | http://www.genome.jp/kegg/ | Altermann and Klaenhammer, 2005; Du et al., 2014 |
| REACTOME | http://www.reactome.org/ | Joshi-Tope et al., 2005; Jupe et al., 2012 |
| DAVID | https://david.ncifcrf.gov/ | Huang et al., 2009 |
| Panther | http://www.pantherdb.org/ | Mi et al., 2016; Mi and Thomas, 2009 |
| | **Commercially available** | |
| Ingenuity Pathways Analysis (IPA) | http://www.ingenuity.com/ | Cameron et al., 2008; Kramer et al., 2014 |
| MetaCore | https://portal.genego.com/ | Ekins et al., 2006; Schuierer et al., 2010 |
| Pathway Studio | https://www.pathwaystudio.com/ | Nikitin et al., 2003; Yuryev et al., 2009 |

Farrington, 2014; Aithal, 2015). IDILI occurs in a minority of patients using a drug, but may cause serious or even life-threatening damage. However, there are limitations that prevent the accurate prediction of the toxicity of idiosyncratic hepatotoxic drugs. To overcome this problem, gene expression profiling has been employed to predict hepatotoxicity. Laifenfeld et al. (2014) attempted to develop a prediction method for idiosyncratic hepatotoxic drugs using the causal relationship with hepatic gene expression. The proposed method was to identify the cellular and molecular mechanisms initiated by idiosyncratic hepatotoxic drugs, and then to verify whether or not the drugs of interest are related to the expression of these genes. Rats were administered either IDILI-inducing or non-hepatotoxic drugs, and the network of altered genes in their livers after administration was analyzed using a microarray experiment. Molecular networks such as mitochondrial damage, inflammation, and endoplasmic reticulum (ER) stress were more closely associated with idiosyncratic hepatotoxicity than non-hepatotoxic drugs. It was also confirmed that the expression of genes involved in mitochondrial damage and ER stress was influenced by idiosyncratic hepatotoxic drugs in rat primary cells. Data suggest that hepatotoxicity of drugs can be predicted through analysis of the expression of genes involved in the network.

In another case study, Lee et al. (2016) performed genomic analysis to identify the molecular mechanism underlying hepatotoxicity induced by a idiosyncratic hepatotoxic drug and identify regulatory genes that lead to hepatotoxicity. Diclofenac, a nonsteroidal anti-inflammatory drug (NSAID), is a representative idiosyncratic hepatotoxic drug. In this study, serum levels of alanine aminotransferase (ALT) and aspartate aminotransferase (AST) significantly increased in mice administered diclofenac (30 mg/kg) for 1 or 3 days. Based on immunohistochemical staining, expression of CD68, macrophage colony-stimulating factor (M-CSF), lipopolysaccharide binding protein (LBP), and Ki67 increased with diclofenac, indicating the activation of Kupffer cells. Gene function analysis revealed that diclofenac affects gene networks involved in inflammation, immune stress and acute phase responses, and master regulatory genes including the leptin receptor (*Lepr*), lipocaline 2 (*Lcn2*), one of the nuclear factors of kappa light polypeptide (*Nfkbiz*), suppressor of cytokine signalling 3 (*Socs3*), serum amyloid P-component (*Apcs*), and cytotoxic T lymphocyte-associated protein 4 (*Ctla4*). In particular, *Stat3* is differentially phosphorylated by diclofenac, induces gene changes involved in the acute response by stimulating IL-6, and is controlled by *Socs3*. The results of this study showed that diclofenac appears to influence the master regulatory protein that controls proinflammatory cytokines and acute response in the liver. Evidence indicated that an imbalance of pro- and anti-inflammatory conditions might be the cause of IDILI.

Recently, human embryonic stem cells (hESCs) have been developed as a useful cell model to predict human toxicity or disease because they can be differentiated into many cell types (Heng et al., 2009; Saha and Jaenisch, 2009; Son et al., 2016). Several investigations reported that gene expression profiling in hESCs permits investigation into toxic mechanisms and the discovery of drug candidates (Qian et al., 2002; Hou et al., 2013; Puppala et al., 2013; Son et al., 2014). van Dartel et al. (2011) reported that embryonic stem cells could be employed to predict developmental toxicity based on gene expression profiling. In this investigation, mouse embryonic stem cells were treated with five developmental toxicants including monobutyl phthalate, methoxyacetic acid, valproic acid, retinoic acid, and 5-fluorouracil, and one non-developmental toxic chemical, penicillin, during differentiation for up to 48 hours. Using PCA of differentially expressed genes, a specific gene panel was identified which distinguished the differentiation status allowing significantly affected gene sets to be determined for each developmental toxicant. Data showed that the gene signature could be used to identify developmental toxicants, and that gene expression profiles from embryonic stem cells enable more rapid drug testing by predicting toxicity at an earlier stage.

Recently, RNA-Seq approaches have been widely used to analyze gene expression patterns as well as to discover novel genes involved in toxicity. Although RNA-Seq provides more detailed information regarding alternative variants and rarely expressed genes, gene expression profiling via microarray analysis can also be used to easily generate consistent expression patterns compared to RT-PCR. Gene expression profiling analysis may lead to a better understanding of molecular mechanisms and may be used to predict toxicity with further statistical analysis.

## *Next-generation sequencing analysis*

Next-generation sequencing (NGS) technologies have significantly grown in capacity and innovation for better investigating the complexities of genomes (Goodwin et al., 2016). These recent improvements in NGS technology include increased read lengths and reduced cost of sequencing. Due to these recent improvements, it is now possible to use sequencing as both a diagnostic and prognostic tool (Kircher and Kelso, 2010). NGS platforms generate vast quantities of data, but error rates are higher and sequences are generally shorter (35–700 bp) (Liu et al., 2012) than those of traditional Sanger sequencing methods; thus, careful examination of results is necessary for variant discovery and clinical applications. Although several long-read sequencing approaches have recently been developed to resolve the length limitation of NGS methods, they are considerably more expensive and have lower throughput than short-read sequencing platforms.

### *Short-read sequencing*

Short-read sequencing approaches can be classified into two categories: sequencing by ligation (SBL; Tomkinson et al., 2006) and sequencing by synthesis (SBS; Metzker, 2010). In SBL approaches, a probe oligonucleotide labeled with fluorescent dyes hybridizes to a DNA fragment, and DNA ligase joins the molecule to an adjacent oligonucleotide. The emission spectrum of the fluorophore indicates the identity of the base or bases complementary to specific positions of the probe sequence. In SBS approaches, a polymerase is used and a signal, such as a fluorophore or a change in ionic concentration, indicates the incorporation of a nucleotide into an elongating strand. In most SBL and SBS approaches, DNA is clonally amplified on a solid surface. Having many thousands of identical copies of a DNA fragment within a defined area ensures that the signal can be distinguished from background noise. Excess parallelization is also facilitated by the creation of many millions of individual SBL or SBS reaction centers, each with its own clonal DNA template. A sequencing platform can collect information from many millions of reaction centers simultaneously, thereby sequencing many millions of DNA molecules in parallel.

*Long-read sequencing*

Long-read sequencing generate reads of several kilobases, thus enabling identification of complex large-scale variations such as long repetitive elements, copy number changes, and structural variation that are relevant to evolution, adaptation, and disease (McCarroll and Altshuler, 2007; Mirkin, 2007; Stankiewicz and Lupski, 2010); however, they are not readily resolved by short-read sequencing. Complex or repetitive regions can be mapped in a single continuous long-read without ambiguity in the positions or size of genomic elements. Long-reads are also useful for identifying gene isoforms because they can span entire mRNA transcripts. Single-molecule real-time sequencing approaches and synthetic approaches based on short-read sequencing are the two main categories of long-read sequencing. Single-molecule approaches do not use the DNA amplification commonly employed for short-read sequencing. Instead, synthetic approaches use computational assembly of short-reads to generate a larger fragment.

*NGS applications*

Whole-genome sequencing (WGS) provides the most comprehensive view of genomic information (Cirulli and Goldstein, 2010). Hence, WGS is frequently used to identify cancer-generating genomic changes (Ellis et al., 2012) and human variability among a large number of people from diverse ethnic populations (Genomes Project Consortium, 2010). The 1000 Genomes Project has analyzed the genomes of 2504 individuals from 26 different ethnic populations (Genomes Project Consortium, 2015; Sudmant et al., 2015) and identified a considerable number of human variations at the population level (Consortium, 2015; Gudbjartsson et al., 2015). Compared to WGS, whole-exome sequencing (WES) (Hodges et al., 2007) can analyze more samples within a sequencing run by only covering the exonic regions with a considerably higher sequencing depth. NGS is also useful for identifying protein–DNA interactions and histone modifications through immunoprecipitation, as in the case of ChIP–seq (Park, 2009). Open chromatin regions can be detected using NGS-based technologies such as DNase-Seq (Boyle et al., 2008) and ATAC-seq (Buenrostro et al., 2013). Genome-wide methylation patterns are also frequently analyzed by methyl-seq (Rauch et al., 2005) or other NGS-based approaches using selective digestion of methylated or unmethylated regions (Oda et al., 2009; Ladd-Acosta et al., 2010). NGS has been increasingly employed for the quantification and characterization of transcriptomes, particularly in toxicogenomic studies (Waters and Fostel, 2004).

## Computational toxicology

Over the last decade, traditional animal tests have been replaced by alternative testing methods using cell culture and genomics. Recent programs for risk assessment and toxicity testing methods have focused on human cell line tests, high-throughput screening, and computational modeling. Some representatives of such programs are USA-Tox21 (Krewski et al., 2010), Japan-Open TG-GATEs (Igarashi et al., 2015), and International-OpenTox (Tcheremenskaia et al., 2012). Based on rapidly increasing toxicity data, computational approaches enable toxicologists to gain new insights into adverse outcomes, to integrate the results from a variety of toxicity tests, and develop a quantitative method of assessing chemical toxicity. It is the aim of this chapter to provide an overview of the methods used to develop computational models of chemical toxicity. Usually, the development of computational models to predict the toxicity of compounds requires the use of strong biological evidence and significant statistical methods. To build a computational toxicity model, the first step is to carefully select large training sets of experimental data regarding both toxic and nontoxic compounds across multiple species and mechanisms of toxicity, because the accuracy of any predictive model depends on its training set (Wang, 2008). The next step is to choose a computational algorithm, such as a rule-based approach, machine learning via artificial neural networks or support vector machines. The predictive model is trained to classify compounds as toxic or nontoxic using this computational algorithm. Because the algorithms all have unique strengths and weaknesses, various learning methodologies should be applied to improve the accuracy of a predictive model. The predictive accuracy of the model is estimated using a testing set of either a gold standard set or an independent portion of the training set (Martin and Yu, 2006). Usually, the gold standard set is preferred to evaluate a predictive model. This step is critical to evaluate the performance of a predictive model.

### Chemical and toxicological databases

To build a predictive model, toxicity data need to be available, either privately through an in-house experiment or publicly through websites and online databases. Usually, these databases are specialized for different purposes. Understanding the focus of each database is necessary for creating an optimal training set from public databases (Table 7.3).

Pubchem (Kim et al., 2016) provides a large repository of information about all of the chemicals that are used in medicine and industry. Because Pubchem is a companion database to the National Center for Biotechnology Information (NCBI)'s other databases, chemicals in PubChem's database have readily available information regarding bioactivity, protein 3D

***Table 7.3*** Resources for building a predictive model

| Name | Description | Website |
|---|---|---|
| Pubchem | Chemical and drug database | http://pubchem.ncbi.nlm.nih.gov |
| DrugBank | Drug and drug target database | http://drugbank.ca/ |
| ToxCast | *In vitro* toxicity database | https://www.epa.gov/chemical-research/toxicity-forecasting |
| ToxRef | *In vivo* toxicity database | ftp://newftp.epa.gov/comptox/High_Throughput_Screening_Data/Animal_Tox_Data |
| DSSTox | Integrated databases between chemical structure and toxicity data using standard format | https://www.epa.gov/chemical-research/distributed-structure-searchable-toxicity-dsstox-database |
| CTD | Chemical-gene-phenotype database | http://ctdbase.org |
| Open TG-GATEs | Toxicant's microarray and pathology database | http://toxico.nibiohn.go.jp/english/index.html |

structures, and literature references, as well as chemical properties and patents. Millions of compound structures and descriptive datasets can be downloaded for free through a web interface and file transfer protocol (FTP). In PubChem, a substance refers to the permanent identifier for a depositor-supplied molecule and a compound is the permanent identifier for a unique chemical structure. In computational toxicology, PubChem is often used to access public biological data regarding compounds of interest for building a predictive model.

DrugBank (Wishart et al., 2008) is an annotated resource about drugs and drug targets. DrugBank contains information on withdrawn drugs and drug candidates as well as FDA-approved drugs. Because these drugs exert some toxicity, referred to as side effects, the drug target and 3D structure could be valuable to understanding the mode of action of a drug-mediated toxicity. ToxCast (Dix et al., 2007) is part of the Tox21 project. Its goal is to produce a large-scale *in vitro* dataset for building predictive models. Users of ToxCast can access *in vitro* assay data on 1800 chemicals from various sources, including both industrial and consumer products. The *in vitro* assay data are produced by high-throughput screening assays, to limit the number of lab animal tests required, while quickly and efficiently testing chemicals for potential health effects. ToxRef (Martin et al., 2009) provides results from thousands of *in vivo* toxicity studies on nearly 800 chemicals, and is also part of the Tox21 project. This database supports access to high-value toxicity information such as No Effect Level (NEL), Lowest Effect Level (LEL), No Observed Adverse Effect Level (NOAEL), and Lowest Observed Adverse Effect Level (LOAEL). The Distributed Structure Searchable Toxicity Database (DSSTox) provides a public chemistry resource of integrated toxicity data (Richard and Williams, 2002). A specialized feature of DSSTox is manual annotation between bioassay and physicochemical property data for toxicants by experts using the standard file format (SDF).

#### *QSAR*

Toxicants have chemical structures with physio-chemical properties that lead to adverse outcomes in the human population. Therefore, the correlation between a toxicant's structural features and toxicity-related data are used to build predictive models using rule-based methods or machine learning algorithms based on the principle that similar chemical structures possess similar properties (Leo et al., 1969). These predictive models are termed *quantitative structure-activity relationships* (QSARs). In toxicology, the activity of QSAR is a proxy for toxicity or adverse outcomes. Basically, a toxicant's structure is displayed as molecular descriptors encoding independent properties of toxicity. QSAR methods have recently become useful, particularly in the prediction of mutagenicity (James, 2012). Because mutagenic compounds share the chemical mechanism of action for mutagenesis, a QSAR model can detect the relationship between substructural features and mutagenicity among the compounds. These substructural features or functional groups that may confer mutagenicity potential on the compounds that contain them are generally referred to as structure alerts. QSAR methods are used both to make predictive models about the behaviors of known structure alerts and to search for new toxicants. QSAR methods use three broad approaches: (i) rule-based modeling; (ii) statistical modeling; and (iii) hybrid modeling (Table 7.4). Rule-based modeling is based on capturing expert knowledge regarding the causes of toxicity. A rule-based model can easily explain the mechanism of toxicity of a queried compound containing structure alerts. The statistical model is not useful for elucidating the mechanism of toxicity, because it is based on statistical analysis of training data to identify patterns associated with toxicity. Statistical models can be used even if there is no evidence of structure alerts in the training set.

#### *Docking simulation*

Originally, docking simulation used computer-aided drug design (CADD) and virtual screening. In the field of toxicology, docking simulation is a

***Table 7.4*** QSAR models

| Method | Program | Available type |
|---|---|---|
| Expert rule-based system | Derek | Commercially |
| | HazardExpert | Commercially |
| | Toxtree | Publicly |
| | OECD toolbox | Publicly |
| Statistical-based system | MultiCASE | Commercially |
| | TOPKAT | Commercially |
| | Lazar | Publicly |
| | CAESAR | Publicly |
| Hybrid system | OASIS TIMES | Commercially |

promising method for predicting the preferred orientation of a toxicant to its target protein when they are bound together in a stable complex. Thus, docking simulation can bring us closer to understanding and predicting the mechanisms of chemical toxicity (Liebler and Guengerich, 2005). For example, docking simulation can search a chemical for unintended receptors such as drug metabolism enzymes (e.g., cytochrome P450) (Baillie, 2008), hormone-mediated receptors (Gronemeyer et al., 2004), and hERG potassium channels (Sanguinetti and Tristani-Firouzi, 2006). Docking simulations have also become important components of the emerging multi-scale toxicity model incorporating structural and functional data at multiple scales (Hunter and Borg, 2003). For docking simulation, the programs DOCK6.3 (Ewing et al., 2001) and AutoDock4.2 (Morris et al., 2009) are publicly available and in wide use. These docking programs use a set of predefined toxicant-binding pockets on the target protein. The docking program then calculates the optimal orientation of the toxicant in the pocket of the target protein using energy functions (Lengauer and Rarey, 1996). The docking score is calculated based on all of the atoms that interact between the toxicant and target protein. The docking score can be interpreted as an approximate binding affinity, where a negative docking score represents a high binding affinity between two molecules. Chemical toxicity can be predicted by comparing the docking score of a new chemical with the docking score of a positive control toxicant. If the new chemical has a more negative score than the known toxicant, the new chemical may exhibit toxicity with the target protein.

## *Proteomics*

Proteomics is the study of the proteome, which is the entire set of proteins in an organism. It is an important component of functional genomics. Proteomics is generally defined as large-scale analysis of the protein response to a toxicant on a cellular level, but it is often specifically used to refer to protein purification and mass spectrometry (MS). Proteomics is more complicated than genomics because an organism's genome is relatively consistent, whereas the proteome differs between cell types. Distinct genes are expressed in different cell types, and the basic set of proteins expressed in all cells still needs to be identified. This phenomenon was previously evaluated using RNA analysis, but protein content was not quantified (Dhingraa et al., 2005; Rogers et al., 2008). It is now known that mRNA is not always translated into protein (Shyu et al., 2008); therefore, proteomic analysis is necessary to confirm the presence of a protein and provide direct quantification of the protein present in a cell.

## *Methods of studying proteins*

In proteomics, there are multiple methods for studying proteins. Generally, antibodies (immunoassays) or MS can be used to detect proteins. Complex biological samples should be subjected to biochemical separation steps, before the detection step, because accurate quantification is not possible when there are too many analytes in the sample.

### *Protein detection with antibodies (immunoassays)*

Biochemistry and cell biology studies used antibodies to particular proteins or to their modified forms. Antibodies are among the most common analytical tools utilized by molecular biologists today. There are several specific techniques and protocols that employ antibodies for protein detection. The enzyme-linked immunosorbent assay (ELISA) has been used to detect and quantitatively measure proteins for decades. The Western blot can be utilized for detection and quantification of individual proteins. A complex protein mixture sample can be separated using SDS-PAGE, and the target protein can be identified using an antibody in an additional step.

### *Mass spectrometry*

Edman degradation, wherein a single peptide is subjected to multiple steps of chemical degradation to resolve its sequence, was introduced in 1967 as one of the earliest methods of protein analysis. More recent methods include MS-based techniques, made possible by development of soft ionization methods such as matrix-assisted laser desorption/ionization (MALDI) and electrospray ionization (ESI). These methods enable the top-down and bottom-up proteomics workflow and often include additional separation before analysis.

*Mass spectrometry and protein profiling*

There are two MS-based methods currently used for protein profiling. The more widespread method uses high resolution two-dimensional electrophoresis for separation, then selection and staining of differentially expressed proteins followed with identification by MS. The second quantitative method uses stable isotope tags to differentially label proteins in complex mixtures. Here, the proteins within a complex mixture are isotopically labeled, and then digested to yield labeled peptides. The labeled mixtures are then combined, and the peptides are separated by multidimensional liquid chromatography and are analyzed by tandem MS. Quantitative proteomics using the stable isotope tagging method is an increasingly useful tool. First, tags for specific sites or proteins have been employed in chemical reactions to probe specific protein functions. Phosphorylated peptides are analyzed using isotopic labeling and selective chemistry to separate the protein fraction. Second, isotopic labeling technology was utilized to differentiate between partially purified or purified macromolecular complexes (e.g., RNA polymerase II pre-initiation complex and the proteins complexed with a transcription factor). Third, isotopic labeling technology was recently combined with chromatin separation to identify and quantify chromatin-associated proteins (Bonaldi et al., 2008).

## *Applications of proteomics*

The identification of potential new drugs for the treatment of disease has been one of the major applications of human genomics and proteomics. Genome and proteome information associated with a disease can be used as targets for new drugs. For example, if a certain protein is related to a specific disease, its 3D structure provides information useful to the design of drugs to interact with the action of the protein. In addition, a xenobiotic that fits the active site of a protein can inactivate the protein and produce disease. This is the basic concept underlying new drug discovery tools or toxic mechanism discovery methods (Vaidyanathan, 2012). Interaction proteomics, expression proteomics, protein networks, and biomarkers are crucial areas of proteomics that could help decipher the mechanistic or holistic toxicity of xenobiotics.

## *Proteomics for systems toxicology*

Development of quantitative proteomics methods enables us to clearly analyze cellular systems. Biological systems are subject to various stresses including xenobiotics. Transcriptional and translational responses to stresses result in functional changes in the proteome on the cellular or organismal level. Quantifying and describing proteomic changes are important for understanding biological effects at this larger, holistic level. In this way, proteomics play a complementary role to genomics, transcriptomics, epigenomics, metabolomics, and other -omics approaches for the more comprehensive integrative analysis of biological responses to a toxicant. The Cancer Proteome Atlas provides quantitative protein expression data for approximately 200 proteins in over 4000 tumor samples with matched transcriptomic and genomic data (Li et al., 2013).

## Toxicometabolomics

Toxicometabolomics is a term that integrates toxicology and metabolomics as suggested by Kim et al. (2010). A metabolome is generally termed as the whole set of small metabolic molecules in a cell, tissue, organ, organism, or species. It includes small circuits of pathway networks. Metabolomics is the method of studying, profiling, and fingerprinting metabolites in various physiological states or in response to stressors (Fiehn, 2002). Metabolic profiling is the primary tool used to analyze a class of metabolites. Metabolomics aims to include all of the classes of endogenous metabolites, and utilizes metabolic fingerprinting to maintain the rapid classification of biological samples according to their origin and biochemical relevance (Nicholson et al., 1999; Lindon et al., 2004). Toxicometabolomic techniques aim to identify and analyze changes to those endogenous molecules induced by xenobiotic toxicity. In toxicological research, toxicometabolomics is also viewed as holding great promise, including use in specific biomarker discovery for clinical diagnostics and toxicological studies.

### Analytical technologies

Currently, metabolomics studies have relied primarily on MS and nuclear magnetic resonance (NMR) spectroscopy as analytical platforms. MS requires a pre-separation procedure for metabolites using gas chromatography (GC) or liquid chromatography (LC). Isolation of metabolites from biological samples requires the preparation of an extract. It is almost impossible to detect the entire population of metabolites in a system using a single analytical method. Table 7.5 briefly summarizes some representative analytical platforms in toxicometabolomics.

### Toxicological applications

Using metabolomic techniques, it is possible to systematically determine metabolite concentrations in a sample. This new technology has

***Table 7.5*** Analytical methods used in metabolomics studies

| Analytical methods | Feature | References |
|---|---|---|
| NMR spectroscopy | • Cheap after initial purchase<br>• Robust and reliable<br>• Minimal sample preparation<br>• High throughput<br>• Significant metabolite overlap<br>• Large initial outlay | Nicholson and Wilson, 1989<br>Raamsdonk et al., 2001<br>Reo, 2002 |
| LC-MS | • Excellent sensitivity<br>• No need to derivatise<br>• More global than NMR or GC-MS<br>• Either specific or global<br>• LC reproducibility is less than GC<br>• Ion suppression can impede some metabolite detection | Fiehn et al., 2000<br>Fiehn, 2002<br>Wilson et al., 2005 |
| GC-MS | • Good sensitivity<br>• Cheap to purchase<br>• Good identification software<br>• Good chromatograms compared to LC-MS | Garcia and Barbas, 2011 |

*Source:* Kim KB, Lee BM, *Toxicol. Res.*, 25, 59–69, 2009b.

the potential for application in the areas of drug discovery/development and preventative screening/diagnostics. Research continues to refine this technology in an effort to put these methods to use as quickly as possible (Lindon et al., 2004). Metabolic profiling of biological samples such as urine or blood can be utilized to determine the biological changes induced by the toxic effects of a chemical or mixture of chemicals (Kim et al., 2008 and 2009a). The metabolic changes observed can be closely related to a specific toxicity (e.g., in hepatic or renal lesions) (Nicholson et al., 1985; Kim et al., 2008, 2010; Park et al., 2009). This is of particular interest to pharmaceutical companies that want to evaluate the toxicity of new drug candidates. If a new compound can be screened for adverse toxicity before it reaches clinical trials, companies can save the enormous cost of these trials (Lindon et al., 2004). Biomarker discovery has been one of the most important applications of toxicometabolomics. Table 7.6 summarizes the toxicometabolomic biomarkers associated with hepatic and renal toxicity.

## *Toxicometabolomics for systems toxicology*

Toxicometabolomics aims to identify and quantify all of the small molecular metabolites in a cell, tissue, biofluid, or whole organism as well as

*Table 7.6* Toxicometabolomic biomarkers associated with target organ toxicity

| Target organ | Toxicants | Biomarkers | Ref. |
|---|---|---|---|
| Liver toxicity | Allyl alcohol | ↑ creatinine, lactate, phenylacetyl glycine<br>↓ *N*-methyl nicotinamide, taurine | Beckwith-Hall et al., 1998 |
| | Acetaminophen | ↑ taurine, phenylacetate | Kim et al., 2008 |
| | D-galactosamine | ↑ allantoin<br>↓ 2-oxoglutarate, lactate, 1-methylnicotinamide, hippurate, benzoate | Kim et al., 2008 |
| | Bromobenzene | ↑ 5-oxoproline, glucose, acetate, lactate<br>↓ citrate, α-ketoglutarate, succinate | Waters et al., 2006 |
| | α-Nephthylisocyanate | ↑ taurine, creatine, glucose<br>↓ citrate, α-ketoglutarate, succinate | Waters et al., 2001 |
| | Methapyrilene | ↑ succinate, triglycerid, dimethylglycine, trimetylamine-*N*-oxide<br>↓ glucose, glycogen | Craig et al., 2006 |
| | Hydrazine | ↑ β-alanine, 3-D-hydroxybutyrate, citrulline, *N*-acetylcitrulline<br>↓ trimethylamine-*N*-oxide | Bollard et al., 2005 |
| Renal toxicity | Gentamicin | ↑ glucose<br>↓ trimethylamine-*N*-oxide | Lenz et al., 2005 |
| | Cisplatin | ↑ histidine<br>↓ 3-hydroxyphenylacetate | Boudonck et al., 2009 |
| | Mercuric chloride | ↑ acetate, amino acids, glucose, organic acids<br>↓ citrate, creatinine, hippurate, α-ketoglutarate, succinate | Nicholson et al., 1985<br>Kim et al., 2010 |

*Source:* Kim KB, Lee BM, *Toxicol. Res.*, 25, 59–69, 2009b.

their response to xenobiotics or toxicants. The cellular metabolome serves as the expression of a biological phenotype influenced by the genome and proteome. Metabolomics can provide a snapshot of the essential biochemistry of a biological sample and its cellular metabolism. Therefore, changes in metabolome can be observed as the result of adverse biological reactions to toxic substances. Most importantly, changes in metabolism can be observed as a result of drug toxicity, which provides rapid information regarding the decision to withdraw or change a medication before the onset of adverse reactions. Toxicometabolomics integrated with toxicogenomics and proteomics could play a crucial role, in terms of systems toxicology, for the successful explanation of the holistic biological response to xenobiotic toxicity.

## References

Aithal GP (2015). Pharmacogenetic testing in idiosyncratic drug-induced liver injury: Current role in clinical practice. *Liver Int.* 35, 1801–8.

Altermann E, Klaenhammer TR (2005). PathwayVoyager: Pathway mapping using the Kyoto Encyclopedia of Genes and Genomes (KEGG) database. *BMC Genomics.* 6, 60.

Baillie TA (2008). Metabolism and toxicity of drugs. Two decades of progress in industrial drug metabolism. *Chem Res Toxicol.* 21, 129–37.

Bayerlova M, Jung K, Kramer F et al. (2015). Comparative study on gene set and pathway topology-based enrichment methods. *BMC Bioinformatics.* 16, 334.

Beckwith-Hall BM, Nicholson JK, Nicholls AW et al. (1998). Nuclear magnetic resonance spectroscopic and principal components analysis investigations into biochemical effects of three model hepatotoxins. *Chem Res Toxicol.* 11, 260–72.

Bollard ME, Keun HC, Beckonert O et al. (2005). Comparative metabonomics of differential hydrazine toxicity in the rat and mouse. *Toxicol Appl Pharmacol.* 204, 135–51.

Bonaldi T, Straub T, Cox J et al. (2008). Combined use of RNAi and quantitative proteomics to study gene function in Drosophila. *Mol Cell.* 31, 762–72.

Boudonck KJ, Mitchell MW, Német L et al. (2009). Discovery of metabolomics biomarkers for early detection of nephrotoxicity. *Toxicol Pathol.* 37, 280–92.

Boyle AP, Davis S, Shulha HP et al. (2008). High-resolution mapping and characterization of open chromatin across the genome. *Cell.* 132, 311–22.

Buenrostro JD, Giresi PG, Zaba LC et al. (2013). Transposition of native chromatin for fast and sensitive epigenomic profiling of open chromatin, DNA-binding proteins and nucleosome position. *Nat Methods.* 10, 1213–8.

Burgoon LD (2006). The need for standards, not guidelines, in biological data reporting and sharing. *Nat Biotechnology.* 24, 1369–73.

Cameron CM, Cameron MJ, Bermejo-Martin JF et al. (2008). Gene expression analysis of host innate immune responses during Lethal H5N1 infection in ferrets. *J Virology.* 82, 11308–17.

Cirulli ET, Goldstein DB (2010). Uncovering the roles of rare variants in common disease through whole-genome sequencing. *Nat Rev Genet.* 11, 415–25.

Consortium UK (2015). The UK 10K project identifies rare variants in health and disease. *Nature*. 526, 82–90.

Craig A, Sidaway J, Holmes E et al. (2006). Systems toxicology: Integrated genomic, proteomic and metabonomic analysis of methapyrilene induced hepatotoxicity in the rat. *J Proteome Res*. 5, 1586–601.

Cunningham ML, Lehman-McKeeman L (2005). Applying toxicogenomics in mechanistic and predictive toxicology. *Toxicol Sci*. 83, 205–6.

D'Haeseleer P (2005). How does gene expression clustering work? *Nat Biotech*. 23, 1499–501.

Dhingraa V, Gupta M, Andacht T et al. (2005). New frontiers in proteomics research: A perspective. *Int J Pharmaceutics*. 299, 1–18.

Dix DJ, Houck KA, Martin MT et al. (2007). The ToxCast program for prioritizing toxicity testing of environmental chemicals. *Toxicol Sci*. 95, 5–12.

Du J, Yuan Z, Ma Z et al. (2014). KEGG-PATH: Kyoto encyclopedia of genes and genomes-based pathway analysis using a path analysis model. *Mol BioSystems*. 10, 2441–7.

Ekins S, Bugrim A, Brovold L et al. (2006). Algorithms for network analysis in systems-ADME/Tox using the MetaCore and MetaDrug platforms. *Xenobiotica*. 36, 877–901.

Ellis MJ, Ding L, Shen D et al. (2012). Whole-genome analysis informs breast cancer response to aromatase inhibition. *Nature*. 486, 353–60.

Enayetallah AE, Puppala D, Ziemek D et al. (2013). Assessing the translatability of in vivo cardiotoxicity mechanisms to in vitro models using causal reasoning. *BMC Pharmacol Toxicol*. 14, 46.

Ewing TJ, Makino S, Skillman AG et al. (2001). DOCK 4.0: Search strategies for automated molecular docking of flexible molecule databases. *J Computer-aided Mol Design*. 15, 411–28.

Fiehn O (2002). Metabolomics—The link between genotypes and phenotypes. *Plant Mol Biol*. 48, 155–71.

Fiehn O, Kopka J, Dormann P et al. (2000). Metabolite profiling for plant functional genomics. *Nat Biotech*. 18, 1157–61.

Garcia A, Barbas C (2011). Gas chromatography-mass spectrometry (GC-MS)-based metabolomics. *Methods Mol Biol*. 708, 191–204.

Genomes Project Consortium (2010). A map of human genome variation from population-scale sequencing. *Nature*. 467, 1061–73.

Genomes Project Consortium (2015). A global reference for human genetic variation. *Nature*. 526, 68–74.

Glaab E, Schneider R (2015). Comparative pathway and network analysis of brain transcriptome changes during adult aging and in Parkinson's disease. *Neurobiol Dis*. 74, 1–13.

Goodwin S, McPherson JD, McCombie WR (2016). Coming of age: Ten years of next-generation sequencing technologies. *Nat Rev Genet*. 17, 333–51.

Gronemeyer H, Gustafsson JA, Laudet V (2004). Principles for modulation of the nuclear receptor superfamily. *Nature Reviews Drug Discovery*. 3, 950–64.

Gudbjartsson DF, Helgason H, Gudjonsson SA et al. (2015). Large-scale whole-genome sequencing of the Icelandic population. *Nat Genet*. 47, 435–44.

Guo L, Lobenhofer EK, Wang C et al. (2006). Rat toxicogenomic study reveals analytical consistency across microarray platforms. *Nat Biotech*. 24, 1162–9.

Heng BC, Richards M, Shu Y, Gribbon P (2009). Induced pluripotent stem cells: A new tool for toxicology screening? *Arch Toxicol*. 83, 641–4.

Hodges E, Xuan Z, Balija V et al. (2007). Genome-wide in situ exon capture for selective resequencing. *Nat Genet*. 39, 1522–7.

Hoeng J, Talikka M, Martin F et al. (2014). Case study: The role of mechanistic network models in systems toxicology. *Drug Discovery Today*. 19, 183–92.

Hou Z, Zhang J, Schwartz MP et al. (2013). A human pluripotent stem cell platform for assessing developmental neural toxicity screening. *Stem Cell Res and Ther*. 4 Suppl 1, S12.

Huang DW, Sherman BT, Lempicki RA (2009). Systematic and integrative analysis of large gene lists using DAVID bioinformatics resources. *Nat Protocols*. 4, 44–57.

Hunter PJ, Borg TK (2003). Integration from proteins to organs: The Physiome Project. *Nature Reviews Mol Cell Biol*. 4, 237–43.

Hussaini SH, Farrington EA (2014). Idiosyncratic drug-induced liver injury: An update on the 2007 overview. *Expert Opinion on Drug Saf*. 13, 67–81.

Igarashi Y, Nakatsu N, Yamashita T et al. (2015). Open TG-GATEs: A large-scale toxicogenomics database. *Nucleic Acids Res*. 43, D921–7.

James P (2012). Genetic toxicology. Principles and methods. Preface II. *Methods Mol Biol*. 817, 7–11.

Joshi-Tope G, Gillespie M, Vastrik I et al. (2005). Reactome: A knowledgebase of biological pathways. *Nucleic Acids Res*. 33, D428–32.

Joyce AR, Palsson BO (2006). The model organism as a system: Integrating 'omics' data sets. *Nat Rev Mol Cell Biol*. 7, 198–210.

Jupe S, Akkerman JW, Soranzo N et al. (2012). Reactome—A curated knowledgebase of biological pathways: Megakaryocytes and platelets. *J Thrombosis Haemostasis*. 10, 2399–402.

Kim KB, Chung MW, Um SY et al. (2008). Metabolomics and biomarker discovery: NMR spectral data of urine and hepatotoxicity by carbon tetrachloride, acetaminophen, and D-galactosamine in rats. *Metabolomics*. 4, 377–92.

Kim KB, Kim SH, Um SY et al. (2009a). Metabolomics approach to risk assessment: Methoxyclor exposure in rats. *J Toxicol Environ Health*. A 72, 1352–68.

Kim KB, Lee BM (2009b). Metabolomics, a new promising technology for toxicological research. *Toxicol Res*. 25, 59–69.

Kim KB, Um SY, Chung MW et al. (2010). Toxicometabolomics approach to urinary biomarkers for mercuric chloride ($HgCl_2$)-induced nephrotoxicity using proton nuclear magnetic resonance ($^1H$ NMR) in rats. *Toxicol Appl Pharmacol*. 249, 114–26.

Kim S, Thiessen PA, Bolton EE et al. (2016). PubChem Substance and Compound databases. *Nucleic Acids Res*. 44, D1202–13.

Kircher M, Kelso J (2010). High-throughput DNA sequencing—Concepts and limitations. *Bioessays*. 32, 524–36.

Kramer A, Green J, Pollard J et al. (2014). Causal analysis approaches in Ingenuity Pathway Analysis. *Bioinformatics*. 30, 523–30.

Krewski D, Acosta D Jr, Andersen M et al. (2010). Toxicity testing in the 21st century: A vision and a strategy. *J Toxicol Environ Health B*. 13, 51–138.

Ladd-Acosta C, Aryee MJ, Ordway JM et al. (2010). Comprehensive high-throughput arrays for relative methylation (CHARM). *Curr Protoc Hum Genet*. 20, 21–19.

Laifenfeld D, Qiu L, Swiss R et al. (2014). Utilization of causal reasoning of hepatic gene expression in rats to identify molecular pathways of idiosyncratic drug-induced liver injury. *Toxicol Sci*. 137, 234–48.

Lee EH, Oh JH, Selvaraj S et al. (2016). Immunogenomics reveal molecular circuits of diclofenac induced liver injury in mice. *Oncotarget*. 7, 14983–5017.

Lengauer T, Rarey M (1996). Computational methods for biomolecular docking. *Current Opinion in Structural Biol*. 6, 402–6.

Lenz EM, Bright J, Knight R et al. (2005). Metabonomics with 1H-NMR spectroscopy and liquid chromatography-mass spectrometry applied to the investigation of metabolic changes caused by gentamicin-induced nephrotoxicity in the rat. *Biomarkers*. 10, 173–87.

Leo A, Hansch C, Church C (1969). Comparison of parameters currently used in the study of structure-activity relationships. *J Med Chem*. 12, 766–71.

Lesack K, Naugler C (2011). An open-source software program for performing Bonferroni and related corrections for multiple comparisons. *J Pathol Informatics*. 2, 52.

Li J, Lu Y, Akbani R et al. (2013). TCPA: A resource for cancer functional proteomics data. *Nat Methods*. 10, 1046–7.

Liebler, DC, Guengerich FP (2005). Elucidating mechanisms of drug-induced toxicity. *Nat Rev Drug Discovery*. 4, 410–20.

Lindon JC, Holmes E, Bollard ME et al. (2004). Metabonomics technologies and their applications in physiological monitoring, drug safety assessment and disease diagnosis. *Biomarkers*. 9, 1–31.

Liu L, Li Y, Li S et al. (2012). Comparison of next-generation sequencing systems. *J Biomed Biotechnol*. 2012, 2513–64.

Mah N, Thelin A, Lu T et al. (2004). A comparison of oligonucleotide and cDNA-based microarray systems. *Physiol Genomics*. 16, 361–70.

Martin MT, Judson RS, Reif DM et al. (2009). Profiling chemicals based on chronic toxicity results from the U.S. EPA ToxRef Database. *Environ Health Persp*. 117, 392–9.

Martin R, Yu K (2006). Assessing performance of prediction rules in machine learning. *Pharmacogenomics*. 7, 543–50.

McCarroll SA, Altshuler DM (2007). Copy-number variation and association studies of human disease. *Nat Genet*. 39, S37–42.

Metzker ML (2010). Sequencing technologies—The next generation. *Nat Rev Genetics*. 11, 31–46.

Mi H, Huang X, Muruganujan A et al. (2016). PANTHER version 11: Expanded annotation data from Gene Ontology and Reactome pathways, and data analysis tool enhancements. *Nucleic Acids Res*. pii:gkw1138 (Epub ahead of print)

Mi H, Thomas P (2009). PANTHER pathway: An ontology-based pathway database coupled with data analysis tools. *Methods Mol Biol*. 563, 123–40.

Mirkin SM (2007). Expandable DNA repeats and human disease. *Nature*. 447, 932–40.

Morris GM, Huey R, Lindstrom W et al. (2009). AutoDock4 and AutoDockTools4: Automated docking with selective receptor flexibility. *J Comput Chem*. 30, 2785–91.

Mortazavi A, Williams BA, McCue K et al. (2008). Mapping and quantifying mammalian transcriptomes by RNA-Seq. *Nat Methods*. 5, 621–8.

Nicholson JK, Lindon JC, Holmes E (1999). 'Metabonomics': Understanding the metabolic responses of living systems to pathophysiological stimuli via multivariate statistical analysis of biological NMR spectroscopic data. *Xenobiotica*. 29, 1181–9.

Nicholson JK, Timbrell JA, Sadler PJ (1985). Proton NMR spectra of urine as indicators of renal damage. Mercury-induced nephrotoxicity in rats. *Mol Pharmacol*. 27, 644–51.

Nicholson JK, Wilson ID (1989). High resolution proton magnetic resonance spectroscopy of biological fluids. *Prog NMR Spectrosc*. 21, 449–501.

Nikitin A, Egorov S, Daraselia N et al. (2003). Pathway studio—The analysis and navigation of molecular networks. *Bioinformatics*. 19, 2155–7.

Oda M, Glass JL, Thompson RF et al. (2009). High-resolution genome-wide cytosine methylation profiling with simultaneous copy number analysis and optimization for limited cell numbers. *Nucleic Acids Res*. 37, 3829–39.

Oh JH, Heo SH, Park HJ et al. (2014). Genomic and proteomic analyses of 1,3-dinitrobenzene-induced testicular toxicity in Sprague-Dawley rats. *Reprod Toxicol*. 43, 45–55.

Park PJ (2009). ChIP-seq: Advantages and challenges of a maturing technology. *Nat Rev Genet*. 10, 669–80.

Park JC, Hong YS, Kim YJ et al. (2009). A metabonomic study on the biochemical effects of doxorubicin in rats using (1)H-NMR spectroscopy. *J Toxicol Environ Health A*. 72, 374–84.

Puppala D, Collis LP, Sun SZ et al. (2013). Comparative gene expression profiling in human-induced pluripotent stem cell—Derived cardiocytes and human and cynomolgus heart tissue. *Tox Sci*. 131, 292–301.

Qian Z, Fernald AA, Godley LA et al. (2002). Expression profiling of CD34+ hematopoietic stem/progenitor cells reveals distinct subtypes of therapy-related acute myeloid leukemia. *Proc Nat Acad Sci*. 99, 14925–30.

Raamsdonk LM, Teusink B, Broadhurst D et al. (2001). A functional genomics strategy that uses metabolome data to reveal the phenotype of silent mutations. *Nat Biotech*. 19, 45–50.

Rauch C, Trieb M, Wibowo FR et al. (2005). Towards an understanding of DNA recognition by the methyl-CpG binding domain 1. *J Biomol Struct Dyn*. 22, 695–706.

Reiner A, Yekutieli D, Benjamini Y (2003). Identifying differentially expressed genes using false discovery rate controlling procedures. *Bioinformatics*. 19, 368–75.

Reo NV (2002). NMR-based metabolomics. *Drug Chem Toxicol*. 25, 375–82.

Richard AM, Williams CR (2002). Distributed structure-searchable toxicity (DSSTox) public database network: A proposal. *Mut Res*. 499, 27–52.

Ringner M (2008). What is principal component analysis? *Nat Biotech*. 26, 303–4.

Roth RA, Ganey PE (2011). Animal models of idiosyncratic drug-induced liver injury—Current status. *Crit Rev Toxicol*. 41, 723–39.

Saha K, Jaenisch R (2009). Technical challenges in using human induced pluripotent stem cells to model disease. *Cell Stem Cell*. 5, 584–95.

Sanguinetti MC, Tristani-Firouzi M (2006). hERG potassium channels and cardiac arrhythmia. *Nature*. 440, 463–9.

Schena M, Shalon D, Davis RW et al. (1995). Quantitative monitoring of gene expression patterns with a complementary DNA microarray. *Science*. 270, 467–70.

Schuierer S, Tranchevent LC, Dengler U et al. (2010). Large-scale benchmark of Endeavour using MetaCore maps. *Bioinformatics*. 26, 1922–3.

Severgnini M, Bicciato S, Mangano E et al. (2006). Strategies for comparing gene expression profiles from different microarray platforms: Application to a case-control experiment. *Anal Biochem*. 353, 43–56.
Shyu AB, Wilkinson MF, van Hoof A. (2008). Messenger RNA regulation: To translate or to degrade. *EMBO J*. 27, 471–81.
Rogers S, Girolami M, Kolch W et al. (2008). Investigating the correspondence between transcriptomic and proteomic expression profiles using coupled cluster models. *Bioinformatics*. 24, 2894–900.
Son MY, Lee MO, Jeon H et al. (2016). Generation and characterization of integration-free induced pluripotent stem cells from patients with autoimmune disease. *Exp Mol Med*. 48, e232.
Son MY, Seol B, Han YM et al. (2014). Comparative receptor tyrosine kinase profiling identifies a novel role for AXL in human stem cell pluripotency. *Hum Mol Gen*. 23, 1802–16.
Stankiewicz P, Lupski JR (2010). Structural variation in the human genome and its role in disease. *Annu Rev Med*. 61, 437–55.
Sudmant PH, Rausch T, Gardner EJ et al. (2015). An integrated map of structural variation in 2,504 human genomes. *Nature*. 526, 75–81.
Tcheremenskaia O, Benigni R, Nikolova I et al. (2012). OpenTox predictive toxicology framework: Toxicological ontology and semantic media wiki-based OpenToxipedia. *J Biom Semantics*. 3 Suppl 1, S7.
Tennant RW (2002). The National Center for Toxicogenomics: Using new technologies to inform mechanistic toxicology. *Environ Health Perspt*. 110, A8-10.
Thomas RS, Rank DR, Penn SG et al. (2001). Identification of toxicologically predictive gene sets using cDNA microarrays. *Mol Pharmacol*. 60, 1189–94.
Tomkinson AE, Vijayakumar S, Pascal JM et al. (2006). DNA ligases: Structure, reaction mechanism, and function. *Chem Rev*. 106, 687–99.
Vaidyanathan G (2012). Redefining clincal trials: The age of personalized medicine. *Cell*. 148, 1079–80.
van Dartel DA, Pennings JL, de la Fonteyne LJ et al. (2011). Evaluation of developmental toxicant identification using gene expression profiling in embryonic stem cell differentiation cultures. *Tox Sci*. 119, 126–34.
Wang F (2008). *Biomarker Methods in Drug Discovery and Development*. Totowa, NJ: Humana Press.
Wang Z, Gerstein M, Snyder M (2009). RNA-Seq: A revolutionary tool for transcriptomics. *Nat Rev Genet*. 10, 57–63.
Waring JF, Jolly RA, Ciurlionis R et al. (2001). Clustering of hepatotoxins based on mechanism of toxicity using gene expression profiles. *Toxicol Appl Pharmacol*. 175, 28–42.
Waters MD, Fostel JM (2004). Toxicogenomics and systems toxicology: Aims and prospects. *Nat Rev Genet*. 5, 936–48.
Waters NJ, Holmes E, Williams A et al. (2001). NMR and pattern recognition studies on the time-related metabolic effects of alpha-naphthylisothiocyanate on liver, urine, and plasma in the rat: An integrative metabonomic approach. *Chem Res Toxicol*. 14, 1401–12.
Waters NJ, Waterfield CJ, Farrant RD et al. (2006). Integrated metabonomic analysis of bromobenzene-induced hepatotoxicity: Novel induction of 5-oxoprolinosis. *J Proteome Res*. 5, 1448–59.

Wilson ID, Plumb R, Granger J et al. (2005). HPLC-MS-based methods for the study of metabonomics. *J Chromatog B*. 817, 67–76.
Wishart DS, Knox C, Guo AC et al. (2008). DrugBank: A knowledgebase for drugs, drug actions and drug targets. *Nucleic Acids Res*. 36, D901–6.
Wu X, Huang H, Wei T et al. (2012). Network expansion and pathway enrichment analysis towards biologically significant findings from microarrays. *J Integrative Bioinformatics*. 9, 213.
Xu J, Kelly R, Fang H et al. (2010). ArrayTrack: A free FDA bioinformatics tool to support emerging biomedical research–An update. *Hum Genomics*. 4, 428–34.
Yuryev A, Kotelnikova E, Daraselia N (2009). Ariadne's ChemEffect and Pathway Studio knowledge base. *Expert Opinion on Drug Discovery*. 4, 1307–18.
Zhao J, Chen J, Yang TH et al. (2012). Insights into the pathogenesis of axial spondyloarthropathy from network and pathway analysis. *BMC Sys Biol*. 6, Suppl 1, S4.

*section two*

---

# *Testing procedures for nontarget organ toxicities*

# *chapter eight*

# *Carcinogenesis*

***Kyung-Soo Chun, Hyung Sik Kim, and Byung-Mu Lee***

*Contents*

# *Introduction*

## *Historical background*

The relationships between cancer and exposure to chemicals have long been noted.

1. In 1761, Hill found that users of tobacco snuff had a high rate of nasal cancer.
2. Sir Percival Pott (1744–1788, English surgeon) observed, in 1775, that exposure to soot by chimney sweeps induced cancer of the scrotum (Pott, 1775).
3. Twenty years later, Sommering noted that cancer of the lip was often associated with pipe smoking.

4. Rehn discovered in 1895 that bladder tumors occurred among workers in aniline dye factories. In the twentieth century, cancers induced by a variety of chemicals under different exposure conditions have been observed.
5. In 1915, Katsusaburo Yamagiwa and Koichi Ichikawa (1918) first succeeded in inducing experimental tumors in the skin of sensitive rabbit ears by applying coal tar (a complex mixture of chemicals) repeatedly to their skin every 2 or 3 days for a period of more than 100 days (Bishop, 1987).
6. Later in 1930, Earnest Kennaway demonstrated that dibenzanthracene, a chemical constituent of coal tar, was able to produce cancer in rats.
7. In 1933, Cook et al. (1933) also showed that benzo(a)pyrene (BaP) isolated from coal tar was carcinogenic in mouse skin.

In view of the seriousness of carcinogenesis, and the rapid development of new chemicals, many governmental agencies, as well as academic and industrial laboratories, have undertaken extensive research and testing in laboratory animals. These endeavors have provided leads for further epidemiological studies.

## Definition and identification

The term *chemical carcinogenesis* is generally defined to indicate the induction or enhancement of neoplasia by chemicals. Although in the strict etymologic sense this term means the induction of carcinomas, it is widely used to indicate tumorigenesis. In other words, it includes not only epithelial malignancies (carcinomas) but also mesenchymal malignant tumors (sarcomas). Leukemias and lymphomas arise from the blood-forming cells and from cells of the immune system, respectively. Tumors are further classified according to tissue of origin (e.g., lung or breast carcinomas) and the type of cell involved. For example, fibrosarcomas arise from fibroblasts, and erythroid leukemias from precursors of erythrocytes (red blood cells). The cells tend to replicate, thereby invading surrounding tissues and metastasizing in remote parts of the body.

A chemical may be identified as a carcinogen based on observations in humans and supported by tests in lab animals. It should be emphasized that chemicals induce tumors in rodents but that these types of tumors do not necessarily occur in humans; for example, solvent-induced renal tumors are dependent on proteins not present in humans. Thus this type of chemical-induced tumor is not relevant for humans. Human data may be derived from clinical observations as noted above. However, the relationship between the development of a cancer and exposure to a chemical is complex. First, there is a long latency, generally in years or decades, between the time of exposure and development of cancer. Further, humans are exposed to a multiplicity of potentially carcinogenic factors; in general, individuals are exposed to mixtures of chemicals where one compound alone may or may not induce carcinogenesis, however, they may be dependent upon each other, in some cases, to produce an effect. In addition, exposure of the female parent to chemicals during pregnancy may result in cancer development in offspring without any evidence of cancer in the mother. In view of these facts, very extensive epidemiological studies are needed. Further, exposure to a certain chemical may not induce cancer until the individual's immune system becomes compromised such as in AIDS.

In addition to human data, lab tests in animals provide valuable supporting evidence. An important example involves chronic exposure of animals to test chemicals. However, animals, as humans, develop cancer even without being exposed to a known carcinogen. In view of this, it is generally agreed (e.g., WHO, 1969) that fulfillment of one or more of the following criteria by the test animals be considered as a positive sign for carcinogenesis:

1. An increase in the frequency of one or several types of tumors that also occur in the controls
2. Development of tumors not seen in the controls
3. Occurrence of tumors earlier than in the controls
4. An elevation in number of tumors in individual animals, compared to controls

### *Weight of evidence*

Evidence of carcinogenicity consists of human and animal data. However, because of interspecies differences in response to chemicals, reliable human data are given much greater weight. In fact, the earliest discoveries of chemical carcinogens were made in humans, as noted earlier. In view of the seriousness of cancer, however, it will be grossly imprudent to wait for relevant results to be generated from long-term human studies to assess each chemical for its carcinogenicity. Consequently, appropriate studies need to be carried out in animals. The significance of the results unfortunately varies greatly among different studies. For example, aflatoxin $B_1$ induces tumors in a variety of animals, with small doses (in ppb) and with a relatively short latency period. On the other hand, saccharin yields positive results inconsistently, with very large doses (in tens of thousands of ppm) and only after very long periods of treatment. Atrazine induces mammary tumors in Sprague–Dawley rats, whose reproductive system does not resemble that of humans in function, thus limiting the biological relevance of these findings to humans. Further, experimental design and conduct of the studies also differ in their adequacy.

To facilitate the evaluation of such diverse findings, a *weight of evidence* scheme has been adopted, taking into account the species used, as interspecies data cannot always be utilized as in the case of atrazine-induced mammary tumors in Sprague–Dawley rats. The findings may be considered "sufficient" when there are benign and malignant tumors in multiple species (or strains, or in multiple experiments), or there are large numbers of tumors (or at an unusual site, or being that of a special type).

"Limited" evidence means positive results in only one species, strain, or experiment, or when the experimental design or conduct is inadequate. "Inadequate" evidence applies to results that are difficult to interpret. Similarly, data obtained in humans vary greatly in their significance as well. Using these criteria, EPA (1996) and IARC (1987) classified chemical carcinogens into five categories (Table 8.1).

In addition, the National Toxicology Program classified them into two categories: Group 1, Known to be human carcinogens (K); Group 2, Reasonably anticipated to be human carcinogens (R). The American Conference of Governmental Industrial Hygienists has five categories: Group A1, Confirmed human carcinogen; Group A2, Suspected human carcinogen; Group A3, Confirmed animal carcinogen with unknown relevance to humans; Group A4, Not Classifiable as a Human Carcinogen, and Group A5, Not Suspected as a Human Carcinogen.

***Table 8.1*** Classification of carcinogens based on "weight of evidence"

| Categories | IARC | EPA | Human data | Animal data |
|---|---|---|---|---|
| Human carcinogen | 1 | A | Sufficient | Sufficient or limited |
| Probable human carcinogen | 2A | B1, B2[a] | Limited or inadequate[b] | Sufficient |
| Possible human carcinogen | 2B | C | Absent or inadequate | Sufficient or limited[b] |
| Not classifiable | 3 | D | Absent or inadequate | Inadequate or absent |
| Not carcinogenic | 4 | E | Absent or extensive negative data | Negative evidence in at least two species |

[a] EPA classifies carcinogens with sufficient animal data as "probable human carcinogen" and places them in category B1 or B2 depending on the weight of human data.
[b] IARC accepts positive genotoxicity in lieu of human data.

### *Hallmarks of cancer*

For many decades, scientists and physicians noted the characteristics of tumors, but did not possess the techniques to understand what was happening at the cellular level. However, as technology improved, cancer research has progressed and it is now established that all cancer types share the common hallmark characteristics reviewed by Hanahan and Weinberg (2011) (Table 8.2).

## *Mode of action*

Chemical carcinogenesis, as shown in Figure 8.1, is a multistage process. Carcinogenic chemicals act by initiating certain genetic changes in a cell (initiation), then by promoting the formation of a benign neoplasm (promotion), and finally converting the benign neoplasm to a malignant cancer (progression), or enhancing the activity of another chemical.

### *Bioactivation*

Most carcinogenic substances are inactive and require metabolic activation, by undergoing bioactivation in the body to form reactive intermediates. A common type of reactive metabolite is epoxide. For example, aflatoxin $B_1$ is converted to aflatoxin-8,9-epoxide. Benzene, vinyl chloride, and a number of polycyclic hydrocarbons also form epoxides. Other carcinogens, such as 2-acetylaminofluorene (AAF) and certain aminoazo dyes form *N*-hydroxy derivatives (see Appendix 3.1).

Certain chemicals are bioactivated to ultimate carcinogens via an intermediary step. An example of this is BaP, which forms BaP-7,8-epoxide, the intermediary carcinogen. The latter then transforms to BaP-7,8-diol-9,10-epoxide, the ultimate carcinogen. Styrene undergoes oxidative metabolism to styrene 7,8-oxide, which is the intermediary carcinogen (Nestmann et al., 2005). Styrene is noncarcinogenic in most animal experiments, after either ingestion or inhalation. As a result, the Dutch Health Council decided to consider it a noncarcinogen. However, its main metabolite, styrene-7,8-epoxide, is highly mutagenic, and most likely carcinogenic in animals *in vivo.* Chromium undergoes reduction to a lower oxidation state to induce carcinogenesis (Shi et al., 1998). Arsenic requires transformation to induce cancer but this only occurs in populations possessing a certain phenotype, indicating that not only bioactivation is crucial but the presence of specific gene material needs to be present for an effect.

***Table 8.2*** Hallmarks of cancer

| Hallmark of cancer | Characteristics |
|---|---|
| 1. Genome instability and mutation | • Cancer cells are genetically unstable.<br>• The gene defects include; (1) detection of DNA damage and activating repair machinery, (2) repair of damaged DNA, and (3) inactivation or interception of mutagenic molecules before interaction with DNA. |
| 2. Tumor-promoting inflammation | • Cancer cells are frequently found in an inflammatory environment.<br>• Inflammation provides growth factor, proangiogenic factors, and extracellular matrix-modifying enzymes that facilitate angiogenesis, invasion, and metastasis. |
| 3. Sustaining proliferative signaling | • Cancer cells grow uncontrollably.<br>• Growth factors independent of cancer cells derive from constitutive activation of components of signaling pathways. |
| 4. Evading growth suppressors | • Cancer cells avoid anti-growth signaling.<br>• Cancer cells with defects in function of RB pathway miss the services of a critical gatekeeper of cell-cycle progression whose absence permits persistent cell proliferation. |
| 5. Resisting cell death | • Loss of apoptosis gatekeeper, protein P53.<br>• Most human cancers have mutated or missing gene for p53. Cancer cells produce anti-apoptotic proteins (Bcl-2, Bcl-XL), but diminish pro-apoptotic proteins (Bax, Bak). |
| 6. Enabling replicative immortality | • Cancer cells require unlimited replicative potential to generate macroscopic tumors.<br>• Elevated levels of telomerase extend the length of telomeres on chromosomes, which delays senescence, and allows cellular proliferation. |
| 7. Reprogramming energy metabolism | • Cancer cells in the presence of $O_2$ reprogram their glucose metabolism by limiting their energy metabolism to glycolysis, leading to an "aerobic glycolysis" state. |
| 8. Evading immune destruction | • Cancer cells destroy body's immune defenses to some degree, allowing them to proliferate and invade other tissues. |
| 9. Inducing angiogenesis | • $O_2$-deprived cells begin to generate chemical signals for new blood flow by releasing VEGF and FGF.<br>• New blood vessels sprout and grow in and around the tumor to supply the needed blood to cancer cells. |
| 10. Activating invasion and metastasis | • Cancer cells invade nearby tissues by releasing enzymes called MMPs. The cells within the tumor lose their adhesiveness and move into other tissues. |

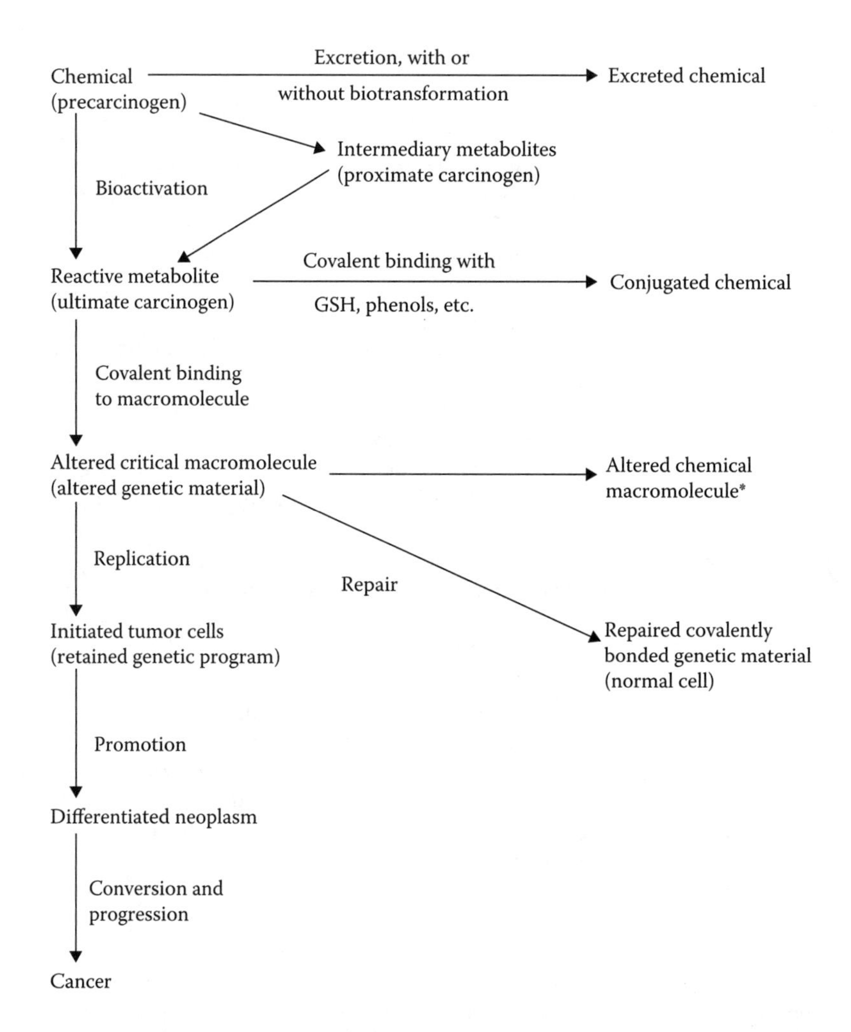


***Figure 8.1*** Schematic diagram depicting the fate of a genotoxic carcinogen and its relation with carcinogenesis. Events in the left-hand column lead to cancer formation, whereas those in the right-hand column are harmless. (*) indicates that the step may be important during other stages of carcinogenesis.

## *Interaction with biomolecules*

The reactive metabolites covalently bind to biomolecules such as DNA, RNA, proteins, and lipids to form DNA-, RNA-, proteins, and lipid adducts, respectively (Poirier et al., 1977; Kwack and Lee, 2000). Some of these components, such as proteins and lipids, may not play a critical role in carcinogenesis, but the biological role of protein adducts and lipid adducts needs to be fully investigated. When DNA is the target, the reaction may lead to point mutation, frameshift mutation, and others. These changes may not persist: they may be reversed by an error-free DNA repair or disappear when the cell dies. However, some of these may persist, not be reversed by an error-prone DNA repair and lead to mutation and cancer.

## Initiation

Initiation is the first stage of the cancer process by induction of a mutation in a critical gene involved in the control of cell proliferation (Figure 8.2). As with mutational events, initiation requires one or more rounds of cell division for "fixation" of the process. If the cell with an altered DNA undergoes mitosis, the alteration is retained. The cell with the altered DNA is termed an "initiated" cell. The endpoint of initiation is "mutation," an alteration in genotype. Further, initiation is irreversible although some initiated cells may eventually die during development of the neoplasm. Depending on the site of the alteration, the cell may be partially or fully preneoplastic. The process generally involves the conversion of proto-oncogenes to oncogenes or tumor suppressor genes inactivation (Table 8.3).

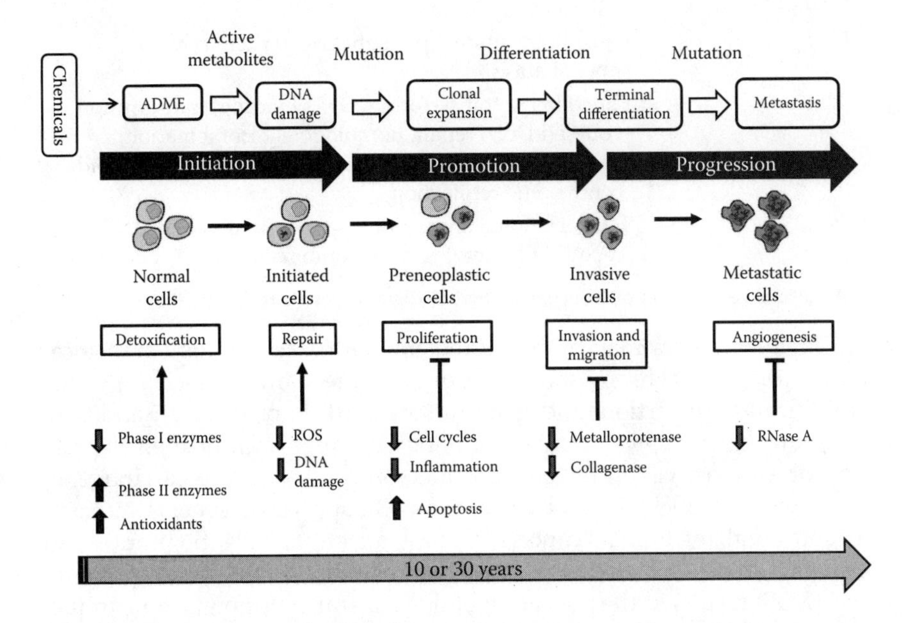


*Figure 8.2* Schematic represents of chemical carcinogens on multiple stage carcinogenesis. (Data quoted from Kim HS, Kacew S, Lee BM, *Arch Toxicol*, 90, 2389–404, 2016. With permission of the authors and the publisher.)

*Table 8.3* Lists of oncogenes and tumor suppressor genes

| Oncogene* | Function |
|---|---|
| *ras* | GTP-binding protein |
| *Raf* | Serine/threonine-specific protein kinase |
| *Jun* | Transcription factor |
| *fos* | Transcription factor |
| *Src* | Tyrosine-specific protein kinase |
| *erbB* | Epidermal growth factor receptor |
| *myc* | Transcription factor |
| *sis* | Platelet-derived growth factor |
| **Tumor-suppressor genes** | **Function** |
| *Rb1* | Cell cycle regulation |
| *P53* | Cell cycle regulation, apoptosis |
| *APC* | Signaling through adhesion molecules to nucleus |
| *WT1* | Transcriptional regulation |
| *NF1* | Catalysis of RAS inactivation |
| *NF2* | Linkage of cell membrane to actin cytoskeleton |
| *P16INK4A* | Cell cycle regulation |
| *PTEN* | Phosphoinositide 3-phosphatase, protein tyrosine phosphatase |
| *BRCA1* | Functions in transcription, DNA binding, transcription coupled DNA repair, homologous recombination, chromosomal stability, ubiquitination of proteins, and centrosome replication |
| *BRCA2* | Transcriptional regulation of genes involved in DNA repair and homologous recombination |

* Abnormal versions of proto-oncogenes that mediate cancerous transformations.

*Proto-oncogenes* may be converted into *oncogenes* through translocation to a different chromosomal site, or other mechanisms such as genetic amplification, insertion, and gene mutation (Bishop, 1987). In addition, there are *tumor suppressor genes* or *antioncogenes*; a lack of their expression or an inactivation of their products may also lead to carcinogenesis (Weinberg, 1989). One of them, the p53 suppressor gene, is mutated in about half of human cancers (Greenblatt et al., 1994; Sugimura and Ushijima, 2000). In the case of silica, the generation of reactive oxygen species (ROS) results in the activation of nuclear transcription factors, induction of oncogene expression, redox regulation of p53 tumor suppressor gene, and induction of apoptosis (Shi et al., 1998, 1999). ROS generation, as a step in the pathway of carcinogenesis, is also involved in cancers caused by cigarette smoking, radon, and polycyclic aromatic hydrocarbons (Vallyathan et al., 1998).

## *Promotion*

Tumor promotion comprises the selective clonal expansion of initiated cells. The initiated cell, with altered genotype, may remain dormant for a long period of time before it becomes a benign tumor through cell proliferation in the presence of *promoters* (Butterworth and Goldworthy, 1991). The dormancy is probably due to the suppressant influence of the surrounding normal cells exerted through certain intercellular communication (Trosko and Chang, 1988).

Tumor promoters are generally nonmutagenic, are not carcinogenic alone, and often (but not always) able to mediate their biologic effects without metabolic activation. These agents are characterized by their ability to reduce the latency period for tumor formation after exposure of a tissue to a tumor initiator, or to increase the number of tumors formed in that tissue. Their influence can be reduced by programmed cell death (apoptosis), cell killing (e.g., from cytotoxic chemicals), cell removal (e.g., partial hepatectomy), growth factors (e.g., hormones), and other factors (Figure 8.2).

While initiation is generally considered to be a permanent process, promotion is not. Further, it is reversible. Therefore, for an initiated cell to continue to replicate, it must be exposed to a promoter more or less continuously. The endpoint of promotion is the formation of a benign tumor with altered genotype and phenotype.

## *Conversion and progression*

Conversion is the transformation of a preneoplastic cell into one that expresses the malignant phenotype. This process requires further genetic changes. Conversion of a fraction of these cells to malignancy may be accelerated in proportion to the rate of cell division and the quantity of dividing cells in the benign tumor or preneoplastic lesion. These are characterized by biochemical and/or morphological changes in the activity or structures of the genome. The mechanism of action is not fully understood, but may involve activation of the initiated cells by exposure to clastogenic agents or complete carcinogens (Pitot et al., 1988). During this period, the neoplasm may convert from benign to malignant tumor, which is invasive and metastatic. Metastasis may also involve the ability of tumor cells to secrete proteases that allow invasion beyond the immediate primary tumor location (Figure 8.2).

Similar to initiation, progression is an irreversible process. Table 8.4 provides a list of the characteristics of initiation, promotion, and progression.

***Table 8.4*** Morphologic and biologic characteristics of the stages of initiation, promotion, and progression in hepatocarcinogenesis in the rat

| Initiation | Promotion | Progression |
|---|---|---|
| Irreversible with "stem cell" potential<br>Genotoxic and rapid | Reversible, epigenetic, slow and long latency | Irreversible<br>Morphologically altered in cell genome's structure |
| Efficacy sensitive to xenobiotic and other chemical factors | Promoted cell population dependent on continued exposure to promotors | |
| Spontaneous occurrence of initiated cells is measurable | Efficiency sensitive to dietary and hormonal factors | Growth of altered cells sensitive to environmental factors during early phase |
| Requires cell division for "fixation" leading to mutation | Cellular proliferation and clonal expansion leading to benign tumor | Conversion of benign into malignant tumor |
| Dose–response does not exhibit a measurable threshold | Threshold exists and maximal effect dependent on dose of initiator | Benign and/or malignant neoplasms seen |
| Effect of initiators depends on quantitation of focal lesions after exposure to promoter | Effectiveness of promoters depends on time and dose rate | "Progressors" act to advance promoted cells into this stage |

*Source:* Adapted from Pitot HC, Beer D, Hendrich S, *Theories of Carcinogenesis*, Hemisphere, Washington, DC, 1988.

# *Categories of carcinogens*

Carcinogens may also be classified according to their *mode of action* into genotoxic and nongenotoxic carcinogens. The term "genotoxic carcinogen" indicates a chemical capable of producing cancer by directly altering the genetic material of target cells, while "nongenotoxic carcinogen" represents a chemical capable of producing cancer by some secondary mechanism not related to direct gene damage.

## *Genotoxic carcinogens*

Genotoxic carcinogens initiate tumors by producing DNA damage (Figure 8.1). There are two types. Most genotoxic carcinogens are electrophiles that interact directly with DNA through the formation of covalent bonds, resulting in DNA–carcinogen complexes (called DNA

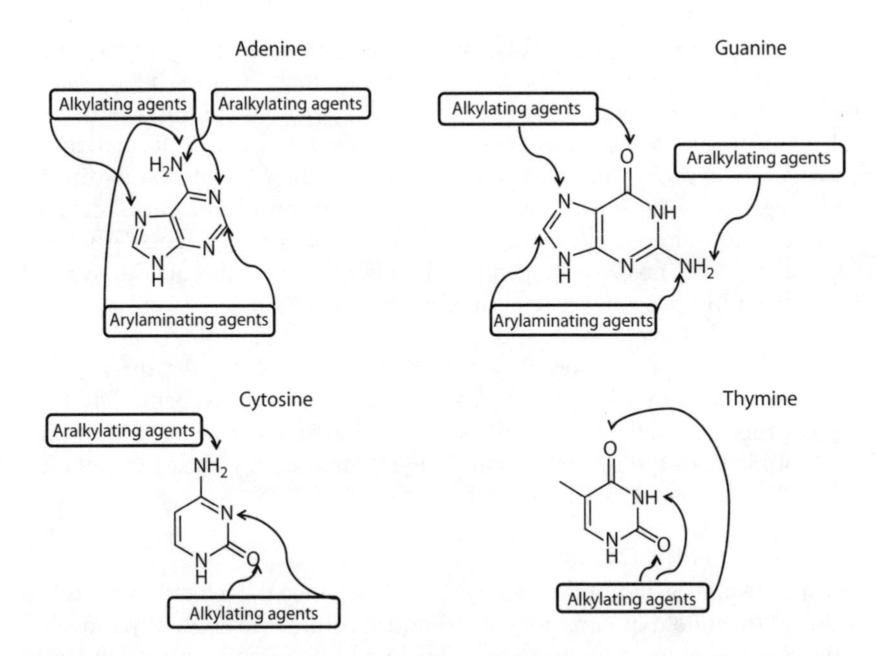


***Figure 8.3*** Types of DNA adduct formation in purine and pyrimidine bases.

adducts). DNA adducts are primary lesions formed by electrophilic genotoxic agents through covalent binding to DNA. The purine and pyrimidine bases guanine, adenine, thymine, and cytosine contain numerous nucleophilic sites (Figure 8.3). Hence, DNA is prone to alterations by electrophiles. DNA-adduct formation is generally considered an important step in chemical carcinogenesis because DNA-adduct formation has been demonstrated for the majority of carcinogens.

*Direct-acting carcinogens*

These chemicals are also known as ultimate carcinogens. They are electrophilic (electron-loving, electron-deficient) and bind to DNA and other macromolecules (electron-rich molecules, nucleophiles). Examples are alkyl and aryl epoxides, lactones, sulfate esters, nitrosamides, nitrosoureas, ochratoxin A (Clark and Snedeker, 2006), arsenic (Bernstam and Nriagu, 2000), benzene (Pyatt et al., 2007), and platinum amine chelators. Because of their high reactivity, these direct-acting carcinogens are often more active *in vitro* but less so *in vivo*.

*Precarcinogens*

They are also known as procarcinogens. They require conversion through bioactivation to become ultimate carcinogens, either directly or via an intermediary stage—the proximate carcinogens. Most of the presently known chemical carcinogens fall into this class. These include the polycyclic aromatic hydrocarbons (PAHs), diesel exhaust particles, aromatic amines, halogenated hydrocarbons, nitrosamines, cycasin, aflatoxin B, pyrrolizidine alkaloids, safrole, and thioamides. Different types of bioactivation (such as formation of epoxides, *N*-hydroxy derivatives) are involved in their conversion to direct-acting agents, as discussed in Chapter 3. These chemicals may also activate proto-oncogene to oncogene and inactivate oncosuppressor genes. Another type of activation involves the generation of ROS, which subsequently stimulates the multistep sequence resulting in carcinogenesis.

As noted above, timely and error-free DNA repair plays, an important part in the prevention of neoplastic transformation. An interesting example is dimethyl nitrosamine, whose damage to hepatocyte DNA is rapidly repaired in the rat but only slowly in the hamster who is thus more susceptible than the rat to this carcinogen. Further, it induces tumors in the rat brain where the repair mechanism is deficient.

*Nongenotoxic carcinogens*

These substances do not damage DNA but enhance the growth of tumors induced by genotoxic carcinogens or induce tumors through other mechanisms such as epigenetic regulation [e.g., DNA methylation, histone modification, nucleosome positioning (physical alteration), and posttranscriptional gene regulation by noncoding RNA (micro-RNAs)] (Ducasse and Brown, 2006; Kanwal and Gupta, 2010). These are briefly described hereafter.

*Cocarcinogens*

These substances, not carcinogenic on their own, enhance the effects of genotoxic carcinogens when given simultaneously. They may act by affecting an increase in the concentration of the initiator, the genotoxic carcinogen itself, or that of the reactive metabolite. This can be achieved either by an increase of the absorption of the carcinogen, via the gastrointestinal tract or the skin, or by enhanced bioactivation. The same result can also be achieved through a decrease of the elimination of the initiator, either by inhibiting the detoxification enzymes, or by depleting the endogenous substrates involved in phase II reactions, such as GSH.

Apart from increasing the concentration of the reactive species at the site of action, cocarcinogens may inhibit the rate or fidelity of DNA repair, or enhance conversion of DNA lesions to permanent alterations.

Tobacco smoke contains relatively small amounts of genotoxic carcinogens, such as PAH and tobacco-specific nitrosamines; its marked carcinogenic effects are perhaps attributed to catechols which act as cocarcinogens.

*Promoters*

These chemicals increase the effects of initiators when given subsequently. The classic example of this phenomenon was provided by studies demonstrating that an initial application, on the mouse skin, of a carcinogenic PAH did not induce skin cancer until after applying, at the same site, phorbol esters from croton oil (Berenblum and Shubik, 1947, 1949). The application of the promoters could be delayed for months or even a year without losing their effect. These studies clearly demonstrate the *two-stage* process of carcinogenesis as well as the persistence of the initiator's effect. Incidentally, croton oil is also cocarcinogenic since it is effective when applied at the same time as the initiator.

The possible mechanisms of action of promoters include the following:

1. Stimulation of cell proliferation through cytotoxicity leading to compensatory regeneration or hormonal effects
2. Inhibition of gap junction intercellular communication, thereby releasing the initiated cells from the restraint exercised by the surrounding normal cells
3. Immunosuppression
4. An increase in cell turnover rates and transformation

*Cytotoxicants*—Such as nitrilotriacetic acid, a non-eutrophying replacement for phosphate in household detergent, produce tumors through cell proliferation resulting from cell injury and death. Unleaded gasoline and a number of other chemicals have been shown to induce renal tubular necrosis resulting from the deposition of $\alpha 2_{\mu}$-globulin in male rats. The cell death and subsequent regeneration are believed to produce kidney tumors in male rats (Swenberg et al., 1989).

*Hormones*—Such as estradiol and diethylstilbestrol have been shown to produce an increase in tumors in animals (e.g., breast cancer in mice) and in humans (e.g., endometrial cancer in menopausal females maintained on estrogen). These substances are not genotoxic but act as promoters. The actual initiators are not known. Androgens have little, if any, carcinogenic effect. The herbicide aminotriazole and certain fungicides induce thyroid tumors through a hormonal mechanism as well (McClain, 1989).

*Gap junction intercellular communication* (GJIC)—This is an important mechanism in regulating cell growth. A number of chemicals interfere with this mechanism, thereby inducing hyperplasia and acting as promoters in carcinogenesis (Trosko and Chang, 1988). Klaunig (1991) listed, among others, a number of pesticides (e.g., chlordane, DDT, dieldrin, endosulfan, and lindane) and pharmaceuticals (phenobarbital and diazepam) as being able to inhibit hepatic gap junctional intercellular communication.

*Immunosuppressive drugs*—Such as cyclosporin A and azathioprine are increasingly being used in conjunction with organ transplantation. They have been shown to produce leukemias and sarcomas in some patients and in mice and rats. The genotoxic agents are likely to be viruses, and these immunosuppressive drugs promote development of tumors through non-genotoxic mechanisms (Ryffel, 1992).

*Peroxisome proliferators*—Consist of a variety of chemicals that have the common property of inducing rodent liver tumors and increasing peroxisomes in liver cells (Melnick, 2001). These chemicals have therefore been considered as a special class of carcinogens (Reddy and Lalwani, 1983). Examples are hypolipidemic drugs, such as clofibrate and fenofibrate; certain phthalate plasticizers, such as di(2-ethylhexyl) phthalate, and the solvent 1,1,2-tricholoroethylene. These chemicals are not genotoxic, but by increasing the number of peroxisomes, they may increase the formation of $H_2O_2$, leading to formation of ROS and thereby enhancing cell replication (Lake, 1995).

### *Solid-state carcinogens*

These are exemplified by asbestos and implanted materials such as plastics, metal, and glass. These substances exert no genotoxic effects, but produce tumors of mesenchymal origin. Although the precise mode of action is not known, the tumors induced are preceded by an exuberant foreign-body reaction including hyperplastic fibrosis with a high frequency of chromosomal changes in the preneoplastic cells (Weisburger and Williams, 1993). In many cases, there is concomitant exposure to the substances in cigarette smoke, and thus the frequency of lung cancer in individuals exposed to asbestos and cigarette smoke is markedly higher than those exposed to asbestos alone. The absence of tumors in subjects exposed to asbestos alone, but the presence of cancer in patients exposed to asbestos and cigarette smoke, is a strong indication that asbestos may be acting as an initiator rather than a direct carcinogen (Vallyathan et al., 1998).

### *Metals and metalloids*

Arsenic, cadmium, chromium, nickel, uranium, and their compounds are carcinogenic in humans. A number of others such as beryllium, cobalt, and lead are considered to be carcinogens in animals (IARC, 1987). Arsenic was thought to be an exception in that it is carcinogenic in humans but not animals (Bernstam and Nriagu, 2000). Recent data, however, show that intratracheal instillation of $As_2O_3$ in Syrian hamsters resulted in an increase in pulmonary adenomas, and after intrauterine exposure, apparently induced lung tumors in mice. Radon and its daughters diffuse into the ambient air, become attached to particles in uranium mines, and upon inhalation produce lung cancer.

The mechanisms underlying metal-induced carcinogenesis are not fully understood, but may involve genotoxic and/or epigenetic activities. Sunderman (1984) listed a number of promising avenues for research. Among them are the formation of crosslinks between DNA and proteins or between adjacent DNA strands, and impairment of the fidelity of DNA replication by altering the conformation of DNA polymerases. Radon was shown to penetrate bronchial epithelial nuclei, resulting in DNA mutation, leading to malignant transformation of cells (Vallyathan et al., 1998). These substances may be classified as genotoxic carcinogens because they alter gene expression in one way or another. In addition, damage of cytoskeleton by certain metals may contribute to their carcinogenicity (Chou, 1989). A probable mechanism of metal carcinogenesis includes an increase in ROS and reactive nitrogen species (RNS) formation through redox cycling reactions by disrupting metal homeostasis (e.g., Fe, Co, Cu, Cr), oxidative stress, and depletion of GSH (e.g., As, Cd, and Pb) (Jomova and Valko, 2011)., Perturbation of DNA methylation and global or gene specific histone modification are reported as epigenetic modes of action (Arita and Costa, 2009).

### *Cell phones*

The U.S. National Toxicology Program (NTP) at the National Institute of Environmental Health Sciences (NIEHS) has carried out carcinogenesis studies of radiofrequency radiation (RFR) at frequencies and modulations used in the U.S. telecommunications industry. According to the NTP report (Wyde et al., 2016), male Harlan Sprague Dawley rats exposed to heavy RF radiation (1.5, 3, and 6 W/kg, whole body exposures) were more likely to develop malignant gliomas in the brain and schwannomas of the heart. However, there was no significant difference in tumor rates among the female rats in the study. Currently, mechanism underlying tumorigenicity of mobile phones is not elucidated. *The FDA's website provides a couple of steps people can take to minimize radiation exposure when using cell phones, including reducing the amount of time spent using a cell phone and using speaker mode or a headset to place more distance between one's head and cell phone.*

### *Perchlorethylene*

Perchloroethylene is a colorless, nonflammable liquid with a sweet, etherlike odor. It is also called tetrachloroethylene, PCE, or PERC ($C_2Cl_4$). PERC is the most commonly used dry cleaning solvent, which is effective for removing stains and dirt from a wide variety of fabrics without shrinking the material or ruining the colors. PERC is also an ingredient in aerosol products, solvent soaps, printing inks, adhesives, sealants, paint removers, paper coatings, leather treatments, automotive cleaners, polishes, lubricants, and silicones. PERC is a volatile organic compound (VOC) and a strongly suspected carcinogen and air pollutant. Studies in humans suggest that exposure to PERC might lead to a higher risk of developing bladder cancer, multiple myeloma, or non-Hodgkin's lymphoma; but the evidence is not sufficient. In animals, PERC produces cancers of the liver, kidneys, and blood. EPA considers PERC likely to be carcinogenic to humans by all routes of exposure (CASRN 127-18-4). The International Agency for Research on Cancer (IARC) considers PERC to probably be carcinogenic to humans. The Department of Health and Human Services (DHHS) considers PERC to be reasonably likely to be a human carcinogen (R).

*Secondary carcinogens*

This term has been used to refer to substances that are not directly carcinogenic but can induce cancer following a distinctly noncarcinogenic effect. For example, polyoxyethylene monostearate (Myrj 45), at high doses, elicited bladder stones that in turn produced bladder tumors. No tumors were observed in any of the animals that had no bladder stones. On the other hand, this term has also been used in connection with those genotoxic carcinogens that require bioactivation.

## *Epigenetic carcinogenesis*

Epigenetic changes also play important roles in the regulation of carcinogenesis. The definition of epigenetics, in this context, is modification of expression of cancer-related genes without alterations in DNA sequences. The molecular mechanism(s) underlying epigenetic modifications are closely associated with DNA methylation, histone protein acetylation, methylation, and phosphorylation (Cedar and Bergman 2009; Kanwal and Gupta 2012). Recently, differential DNA methylation and altered histone modifications have been found to be implicated. For example, the environmental contaminant arsenic is known to produce repression of tumor suppressor genes via methylation and to drive global DNA hypomethylation, a phenomenon frequently associated with cancer (Arita and Costa, 2009). These genetic and epigenetic alterations interact at all stages of cancer development, working together to promote cancer progression (Jones and Laird, 1999). The epigenetic alterations may be the key initiating events in some forms of cancer (Feinberg et al., 2006). The fact that epigenetic aberrations are potentially reversible and can be restored to their normal state by epigenetic therapy makes such initiatives promising and therapeutically relevant (Yoo and Jones, 2006).

Epigenetic regulation of target genes contributes to cellular defects including the silencing of tumor suppressor genes, cell cycle regulators, apoptotic cell death-related factors, and DNA repair genes. Further, nuclear receptors and transcription factors are altered through DNA hypermethylation in promoter CpG islands, the acetylation/deacetylation of histones, and acetylation or methylation of nonhistone proteins, such as p53, NF-κB, and HSP90 (Alam et al., 2015; Kanwal and Gupta, 2012).

## *Some human carcinogens/target organs*

As noted above, the designation of a chemical, or mixture, as a human carcinogen is based on sufficient human data and, as a rule, some animal data. Human carcinogens induce cancers in different organs or systems. Table 8.5 lists the target organs of some human carcinogens, grouped by the "reason"/site of exposure.

In addition to the carcinogens related to diet and lifestyle, it is generally recognized that high intake of fat and/or calories and deficiencies in vitamins A and E pose risks of increasing certain cancers. However, these factors, in the strict sense, are not carcinogens but modify/promote carcinogenesis by certain indirect mechanisms. Caloric restriction reduces carcinogenesis and increases the survival time.

As noted above, certain biochemical changes occur in the body after exposure to a carcinogen. Some of these changes can be detected in biological samples. Clinically, they may serve to monitor such exposure, or to assess the progress of cancer and progress of treatment. Appendix 8.1 describes a few examples to illustrate their uses.

## *Tests for carcinogenicity*

### *Short-term tests for mutagenesis/carcinogenesis*

In recent years, a number of relatively simple and much shorter tests have been devised and employed to detect the mutagenic activity of chemicals. These tests utilize a variety of systems including microbes, insects, and mammalian cells, as well as a battery of parameters such as gene mutation, chromosomal aberration, and DNA repair. These mutagenesis tests and tests using cell transformation as endpoints will be described and discussed in the next chapter.

Although not all mutagens are carcinogenic, nor vice versa, the relationship between these two activities is nevertheless so close that mutagenesis tests are performed frequently as a rapid screening of chemicals

*Table 8.5* Some human carcinogens and their target organs

| | |
|---|---|
| **Dietary and lifestyle** | |
| Aflatoxin | Liver |
| Alcoholic beverages | Pharynx, esophagus, liver, larynx, oral cavity |
| Betel chewing | Mouth, pharynx, larynx |
| Tobacco smoke | Lung, larynx, oral cavity, pharynx, esophagus, pancreas, kidney, urothelial |
| **Industrial and environmental** | |
| 4-Aminobiphenyl | Bladder |
| Aromatic amines | Bladder |
| Azo dyes | Bladder |
| Arsenic | Skin, bronchus, liver |
| Asbestos | Lung, pleura, peritoneum |
| Benzene | Bone marrow |
| Benzidine | Bladder |
| Cadmium | Lung, prostate |
| Chromium (VI) compounds | Respiratory tract |
| 2-Naphthylamine | Bladder |
| Nickel compounds | Nasal sinus, bronchus |
| Polynuclear aromatic hydrocarbons, from coke, coal, tar, etc. | Skin, bronchus, stomach |
| Vinyl chloride monomer | Liver, hemangiosarcoma |
| Wood dust | Nasal sinus |
| **Manufacturing** | |
| Anthraquinone dyes | Kidney, liver, urinary bladder |
| Aluminum production | Lung, bladder |
| Auramine manufacture | Bladder |
| Boot and shoe manufacture | Nasal cavity, hematopoietic system |
| Coke production | Skin, lung, kidney |
| Iron and steel founding | Nasal cavity |
| Magenta manufacture | Bladder |
| Painting | Lung |
| Rubber industry | Bladder, hematopoietic system |
| **Medicinal** | |
| Azathioprine | Lymph node, skin |
| Cyclophosphamide | Bladder, bone marrow |
| Estrogens | Cervix, uterus, breast |
| Methoxsalen (8-methoxypsoralen) with UV radiation | Skin |
| Phenacetin | Renal pelvis, bladder |
| Thorotrast (thorium-232) | Liver, bile duct |

for their potential carcinogenicity. To improve the reliability of the results, a battery of these tests is usually conducted (e.g., U.S. ISGC, 1986). Weisburger and Williams (1993) recommended the following short-term *in vitro* tests:

1. Bacterial mutagenesis
2. Mammalian mutagenesis
3. Mammalian cell DNA repair
4. Chromosome integrity
5. Cell transformation

The results of these tests are also useful in defining the mechanism of action. Descriptions of these tests are provided in Chapter 9.

## *Limited carcinogenicity tests*

Limited carcinogenicity tests are superior to the mutagenesis tests in that the endpoint is tumor formation. Further, the duration of these tests is shorter than that of the long-term carcinogenicity studies.

### *Skin tumors in mice*

Mouse skin responds to topical application of chemicals such as PAH and crude products (such as tar from coal and petroleum), by formation of papillomas and carcinomas. This procedure, introduced by Berenblum and Shubik (1947), has been widely used. Mouse skin responds positively because it apparently has the enzymes that convert the substances into active metabolites.

Some chemicals act as both initiators and promoters; they may, therefore, be referred to as complete carcinogens. Others act mainly or exclusively as initiators. Their carcinogenicity is revealed only after the application of a promoter, which is an incomplete carcinogen. Pereira (1982) compiled reports in the literature of the results obtained, through the mouse skin test, on the effects of chemicals as initiators and as promoters.

### *Pulmonary tumors in mice*

Strain A mice spontaneously have an essentially 100% lung tumor incidence by 24 months of age. Positive results from carcinogens can be obtained in about 24 weeks when few controls have tumors. With some chemicals, the test can be completed in 12 weeks.

### *Altered foci in rodent livers*

It has been demonstrated that distinct liver foci appear before the development of hepatocarcinoma. These foci are resistant to iron accumulation, a phenomenon that can be identified histochemically. There are also abnormalities in certain enzymes, which can be demonstrated histochemically. The latter alteration occurs in rats but not mice. These foci can be detected within 3 weeks of exposure and occur in large numbers after 12–16 weeks (Goldfarb and Pugh, 1982).

*Breast cancer in female rats*

Polycyclic hydrocarbons induce breast cancers in young female Sprague–Dawley and Wistar rats. The tumors develop in less than 6 months (Huggins et al., 1959). The Sprague–Dawley rat lacks progesterone but has high estrogen levels.

## *Long-term carcinogenicity studies*

These studies are designed to provide definitive information on the carcinogenic effects of chemicals on the animals. Because of the great expense and time required, they are usually undertaken after a review of other data, such as the chemical structure and results from short-term mutagenesis tests and long-term chronic toxicity studies, which are described, respectively, hereafter and in Chapter 6.

Guidelines on the long-term carcinogenicity studies are outlined in this section. More detailed descriptions and references to some comments are provided in a number of papers (WHO, 1969; OECD, 1981; U.S. ISGC, 1986).

*Animals*

Rats and mice are generally preferred because of their small size, short life span, ready availability, and the relative abundance of information on their response to other carcinogens. Hamsters are also used, especially in studies on cancers of the bladder, breast, gastrointestinal tract, and respiratory tract. Dogs and nonhuman primates are occasionally used for their positive response to 2-naphthylamine; the latter is also used for their higher phylogenetic order. But their use is limited because of their large size and relatively long life span, thereby requiring a 7- to 10-year exposure to the chemical on test.

The characteristics of a preferred strain are as follows:

1. Known sensitivity to substances of similar chemical structure
2. Low incidence of spontaneous tumors
3. Similarity of its rate and pattern of biotransformation and those of humans, if known

Both genders need to be included in these studies; differences in response to the carcinogenic activity of chemicals are well documented. To provide a sufficient number of animals for statistical analysis, which survive until the appearance of tumors, it is a common practice to start the tests with at least 50 animals of each gender per dose group, including controls.

*Inception and duration*

The studies are generally started shortly after weaning the animals to allow maximum duration of exposure. The duration of the studies is generally 24 months in rats and 18 months in mice. If the animals are in good condition, the duration may be extended to 30 and 24 months, respectively.

*Route of administration*

The chemical under test should be given to the animals by the route of human exposure, which is usually oral. This principle readily applies to food additives and contaminants as well as most drugs. For industrial and environmental chemicals, the main route of entry is inhalation. Alternatively, the test chemical may be instilled intratracheally.

*Doses and treatment groups*

Usually two or three dose levels are included in such studies. In addition, control groups are also included for comparison. The doses are selected on the basis of the short-term studies and metabolism data, with the aim that the high dose would produce some minor signs of toxicity but not significantly reduce the life span of the animals. The two lower doses are generally some fractions of the high dose (e.g., one-half and one-quarter) and are expected to permit the animals to survive in good health, or until a tumor develops.

The "maximally tolerated dose" (MTD) is generally used as the high dose in long-term carcinogenicity study. It is estimated from 90-day studies and defined as one that would (i) not produce morphologic evidence of toxicity of a severity that interferes with the interpretation of the long-term study, and (ii) not comprise so large a fraction of the animal's diet that it might lead to nutritional imbalance (U.S. ISGC, 1986), and (iii) not produce toxic effects without causing death and to decrease body weight gain by no more than 10% relative to controls (OECD, 2002). Ideally, the MTD should provide some signs of toxicity without causing tissue necrosis or metabolic saturation, and without substantially altering normal life span due to effects other than tumors. However, the use of MTD has been criticized, especially when it is much higher than the expected human exposure; there is the possibility of alteration of metabolic pattern by "overloading" the animals (Mermelstein et al., 1994).

An untreated group consisting of the same number, or a larger number, of animals as each dose group is included. In addition to these negative controls, another group of animals is often incorporated that is given a known carcinogen at a dose level that has been shown to be carcinogenic. The positive controls provide more confidence in the results on the test chemical by serving as a check on the sensitivity of the particular lot of animals used, as well as the adequacy of the facilities and procedures in the specific laboratory. It will also provide some indication of the relative potency of the test chemical. If a vehicle, such as acetone or dimethyl sulfoxide, is to be used, its possible effect should also be tested in a group of animals as vehicle control.

#### *Observations and examinations*

The animals need to be examined daily for mortality and morbidity. Dead and moribund animals need to be removed from cages for gross and microscopic examinations whenever the condition of the tissues permits. The onset, location, size, and growth of any unusual tissue masses needs to be carefully examined and recorded. Signs of toxicity should also be noted. All animals found dead or dying should be subjected to gross autopsy. The survivors at the end of the study should be sacrificed and examined. In addition, a number of organs need to be weighed, including the liver, kidneys, heart, testes, ovaries, and brain. Samples of all tissues need to be preserved for histologic examination. Microscopic examinations need to be conducted on all tumor growths and all tissues showing gross abnormalities.

#### *Reporting of tumors*

As carcinogenesis can manifest itself in a variety of forms (see the section "Definition and Identification"), it is necessary to record the following:

1. Number of various types of tumors (both benign and malignant) and any unusual tumors
2. Number of tumor-bearing animals
3. Number of tumors in each animal
4. Onset of tumors whenever determinable

## *Evaluation*

### *Preliminary assessment*

#### *Chemical structure*

A number of chemicals are known to be carcinogenic. A list of known human carcinogens is presented in Table 8.3. In addition, a large number of chemicals have been shown to be carcinogenic in animals (see the section "Genotoxic Carcinogens"). As chemicals that have structures similar to any of these or other carcinogens/mutagens are not necessarily carcinogens, they should nevertheless be assigned a high priority in carcinogenicity testing programs. In fact, certain chemical structures have been shown to be correlated with carcinogenicity (Ashby and Tennant, 1988). Doi et al. (2005) demonstrated that substitution of a functional group in the anthraquinone dye resulted in the presence of carcinogenicity, or the absence, or development at a different site. Amino substitutions diminished while bromine substitutions enhanced the carcinogenicity and extended the target tissues to the forestomach and lungs, as well as the kidneys and liver.

#### *Mutagenicity*

Mutagenic agents produce heritable genetic changes essentially through effects on DNA. The mutagenicity tests also provide information on the mode of action as well as on the question as to whether metabolic activation is required for the mutagenicity. Although positive results from these tests do not constitute positive evidence that the chemical is carcinogenic, they do indicate that extensive testing is required. Further, mutagenesis data are useful in the risk assessment of the chemical in question. On the other hand, negative results do not establish the safety of the chemical.

#### *Limited carcinogenicity tests*

The endpoint in these tests is tumor formation. Therefore, certain chemicals, such as cocarcinogens that yield negative results in mutagenesis tests, may be positive in these tests. Positive results from more than one of these limited carcinogenicity tests may be considered unequivocal qualitative evidence of carcinogenicity.

### *Definitive assessment*

Data from well-designed and properly executed long-term carcinogenicity studies generally provide a reliable basis for assessment of carcinogenic potential.

#### *General considerations*

Results from these studies are generally more reliable than those from rapid screening tests. However, the conclusiveness of the results depends upon a number of factors. For example, too few animals surviving until tumor development may preclude statistical analysis of data. This event may occur as a result of insufficient animals placed in each dosage group and/or excessive mortality resulting from improper husbandry, or from competing toxicity of the chemical given at inordinately high-dose levels. The thoroughness of the postmortem examination also plays an important role. This applies to the gross and the microscopic examinations.

#### *Tumor incidence*

As noted at the beginning of the chapter, carcinogenesis may manifest itself in one of four ways, or any combination thereof. An appreciable increase in the tumor-bearing animals is the most common fashion. The occurrence of unusual tumors is an important phenomenon if there are a significant number of them; when one or only a few of them are detected, further critical examination is required. An increase in the number of tumors per animal, without a concomitant elevation in tumor-bearing animals, usually indicates cocarcinogenicity only. The tumors in the experimental animals may not be at the same stage of development. The stages may include, for example, atypical hyperplasia, benign tumors, carcinomas in situ, invasion of adjacent tissues, and metastasis to other parts of the body. Although tumors of the same type but at different stages need to be separately tabulated, these should be combined for statistical analysis.

#### *Dose–response relationship*

Generally, a positive dose–response relationship is apparent. However, there may be a lower tumor incidence in a high-dose group. This phenomenon usually results from poor survival among these animals, which succumb to competing toxic effects of the chemical.

#### *Reproducibility of the results*

The confidence in a carcinogenicity study is enhanced if the results are produced in another strain of animals, as reproducibility in another species is even more significant. However, if negative results are obtained in another species, this fact may not nullify the positive findings but does justify further investigation.

## *Evaluation of safety/risks*

The various approaches used in the evaluation of the safety/risk of carcinogens are discussed in Chapter 30. The following points, however, are worth emphasizing.

First, while the tests enumerated above are a valuable basis for risk/safety assessment, other data relating to the mechanism of action and influences of modifying factors are also essential (U.S. ISGC, 1986). The significant differences between genotoxic and nongenotoxic carcinogens are also considered as valid reasons for assessing their risks differently: it is generally presumed that genotoxic carcinogens exhibit no threshold, whereas nongenotoxic carcinogens induce cancer secondary to other biological effects which are likely to show no-effect dose levels. However, a chemical, such as chloroform, may act as an epigenetic as well as a genotoxic carcinogen.

Further, there are chemicals with carcinogenicity secondary to noncarcinogenic biologic or physical effects that are elicited only at dose levels that could never be approached in realistic human exposure situations. There was general consensus that there are threshold doses for such secondary carcinogens (Lu, 1976; Munro, 1988). The U.S. ISGC (1986) also cautions that extremely high doses of a toxicant may exhibit *qualitatively* different distribution, detoxication, and elimination of the toxicant. The response at such doses, therefore, may not be applicable to more realistic exposure conditions. In addition, evidence of extensive tissue damage, disruption of hormonal function, formation of urinary stones, and saturation of DNA repair function need to be carefully reviewed.

Carcinogens also differ in their potency and latency periods. Some carcinogens are active in a particular species, whereas others affect several species and strains of animals. All these factors must be taken into account in evaluating the safety/risk of carcinogens. The type of tumor observed needs to be taken into account if one is comparing rodent to human data, especially if the tumor is species-dependent and does not have relevance for humans.

Finally, it is important to bear in mind that chemicals differ tremendously in their value to humans. For example, the use of a food color can often be suspended on the basis of suggestive carcinogenicity data. On the other hand, life-saving drugs, even when there is evidence of their carcinogenicity in humans, may still be used clinically. There are also environmental carcinogens, including those in food, that cannot be eliminated with present technology (see also Ames, 1989). The concentration of chemical is crucial in the decision making process if one is to ban a chemical due to its carcinogenic properties.

## *Appendix 8.1 Biomarkers of carcinogenesis/ human cancers*

### *Biomarkers of exposure and initiation*

Initiation is associated with covalent binding of electrophilic carcinogens or their reactive metabolites to DNA. The carcinogen–DNA adduct can be demonstrated and quantified to indicate exposure and effect of the carcinogen. This procedure has been applied to situations wherein human exposure to a particular carcinogen is suspected, for example, in the determination of exposure to aflatoxin $B_1$ and its relationship to hepatocellular carcinoma (Qian et al., 1994).

### *Biomarker of promotion*

Promotion has been most extensively studied in skin carcinogenesis. A variety of biochemical changes have been noted in initiated as well as normal cells on treatment with promoters, the most active of which is TPA (12-*o*-tetradecanoyl phorbol-13-acetate). The changes include accumulation of plasminogen activator and increased prostaglandin synthesis. Growth factors, protein kinase C, TPA- and dioxin-responsive elements in genes, interaction of promoters with oncogenes, and/or suppressor genes are being studied to determine their role as markers of preneoplasia in the liver.

### *Tumor markers*

α-Fetoprotein (AFP) is a product of fetal liver and hepatocarcinoma. AFP had, therefore, been used to screen large populations for hepatocellular carcinomas, allowing early detection and treatment. However, it has been shown to be nonspecific. Human chorionic gonadotropin (HCG) is a sensitive marker and can be used to detect cancers of male and female sex organs at a subclinical phase. Carcinoembryonic antigen (CEA) is found in patients with carcinoma of the colon and rectum. Prostate-specific antigen (PSA) has been shown to be a useful biomarker of tumor and other lesions of the prostate. CA 125 is useful in diagnosing and monitoring treatment of ovarian cancer. Telomerase is a ribonucleoprotein enzyme that adds TTAGGG repeats onto telomeres to compensate for shortening and instability of desmosomes. Telomerase is detected in most cancers and immortal cell lines. Oncogene expression, tumor suppressor gene inactivation, formation of DNA and protein adducts, and endogenous production of paraneoplastic hormones by the tumor are all potential useful tools for the determination of which specific agents interact with cells to produce tumors.

### *Biomarkers of susceptibility*

Individuals with certain genetic disposition may be more susceptible to carcinogenesis. For example, those with xeroderma pigmentosa are prone to skin cancer. Polymorphism of x-oxidation has been linked to susceptibility to colon cancer (Kadlubar et al., 1992) and polymorphism in glutathione S-transferase to increased lung cancer (Seidegard et al., 1990). In the case of arsenic-induced carcinogenesis, polymorphism in the genes encoding the enzymes involved in the methylation of arsenic can lead to increased frequency of skin cancer (Steinmaus et al., 2007). A single nucleotide polymorphism in the JWA gene was found to be associated with a higher frequency of leukemia in the Chinese population (Zhu et al., 2007).

Genetic polymorphisms in various metabolic enzymes were attributed to result in a higher frequency of benzene-induced carcinogenesis in China (Gu et al., 2007).

## Further reading

WHO (1993). Biomarkers and Risk Assessment: Concepts and Principles. Environ Health Criteria 155. Geneva: World Health Organization.

## References

Alam H, Gu B, Lee MG (2015). Histone methylation modifiers in cellular signaling pathways. *Cell Mol Life Sci.* 72, 4577–92.

Ames, BN (1989). What are the major carcinogens in the etiology of human cancer? Environmental pollution, natural carcinogens, and the causes of human cancer: Six errors. In: De Vita VT Jr et al. eds. *Important Advances in Oncology.* Philadelphia, PA: J. P. Lippincott.

Arita A, Costa M (2009). Epigenetics in metal carcinogenesis: Nickel, arsenic, chromium and cadmium. *Metallomics.* 1, 222–8.

Ashby J, Tennant RW (1988). Chemical structure, Salmonella mutagenicity and extent of carcinogenicity among 222 chemicals tested in rodents by the U.S. NCI/NTP. *Mutat Res.* 204, 17–115.

Berenblum I, Shubik P (1947). A new quantitative approach to the study of the stages of chemical carcinogenesis in the mouse's skin. *Br J Cancer.* 1, 383–91.

Berenblum I, Shubik P (1949). An experimental study of the initiating stage of carcinogenesis, and a re-examination of the somatic cell mutation theory of cancer. *Br J Cancer.* 3, 109–18.

Bernstam L, Nriagu J (2000). Molecular aspects of arsenic stress. *J Toxicol Environ Health B.* 3, 293–322.

Bishop JM (1987). The molecular genetics of cancer. *Science.* 235, 305–11.

Butterworth BE, Goldworthy TL (1991). The role of cell proliferation in multistage carcinogenesis. *Proc Soc Exp Biol Med.* 198, 683–7.

Cedar H, Bergman Y (2009). Linking DNA methylation and histone modification: Patterns and paradigms. *Nature Rev Genetics.* 10, 295–304.

Chou IN (1989). Distinct cytoskeletal injuries induced by As, Cd, Co, Cr, and Ni compounds. *Biomed Environ Sci.* 2, 358–65.

Clark HA, Snedeker SM (2006). Ochratoxin A: Its cancer risk and potential for exposure. *J Toxicol Environ Health B.* 9, 265–96.

Cook JW, Hewett CL, Hieger I (1933). The isolation of a cancer-producing hydrocarbon from coal tar. Parts I, II and III. *J Chem Soc.* 24, 395–405.

Doi AM, Irwin RD, Bucher JR (2005). Influence of functional group substitutions on the carcinogenicity of anthraquinone in rats and mice: Analysis of long-term bioassays by the National Cancer Institute and the National Toxicology Program. *J Toxicol Environ Health B.* 8: 109–26.

Ducasse M, Brown MA (2006). Epigenetic aberrations and cancer. *Mol Cancer* 5, 60.

Environmental Protection Agency (EPA). (1996). Guidelines for Carcinogen Risk Assessment. Fed Reg 61, 17957–8010.

Feinberg AP, Ohlsson R, Henikoff S (2006). The epigenetic progenitor origin of human cancer. *Nat Rev Genet*. 7, 21–33.

Goldfarb S, Pugh MB (1982). The origin and significance of hyperplastic hepatocellular islands and nodules in hepatic carcinogenesis. *J Am Coll Toxicol*. 1, 119–44.

Greenblatt MS, Bennett NP, Hollstein M et al. (1994). Mutations in the p53 tumor suppressor gene: Clues to cancer etiology and molecular pathogenesis. *Cancer Res*. 55, 4855–78.

Gu S-Y, Zhang Z-B, Wan J-X et al. (2007). Genetic polymorphism in CYP1A1, CYP2D6, UGT1A6, UGT1A7 and SULT1A1 genes and correlation with benzene exposure in a Chinese occupational population. *J Toxicol Environ Health A*. 70, 916–24.

Hanahan D, Weinberg RA (2011). Hallmarks of cancer: The next generation. *Cell*. 144, 646–74.

Huggins C, Briziarelli G, Sutton H Jr. (1959). Rapid induction of mammary carcinoma in the rat and the influence of hormones on the tumors. *J Exp Med*. 109, 25–41.

IARC. (1987). Monographs for Carcinogenic Chemicals: Overall Evaluation of Carcinogenicity: An Updating of IARC Monographs. Vols. 1–42 (suppl. 7). Lyon, France: International Agency for Research on Cancer.

Jomova K, Valko M (2011). Advances in metal-induced oxidative stress and human disease. *Toxicology*. 283, 65–87.

Jones PA, Laird PW (1999). Cancer epigenetics comes of age. *Nat Genet*. 21, 163–167.

Kadlubar FF, Butler MA, Kaderlick KR et al. (1992). Polymorphisms for aromatic amine metabolism in humans: Relevance for human carcinogenesis. *Environ Health Perspect*. 98, 69–74.

Kanwal R, Gupta S (2010). Epigenetics and cancer. *J Appl Physiol*. 109, 598–605.

Kanwal R, Gupta S (2012). Epigenetic modifications in cancer. *Clin Genetics*. 81, 303–11.

Kim HS, Kacew S, Lee BM (2016). Genetic and epigenetic cancer chemoprevention on molecular targets during multistage carcinogenesis. *Arch Toxicol*. 90, 2389–404.

Klaunig JE (1991). Alterations in intercellular communication during the stage of promotion. *Proc Soc Exp Biol Med*. 198, 688–92.

Kwack SJ, Lee BM (2000). Correlation between DNA or protein adducts and benzo(a) pyrene diol epoxide I-triglyceride adduct detected in vitro and in vivo. *Carcinogenesis*. 21, 629–32.

Lake BG (1995). Mechanisms of hepatocarcinogenicity of peroxisome-proliferating drugs and chemicals. *Ann Rev Pharmacol Toxicol*. 35, 483–507.

Lu FC (1976). Threshold doses in chemical carcinogenesis: Introductory remarks. *Oncology*. 33, 50.

McClain, RM (1989). The significance of hepatic microsomal enzyme induction and altered thyroid function in rats: Implications for thyroid gland neoplasia. *Toxicol Pathol*. 17, 294–306.

Melnick RL (2001). Is peroxisome proliferation an obligatory precursor step in the carcinogenicity of di(2-ethylhexyl)phthalate (DEHP)? *Environ Health Perspect*. 109, 437–42.

Mermelstein R, Marrow PE, Christian MS (1994). Organ or system overload and its regulatory implications. *J Am Col Toxicol*. 13, 143–7.

Munro IC (1988). Risk assessment of carcinogens: Present status and future directions. *Biomed Environ Sci*. 1, 51–8.

Nestmann ER, Lynch BS, Ratpan F (2005). Perspectives on the genotoxic risk of styrene. *J Toxicol Environ Health B*. 8, 95–107.

OECD. (1981). OECD Guidelines for Testing of Chemicals. Paris, France: Organization for Economic Cooperation and Development.

OECD. (2002). Guidance notes for analysis and evaluation of chronic toxicity and carcinogenicity studies. OECD series on testing and assessment no. 35, OECD, Paris. Online. Available from: http://www.olis.oecd.org/olis/2002doc.nsf/LinkTo/NT00002BE2/$FILE/JT00130828.PDF.

Pereira MA (1982). Mouse skin bioassay for chemical carcinogens. *J Am Coll Toxicol*. 1, 47–82.

Pitot HC, Beer D, Hendrich S (1988). Multistage carcinogenesis: The phenomenon underlying the theories. In: Iversen OH, ed. *Theories of Carcinogenesis*. Washington, DC: Hemisphere.

Poirier MC, Yuspa SH, Weinstein IB et al. (1977). Detection of carcinogen-DNA adducts by radioimmunoassay. *Nature*. 270, 186–8.

Pott P (1775). Cancer scroti. In: *Chirurgical Observations Relative to the Cataract, the Polypus of the Nose, the Cancer of the Scrotum, the Different Kinds of Ruptures, and the Modification of the Toes and Feet*. London: Hawes: Clarke, Collins, pp. 63–8.

Pyatt DW, Aylward LL, Hays SM (2007). Is age an independent risk factor for chemically induced acute myelogenous leukemia in children? *J Toxicol Environ Health B*. 10, 379–400.

Qian GS, Ross RK, Yu MC et al. (1994). A follow-up study of urinary markers of aflatoxin exposure and liver cancer risk in Shanghai, China. *Cancer Epidemiol Biomarkers Prev*. 3, 3–10.

Reddy JK, Lalwani ND (1983). Carcinogenesis by hepatic peroxisome proliferators: Evaluation of the risk of hyperlipidemic drugs and industrial plasticizers to humans. *CRC Crit Rev Toxicol*. 12, 1–58.

Ryffel B (1992). The carcinogenicity of cyclosporin. *Toxicology*. 73, 1–22.

Seidegard J, Pero RW, Markowitz MM et al. (1990). Isoenzyme(s) of glutathione transferase (class mu) as a marker for susceptibility to lung cancer: A follow-up study. *Carcinogenesis*. 11, 33–6.

Shi X, Castranova V, Halliwell B et al. (1998). Reactive oxygen species and silica-induced carcinogenesis. *J Toxicol Environ Health B*. 1, 181–97.

Shi X, Chiu A, Chen CT et al. (1999). Reduction of chromium (VI) and its relationship to carcinogenesis. *J Toxicol Environ Health B*. 2, 87–104.

Steinmaus C, Moore LE, Shipp M et al. (2007). Genetic polymorphism in MTHFR 677 and 1298, GSTM1 and T1 and metabolism of arsenic. *J Toxicol Environ Health A*. 70, 159–70.

Sugimura T, Ushijima T (2000). Genetic and epigenetic alterations in carcinogenesis. *Mutat Res*. 462, 235–46.

Sunderman FW Jr (1984). Recent advances in metal carcinogenesis. *Am Clin Lab Sci*. 14, 93–122.

Swenberg JA, Short B, Borghoff S et al. (1989). The comparative pathobiology of $\alpha 2_{\mu}$-globulin nephropathy. *Toxicol Appl Pharmacol*. 97, 35–46.

Trosko JE, Chang CC (1988). Chemical and oncogene modulation of gap junctional intercellular communication. In: Langenbach R et al. eds. *Tumor Promoters: Biological Approaches for Mechanistic Studies and Assay Systems*. New York: Raven Press.

U.S. ISGC (1986). Chemical carcinogens: A review of the science and its associated principles. U.S. Interagency Staff on Carcinogens. *Environ Health Persp.* 67, 201–82.

Vallyathan V, Green F, Ducatman B et al. (1998). Roles of epidemiology, pathology, molecular biology, and biomarkers in the investigation of occupational lung cancer. *J Toxicol Environ Health B.* 1, 91–116.

WHO (1969). Principles for the testing and evaluation of drugs for carcinogenicity. *WHO Tech Rep Ser.* 426, 5–26.

Weinberg RA (1989). Oncogenes, antioncogenes, and the molecular bases of multistep carcinogenesis. *Cancer Res.* 49, 3713–21.

Weisburger JH, Williams GM (1993). Chemical carcinogenesis. In: Amdur MO, Doull J, Klaassen CD, eds. *Casarett and Doull's Toxicology.* New York: McGraw-Hill, pp. 127–200.

Wyde M, Cesta M, Blystone C et al. (2016). Report of Partial findings from the National Toxicology Program Carcinogenesis Studies of Cell Phone Radiofrequency Radiation in Hsd: Sprague Dawley® SD rats (Whole Body Exposure). bioRxiv, doi: http://dx.doi.org/10.1101/055699.

Yamagiwa K, Ichikawa K (1918). Experimental study of the pathogenesis of carcinoma. *J Cancer Res.* 3, 1–21.

Yoo CB, Jones PA (2006). Epigenetic therapy of cancer: Past, present and future. *Nat. Rev. Drug Discov.* 5, 37–50.

Zhu Y-J, Li C-P, Tang W-Y et al. (2007). Single nucleotide polymorphism of the JWA gene is associated with risk of leukemia: A case-control study in a Chinese population. *J Toxicol Environ Health A.* 70, 895–900.

# chapter nine

# Mutagenesis

**Kyung-Soo Chun and Hyung Sik Kim**

Contents

## Introduction

Mutagenesis can occur as a result of interaction between mutagenic agents (mutagens) and genetic materials present in organisms. Although spontaneous mutations and natural selection are the major means of evolution, in recent decades, a number of toxicants have been found to induce mutagenic effects in a variety of organisms. Mutations can be produced by external factors (e.g., high temperatures), toxic chemicals (most carcinogens, etc.), radiation (ionizing and nonionizing), as well as internal factors (e.g., cellular metabolism and respiration, reactive oxygen species, and reactive nitrogen species), and DNA replication/transcription error. Electromagnetic fields and free radicals generated from electronic equipment/devices, medical devices (e.g., x-ray, MRI, etc.), electricity, microwaves, radar, and cellular phones could be sources of mutations. Mutations are classified into microlesions (e.g., gene mutation: frame shift and base substitution) and macro lesions (e.g., chromosomal abnormalities: gap, fragments, deletion, ring, translocation, and numerical change). Some individuals exhibit mutations in skin cells or other tissues, termed somatic mutations. In contrast, germ mutations occur only in the sex cells and are more threatening because they are transmitted to subsequent generations.

## Health hazards in humans

The hereditary effects of human exposure to these mutagenic substances cannot be ascertained at present. However, some spontaneous abortions, stillbirths, and heritable diseases have been shown to be related to changes in DNA molecules and chromosomal aberrations. There are approximately 1000 dominant gene mutations responsible for various illnesses, including hereditary neoplasms such as bilateral retinoblastoma, and about the same number of recessive gene disorders such as sickle-cell anemia, cystic fibrosis, and Tay–Sachs disease. In addition, abnormal chromosomal numbers are associated with diseases such as Down's syndrome, Klinefelter syndrome, and Edward's syndrome. These have been estimated to occur with an incidence of 0.5% among the live births in the United States. The true effects of any additional mutagen in the environment can only be manifested after a lapse of several generations. The seriousness of this matter, therefore, warrants extensive investigations in various fields of mutagenesis. It is also worth noting that various gene mutations and chromosomal abnormalities have been detected in human tumors. Some examples are listed in Table 9.1. For more information on this topic, see Rabbitts' review (1994).

A number of human diseases are the result of defects of the DNA repair systems. These defects often lead to an increased incidence of cancer. Table 9.2 summarizes information about these diseases, which are

***Table 9.1*** Examples of chromosomal abnormalities associated with human cancers

| Neoplasm | Abnormality of chromosome |
|---|---|
| Chronic myelogenous leukemia | Translocation of chromosomes 9 and 22 |
| Acute monocytic leukemia | Loss of long arm of chromosome 11 |
| Small-cell lung cancer | Loss of short arm of chromosome 6 |
| Myeloproliferative diseases | Extra chromosome 1 |
| Retinoblastoma | Deletion of chromosome 13 |
| Down's syndrome | Trisomy 21 |
| Edward's syndrome | Trisomy 18 |
| Turner syndrome | Only one sex chromosome, an X |
| Klinefelter syndrome | Translocation of chromosomes 21 and 22 |
| Ewing's sarcoma | Translocation of chromosomes 1 and 22 |
| Acute megakaryoblastic leukemia | Translocation of chromosomes 2 and 3 |
| Burkitt's lymphoma | Translocation of chromosomes (8;14),(2;8),(8;22) |

***Table 9.2*** Examples of human diseases with DNA-repair defects

| Disease | Cancer susceptibility | Symptoms |
|---|---|---|
| Ataxia telangiectasia | Lymphomas | Ataxia, dilation of blood vessels (telangiectases) in skin and eyes, chromosome aberrations, immune dysfunction |
| Bloom's syndrome | Carcinomas, leukemias, lymphomas | Photosensitivity, facial telangiectases, chromosome alterations |
| Cockayne syndrome | Mental retardation, (normally no cancer is associated) | Dwarfism, retinal atrophy, photosensitivity, progeria, deafness, trisomy 10 |
| Fanconi's anemia | Leukemias | Hypoplastic pancytopenia, congenital anomalies |
| Xeroderma pigmentosum | Skin carcinomas and melanomas | Skin and eye photosensitivity, keratoses |

*Source:* Kornberg A, Baker T, *DNA replication*, 2nd ed. W.H. Freeman, Oxford, UK, 1992.

usually autosomal recessive disorders. For example, patients with xeroderma pigmentosa are deficient in excision repair in the skin; they are susceptible to ultraviolet light and many chemical carcinogens and thus are prone to developing skin tumors. Those with ataxia telangiectasia have such deficiencies in the lymphoid system and are susceptible to x-rays and the carcinogen methyl nitro-nitrosoguanidine. Fanconi's anemia is associated with defective DNA repair in the blood and skeleton. Cockayne syndrome patients are also sun sensitive but exhibit distinctive congenital neurological and skeletal abnormalities, including mental deficiency and dwarfism (Nance and Berry, 1992). Cells from these patients are sensitive to UV irradiation and have a defective RNA synthesis after UV. The afflicted persons are susceptible to mitomycin C and psoralens.

On the other hand, tests for mutagenicity have become more widely used in recent years because of their value as a rapid screening for carcinogenicity (see Chapter 8). This development stems mainly from the fact that most mutagens have been found to be carcinogens. Further, these tests, with a variety of endpoints, are useful in the elaboration of the mode of action of carcinogens.

## *Categories of mutagenesis and their tests*

Attempts to identify human carcinogens by short-term tests began with the use of a bacterial mutagenesis assay. It is well known that DNA, consisting of nucleotide bases, plays a key role in genetics. First, it transmits the genetic information from one generation of cells to the next through self-replication. This is done by the separation of the double strands of the DNA molecule and the synthesis of new daughter strands. Second, the genetic information coded in the DNA molecule is expressed through the transcription of a complementary RNA strand from one strand of DNA, which serves as a template, and the subsequent translation of the information from the RNA to the amino acids in proteins. Every set of three nucleotide bases, a codon, specifies an amino acid. Derangement of the bases, therefore, alters the amino acid content of the protein synthesized.

In earlier studies, mutagenic activity was demonstrated mainly in fruit flies and onion root tips because of the simpler techniques involved. More recently, many new test systems have been developed. These range in complexity from microorganisms to intact mammals. The use of such widely different organisms is based on the fact that all double-stranded DNA share the same biochemical characteristics, which are listed in Table 9.3.

At present, there are more than 100 test systems. A number of exemplary tests are outlined in this chapter under four major categories, namely, gene mutation, chromosomal effects, DNA repair, and recombination, as

***Table 9.3*** Basic biochemical characteristics of all double-stranded DNA

1. DNA consists of two different purines (G, A) and two different pyrimidines (T, C).
2. A nucleotide pair consists of one purine and one pyrimidine [adenine/thymine (A–T) or guanine/cytosine (G–C)].
3. Nucleotide pairs are connected to a double helix molecule by sugar-phosphate backbone linkages and hydrogen bonding.
4. The A–T base pair is held by two hydrogen bonds, while the G–C is held by three.
5. The distance between each base pair in a molecule is 3.4 Å, producing 10 nucleotide pairs per turn of the DNA helix.
6. The number of adenine molecules must equal the number of thymine molecules in a DNA molecule. The same relationship exists for guanine and cytosine molecules. However, the ratio of A–T to G–C base pairs may vary in DNA from species to species.
7. The two strands of the double helix are complementary and antiparallel with respect to the polarity of the two sugar-phosphate backbones, one strand being 3′–5′ and the other being 5′–3′ with respect to the terminal OH group on the ribose sugar.
8. DNA replicates by a semiconservative method in which the two strands separate and each is used as a template for the synthesis of a new complementary strand.
9. The rate of DNA nucleotide polymerization during replication is approximately 600 nucleotides per second. The helix must unwind to form templates at a rate of 3600 rpm to accommodate this replication rate.
10. The DNA content of cells is variable ($1.8 \times 10^9$ Da for *Escherichia coli* to $1.9 \times 10^{11}$ Da for human cells).

*Source:* Brusick DJ, *Principles of Genetic Toxicology*, 2nd ed. Plenum Press, New York, 1987.

well as others designed to confirm carcinogenicity. Because of the brevity of their description, at least one reference is cited for each test. Additional references and more details are given elsewhere on these and other tests (OECD, 1987; EPA, 1994; Hoffmann, 1996).

It is worth noting that gene mutation may be detected in all organisms including bacteria. On the other hand, effects related to chromosomes (aberrations, aneuploidy, and DNA repair) can be detected only in higher organisms, that is, those with chromosomes.

## *Gene mutations*

Gene mutations involve additions or deletions of base pairs or substitution of a wrong base pair in DNA molecules. Substitutions consist of transitions and transversions. The former involve the replacement of a purine (adenine, guanine) by another or a pyrimidine (cytosine, thymine) by another. With transversion, a purine is replaced by a pyrimidine, or vice versa. When the number of base pairs added or deleted is not a multiple of three, the amino acid sequence of the protein coded distal to the addition or deletion will be altered. This phenomenon is called frameshift mutation and is likely to affect the biological property of the protein. Figure 9.1 clearly illustrates the effects of a deletion and an addition of a nucleotide base.

In addition, a mutagenic chemical, or a part of it, may be incorporated into the DNA molecule. For example, a number of electrophilic compounds react with DNA forming covalent addition products, known as "DNA adducts." Thus acetyl aminofluorene (AAF) binds specifically to the carbon at the eight position of guanine. For a partial list of such chemicals, see discussions on procarcinogens in "Categories of Carcinogens" in Chapter 8. Alkylating agents, such as ethylnitrosourea and diethyl sulfate, donate an alkyl group to DNA. Further, each mutagenic agent shows a predilection for damaging specific nucleotides, which produce recognizable patterns of DNA base pairs. DNA substitution mutations are of two types. Transitions are interchanges of two-ring purines (A<->G) or of one-ring pyrimidines (C<->T): they therefore involve bases of similar shape. Transversions are interchanges of purine for pyrimidine bases,

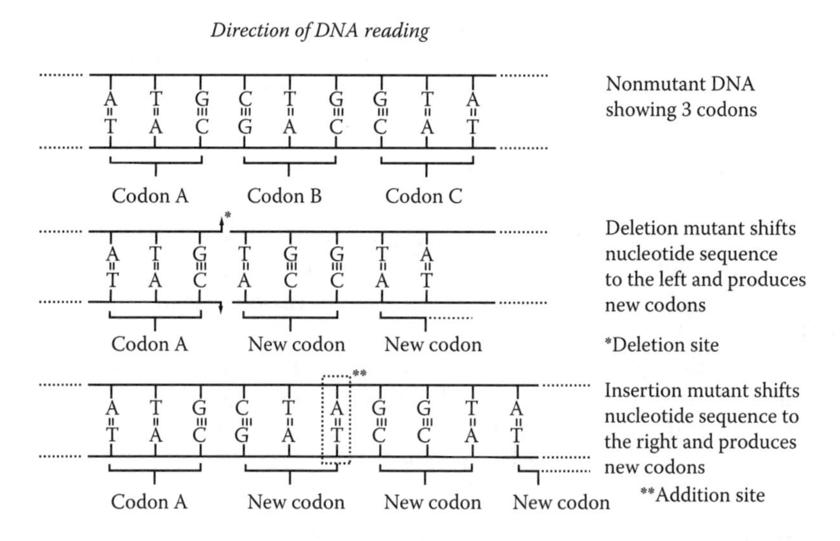


***Figure 9.1*** Frameshift mutations resulting from deletion or insertion of a nucleotide base. A series of new codons is formed distal to the deletion or insertion, and hence new amino acids in the protein synthesized. (From Brusick DJ, *Principles of Genetic Toxicology*, 2nd ed. Plenum Press, New York, 1987.)

***Table 9.4*** Mutations induced by DNA damaging agents[a]

| Modifying agents | Example | Recognized base | Base pairing Old | Base pairing New |
|---|---|---|---|---|
| Small adduct | G -> Me.G | A | G:C | A:T |
| Large adduct | G -> G.B(a)P | T | G:C | T:A |
| UV light | Cytosine dimers | T | G:C | A:T |
| Oxidants | G -> 8-OHdG | T | G:C | T:A |
| Oxidants | Strand breaks | | Deletions | |
| Ionizing radiation | Strand breaks | | Deletions | |
| Spontaneous | C/MeC deamination | T | G:C | A:T |

*Note:* A, G, C, T, DNA bases; Me.G, methylguanine; B(a)P, benzo(a)pyrene.

[a] There are the major mutations; others occur with each agent.

which therefore involve the exchange of one-ring and two-ring structures. The imino tautomer of adenine can pair with cytosine, eventually leading to a transition from A-T to G-C (Table 9.4).

These various changes in the DNA molecule may cause the substitution of a new amino acid in the subsequently coded protein molecule or result in a different sequence of amino acids in the protein synthesized. Further, a protein synthesis termination codon may be formed, yielding a shortened protein. While the first type of effect may or may not result in a modification of the biological property of the protein molecule, the latter two types almost invariably do.

## *Mitochondrial mutagenesis*

Even though the mitochondrial genome is considerably shorter in comparison with nuclear DNA (nDNA) ($3 \times 10^9$ bp), it is important for maintenance of stable respiratory functions of each individual cell and therefore of a whole organism. Despite the smaller number of genes in mitochondria, the mutation rate is 10 to 16-fold higher than nuclear mutations (Chinnery and Samuels, 1999). There are several factors that produce damage to mitochondria and their genome (Paraskevaidi, 2016). First, mitochondrial DNA (mtDNA) is adversely affected by its closeness to the electron transfer chain system, where high levels of ROS are produced, as well as by its histone-free packaging and insufficiency of repair mechanisms, compared with nDNA. Second, it is possible for various environmental contaminants, such as lipophilic compounds (e.g., PAHs) or heavy metals (e.g., Hg, Pb, or Cd), to accumulate in the phospholipid membranes of mitochondria, which results in dysfunctionality. Finally, another potential reason for mitochondrial impairment is the contribution of cytochrome P450 (CYPs), which bioactivates inert chemicals accumulated in mitochondrial membranes, such as environmental toxicants, and transform them to their toxic metabolite form.

Epigenetic changes on mtDNA such as methylation and hydroxymethylation, produced by environmental factors, alter mtDNA expression and subsequently lead to further alterations of nDNA (Shock et al. 2011). These events result in modification of genome, which may initiate a variety of diseases. Dysfunctionality of mitochondria jeopardizes cell energy production, and this limits energy and affects the function of all organs and especially those with high energy demands such as the brain, muscle, liver, heart, and kidneys (Chinnery et al., 1999).

## *Microbial tests* in vitro

These involve prokaryotic and eukaryotic microorganisms. Prokaryotic microorganisms consist of various strains of bacteria. For the detection of point mutations, the most commonly used bacteria are *Salmonella typhimurium* and *Escherichia coli*. Most bacterial systems are intended to detect reverse mutation. For example, the Ames test (Ames, 1971) measures the reversion of histidine-dependent mutants (His–, auxotroph) of *S. typhimurium* to the histidine-independent wild type (His+, autotroph). The mutants are incubated in a medium that contains insufficient histidine to permit visible growth. If the toxicant added to the culture medium is capable of inducing reverse mutation, then the bacteria can become histidine-independent and grow appreciably in the histidine-deficient medium (Figure 9.2). It is customary to use several strains because of their specificity. Their mutation to histidine independency results from either frameshift or base-pair substitution; different mutagens may affect one strain but not the other.

A number of strains of *S. typhimurium* have been rendered more sensitive to the effects of mutagens through alterations in the permeability of their cell walls (deficient in lipopolysaccharide) and in their DNA excision repair capabilities (through a specific deletion in the DNA molecule) and through the bearing of an ampicillin-resistance factor (Ames et al., 1975; McCann et al., 1975). These various tester strains (e.g., TA 98, 100, 1535, 1537, and 1538) may be susceptible to different mutagens.

As many mutagens are inactive before bioactivation, the test can be carried out with a bioactivating system included in the *in vitro* procedure. The bioactivating system, called S-9, usually consists of the microsomal fraction (containing the mixed-function oxidase system) of the liver of the rat or other animals, although human liver is also used for special purposes. The activity of the microsomal enzyme is usually enhanced by pretreating the animal with an inducing agent, such as 3-methylcholanthrene,

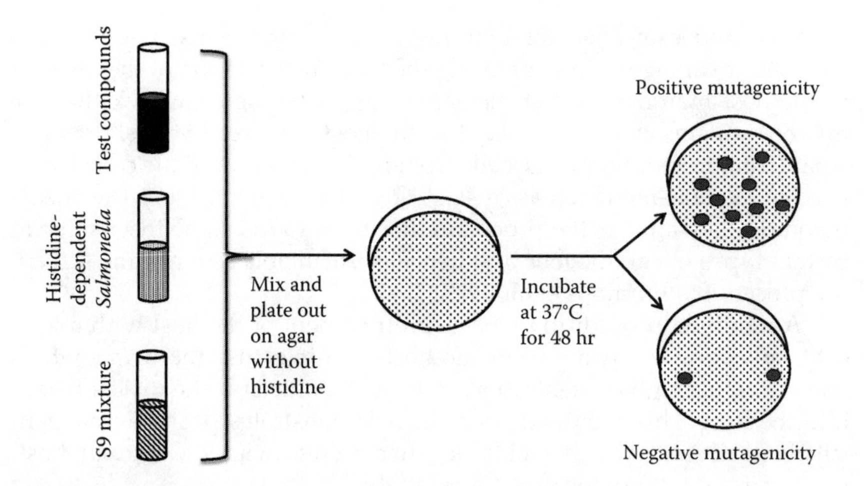


***Figure 9.2*** The Ames test for mutagenicity is commonly used as a first step for assessing carcinogens. (From Brusick DJ, *Principles of Genetic Toxicology,* 2nd ed. Plenum Press, New York, 1987.)

phenobarbital, or polychlorinated biphenyls. Appropriate cofactors are also added to the mixture prior to incubation. Strains of *E. coli* that are tryptophan-dependent are also used to detect reverse mutation. Mutagenic changes result in tryptophan-independent strains (Ames et al., 1975).

## *Eukaryotic microorganisms*

Certain strains of *Saccharomyces, Schizosaccharomyces, Neurospora,* and *Aspergillus* have been developed mainly to detect reverse mutations and, to a limited extent, forward mutations. Similar to bacterial systems, these systems in general also include bioactivating enzymes and cofactors. For example, a type of mutant of *Saccharomyces cerevisiae* requires adenine and produces red-pigmented colonies, whereas the wild-type microorganisms are adenine-independent and produce white colonies. Thus, the reverse mutation can be determined by the prevalence of white colonies (Brusick and Mayer, 1973).

## *Microbial tests:* In vivo *(host-mediated assay)*

In this type of test, the microorganisms are injected into the peritoneal cavity of the host mammal (usually the mouse). They can also be injected into the circulatory system or the testes. The toxicant is injected into the host, usually prior to the introduction of the microorganisms. After an elapse of a few hours, the host is sacrificed. The microorganisms are then collected and examined for manifestations of mutations. These assays have the advantage of incorporating the biotransformation of the toxicant in the host mammal, but at the same time have the drawback that the microorganisms can only be kept in the host for a relatively short time. Apart from microorganisms, cells from multicellular animals can also be used in the host-mediated assay (Gabridge and Legator, 1969). Despite its theoretical advantage, the procedure has been found to be insensitive to certain types of carcinogens and hence is unsuitable as a routine screening procedure (Simmons et al., 1979).

A modified procedure involves pretreatment of the host with a toxicant, collecting the urine from the host, and injecting the urine, which may contain a high concentration of the metabolite(s) of the toxicant, back into the host. This modified procedure demonstrates positive mutagenicity with 2-AAF, which yields negative results with the regular host-mediated assay (Durston and Ames, 1974).

### *Insects*

The fruit fly *Drosophila melanogaster* is the most commonly used insect. It is well characterized genetically. It has an advantage over microorganisms in that it metabolizes toxicants in a manner that is similar to mammals. Further, it is superior to mammals in two respects, namely, its generation time is only 12–14 days and it can be tested in sufficient numbers at a much lower cost.

The sex-linked recessive lethal test measures the lethal effect on the $F_2$ males after exposing the males of the parental generation. It is the preferred procedure because the X chromosome represents about 20% of the total genome, and it is capable of screening for point mutations and short deletions at about 800 loci on the X chromosome (Lee et al., 1983).

### *Mammalian cells in culture*

The most commonly used systems include cells from the mouse lymphoma, human lymphoblasts, and cells from the lung, ovary, and other tissues of Chinese hamsters. These cells usually maintain a near-diploid chromosome number, grow actively, and have high cloning efficiency. Both forward and reverse mutations may occur, and mutants respond selectively to nutritional, biochemical, serological, and drug-resistant growth manipulations. For example, cells from mouse lymphoma, which are heterozygous at the thymidine kinase locus (TK+/–), may undergo forward mutation, for example, via the action of a mutagen, and become TK–/–. Both genotype TK+/– and TK–/– grow in a normal medium, but TK–/– also grow in a medium containing 5-bromo-2′-deoxyuridine (BrdU). The mutagenicity of a toxicant may thus be determined by comparing growth of lymphoma cells in the presence and absence of toxicant both in a medium containing BrdU and in a normal medium (DeMarini et al., 1989).

In Chinese hamsters, as in humans, the use of preformed hypoxanthine and guanine is controlled by an X-linked gene. Mutant cells at these loci are deficient in the enzyme hypoxanthine-guanine phosphoribosyl transferase, and are identified by their resistance to toxic purine analogs, such as 8-azaguanine or 6-thioguanine, which kill the cells that utilize these analogs (DeMarini et al., 1989).

These cell lines are generally deficient in metabolizing enzymes. Therefore, such enzyme systems are often added (*microsome mediated*). Alternatively, these cells can be cocultivated with other cells that possess greater ability to biotransform toxicants. Such a *cell-mediated* system involves the use of freshly isolated hepatocytes as a feeder system (Williams, 1979). It offers an additional advantage of displaying capabilities to conjugate as well as to degrade toxicants.

## *Gene mutation tests in mice*

### *The mouse spot test*

This test is designed to detect gene mutation in somatic cells. Basically, it involves treating the pregnant mouse whose embryos are heterozygous at specific coat color loci and examining the newborn for any mosaic patches in its fur. Such patches indicate the formation of clones of mutant cells that are responsible for the color of the fur. This test is relatively inexpensive and takes only a few weeks to complete. Although it may yield false-positive results, it has not yet yielded false-negative results. The spot test is, therefore, a useful prescreen for heritable germinal mutations in mammals (Russell, 1978).

### *The specific locus test*

The specific locus test was developed for determining mutagenicity of ionizing radiation in germ cells. This procedure was later adapted to assess mutagenicity of chemicals (Searle, 1975). It has the advantage of directly detecting in intact mammals the mutagenic effects of toxicants in the germ cells, but it usually requires a large number of animals.

It involves exposing nonmutant mice to the chemical and subsequently mating them to a multiple-recessive stock. The mutant offspring has an altered phenotype expressed in hair color, hair structure, eye color, ear length, and other traits. Some mutants are mosaic rather than the whole animal. Mutations can also be detected by the rejection or acceptance of skin grafts made between first-generation offsprings. It can be further characterized immunogenetically (Russell and Shelby, 1985).

## Chromosomal effects

The effect of a toxicant on chromosomes may be sufficient to be visible microscopically, and may manifest itself as structural aberrations or as changes in number. The former, *aberrations*, include deletions, duplications, and translocations. The latter, *aneuploidy* (45 or 47 chromosomes), involve a decrease or an increase in the number of the chromosomes (euploid, 2n = 46 chromosomes) Another type of aneupolidy is triploid (3n = 69, three haploid sets of 23 chromosomes), or tetrapolid (4n = 92, in plants), called *polyploidy*. Some of the effects are heritable.

The mode of action underlying these effects may involve molecular cross-linkage, which may induce an arrest of the synthesis of DNA, thereby leaving a gap in the chromosome. An unsuccessful repair of the DNA damage may also be responsible. Nondisjunction (failure of a pair of chromosomes to separate during mitotic division) can lead to mosaicism. A nondisjunction during gametogenesis (meiotic nondisjunction) gives rise to daughter cells that contain either one extra chromosome or one less than normal. The former is known as *trisomy* (e.g., Down's syndrome associated with mental retardation and heart problems, caused by an extra copy of chromosome 21, also known as trisomy 21) and the latter as *monosomy*. Babies born with trisomy 18 have severe mental retardation/other birth defects and they do not survive for more than the first few months of life. Babies with monosomy most commonly do not survive during prenatal development. Turner syndrome is caused by the absence of one sex chromosome, also known as 45, XO. About 99% of pregnancies affected with Turner syndrome are miscarried. The estimated chances for a woman to deliver a child with an aneuploidy dramatically increase with maternal age.

A number of test systems have been developed to determine the chromosomal effects. The following are the major systems.

### Insects

*Drosophila melanogaster* has the advantage in that the chromosomes of some of its cells are superior in size and morphology. In addition, the chromosomal effects can be readily confirmed genetically, such as the sex-linked recessive lethality. The chromosomal effects include loss of X and Y chromosomes and *trans* locations of fragments between second and third chromosomes.

Effects on the sex chromosome can also be detected by phenotypic changes, such as body color, eye color, and shape of the eye (National Research Council, 1983).

## *Cytogenetic studies with mammalian cell* in vitro *tests*

For cytogenetic tests, the commonly used cells are derived from Chinese hamster ovaries and human lymphocytes. These cells are cultured in a suitable medium. They are then exposed to different concentrations of the test chemical in the presence or absence of a bioactivator system (usually the microsomal fraction of the rat liver homogenate). The test generally includes two positive control mutagens, namely, ethylmethane sulfonate, which is direct acting, and dimethyl nitrosamine, which requires bioactivation. After an appropriate incubation period, cell division is arrested by addition of colchicine. The cells are then mounted, stained, and scored (Preston et al., 1981).

An example of scoring of *aberrations* is shown below: chromatid gap, chromatid break, chromosome gap, chromosome break, chromatid deletion, fragment, acentric fragment, translocation, triradial chromosome, quadriradial chromosome, pulverized chromosome, pulverized cells, ring chromosome, dicentric chromosome, minute chromosome, greater than 10 aberrations, polyploid, and hyperploid (Brusick, 1987).

Fluorescent in situ hybridization, a sensitive cytogenetic technique, was also introduced to analyze the presence or absence of specific DNA sequences on chromosomes by fluorescence microscopy.

## In vivo *tests*

Mammalian cells used in the *in vivo* study of chromosomal effects include germ cells and somatic tissues. The chemical to be tested is administered to intact animals, such as rodents and humans. The somatic tissues most commonly used are bone marrow and peripheral lymphocytes. A classic protocol using bone marrow from mice, rats, or hamsters has been provided by the Ad Hoc Committee of the Environmental Mutagen Society and the Institute for Medical Research (1972). The scoring is the same as in the *in vitro* test.

The *micronucleus* test is a somewhat simpler *in vivo* procedure. It involves the use of polychromatic erythrocyte stem cells of CD-1 mice. Six hours after two treatments with the test chemical, given 24 hours apart, animals are sacrificed and bone marrow is collected from the femur of the mice that have undergone the two treatments. An increase in the number of micronucleated cells over the controls (about 0.5%) is considered positive (Schmid, 1976). Many other types of cells may also be used. These micronuclei represent fragments of chromosome and chromatid resulting from spindle/centromere dysfunction.

The male animal is usually used for tests on *germ cells*. In order to allow cells of different stages of spermatogenesis to be exposed, the chemical is given daily for 5 days and animals are sacrificed 1, 3, and 5 weeks following the last dose. The sperm is collected surgically from the cauda epididymides. After mounting and staining, the incidence of abnormal sperm heads is determined, and compared with the negative and positive controls (Wyrobek and Bruce, 1975).

### *Sister chromatid exchange*

This test measures a reciprocal exchange of DNA between two sister chromatids of a duplicating chromosome. The exchange takes place because of a breakage and reunion of DNA during its replication. The test can be done with mouse lymphoma cells, Chinese hamster ovary cells, and human lymphocytes. It may also be conducted *in vivo* by collecting cells from treated animals. The procedure involves labeling of cells with 5-BrdU (5-bromo-deoxyuridine), and after two cycles of replication, the cells are stained with a fluorescent-plus-Giemsa technique. The frequency of sister chromatid exchange per cell and per chromosome is scored and compared. The exchange is visible because, in one chromatid, the semi-conservative replication of DNA results in a substitution of BrdU in *one* polynucleotide strand; in the other chromatid, the BrdU is substituted in *both* polynucleotide strands (Wolff, 1977).

Although the mechanism underlying the sister chromatid exchange is not fully understood, it shows that a chemical has attacked the chromosomes or impaired their replication. The test has the advantage of being simple to perform. Further, its endpoint is often observed at concentrations lower than those required for other tests (NRC, 1983).

### *Dominant lethal test in rodents*

This test is designed to demonstrate toxic effects on germ cells in the intact male animal, usually the mouse or rat. The effects can manifest themselves in the mated females as dead implantations and/or preimplantation losses (the difference between the number of corpora lutea and the number of implantations). These effects are generally due to chromosomal damage, which lead to developmental errors that are fatal to the zygote. However, other cytotoxic effects can also result in early fetal death (see also Chapter 20).

### *Heritable translocation test in mice*

This test is intended to detect the heritability of chromosomal damage. The damage, consisting of reciprocal translocation in the germ line cells of the treated male mice, are transmitted to the offspring. By mating the male $F_1$ progeny with untreated female mice, the chromosomal effects are revealed by a reduction of viable fetuses. The presence of these reciprocal translocations can be verified by the presence of translocation figures among the double tetrads at meiosis (Adler, 1980).

## *DNA repair and recombination*

These biological processes are not mutations per se, but occur after DNA damage. These phenomena, therefore, indicate the existence of DNA damage, which are caused essentially by mutagens. There are three main types of DNA damage that can be repaired: missing, incorrect, or altered bases; interstrand crosslinks; and strand breaks.

### *Bacteria*

Among *E. coli* there are those with normal DNA polymerase I enzyme, which is capable of repairing DNA damage, and those deficient in this enzyme. Mutagens induce DNA damage and thereby impair the growth of the *E. coli* that is deficient in the repair enzyme, whereas the growth of those with this enzyme is not affected. The DNA repair-efficient strain is included to rule out the effect of cytotoxicity (Rosenkranz et al., 1976).

Similarly, there are also recombination efficient and deficient strains of *Bacillus subtilis*. Damage to DNA is repaired in the former strain through recombination but not the latter. Mutagens thus inhibit the growth of the latter but not former.

### *Yeasts*

Various eukaryotic microorganisms, such as *Saccharomyces cerevisiae*, have been used to test the mutagenicity of chemicals by the induced mitotic crossing-over and mitotic gene conversion. These effects on DNA result in the growth of colonies with different colors (Zimmermann et al., 1984).

### *Mammalian cells/UDS*

Unscheduled DNA synthesis (UDS) is an indication of DNA repair. It can be detected in human cells in culture. The synthesis is determined by the amount of radioactive thymidine incorporated per unit weight of DNA over the control value. This is done both in the presence and absence of an added activator system (Stich and Laishes, 1973). Such synthesis can also be determined in primary rat hepatocytes. The extent of DNA synthesis is determined using an autoradiographic method. Since these cells have sufficient metabolic activity, there is no need to add an activator system (Williams, 1979).

Because of their greater relevance to genetic risk, germ cells have also been used in UDS tests: male mice are treated with a suspected mutagen, and [$^3$H]-thymidine ([$^3$H]-dT) is injected intratesticularly. Any incorporation of [$^3$H]-dT into the DNA of meiotic and postmeiotic germ cells indicates the production of repairable damage to the DNA (Russell and Shelby, 1985).

## *Other tests*

As noted in Chapter 8, a number of related mutagenesis tests are used to determine carcinogenicity.

### In vitro *transformation of mammalian cells*

Cells from the BALB/3T3 mouse are most commonly used in this test. Others include Syrian hamster embryo cells, mouse 10T1/2 cells, and human cells. Normally these cells grow in the culture medium to form a monolayer. Those treated with a carcinogen, however, reproduce without being attached to a solid surface and grow over the monolayer. The appearance of such multilayered colonies indicates malignant transformation. This endpoint can be confirmed by injecting these cells into syngeneic animals. In general, malignant tumors develop if cells have undergone transformation (Kakunaga, 1973). Therefore, in general, positive results from this test are especially significant.

### *Nuclear enlargement test*

HeLa cells are grown in culture medium and treated with different concentrations of the chemical on test. After an appropriate duration, cells are harvested and counted. They are then stripped of their cytoplasmic material and size of the nucleus is determined with a particle counter. An increase in the nuclear size indicates the carcinogenicity of the chemical (Finch et al., 1980).

## *Evaluation*

### *Selection of test systems*

Since mutagens affect the genetic material in different ways, they may yield negative results in one test but positive results in others. To rule out false negatives (and false positives), it is advisable to conduct several tests, preferably of different categories. OECD (1987) recommended a series of tests for screening, confirmation, and risk assessment (Table 9.5). Ideally,

*Table 9.5* Utility and application of assays

| |
|---|
| **A. Assays that may be used for mutagen and carcinogen screening** |
| *Salmonella typhimurium* reverse mutation assay |
| *Escherichia coli* reverse mutation assay |
| Gene mutation in mammalian cells in culture |
| Gene mutation in *Saccharomyces cerevisiae* |
| *In vitro* cytogenetics assay |
| Unscheduled DNA synthesis (UDS) *in vitro* |
| *In vitro* sister chromatid exchange (SCE) assay |
| Mitotic recombination in *S. cerevisiae* |
| *In vitro* cytogenetics assay |
| Micronucleus (MN) test |
| *Drosophila* sex-linked recessive lethal test |
| **B. Assays that confirm *in vitro* activity** |
| *In vitro* cytogenetics assay |
| Micronucleus test |
| Mouse spot test |
| *Drosophila* sex-linked recessive lethal test |
| **C. Assays that assess effects on germ cells and that are applicable for estimating** |
| Genetic risk |
| Dominant lethal assay |
| Heritable translocation assay |
| Mammalian germ cell cytogenetic assay |

*Source:* OECD, OECD Guidelines for Testing Chemicals, OECD Publications and Information Center, Washington, DC, 1987.

test systems with both high sensitivity and specificity constitute the best choice.

The Committee on Chemical Environmental Mutagens of the National Research Council recommended a mutagen assessment program (National Research Council, 1983). It suggests that the mutagenesis tests be placed in three tiers. Tier I consists of (i) the *Salmonella*/microsome gene-mutation test, (ii) a mammalian cell gene-mutation test, and (iii) a mammalian cell chromsomal breakage test. If all tests are negative, the chemical is considered a presumed mammalian nonmutagen. If two of these tests are positive, it is classified as a presumed mammalian mutagen. If only one is positive, then the Tier II test (*Drosophila* sex-linked lethal mutation) is conducted. For further screening of the most crucial chemicals, supplemental tests are undertaken. A specific-locus test is recommended for chemicals with a potential mutagenicity in mammalian germ cells, and a dominant lethal test needs to be performed for those having chromosomal effects (see also WHO, 1990).

Many chemicals have been tested for genotoxicity (mutagenicity, carcinogenicity, and developmental toxicity) using a multiplicity of tests. To facilitate the task of a "weight-of-evidence" analysis of the genotoxicity of the chemicals and an analysis of the merit of the tests used in generating the data, a method has been proposed by the International Commission for Protection against Environmental Mutagens and Carcinogens (ICPEMC, 1992).

## *Significance of results*

### *Relation between mutagenicity and carcinogenicity*

A number of investigators have shown the association between carcinogens and mutagens. For example, McCann et al. (1975) reported in their study of 300 substances for mutagenicity in the *Salmonella*/microsome test. The results were compared with the reported carcinogenicity or noncarcinogenicity of these substances. The authors demonstrated a high correlation between these toxic effects: 90% (156/175) of carcinogens are mutagenic in the test, while 87% (94/108) of the noncarcinogens showed any degree of mutagenicity. The test has been independently validated in other studies. Results reported a 72–91% correlation between mutagenicity and carcinogenicity (Table 9.6). Mason et al. (1990) compiled information on the correlation between carcinogenicity in rodents and mutagenicity as determined by *S. typhimurium*. The correlations varied between 55% and 93%.

***Table 9.6*** Summary of validation studies in *Salmonella* with organic chemical carcinogens and noncarcinogens

| Carcinogens | | | Noncarcinogens | | | |
|---|---|---|---|---|---|---|
| Number tested | Mutagenicity in Ames test (+) | Mutagenicity in Ames test (–) | Number tested | Mutagenicity in Ames test (+) | Mutagenicity in Ames test (–) | References |
| 174 | 90% | 10% | 108 | 13% | 87% | McCann et al. (1975) |
| 167 | 85% | 15% | 86 | 26% | 74% | Sugimura et al. (1977) |
| 58 | 91% | 9% | 62 | 6% | 94% | Purchase et al. (1978) |
| 38 | 72% | 28% | 16 | 19% | 81% | Heddle and Bruce (1977) |
| 63 | 76% | 24% | | | | Dunkel et al. (1985) |

It is of interest to note that many studies demonstrated that certain human leukemias, lymphomas, and solid tumors are associated with specific chromosomal alterations, some of which are listed in Table 9.1. Further, gene mutations and chromosomal damage might convert proto-oncogenes to active oncogenes (Bishop, 1991; Barrett, 1993). For further discussions on the effects of such conversion, see the section on "Mode of Action" of carcinogenesis in Chapter 8.

### *Heritable effects*

At present there is no direct correlation between lab tests for heritable mutations induced by chemical toxicants and human experience. Nevertheless, if a substance has been shown to be mutagenic in a variety of test systems including heritable mutations in intact mammals, it needs to be considered as a mutagen in humans unless there is convincing evidence to the contrary. Fortunately, for many chemicals, such as food additives, pesticides, cosmetics, and most drugs, where human exposure can be avoided, any incidence of mutagenicity will be sufficient to warrant suspension of their use (Flamm, 1977). For environmental pollutants and occupational toxicants that are mutagenic, every effort needs to be made to reduce human exposure to them.

## *References*

Ad Hoc Committee of the Environmental Mutagen Society and the Institute of Medical Research (1972). Chromosome methodologies in mutagen testing. *Toxicol Appl Pharmacol*. 22, 269–75.

Adler ID (1980). New approaches to mutagenicity studies in animals for carcinogenic and mutagenic agents. I. Modification of heritable translocation test. *Teratogen Carcinogen Mutagen*. 1, 75–86.

Ames BN (1971). The detection of chemical mutagens with enteric bacteria. In: Hollander A, ed. *Chemical Mutagens: Principles and Methods for Their Detection, vol. 1.* New York: Plenum Press, 267–82.

Ames BN, McCann J, Yamasaki E (1975). Methods for detecting carcinogens and mutagens with the Salmonella/mammalian-microsome mutagenicity test. *Mutat Res*. 31, 347–64.

Barrett JC (1993). Mechanisms of multistep carcinogenesis and carcinogen risk assessment. *Environ Health Perspect*. 100, 9–20.

Bishop JM (1991). Molecular themes in oncogenesis. *Cell*. 64, 235–48.

Brusick DJ, Mayer VW (1973). New developments in mutagenicity screening techniques with yeast. *Environ Health Perspect*. 6, 83–96.

Brusick DJ (1987). *Principles of Genetic Toxicology*, 2nd ed. New York: Plenum Press.

Chinnery PF, Samuels DC (1999). Relaxed replication of mtDNA: A model with implications for the expression of disease. *Am J Hum Genet*. 64, 1158–65.

Chinnery PF, Howell N, Andrews R, Turnbull D (1999). Clinical mitochondrial genetics. *J Med Genet*. 36, 425–36.

DeMarini DM, Brockman HE, deSerres FJ et al. (1989). Specific-locus induced in eukaryotes (especially mammalian cells) by radiation and chemicals: A perspective. *Mutat Res.* 220, 11–29.

Dunkel VC, Zeiger E, Brusick D et al. (1985). Reproducibility of microbial mutagenicity assays: II. Testing of carcinogens and noncarcinogens in Salmonella typhimurium and Escherichia coli. *Environ Mutagen.* 5, 1–248.

Durston WE, Ames BN (1974). Simple method for the detection of mutagens in urine: Studies with the carcinogen 2-acetylaminofluorene. *Proc Natl Acad Sci USA.* 71, 737–41.

EPA. (1994). Health Effects Test Guidelines, Title 40, Part 798. Washington, DC: U.S. Environmental Protection Agency.

Finch RA, Evans IM, Bosmann HB (1980). Chemical carcinogen in vitro testing: A method for sizing cell nuclei in the nuclear enlargement assay. *Toxicology.* 15, 145–54.

Flamm WG (Chairman, DHEW Working Group on Mutagenicity Testing) (1977). Approaches to determining the mutagenic properties of chemicals: Risk to future generations. *J Environ Pathol Toxicol.* 1, 301–52.

Gabridge MG, Legator MS (1969). A host-mediated microbial assay for the detection of mutagenic compounds. *Proc Soc Exp Biol Med.* 130, 831–4.

Heddle JA, Bruce WR (1977). Comparison of tests for mutagenicity or carcinogenicity using assays for sperm abnormalities, formation of micronuclei, and mutations in *Salmonella*. In: Hiatt HH, Watson JD, Winstein JA eds. *Origins of Human Cancer*, Book C, Cold Harber Conferences on Cell Proliferation, Vol. 4, pp. 1549–57.

Hoffmann GR (1996). Genetic toxicology. In: Klaassen CD, ed. *Casarett and Doull's Toxicology*. New York: McGraw-Hill, 269–300.

ICPEMC. (1992). A method for combining and comparing short-term genotoxicity test data. The basic system. *Mutat Res.* 266, 7–25.

Kakunaga T (1973). A quantitative system for assay of malignant transformation by chemical carcinogens using a clone derived from BALB/3T3. *Int J Cancer.* 12, 463–73.

Kornberg A, Baker T (1992). *DNA Replication*. Oxford, UK, 2nd ed. W.H. Freeman.

Lee WR, Abrahamson S, Valencia R et al. (1983). The sex-linked recessive lethal test for mutagenesis in Drosophila melanogaster: A report of the U.S. EPA Gene-Tox Program. *Mutat Res.* 123, 183–279.

Mason JM, Langenbach R, Sheldby MD et al. (1990). Ability of short term tests to predict carcinogenesis in rodents. *Annu Rev Pharmacol Toxicol.* 30, 149–68.

McCann J, Choi E, Yamasaki E et al. (1975). Detection of carcinogens as mutagens in the Salmonella/microsome tests assay of 300 chemicals. *Proc Natl Acad Sci USA.* 72, 5135–9.

Nance MA, Berry AS (1992). Cockayne syndrome: Review of 140 cases. *Am J Med Genet.* 42, 68–84.

National Research Council (NRC) (1983). Identifying and Estimating the Genetic Impact of Chemical Mutagens. A Report of the Committee on Chemical Environmental Mutagens, National Research Council. Washington, DC: National Academy Press.

OECD. (1987). OECD Guidelines for Testing Chemicals. Washington, DC: OECD Publications and Information Center.

Paraskevaidi M, Martin-Hirsch PL, Kyrgiou M, Martin FL (2016). Underlying role of mitochondrial mutagenesis in the pathogenesis of a disease and current approaches for translational research. *Mutagenesis*. [Epub ahead of print].
Preston RJ, Au W, Bender MA et al. (1981). Mammalian in vivo and in vitro cytogenetic assays: A report of the U.S. EPA Gene-Tox Program. *Mutat Res*. 87, 143–88.
Purchase IF, Longstaff E, Ashby J (1978). An evaluation of 6 short-term tests for detecting organic chemical carcinogens. *Br J Cancer*. 37, 873–903.
Rabbitts TH (1994). Translocations in human cancer. *Nature*. 372, 143–49.
Rosenkranz HS, Gutter G, Spek WJ (1976). Mutagenicity and DNA-modifying activity: A comparison of two microbial assays. *Mutat Res*. 41, 61–70.
Russell LB (1978). Somatic cells as indicators of germinal mutations in the mouse. *Environ Health Perspect*. 24, 113–16.
Russell LB, Shelby MD (1985). Tests for heritable genetic damage and for evidence of gonadal exposure in mammals. *Mutat Res*. 154, 69–84.
Schmid W (1976). The micronucleus test. *Mutat Res*. 31, 9–15.
Searle AG (1975). The specific locus test in the mouse. *Mutat Res*. 31, 277–90.
Shock LS, Thakkar PV, Peterson EJ, Moran RG, Taylor SM (2011). DNA methyltransferase 1, cytosine methylation, and cytosine hydroxymethylation in mammalian mitochondria. *Proc Natl Acad Sci USA*. 108, 3630–5.
Simmons VF, Rozenkranz HS, Zeiger E et al. (1979). Mutagenic activity of chemical carcinogens and related compounds in the intraperitoneal host-mediated assay. *J Natl Cancer Inst*. 62, 911–8.
Stich HF, Laishes BA (1973). DNA repair and chemical carcinogens. *Pathobiol Annu*. 3, 341–76.
Sugimura T, Nagao M, Kawachi T, Honda M, Yahagi T, Seino Y, Sato S, Matsukura N (1977). Mutagen-carcinogens in food, with special reference to highly mutagenic pyrolytic products in broiled food. In: Hiatt HH, Watson JD, Winsten JA, eds. *Origins of Human Cancer*. New York: Cold Spring Harbor Laboratory Press, p. 1561.
WHO. (1990). Summary Report on the Evaluation of Short-term Tests for Carcinogenesis. WHO Environ Health Criteria 109.
Williams GM (1979). The status of in vitro test systems utilizing DNA damage and repair for the screening of chemical carcinogens. *J Assoc Anal Chem*. 63, 857–63.
Wolff S (1977). Sister chromatid exchange. *Annu Rev Genet*. 11, 183–201.
Wyrobek AJ, Bruce WR (1975). Chemical induction of sperm abnormalities in mice. *Proc Natl Acad Sci USA*. 72, 4425–9.
Zimmermann FK, von Borstel RC, von Halle ES et al. (1984). Testing of chemicals for genetic activity with *Saccharomyces cerevisiae*: A report of the U.S. EPA Gene-Tox Program. *Mutat Res*. 133, 199–244.

# chapter ten

# Developmental toxicology

**Helen E. Ritchie and William S. Webster**

Contents

## *What is developmental toxicology?*

Developmental toxicology is the identification and study of hazards for pregnant women that might produce adverse outcomes in pregnancy. Hazards of popular concern include therapeutic and recreational drugs, pesticides, and environmental pollution. Testing drugs and other chemicals for developmental toxicity is an important industry and is subject to extensive national and international regulation. The difference between hazard and risk is frequently ignored in the popular press and this often leads to exaggerated interpretation of developmental toxicity. It is worth restating that in toxicology a hazard is anything that can produce harm, whereas risk is the potential for a hazard to produce harm. A hazard will not pose any risk to a pregnant woman or embryo unless they are exposed to a sufficient amount of that hazard to initiate harm.

## *Methylmercury and thalidomide*

### *Methylmercury (MeHg)*

Modern ideas regarding developmental toxicity have been significantly influenced by two events that occurred over 50 years ago. The first, in 1956 in Minamata City, Japan, involved the poisoning of people by ingestion of fish and shellfish contaminated by methylmercury (MeHg) which had been discharged into the sea from a chemical plant (Hachiya, 2006). The MeHg damaged the brains of people who ingested it, causing severe neurological symptoms and sometimes death.

A number of pregnant women were also exposed. The MeHg affected the developing brain of the embryo inducing mental retardation and a type of cerebral palsy in the newborn (Harada, 1995). The developing fetus proved to be roughly 5–10 times more sensitive than adults (Clarkson, 1992). This was the first clear demonstration that an environmental pollutant affected the developing human embryo and has influenced attitudes ever since. It is now recognized that low level MeHg contamination of fish is widespread and there are guidelines about acceptable daily intake (Rice et al., 2003).

### *Thalidomide*

The second major event was the marketing, in 1957, of the drug thalidomide. In advertisements it was described as a sedative and hypnotic, an "outstandingly safe" alternative to barbiturates that were used as sedatives and sleeping tablets that had produced many deaths from overdoses. Thalidomide appeared to be safe since it was not possible to establish a lethal dose in rats. The drug was promoted around the world and was subsequently prescribed by some doctors to treat morning sickness in pregnancy. In the next few years, it became apparent that thalidomide use during early pregnancy damaged the embryo producing severe limb and other defects. It has been estimated that worldwide over 10,000 infants were born with malformations after their mothers were treated with thalidomide in pregnancy (Schardein, 2000). The drug usually produced no adverse effects in the treated mothers leaving them unaware of the effect on the embryo. A chemical or drug, such as thalidomide, that induces a birth defect is called a teratogen.

The thalidomide and MeHg experiences confirmed that the placenta is not a barrier and does not protect the embryo from exposure to drugs and other chemicals ingested by the mother. The degree of placental transfer varies with molecular weight, lipophilicity, and other physicochemical properties (Griffiths and Campbell, 2014) but in general drugs taken by the mother reach the embryo. The term "thalidomide" is now often used synonymously with scientific/medical failure. It has left the general and medical population with a deep suspicion of any drug use during pregnancy.

## *What is meant by an adverse outcome in pregnancy?*

### *Pregnancy loss*

Human embryonic development is the self-assembly of a human. It is a complex process and frequently goes wrong. There is evidence that over 50% of pregnancies are lost before a woman knows she is pregnant (Macklon et al., 2002). Of clinically recognized pregnancies 10–15% end in spontaneous abortion, mostly in the first 12 weeks of pregnancy (first trimester) (March of Dimes, 2012) (Figure 10.1). A further 1% die (stillbirth) before or at birth (Macdorman and Gregory, 2015).

### *Low birth weight and prematurity*

Based on U.S. data (Hamilton et al., 2015), about 8% of infants have a low birth weight of less than 2500 g compared with a mean of 3389 g. Most are premature infants (~6%). The remainder (~2%) have a normal gestation but show fetal growth retardation (March of Dimes, 2014). Prematurity refers to infants born less than 34 weeks from conception compared with the normal 38 weeks. Birth weight is an important indicator of infant health as there is a close relationship between low birth weight and infant morbidity and mortality (OECD, 2014).

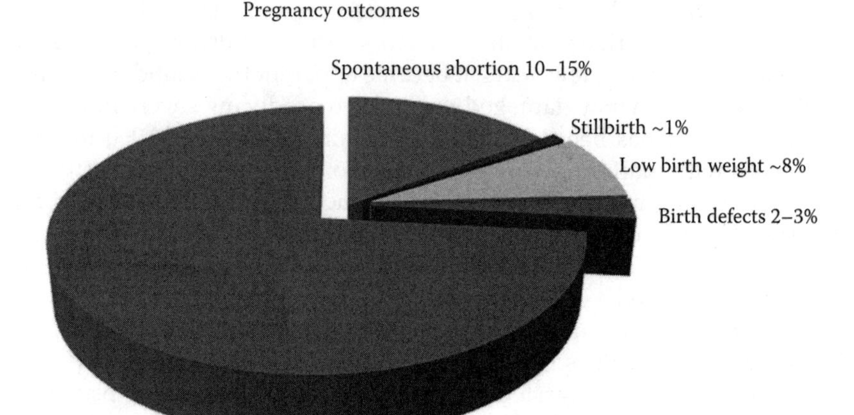


***Figure 10.1*** Outcomes following recognition of clinical pregnancy.

### *Birth defects*

Of all newborn infants, ~2% have a birth defect of surgical, medical, or cosmetic importance. This increases to ~3% at 1 year of age as additional abnormalities such as heart defects are identified (Holmes, 2010). Some of these babies also have low birth weight.

### *Overall*

These figures indicate that for clinically recognized pregnancies only ~70% result in a normal outcome. The frequency of adverse outcomes of pregnancy varies in different countries (Kramer, 2003). Poor nutrition, infections, cigarette smoking, incomplete data collection, race, and ethnicity contribute to this variation (Canfield et al., 2014).

## *What causes these adverse outcomes in human pregnancy?*

Many of these adverse outcomes (particularly spontaneous abortion and birth defects) are due to genetic abnormalities of the developing embryo and are not readily preventable. For example, over 50% of both pre- and post-implantation pregnancy losses are associated with chromosomal abnormalities (Macklon et al., 2002).

In a report on the global impact of birth defects (March of Dimes Foundation, 2006), it was estimated that ~15% of birth defects have a clear genetic origin, either a mutated gene (7–8%) or chromosomal abnormality (6%) (most common is Trisomy 21—Down syndrome) (Table 10.1). Except in rare cases, these genetic defects or mutations occur before conception in either the sperm or the egg. Another 20–25% of birth defects are described as multifactorial, a complex genetic–environmental interaction. These are mostly isolated malformations of the heart, central nervous system, face, and genitourinary system. Only 5–10% of birth defects have an identified exogenous and potentially preventable cause. These hazards include maternal diabetes, associated with about 3% of birth defects, and maternal infections (rubella, cytomegalovirus, varicella, toxoplasmosis, and more recently the Zika virus) associated with ~4% of birth defects. Therapeutic drugs are thought to be responsible for only ~1% of birth defects. Importantly, for over 50% of birth defects the causes are unknown. It is possible that as our knowledge of the complex interactions between genes and the environment increases, more preventable causes will be recognized. However, it is also likely that the cause of some birth defects may never be known as these may represent spontaneous and unpreventable errors in development that might be expected in such a complicated process as embryonic development.

The low contribution of therapeutic drugs and nondetectable contribution of environmental pollution to birth defects is in sharp contrast to popular belief. Legal and illegal recreational drugs are often thought to be hazardous in pregnancy but it is only maternal alcohol abuse that is clearly linked with birth defects and mental retardation. Addictive drugs such as heroin may produce withdrawal symptoms in the newborn and poor postnatal development, but these agents do not appear to initiate birth defects. This breakdown of causes of birth defects may be most typical of western industrialized societies. The prevalence of malaria, zika virus, social custom of consanguineous marriage, advanced parental age, poverty, poor nutrition including iodine deficiency, alcohol abuse, obesity, diabetes, and poor health care including low immunization rates (e.g., rubella) are just some of the parameters that vary greatly between

***Table 10.1*** Causes of birth defects

| Genetic causes | | Example |
|---|---|---|
| Single gene | 7–8% | Achrondroplasia |
| Chromosomal | 6% | Trisomy 21—Down syndrome |
| Multifactorial | 20–25% | Familial cleft lip and palate |
| Exogenous | 5–10% | Diabetes, rubella, thalidomide, varicella, alcohol |
| Unknown | >50% | |

countries and lead to adverse pregnancy outcomes (March of Dimes Foundation, 2006).

## *Normal embryonic development*

With respect to developmental toxicology, human embryonic development may be divided into three basic stages:

*Weeks 1–2* encompass fertilization to implantation of the embryo into the uterine wall. At the end of week 2 the embryo is a flat disc only a couple of millimeters (mm) in length. Studies in rats, mice, and rabbits indicate that toxic events during this developmental period tend to result in death of the embryo rather than abnormal development.

*Weeks 3–8* are known as the organogenic period of human development. The human embryo increases in length from a few millimeters at 3 weeks to ~30 mm at 8 weeks (Figure 10.2). During this time period, the embryo takes on a three-dimensional appearance and all organ systems begin to develop. Each organ has a period of maximum sensitivity during this time period when damage might result in a permanent malformation of that organ. Most severe birth defects result from damage to the embryo during this period (Czeizel, 2008). Thalidomide produced a wide range of defects, but only after exposure between days 21 to 36 of pregnancy. Within that period different structures were sensitive at different times. For example, upper limb defects occurred after exposure 24–32 days after fertilization while lower limb defects occurred 27–34 days postfertilization (Kim and Scialli, 2011). This reflects the fact that upper limbs develop a few days earlier than lower limbs. By 8 weeks, the human embryo has completed the major morphological development of all the major organs such as the heart, liver, brain, and intestines. The major morphological development of the internal genitalia is not completed until ~12 weeks gestation. Development of external genitalia continues to be sensitive throughout gestation.

*Weeks 9–38* of gestation are known as the fetal period of development. During this time, there is mostly growth of the fetus and maturation of the organ systems. Complications during this period of development result in fetal growth retardation. Brain maturation is an especially complex process that continues throughout the fetal period as well as postnatally. Damage to the developing brain may occur at any time during the fetal period resulting in microcephaly, mental retardation and/or behavioral abnormalities. These conditions are not always regarded as structural malformations or birth defects but have major impact on quality of life and family.

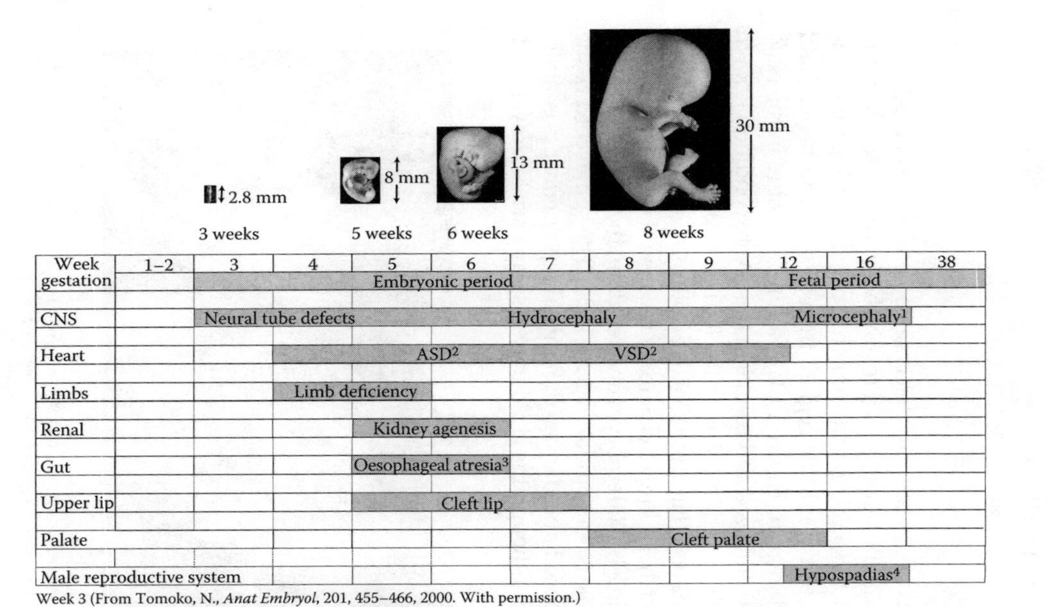


Week 3 (From Tomoko, N., *Anat Embryol*, 201, 455–466, 2000. With permission.)

Weeks 5–8: Embryo #7394, 8097, 4570, Human Developmental Anatomy Collection, National Museum of Health and Medicine, Silver Sping MD. (Data derived from Czeizel, A.E., *Congen Anom*, 48, 103–9, 2008.)

[1] Primary; [2] atrial septal defect, ventricular septal defect; [3] coesophageal atesia/stenosis with/out fistula; [4] without coronal type.

***Figure 10.2*** The critical periods of organ development. Each organ system undergoes aperiod when it is most sensitive to damage that can result in a birth defect. The gray bars show these sensitive periods, which mostly occur during weeks 2–8 of gestation, the organogenic period. Damage can still occur after these sensitive periods and result in less severe defects. The embryo images show that, during the organogenic period, the embryo grows from about 3 mm in length to 30 mm in length. Note that at 4–5 weeks the limbs are incompletely formed and can be malformed by insults at this time. By 8 weeks, the limbs are well developed, with fingers and toes present, and are much less susceptible to damage.

## What is a birth defect?

Birth defects affect any part of the body. Heart defects are the most common, affecting 15% of children with birth defects, perhaps reflecting the complexity of heart development. Other important and common defects are neural tube defects and cleft lip.

### Neural tube defects

One of the most serious types of birth defects is a neural tube defect. The brain and spinal cord initially develop as a relatively flat disc that rolls up to form a tube (the neural tube) during the fourth week of development. The neural tube closes first in the middle region, then in the head region, and finally in the lower back region (Figure 10.3a). Failure of closure in the head region occurs in ~1/1000 embryos and results in the severe condition known as anencephaly in which the brain tissue of the fetus is exposed and largely destroyed during pregnancy (Figure 10.3b). Newborns with this condition usually die soon after birth. Failure of closure of the neural tube in the lower back region also occurs in ~1/1000 embryos and results in the nonlethal condition of myelomeningocele (spina bifida) (Figure 10.3c). The spinal cord tissue in the lower back is exposed and damaged. Surgical repair either prenatally or after birth is possible, although the child may display variable lower limb

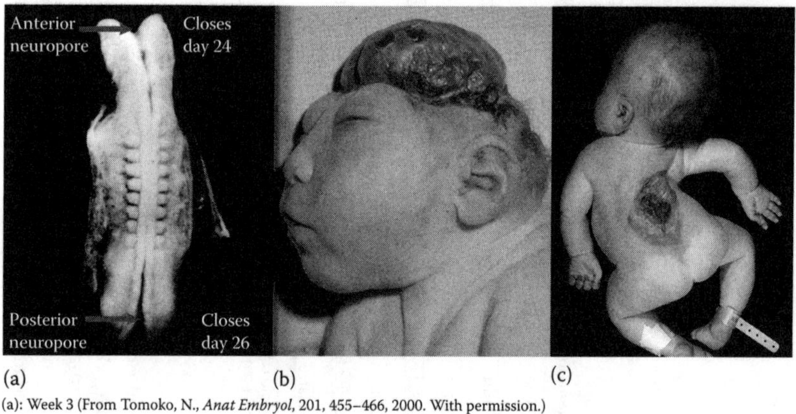


(a): Week 3 (From Tomoko, N., *Anat Embryol*, 201, 455–466, 2000. With permission.)
(b, c): (From Agamanolis, D. P., http://neuropathology-web.org. With permission.)

***Figure 10.3*** Development of brain and spinal cord. (a) Human embryo at ~22 days gestation showing neural tube is closed in the middle region but still open in the head (anterior neuropore) and tail (posterior neuropore regions). (b) Failure of neural tube closure at the anterior neuropore leads to anencephaly. (c) Failure of neural tube closure at the posterior neuropore leads to myelomeningocele.

paralysis as well as poor bowel and bladder control. The prevalence of neural tube defects varies greatly around the world, and there is evidence that prenatal folic acid supplementation markedly reduces the prevalence (De-Regil et al., 2015). To date, 61 countries have mandated folate supplementation of wheat products (Food Fortification Initiative, 2016) with reliable evidence of reduction in prevalence of spina bifida (Atta et al., 2016). Since the neural tube closes before most women are aware they are pregnant, it is recommended that all women of childbearing age consume 0.4 mg of folic acid every day, even if they are not planning a pregnancy any time soon.

## *Cleft lip*

Another common type of birth defect is cleft lip. The upper lip of the embryo develops during the fifth–seventh week after fertilization and is formed by fusion and merging of three pairs of facial prominences. Figure 10.4a shows a 7-week human fetus. The nostrils are enclosed by medial and lateral nasal prominences (MNP and LNP). Although the gap between the two MNP appears large in the embryo, they nearly always merge and midline clefts are rare. The rest of the upper lip involves fusion of MNP and the LNP under the nostril and fusion with the more lateral maxillary prominence (MaxProc). This failure of fusion results in cleft lip which may be unilateral or bilateral and occurs in about 1:750 newborn (Figure 10.4b). Again the incidence of cleft lip varies widely between countries. Although the malformation at birth appears severe and disfiguring it may be surgically repaired to give a normal appearance (Figure 10.4c).

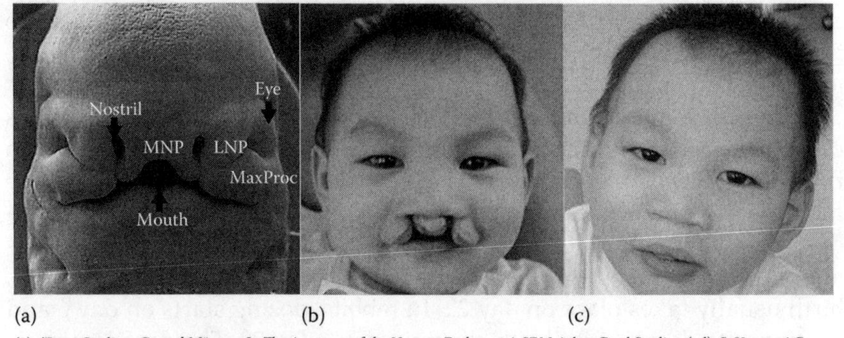


(a): (From Steding, C., and Männer, J., *The Anatomy of the Human Embryo - A SEM Atlas*, Gerd Steding (ed), S. Karger AG, Basel, 2009, p25. With permission.)
(b): (From *Operation restore Hope Australia*. With permission.)

***Figure 10.4*** Development of upper lip and face. (a) Scanning electron microscope image of the face of a 7-week human embryo. (b) Child with bilateral cleft lip, before and (c) after reconstructive surgery.

## *Testing drugs and other chemicals for developmental toxicity*

Drug regulators responded to the thalidomide experience by introducing regulations to ensure that new drugs were tested in pregnant animals before they were licensed for use in humans. While there is still limited understanding of how a chemical such as thalidomide produces birth defects there is greater understanding of the parameters necessary for a chemical to cause birth defects. A teratogenic effect is like other toxic effects, the chemical needs to be present above a threshold level for a minimum duration and (unique to teratogens) needs to be present during organogenesis. Unless these criteria are met, the risk that the chemical will initiate a birth defect is not different than if no chemical exposure had occurred. This knowledge has determined the experimental design of developmental toxicology studies.

### *Testing of therapeutic drugs*

Since pharmaceutical drugs tend to be marketed around the world, there have been attempts to reduce or eliminate the need to duplicate reproductive toxicity testing in different countries. The International Council for Harmonisation of Technical Requirements for Pharmaceuticals for Human Use (ICH) produced guidelines for reproductive toxicity testing required by the European Union, Japan, and the United States for new drug registration (ICH, 2005). These guidelines are generally accepted by other countries; including Australia, Canada, China, Chinese Taipei, India, Singapore, and South Korea. A further revision of the guidelines is currently underway (ICH, 2015). The guidelines specify separate tests to investigate the effect of drugs on (1) fertility, (2) embryonic development, and (3) lactation.

The conventional embryo-fetal developmental toxicity study involves dosing pregnant animals from the time of implantation of the embryo into the uterine wall to closure of the hard palate that forms the roof of the mouth of the embryo. This encompasses the organogenic period of development. Only mammals are used for these definitive safety tests, usually the rat and rabbit. In pregnant rats, this is days 6 to 17 of pregnancy, birth usually takes place on day 22. In rabbits, dosing starts on day 6 and continues to day 19 with birth occurring on ~day 29. The dosed animals are killed shortly before birth and the fetuses examined for internal and external malformations. At least three dosage levels are used. Dosages to be tested include a high dose that should produce some minimal developmental and/or maternal toxicity (for example reduced maternal body weight gain during pregnancy). Excessive maternal toxicity is not recommended since it is thought to adversely affect the offspring leading to inappropriate risk classification (Buschmann, 2013). Other studies require dosing from implantation through to weaning. This additional exposure time covers development of the reproductive system and brain. The offspring of the treated animals then undergo neurobehavioral testing of reflexes, motor activity, learning, and memory. A more complete discussion of these requirements and tests is available (Wise, 2013).

### *Testing of other chemicals*

There are an estimated 100,000 chemicals present in the environment (Egeghy et al., 2012) to which pregnant women may be exposed. These include pesticides, food additives, cosmetics, as well as chemicals used in industry, and environmental pollutants. The vast number and variety of chemicals together with financial costs preclude systematic reproductive toxicity testing in the same way that new therapeutic drugs are tested. There is also ongoing pressure to reduce the number of animals used in safety testing (EU, 2009). This has resulted in development of modified reproductive toxicity tests, which are shorter in duration and use fewer animals. More details on these emerging tests are available (Buschmann, 2013). There have also been regulatory attempts to prioritize which chemicals need to be tested, for developmental and other toxicity studies, based on structural analogy to known toxic chemicals, tonnage of chemical produced, and potential for human exposure (Barton, 2013).

## *Interpretation of developmental toxicity studies*

The interpretation of the results of developmental toxicity is often difficult and sometimes controversial. Many thousands of chemicals have undergone developmental toxicity testing in animals and, based on the results of these tests, several thousand have been identified as hazardous to reproduction and are included in a catalog of teratogenic agents (Shepard, 2010). This is in sharp contrast to the 20 or so chemical groups (mostly drugs) that are known to be a teratogenic risk in humans (Webster and Freeman, 2003) (Table 10.2). This emphasizes the fact that developmental toxicity testing identifies hazard but does not determine risk. In most cases, the exposure level to these hazards in humans during pregnancy is insufficient to produce harm.

Sometimes, developmental toxicity studies show no effect even at the highest concentration tested. This can be reassuring for humans, providing there is evidence that the pregnant animals and their embryos were exposed to the same chemical and metabolites, and at the same concentrations and for the same duration of development as is likely to occur in humans. Such conditions are rarely fulfilled. When thalidomide was

***Table 10.2*** Known human teratogens

| | | |
|---|---|---|
| Pharmaceuticals | Anticonvulsants | Hydantoin (e.g., Phenytoin) |
| | | Primidone |
| | | Diones (e.g., Trimethadione) |
| | | Phenobarbital |
| | | Valproic acid |
| | | Carbamazepine |
| | Anticancer agents | Alkylating agents |
| | | Busulfan |
| | | Cyclophosphamide |
| | | Chlorambucil |
| | | Mechloethamine |
| | | Antimetabolites |
| | | Aminopterin |
| | | Methotrexate |
| | | Cytarabine |
| | Coumarin anticoagulants | (e.g., Warfarin) |
| | Retinoic acids | Isotretinoin |
| | | Etretrinate |
| | | Acitretin |
| | Androgenic hormones | (e.g., Danazol) |
| | Other drugs | Diethylstilbestrol |
| | | Thalidomide |
| | | Lithium |
| | | Penicillamine |
| | | Fluconazole |
| | | Misoprosotol |
| Maternal infections and diseases | | Diabetes |
| | | Rubella, Cytomegalovirus Toxoplasmosis, Zika virus |
| Environmental | | Ionizing radiation[a] |
| | | Methylmercury |
| Other chemicals | | Alcohol |

[a] Ionizing radiation is an established teratogen in both experimental animals and in humans. Exposure of pregnant women to radiation from atomic bomb explosions and therapeutic use in cancer therapy has caused microencephaly in their offspring. Low-level exposure from diagnostic imaging is not normally considered a risk.

tested in pregnant rats and mice, this drug showed little developmental toxicity while in pregnant rabbits and monkeys it produced similar malformations to those seen in the human (Schardein, 2000; Ridings, 2013). The insensitivity of the rodents to thalidomide is thought to be due to metabolic differences between species, but this is unproven.

## *Risk assessment*

When considering dosages used in toxicology testing, it is a common error to equate dose with exposure level. Embryonic exposure levels can rarely be measured; hence, maternal blood concentration of the chemical is used as a surrogate in risk assessments. Most therapeutic drugs are designed to yield relatively constant blood levels (exposure) in the human over a prolonged period of time (drug has a long half-life). Rats and rabbits usually have a higher metabolic rate than humans, so the equivalent dose administered to these animals results in a shorter exposure duration (drug has a short half-life), often minutes compared with hours in the human. To achieve prolonged exposure above anticipated human levels experimental animals are usually given higher doses than humans. An unwanted consequence of this compromise is that the drug in the experimental animals reaches higher peak concentrations compared with levels seen in humans. This makes interpretation of results more difficult and is thought to result in many false-positive results in reproductive toxicity testing.

## *Pharmaceutical drugs—Benefit-risk assessment*

There is a complex benefit-risk assessment for pharmaceutical drug use in pregnancy (Webster and Freeman, 2001). The benefit is the therapeutic gain for the patient and it may be significant. The risk is a possible increased chance of damage to the embryo (and mother). The risk is considered low if developmental toxicity only occurs in animals at exposure levels that are unlikely to occur in humans. However, if exposure levels are similar, then the risk is high. Even when the risk is high the benefit may be considered to be more important. For instance, some drugs used to treat epilepsy, such as valproic acid, are teratogenic in both experimental animals and humans but they are still used in human pregnancy. The rationale is that the drug may be the only available treatment to prevent potentially fatal convulsions in the mother during pregnancy—this is an obvious benefit. The increased risk of an adverse outcome in the pregnancy may be considered acceptable in view of the benefit. The use of decreased dosages of valproic acid during pregnancy reduces the risk of an adverse pregnancy outcome but increases the risk of maternal seizures.

There are many other pharmaceutical drugs that are of concern in pregnancy, not because they produce birth defects, but because these chemicals exert other adverse effects on the embryo (Webster and Freeman, 2003). For instance, maternal use of opioid analgesics might induce opioid dependence in the newborn, known as neonatal abstinence syndrome. These drugs exert their effects mostly in the second and third trimesters.

### Other chemicals

Pesticides, herbicides, industrial chemicals, and environmental pollutants are treated rather differently if they show evidence of developmental toxicity. There is rarely sufficient data on blood levels in animal studies and humans to make a valid comparison. There is also little or no attempt to include benefit in the assessment since, unlike therapeutic drugs, there is no direct benefit to the human. Instead, the chemical is tested at different exposure levels until a no-observable adverse effect level (NOAEL) is established. A 100 or 1000 × safety factor is then applied to the NOAEL to account for interspecies, intraspecies, and individual differences. From this an acceptable daily intake (ADI) is calculated. This is a highly conservative approach to protect human health.

## Recent challenges in developmental toxicology

### Biologic drugs

Although the current methodology of testing for developmental toxicity appears to be largely successful in identifying possible reproductive hazards, some additional challenges have arisen. There has been a significant increase in the so-called "biologic drugs." These are generally proteins and peptides that have a high specificity for human targets. As such, these agents are inappropriate to test in rats and rabbits and sometimes even in monkeys, since they often lack cross-reactivity and may be neutralized by the formation of antibodies. It may not be possible to adequately test these drugs prior to human exposure.

### Neurobehavioral testing

Although neurobehavioral testing of offspring after prenatal drug exposure has been performed for many years, the interpretation of results and regulatory consequences are uncertain. Many pregnant women are prescribed drugs that modulate brain neurotransmitters. These include drugs to treat anxiety, depression, and schizophrenia. It is likely that these drugs also exert an effect on the brain of the embryo with unknown consequences.

### Endocrine disruptors

In recent years, there has been a lot of attention given to groups of chemicals that show weak estrogenic activity and when given to laboratory animals produce abnormalities in genital development. Bisphenol A, often found in plastic bottles, is an example of an endocrine disruptor.

The significance of the animal studies is often uncertain due to the high exposure levels used and marked variations in estrogenic receptors and binding proteins between species.

### Transplacental carcinogens

In the 1950s, diethylstilbestrol (DES), a synthetic estrogen, was used in an attempt to prevent miscarriage. However, DES acted as a transplacental carcinogen producing an increased risk of a rare form of vaginal cancer in female offsprings (Schrager and Potter, 2004). Standard animal testing is not designed to detect transplacental carcinogens.

### Paternal exposure

Although developmental toxicity primarily concentrates on maternal exposure to chemicals there is also some concern regarding paternal exposure. It is possible that males may be exposed, preconceptually, to drugs or other chemicals that damage the DNA of their sperm resulting in birth defects or other adverse outcome in their offspring. This is a particular concern for both male and female cancer survivors who are often treated with drugs that damage DNA. This increases the chance of mutations in their sperm or ova. Another concern is that drugs or chemicals may accumulate in male semen. The embryo could then be exposed to the chemical if intercourse occurred during critical stages of pregnancy. Although this remains a theoretical concern it has been concluded that drug and chemical levels in semen are so low that there is a large safety factor (Klemmt and Scialli, 2005).

## Mechanisms of teratogenesis

It is estimated that there have been more than 30 different theories attempting to explain the mechanisms underlying thalidomide embryopathy, yet with little consensus (Vargesson, 2015). Similarly, the mechanism of action is poorly understood for many other known human teratogens. Unlike traditional toxicants, an adverse outcome induced by a teratogen is the result of interactions between chemical, dose, mother, placenta, and stage of gestation of developing embryo, making it difficult to pinpoint unifying mechanisms (reviewed by van Gelder et al., 2014). Similar to other toxicants, the mechanism of action of a teratogen ultimately involves the interaction of the chemical with a target molecule. This interaction results in cell dysfunction, and sometimes cell death, either by interfering with cell regulation or cell maintenance. For instance, a number of anticancer drugs are human teratogens. These are drugs designed to kill dividing cells and exert a similar effect in the embryo. Another example is retinoids that are used in the embryo for cell signaling. Therapeutic retinoids have proven to be potent human teratogens. The mechanisms underlying teratogenesis for other teratogens, such as those drugs most commonly used to treat epilepsy, remain unknown.

## References

Atta CAM, Fiest KM, Frolkis AD, Jette N, Pringsheim T, St Germaine-Smith C, Rajapakse T et al. (2016). Global birth prevalence of spina bifida by folic acid fortification status: A systematic review and meta-analysis. *Am J Public Health*. 106, 159.

Barton S (2013). Teratology testing under REACH. *Methods Mol Biol*. 947, 57–72.

Buschmann J (2013). The OECD guidelines for the testing of chemicals and pesticides. *Methods in Molecular Biology*. 947, 37–56.

Canfield MA, Mai CT, Wang Y, O'Halloran A, Marengo LK, Olney RS, and National Birth Defects Prevention Network (2014). The association between race/ethnicity and major birth defects in the United States, 1999–2007. *Am J Public Health*. 104, E14–E23.

Clarkson TW (1992). Mercury, major issues in environmental health. *Environ Health Perspect*. 100, 31–8.

Czeilzel AE (2008). Specified critical period of different congenital abnormalities: A new approach for human teratological studies. *Congen Anom*. 48, 103–9.

De-Regil L, Peña-Rosas J, Fernández-Gaxiola AC, Rayco-Solon P (2015). Effects and safety of periconceptional oral folate supplementation for preventing birth defects. Cochrane Database of Systematic Reviews. Issue 12. Art. No.: CD007950.

Egeghy PP, Judson R, Gangwal S, Mosher S, Smith D, Vail J, Cohen Hubal EA (2012). The exposure data landscape for manufactured chemicals. *Sci Total Environ*. 414, 159–66.

EU. (2009). Accessed 15 August 2016. http://europa.eu/rapid/press-release_IP-09-643_en.htm?locale=en.

Food Fortification Initiative. (2016). Enhancing Grains for Healthier Lives. Country profiles. Accessed 15 August 2016. http://www.ffinetwork.org/regional_activity/index.php.

Griffiths SK, Campbell JP (2014). Placental structure, function and drug transfer. *Contin Educ Anaesth Criti Care Pain*. 15, 84–9.

Hachiya NT (2006). The history and the present of Minamata disease—Entering the second half a century. *JMAJ*. 49, 112–8.

Hamilton BE, Martin JA, Osterman MJK, Curtin SC, Mathews TJ (2015). Births: Final Data for 2014. National Center for Health Statistics ed. Hyattsville, MD.

Harada M (1995). Minamata disease: Methylmercury poisoning in Japan caused by environmental pollution. *Crit Rev Tox*. 25, 1–24.

Holmes LB (2010). What birth defects are common in humans? How are they diagnosed at birth? In: *Teratology Primer*. Hales B, Scialli A, Tassinari MS eds. The Teratology Society.

ICH. (2015). S5(R3): Harmonised Tripartite Guidelines. Detection of toxicity to reproduction for medicinal products & toxicity to male fertility. http://www.ich.org/fileadmin/Public_Web_Site/ICH_Products/Guidelines/Safety/S5/S5_R3__Final_Concept_Paper_27Mar2015.pdf.

Kim, JH, Scialli AR (2011). Thalidomide: The tragedy of birth defects and the effective treatment of disease. *Toxicol Sci.* 122, 1–6.

Klemmt L, Scialli AR (2005). The transport of chemicals in semen. *Birth Defects Res B: Devl Reprod Toxicol.* 74, 119–31.

Kramer MS (2003). The epidemiology of adverse pregnancy outcomes: An overview. *J Nutr.* 133 (5 Suppl 2), 1592S–6S.

Macdorman MF, Gregory ECW (2015). Fetal and perinatal mortality 2013. National vital statistics reports ed. Hyattsville, MD: National Center for Health Statistics.

Macklon NS, Geraedts JPM, Fauser BCJM (2002). Conception to ongoing pregnancy: The 'black box' of early pregnancy loss. *Hum Reprod Update.* 8, 333–43.

March of Dimes. (2012). Miscarriage. Last modified July 2012 Accessed 23 August 2016. http://www.marchofdimes.org/complications/miscarriage.aspx.

March of Dimes. (2014). Low birthweight. mast Modified October 2014 Accessed 23 August 2016. http://www.marchofdimes.org/complications/low-birthweight.aspx.

March of Dimes Foundation. (2006). Global Report on Birth Defect: The Hidden Toll of Dying and Disabled Children. White Plains, NY: March of Dimes Birth Defects Foundation.

OECD. (2014). Health at a Glance: Europe 2014. http://dx.doi.org/10.1787/health_glance_eur-2014-en: OECD Publishing.

Rice DC, Schoeny R, Mahaffey K (2003). Methods and rationale for derivation of a reference dose for methylmercury by the U.S. EPA. *Risk analysis.* 23, 107–15.

Ridings JE (2013). The thalidomide disaster, lessons from the past. *Methods Mol Biol.* 947, 575–86.

Schardein J (2000). *Chemically-Induced Birth Defects.* New York: Marcel Dekker.

Schrager S, Potter BE (2004). Diethylstilbestrol exposure. *Am Fam Physician.* 69, 2395–400.

Shepard TH (2010). *Catalog of Teratogenic Agents,* 13th ed. Baltimore, MD: John Hopkins University Press.

van Gelder MM, van Rooij IA, de Jong-van den Berg LT, Roeleveld N (2014). Teratogenic mechanisms associated with prenatal medication exposure. *Therapie.* 69, 13–24.

Vargesson N (2015). Thalidomide-induced teratogenesis: History and mechanisms. *Birth Defects Res C Embryo Today.* 105, 140–56.

Webster WS, Freeman JA (2001). Is this drug safe in pregnancy? *Reprod Toxicol.* 15, 619–29.

Webster WS, Freeman JA (2003). Prescription drugs and pregnancy. *Expert Opin Pharmacother.* 4, 949–61.

Wise LD (2013). The ICH S5(R2) guideline for the testing of medicinal agents. *Methods Mol Biol.* 947, 1–11.

# *chapter eleven*

# *Toxicology of lactation*

**Ok-Nam Bae**

*Contents*



## *General remarks*

The term *lactation* is used to refer to the biological state during which a mammary gland produces and excretes milk, as a balanced mixture of nutrients. The term *breastfeeding* implies all human milk feeding situations when an infant or a child is fed with human milk directly from the breast or as expressed milk (AAPPS, 2012; U.S. FDA, 2015). In terms of toxicological consideration, two different approaches are considered: (1) information on the effects of a chemical and its metabolite(s) on the process of milk production, and (2) data on the presence of a chemical and/or its metabolite(s) in human milk and potential adverse effects on the breastfed child. Although these two approaches have slightly different implications regarding the target of toxicity (for example, a maternally exposed toxicant might affect either the maternal lactation system or the breastfed child through the secreted breast milk), they will be covered as toxicological effects related to lactation.

In most cases, the major concern is focusing on the presence of chemicals in human milk following exposure of the mother, and the potential adverse effects on the breastfed infant or child attributed to exposure to the chemicals through human milk. Prior to discussing the potential toxic effects of chemicals existing in breast milk, we will first introduce the advantages of breastfeeding.

## *Benefits of breastfeeding*

Following birth, the fetal stage develops into the neonate or infant. Exposure to drugs and environmental agents may be either direct through inhalation, ingestion, dermal or a combination of these routes or indirectly via the mother's milk. The importance and necessity of breast milk in the developing neonate have been clearly shown (Kacew, 1994; Berlin and Kacew, 1997). Breastfeeding confers certain benefits on infants, which are summarized in Table 11.1 and discussed in the following sections. The frequency of some disease conditions was clearly diminished in breastfed infants. Outcomes from a systematic review, with meta-analysis on the long-term effects of breastfeeding (Horta et al., 2007), have also been incorporated in Table 11.2.

Breastfeeding has distinct advantages nutritionally, immunologically, and psychologically and should be encouraged despite the presence of environmental toxins. At present, it should be stressed that human milk remains the best nutrient source for the healthy term infant (Redel and Shulman, 1994). Meta-analyses of chronic effects of breastfeeding also demonstrated that the prevalence of overweight/obesity/type-2 diabetes is lower in breastfed subjects (Horta et al., 2007). Not only beneficial to the breastfed child or infants, breastfeeding has also beneficial effects to the nursing mothers. Women who have breastfed for a lifetime total of at least 2 years are associated with a 23% lower risk of coronary heart disease than those who never breastfed (Stuebe et al., 2009). However, the breastfeeding mother is subject to exposure from environmental contaminants including heavy metals, xenoestrogens, pesticides, and solvents, and these pollutants may be present in the milk (Massart et al., 2005). In the majority of cases, it is still more beneficial to breastfeed despite the presence of such contaminants. Recently, the use of plastic baby bottles containing a chemical, bisphenol A (BPA), was linked to the development of abnormal endocrine functions in animals. Although excessive concentrations of BPA produced these changes in nonhuman organisms, regulatory agencies in

**Table 11.1** Adverse infant conditions protected by breastfeeding

| |
|---|
| Infant mortality |
| Sudden infant death syndrome |
| Respiratory tract disease |
| Food allergies |
| Atopic dermatitis |
| Otitis media |
| Asthma |
| Immune system disorders |
| Lymphomas |
| Celiac disease |
| Insulin-dependent diabetes mellitus |
| Inflammatory bowel disease |
| Crohn's disease |
| HIV-related mortality |
| Cholera |
| *Giardia lamblia* diarrhea |
| Rotavirus diarrhea |
| Shigellosis |
| Bacteremia and meningitis |
| Chronic liver disease |

*Source:* Kacew S, *Biomed Environ Sci*, 7, 307–319, 1994. Kacew S, *General and Applied Toxicology*, Macmillan, New York, 2000.

some countries banned the use of this chemical in baby bottles. In the case of breastfeeding, there was no exposure of lactating infants to BPA, again pointing out an advantage for breast versus bottle-feeding.

## *Immune system*

The beneficial effects of breastfeeding against immune system disorders are well established (Davis et al., 1988; Mayer et al., 1988; Kramer, 1988). The finding that lead (Pb) interferes with the immune system indicates that the presence of this metal in milk may prevent protection in Pb-exposed mothers. It should also be noted that in the presence of environmental toxicants and a condition of malnourishment, the immune system is further compromised, as there is an increased sensitivity to viral infection. The transmission of human immunodeficiency virus (HIV) during breastfeeding from infected mothers to suckling infants is well documented (Oxtoby, 1988). Based on this knowledge, the question arises as to the advantages of bottle-feeding in HIV-infected

***Table 11.2*** Evidence on the long-term effects of breastfeeding

| | Range of effect of other public health interventions in later life | | | | Breastfeeding | |
|---|---|---|---|---|---|---|
| Outcome | Diet/dietary advice | Exercise | Multiple risk factor intervention | Modest salt restriction | Pooled effect size (95% I) | Conclusion |
| Overweight or obesity | *Diet/dietary advice & exercise*: 5/6 studies showed no effect on childhood obesity. Meta-analysis not done because of heterogeneity between studies. | | | | Odds ratio 0.78 (0.72–0.84) | Significant (22% reduction), while other interventions showed no effect. |
| Type II diabetes | *Diet/dietary advice & exercise*: 31–46% reduction in risk in persons with impaired glucose tolerance. | | | | Odds ratio 0.63 (0.45–0.89) | Significant (37% reduction) and of similar magnitude to the effect of other interventions. |
| Intelligence test score | | | | | Mean difference 4.9 points (2.97–6.92) | Significant, with a substantial effect size. |

*Source:* Adapted from Horta BL et al., World Health Organization, Geneva, Switzerland, 2007.

mothers. In an extensive study, Lederman (1992) demonstrated that exclusive breastfeeding, even in situations where mothers were HIV infected, produced a decrease in the estimated infant mortality rate, especially in population areas where HIV prevalence was low. Although lactation does not protect against HIV transmission, breastfeeding is clearly beneficial in reducing infant mortality. In a population where HIV infection is exceedingly high, bottle-feeding is preferable. Bearing this in mind, the benefits of breastfeeding substantially outweigh HIV transmission, as one must consider infant mortality. In general, once a mother is infected, antibodies and numerous protective factors are produced in the mother's body and these are secreted in milk to protect babies (Jackson and Nazar, 2006). Clearly, breastfeeding protects against infant mortality regardless of the cause and this physiological process should not be discontinued.

## *Cancer*

The beneficial effects of protecting breastfed infants against lymphoid hypertrophy and lymphomas have been documented (Davis et al., 1988). This protective antineoplastic effect was found to extend to the mother, where lactation for prolonged periods was correlated with a reduction in breast cancer (McTiernan and Thomas, 1986). Although Kvale and Heuch (1988) failed to demonstrate any association in a large cohort study, the more extensive investigation by Newcomb et al. (1994) produced a positive inverse correlation between lactation and risk of breast cancer in premenopausal women. However, no marked reduction in the risk of breast cancer was found in postmenopausal women with a history of lactation. Regardless of the fact that breast cancer occurs in less than one quarter of all cases reported and that lactation provides a slight protective effect, it was concluded that any factor which reduces the incidence of breast cancer should be encouraged.

## *Avoidance of food allergies*

In the case of food allergies or atopic dermatitis, it is generally accepted that breastfeeding delays the development of these disorders (Lucas et al., 1990). Although Kramer (1988) suggested that breastfeeding provided protection against allergic diseases, these manifestations occurred in exclusively breastfed infants. However, it should be noted that the incidence of food allergies decreased dramatically in exclusively breastfed infants. In recent studies, the maternal diet was found to be a critical factor in the development of allergic manifestations in lactating infants. Ingestion of a maternal hypoallergenic diet devoid of cow's milk, eggs, and fish during lactation lowered the cumulative incidence and current prevalence of atopic dermatitis during the first 6 months of age with continuation to the age 4 years old (Chandra et al., 1989; Sigurs et al., 1992). Breastfeeding per se is effective in protecting against allergic disorders provided the offending stimulus is not ingested by the mother and transmitted to the infant via the milk.

### *Psychological bonding*

Breastfeeding is known to create a special psychological bond between an infant and a mother that ultimately leads to a socially healthier child. In addition, lactation enhances maternal postpartum recovery and body weight returns to prepartum levels more rapidly. The physiological process of breastfeeding plays a critical role in human growth and development. The use of bottles to feed nursing infants with milk formula, in developing countries, was found to enhance morbidity and mortality. In addition, with the knowledge that bottles contain BPA, the potential for endocrine disruption was eliminated through breastfeeding. In affluent nations, inadequate knowledge on growth patterns between breastfed and bottle-fed infants resulted in inappropriate counseling against lactation. In an extensive study, Dewey et al. (1992) demonstrated that the growth pattern was equivalent between breastfed and formula-fed infants from birth to the first 3 months. However, breastfed infants gained significantly less weight from 3 to 12 months without any deleterious effects on nutrition, morbidity, motor activity level, or behavioral development. It is evident that breastfed infants are leaner and do not display a faltering growth pattern; women should be encouraged to continue the lactational process beyond 3 months. With the knowledge that growth in breastfed infants is generally less than in formula-fed, growth per se as an index of toxicity in the first year of life is not appropriate.

Maternal nutrient intake is an important factor in the growth pattern of the infant. If a deficiency of zinc (Zn) exists, there may be a delay in infant growth. Thus, in conditions of adequate maternal Zn concentrations, lactation should be encouraged despite a decreased infant growth pattern. A maternal diet deficient in essential nutrients, such as iron or calcium, results in a greater bioavailability of mammary Pb, with consequent developmental delay.

## *Toxic effects of chemicals in breast milk to nursing infant/child*

Despite the advantages of breastfeeding both to the nursing mother and the breastfed infant/child, there is an increasing concern that the effects of chemicals exposed to nursing mothers could ultimately induce adverse health outcomes in breastfed infants or children. Chemicals absorbed in the plasma of nursing mothers pass into breast milk primarily by passive diffusion. Therefore, several factors affecting absorption, distribution, and excretion of chemicals may be determining factors for the available amount of chemical toxicants in breast milk. Oral bioavailability, plasma half-life, lipid solubility, molecular weight, ionization state, and percentage of maternal protein binding are the representative factors influencing the transfer of chemicals into breast milk (Berlin and Briggs, 2005). Milk composition also affects the extent of transfer of chemicals. Milk at the end of feed, namely hindmilk, contains more concentrated fat-soluble chemicals since it has more fat than foremilk.

## *Biomarkers of exposure*

It is clear that chemicals are present in milk and that these agents may affect the suckling infant. However, limited data are available to determine whether the presence of the chemical is sufficient to exert an adverse effect. There have been trials to identify biomarkers of chemical exposure to address whether chemicals excreted via breast milk might affect the nursing child. Diehl-Jones and Bols (2000), using dioxin, established the criteria or biomarkers of exposure. In essence, alterations in certain milk constituents provide evidence for a dioxin-like effect. Examples of biomarkers in milk include lysosyme, cathepsin; vitamins A to K; cytokines interleukin 1 or tumor necrosis factor; and hormones including estrogen, thyroxine, or prolactin. The determination of these biomarkers could then be used to ascertain the degree of exposure. The cellular modifications that one measures include cytochrome P-450 induction, DNA adducts, apoptosis, and chemokinesis. This may prove crucial in terms of therapeutic intervention following an exposure.

## *Toxicants*

The nursing mother can serve as a source of neonatal exposure to drugs or chemicals (Wang and Needham, 2007). No matter whether the agent is an over-the-counter medication or prescribed by a physician, most drugs are detectable in breast milk. The presence of a drug in maternal milk may be construed as a potential hazard to the infant even though only 1–2% of the total intake is likely to be found there. The basis for this observation is the fact that drug metabolizing enzymes involved in degrading and eliminating the drugs are not fully developed in the lactating neonate, resulting in excess amounts of chemical present in the infant. Hence, the primary consideration in maternal drug therapy is the risk to the nursing infant rather than the mere presence of xenobiotic in the milk. Based

***Table 11.3*** Toxicants identified in human breast milk and their adverse infant effects

| Chemical | Effect |
|---|---|
| Silicone | Esophageal dysfunction |
| Hexachlorobenzene | Porphyria cutanea tarda |
| Polychlorinated biphenyls | Abnormal skin pigmentation, bone defects, growth retardation, hypotonia |
| Perchloroethylene | Obstructive jaundice |
| Methylmercury | Developmental delay, abnormal muscle tone, mental retardation, decreased suckling response |
| Lead | Poor mental performance, central nervous system toxicosis |
| Nicotine | Decreased weight gain |
| Cadmium | Low birth weight |

*Source:* Kacew S, *Biomed Environ Sci,* 7, 307–319, 1994. Berlin CM Jr, Kacew S, *Environmental Toxicology and Pharmacology of Human Development,* Taylor & Francis, Washington, DC. 1997; Berlin CM et al., *J Toxicol Environ Health.,* A 65, 1839–1851, 2002.

on the numerous advantages of breastfeeding, the benefit of this physiological process, in the majority of cases, far exceeds the potential risk. Although it may be inadvertent, the suckling infant also derives environmental chemicals from the mother. These chemicals are excreted in breast milk and pose a serious potential hazard to the infant (Berlin et al., 2002) (Table 11.3). Unlike drug therapy, which can be voluntarily terminated, environmental exposure may be chronic and, consequently, more toxic. Emphasis on risk assessment of chemicals in breast milk via infant exposure has increased since human milk is known to concentrate persistent, bioaccumulative, and toxic (PBT) chemicals (LaKind et al., 2004). PBTs accumulate in the lipids of humans and they are not likely to be eliminated easily via urinary or fecal excretion. Generally, the levels of PBTs in breast milk are in positive relationship with the mother's age (Albers et al., 1996), since the levels of these compounds increase with age, and the breast milk is a major route of elimination of maternal PBTs. In addition, both environmental chemicals and drugs present in milk might enter the infant to exert a synergistic adverse effect. Some of these are discussed in the following sections:

## *Silicone*

Silicone is a polymeric substance, which is inert and is unlikely to produce a toxic manifestation. Based on these properties, the use of silicone for breast implantation was considered ideal; however, retrospective studies revealed an increased incidence of rheumatological disorders, in particular, scleroderma and arthritis. Levin and Ilowite (1994) reported that in infants of breastfeeding mothers with silicone implants, there was a decreased lower sphincter pressure and abnormal esophageal wave propagation. Clearly, the inert material silicone was associated with infant esophageal disease as a result of lactational exposure. It has been suggested that leakage from the implant produces immunological substances that lead to scleroderma development. However, it should be noted that silicon concentrations in cows' milk exceed those in human breast milk by a factor of 10 and are even higher in infant formula (Semple et al., 1998). Normally human milk contains immunological components, which provide protection against diseases. In the presence of silicone, the breast milk would contain components that may immunologically compromise the infant not only with esophageal dysfunction but also with increased susceptibility to other immune-related diseases.

## *Mercury*

Lactational exposure of human infants to metals is a concern and raises the issue of risks versus benefits in the maintenance of the breastfeeding process. Mercury (Hg) levels in milk are usually low (<1 ng/mL), but in environmental disasters such as in Minamata, Japan, the levels reached 50 ng/mL. Numerous studies exist on the effects of either prenatal or during both pregnancy and postnatal exposure to metals on developing infants, but few reports are available on the consequences of the presence of metals exclusively in breast milk on children. Bearing in mind the consequences of methylmercury (MeHg) poisoning, especially in Minamata, Japan, consideration should be given to the contribution of lactational exposure to the observed neuronal disturbances in cases where nursing mothers, ingesting Hg-contaminated fish, were found to have severe neurological disorders in their infants (Matsumoto et al., 1965). Takeuchi (1968) clearly demonstrated the effects of epidemic MeHg exposure on fetal and newborn development. Industrial release of MeHg into Minamata Bay, followed by accumulation in edible fish and ingestion by lactating females, resulted in the transfer of metal to the suckling human infant. Similarly, Amin-Zaki et al. (1974) demonstrated that ingestion of homemade bread, prepared from wheat treated with the fungicide MeHg, by lactating mothers produced a significant rise in human infant metal levels. Maternal ingestion of Hg-contaminated food during pregnancy and lactation among fish-eating populations in Canada resulted in abnormal muscle tone and reflexes in boys only (McKeown-Eyssen et al., 1983). In a New Zealand study, Kjellstrom et al. (1989) reported developmental retardation in 4-year-old children of mothers eating Hg-contaminated fish during pregnancy and lactation. Although emphasis was placed on the consequences of prenatal exposure in the Canadian and New Zealand studies, the contribution of milk Hg to toxic outcome was neglected. It should be noted that in some patients with Minamata disease, the neurological symptoms did not develop at the time of exposure but years later. Further, the reported number of cases where children born in a Hg-contaminated area in Japan were healthy yet developed neuropathy in childhood. The contribution of breast milk Hg to late-onset Minamata disease remains to be resolved. Mammary transfer of MeHg to suckling infants has been reported to produce neurological lesions. This finding clearly indicates a positive correlation between exposure to high concentrations of metal in mammary tissue and toxicity in suckling infants.

Although the precise contribution of mammary-derived MeHg to the observed adverse effects on neurological and behavioral changes in suckling pups is not known, it was found that postnatal exposure to this metal produced ocular defects. In contrast, there was a lack of an ocular effect in fetuses of prenatal exposed dams, suggesting that lactation methylmercury may in part contribute to the observed toxicity. It is well known that MeHg is secreted more readily in the maternal colostrum, the period during which eye defects are reported, and passes onto the suckling infant. Mercury itself decreases the suckling response in human infants. Because milk contains essential nutrients for neurological and behavioral development, it is conceivable that less suckling and feeding would contribute to the Hg-induced nervous disorders, as there is less nutritional supply, and this is associated with delayed growth processes.

### *Lead*

The content of Pb in human milk ranged from 5 to 68 ng/mL in a number of studies conducted in the United States and Europe, (Rabinowitz et al., 1985). Levels in Boston averaged 1.7 ng/mL in 1979. Dillon (1974) found Pb levels of approximately 26 ng/mL in seven different U.S. cities. In Mexico City, milk Pb levels reached 45 ng/mL (Berlin and Kacew, 1997; Berlin et al., 2002). It is not surprising that upon examination of the source of infant Pb intoxication, breast milk contained far less metal than either formula or environmental sources such as ceramic-leachable kitchenware, or paint chips (Rabinowitz et al., 1985). There is evidence to suggest a correlation between poor mental performance, as evidenced by the Bayley Infant Assessment Test, and increased Pb level (Needleman et al., 1983). These findings prompted Newman (1993) to recommend the promotion of breastfeeding, as human milk was a less suitable transmission vehicle for Pb contamination compared with formula feeding. Further, it should be stressed that the best source for daily nutrition among infants is human milk.

There is evidence to suggest that the presence of lactational metal results in newborn toxicity, although the contribution of only mammary Pb exposure to observed toxic effects on the central nervous system (CNS) remain unclear. Direct application of topical Pb ointment on the breast was reported to produce CNS toxicosis in the human infant (Dillon, 1974). The presence of Pb in mammary tissue alters the nutritional value of milk as reflected by decreases in the essential elements copper, zinc, and iron, which are required for mammalian metabolism and CNS function. Pb affects the absorption of calcium, iron, and vitamin D. In conditions of diets deficient in essential elements, Pb absorption and toxicity is enhanced in infants. Because breast milk is a source of Pb for suckling infants, it is conceivable that during iron-deficiency anemia or calcium-deficient dietary intake in mothers, the bioavailability of milk Pb is increased, resulting in greater toxicity. Evidence suggests that Pb exposure may interfere with maternal metabolic pathways, resulting in decreased utilization of nutrients in the diet, and thus an absence of nutritional components present in milk. This altered milk composition will consequently adversely affect newborn development.

## *Halogenated hydrocarbons*

Chemical exposure, via accidents and hazardous waste sites, resulted in toxicant accumulation in breast milk. The human maternal ingestion of a fungicide, hexachlorobenzene-treated wheat resulted in chemical accumulation in breast milk. Suckling infants subsequently developed symptoms of a disease, pembe yara, and a condition of prophyria cutanea tarda (Peters et al., 1982). Exposure to organophosphate pesticides such as chlorpyrifos and malathion is worthy of mention, as these compounds have been identified in breast milk (Berlin and Kacew, 1997). Ingestion of chlorpyrifos by a 3-year-old infant resulted in delayed polyneuropathy with transient bilateral vocal paralysis (Aiuto et al., 1993). Although lactation per se was not involved in this specific case, the importance lies in the fact that the manifestations of exposure did not occur until 1 to 3 weeks later. One should be aware that the consequences of lactational exposure to toxicants may also be delayed. This is supported by the reports of a mother who was exposed to 2,4-diphenoxyacetic acid (2,4-D) spray during pregnancy and lactation. Examination of the infant at 5 and 24 months of age revealed multiple malformations and severe mental retardation. Although mammary tissue content of 2,4-D was not determined, prolonged maternal exposure with consequent transmission to the infant was suggested as the cause of the observed toxicity. The fact that lactational-derived organophosphate pesticides alter suckling infant metabolism and that toxicity may be delayed suggests that breastfeeding in severe exposure conditions should be minimized.

Ingestion of polychlorinated biphenyl (PCB)-contaminated rice oil by nursing mothers was found to produce low-birth weight human infants, growth retardation, abnormal skin pigmentation as well as bone and tooth defects (Yamaguchi et al., 1971). In extensive studies in North Carolina, Rogan et al. (1986) measured the levels of PCB in human milk and found an associated hypotonicity and hyporeflexia in nursing infants. Organochlorine pesticides including DDT, aldrin, and dieldrin have been identified in human milk (Berlin and Kacew, 1997; Wang and Needham, 2007). However, it is surprising that manifestations of toxicity in suckling infants following maternal organochlorine exposure have not been reported. This should not be considered proof that the presence of organochlorine contaminants in breast milk fails to affect the infant, as these environmental toxicants induce mammary carcinoma and may act as cocarcinogens. It is well known that suckling infants of cigarette smoking mothers are more prone to respiratory irritation and infections. However, cigarette smoking in the presence of atmospheric pollutants exerts an additive toxic effect on the mother. Conceivably, the presence of organochlorine compounds and nicotine in breast milk may increase infant toxicity as the hydrocarbons act as cocarcinogens. Hence, in susceptible suckling infants, these compounds may precipitate autoimmune diseases or lymphomas.

### *Ethanol (alcohol)*

Alcohol ingestion during pregnancy is known to result in congenital anomalies termed "fetal alcohol syndrome" (FAS). FAS is characterized by mental deficiency, microcephaly, irritability, and poor muscle coordination in the affected subjects. This syndrome is associated with alcoholic women who drank heavily and chronically during pregnancy. Although the contribution of alcohol during lactation to FAS has not been established, it is known that the severity of manifestations in infants is correlated with the amount consumed. Hence, alcohol in breast milk could worsen the already adverse infant development initiated during pregnancy. There are some studies inferring that alcohol exposure during lactation may increase the susceptibility of the infant to develop cancer (Infante-Rivard and El-Zein, 2007).

### *Solvents*

The aromatic hydrocarbon toluene is utilized as a solvent or thinner in numerous industrial products including paints, glue, and resins. The lipophilic property of toluene is of interest in light of the physicochemical properties of breast tissue. Hersh et al. (1985) demonstrated that in infants of approximately 4 years of age, maternal exposure to toluene throughout pregnancy, via glue sniffing, produced embryopathy, mental deficiency, and postnatal growth delay. There is no doubt that *in utero* exposure to toluene was manifested in teratogenesis. However, as there was evidence of postnatal growth deficiency and that toluene has a high affinity for fat, it is also possible that these infants were exposed to this solvent via the mother's milk. This is supported by the finding that obstructive jaundice developed in infants of lactating mothers exposed to the dry cleaning solvent perchloroethylene (Bagnell and Ellenberg, 1977). It is well established that exposure to the organic solvents during pregnancy results in toxemia and anemia. Unfortunately, infants born to these mothers were not followed clinically during lactation. However, as these environmental chemicals accumulate in breast milk and produce metabolic maternal alterations, it is conceivable that solvents may alter infant development. The release of organic solvents from breast milk fat needs to be considered among solvent abusers in light of adverse effects reported in children (Schreiber, 1997).

## *Pharmacological agents*

In certain cases, nursing mothers are required to take medication during breastfeeding. Basically, all drugs transfer into breast milk and might potentially affect the breastfed infant/child, and efforts need to be made to minimize the risk by reducing drug exposure, with the lowest effective dose for the shortest duration. Several factors, such as pharmacokinetic and the intrinsic toxicity of the drug, could ultimately determine the risk of drug to breastfed infant/child. Drugs with greater inherent toxicity or high infant exposure are contraindicated during breastfeeding, as listed in Table 11.4 (Bertino et al., 2012; New Zealand Government, 2015). Drugs to avoid in the newborn and in infants less than 6 months of age, as suggested by Berlin and Briggs (2005), are also included in Table 11.4. Nevertheless, most medicines are considered to be compatible and may be used during breastfeeding, therefore the benefits and risks of treatment, in both nursing mother and the breastfed infant, need to be carefully considered (Berlin and Briggs, 2005). In an attempt to provide more up-to-date information for safe usage of medicines during breastfeeding, a database of medicine levels in breast milk and infant blood and possible adverse reactions in the nursing infant is available to the public at LactMed website (www.toxnet.nlm.nih.gov/newtoxnet/lactmed.htm). In guidance for the Lactation subsection of labeling for human prescription drug and biological products, the U.S. FDA recommends to provide the information on the presence of a drug and/or its active metabolite(s) in human milk, the effects of a drug and/or its active metabolite(s) on the breastfed child, and the effects of a drug and/or its active metabolite(s) on milk production (U.S. FDA, 2015).

***Table 11.4*** Drugs that require caution during breastfeeding

| Contraindicated medicines in breastfeeding | |
|---|---|
| Antineoplastic drugs | Bleomycin |
| | Cyclophosphamide |
| | Methotrexate |
| | Doxorubicin |
| Radionuclides | |
| Psychotropic drugs | Lithium |
| Ergotamine | |
| Immunosuppressive agents | Azathioprine |
| | Ciclosporin |
| Amiodarone | |
| Hormones and antihormones | Testosterone |
| | Tamoxifen |
| Gold salts | |
| Isotretinoin | |
| **Drugs to avoid in the newborn and in infant <6 months of age** | |
| β-Blocking agents | Acebutolol |
| | Atenolol |
| | Labetalol |
| | Propranolol |
| | Sotalol |
| Salicylates | |
| Antineoplatstic agents | |
| Drugs of abuse | Cocaine |
| | Narcotics |
| | Amphetamines |
| | Phencyclidine |

*Source:* Berlin CM, Briggs GG, *Semin Fetal Neonatal Med.*, 10, 149–159, 2005. Bertino E et al., *J Matern Fetal Neonatal Med.*, 25 Suppl 4, 78–80, 2012. New Zealand Government, Medicines use in lactation, *Prescriber Update* 36, 22–5, 2015. WHO, Breastfeeding and Maternal medication: Recommendations for Drugs in the Eleventh WHO Model List of Essential Drugs, 2002.

## *Toxic effects on milk production*

Xenobiotics exposure of nursing mothers might alter the processes of milk production or excretion, that is, lactation. Potential targets for toxicological effects on the lactation system include development/maturation of the mammary tissue, milk secretion and/or regulation of hormones including oxytocin or prolactin (Hood, 2016). These effects might possibly lead to starvation in offspring. Among environmental toxicants, DDT, cigarette smoking, TCDD, PCBs, and ethanol are known to have the potential to affect the normal processes of lactation (Neville, 1995). 2,4-D is known to alter the composition of milk (Stürtz et al., 2000). Several medications may also affect lactation system mediated by alterations in the level of prolactin. Dopaminergic antagonists, antihypertensive drugs, and antiemetic drugs are known to stimulate milk production through increased release of prolactin, while diuretics, dopaminergic agonists, and estrogen have been shown to decrease prolactin levels resulting in reduced secretion of milk (Coker and Taylor, 2010; Schaefer et al., 2007).

## References

Aiuto LA, Pavlakis SG, Boxer RA (1993). Life-threatening organophosphate-induced delayed polyneuropathy in a child after accidental chlorpyrifos. *J Pediatr.* 122, 658–60.

Albers JM, Kreis IA, Liem AK, van Zoonen P (1996). Factors that influence the level of contamination of human milk with poly-chlorinated organic compounds. *Arch Environ Contam Toxicol.* 30, 285–91.

American Academy of Pediatrics Policy Statement (AAPPS) (2012). Breastfeeding and the use of human milk. *Pediatrics.* 129, e827–41.

Amin-Zaki L, Elhassini S, Majeed MA et al. (1974). Studies of infants postnatally exposed to methylmercury. *J Pediatr.* 85, 81–4.

Bagnell PC, Ellenberg HA (1977). Obstructive jaundice due to a chlorinated hydrocarbon in breast milk. *Can Med Assoc J.* 117, 1047–8.

Berlin CM, Briggs GG (2005). Drugs and chemicals in human milk. *Semin Fetal Neonatal Med.* 10, 149–59.

Berlin CM Jr, Kacew S, Lawrence R et al. (2002). Criteria for chemical selection for programs on human milk surveillance and research for environmental chemicals. *J Toxicol Environ Health A.* 65, 1839–51.

Berlin CM Jr, Kacew S (1997). Environmental contamination human milk. In: Kacew S, Lambert GH, eds. *Environmental Toxicology and Pharmacology of Human Development*. Washington, DC: Taylor & Francis.

Bertino E, Varalda A, Di Nicola P, Coscia A, Occhi L, Vagliano L, Soldi A et al. (2012). Drugs and breastfeeding: Instructions for use. *J Matern Fetal Neonatal Med.* 25 Suppl 4, 78–80.

Chandra RK, Puri S, Hamed A (1989). Influence of maternal diet during lactation and use of formula feeds on development of atopic eczema in high risk infants. *Br Med J.* 299, 228–30.

Coker F, Taylor D (2010). Antidepressant-induced hyperprolactinaemia: Incidence, mechanisms and management. *CNS Drugs.* 24, 563–74.

Davis MK, Savitz DA, Graubard BI (1988). Infant feeding and childhood cancer. *Lancet* 2. 365–8.

Dewey KG, Heining MJ, Nommsen LA et al. (1992). Growth of breastfed and formula-fed infants from 0 to 18 months: The DARLING study. *Pediatrics.* 89, 1035–41.

Diehl-Jones WL, Bols NC (2000). Use of response biomarkers in milk for assessing exposure to environmental contaminants: The case for dioxin-like compounds. *J Toxicol Environ Health B*. 3, 79–107.

Dillon HK (1974). Lead concentration in human milk. *Am J Dis Child*. 128, 491–492.

Hersh JH, Podruch PE, Rogers G et al. (1985). Toluene embryopathy. *J Pediatr*. 106, 922–7.

Hood RD (2016). *Developmental and Reproductive Toxicology: A Practical Approach, 3rd Ed*. Informa Healthcare, Boca Raton: CRC Press.

Horta BL, Bahl R, Martines JC, Victora CG (2007). Evidence on the long-term effects of breastfeeding: Systematic reviews and meta-analyses. Geneva, Switzerland: World Health Organization. ISBN 9789241595230. http://whqlibdoc.who.int/publications/2007/9789241595230_eng.pdf. Retrieved 2011-09-18.

Infante-Rivard C, El-Zein M (2007). Parental alcohol consumption and childhood cancers: A review. *J Toxicol Environ Health B*. 10, 101–29.

Jackson KM, Nazar AM (2006). Breastfeeding, the immune response, and long-term health. *J Am Osteopath Assoc*. 106, 203–7.

Kacew S (1994). Current issues in lactation: Advantages, environment, silicone. *Biomed Environ Sci*. 7, 307–19.

Kacew S (2000). Neonatal toxicology. In: Ballantyne B, Marrs T, Syversen T, eds. *General and Applied Toxicology*. New York: Macmillan.

Kjellstrom T, Kennedy P, Wallis S et al. (1989). Physical and mental development of children with prenatal exposure to mercury from fish. Stage 2. Interviews and psychological tests at age 6, Solna, National Swedish Environmental Board, 112 (Report no. 3642).

Kramer MS (1988). Does breastfeeding help protect against atopic disease? Biology, methodology and a golden jubilee of controversy. *J Pediatr*. 112, 181–90.

Kvale G, Heuch I (1988). Lactation and cancer risk: Is there a relation specific to breast cancer? *J Epidemiol Community Health*. 42, 30–7.

LactMed (www.toxnet.nlm.nih.gov/newtoxnet/lactmed.htm).

LaKind JS, Amina Wilkins A, Berlin CM Jr. (2004). Environmental chemicals in human milk: A review of levels, infant exposures and health, and guidance for future research. *Toxicol Appl Pharmacol*. 198, 184–208.

Lederman SA (1992). Estimating infant mortality from human immunodeficiency virus and other causes in breastfeeding and bottle-feeding populations. *Pediatrics*. 89, 290–6.

Levine JJ, Ilowite NT (1994). Scleroderma like esophageal disease in children breastfed by mothers with silicone breast implants. *J Am Med Assoc*. 271, 213–6.

Lucas A, Brooke OG, Morley R et al. (1990). Early diet of preterm infants and development of allergic or atopic disease: Randomized prospective study. *Br Med J*. 300, 837–40.

Massart F, Harrell JC, Federico G et al. (2005). Human breast milk and xenoestrogen exposure: A possible impact on human health. *J Perinatol*. 25, 282–8.

Matsumoto M, Koya G, Takeuchi T (1965). Fetal Minamata disease. *J Neuropathol Exp Neurol*. 24, 563–74.

Mayer EJ, Hamman RF, Gay EC et al. (1988). Reduced risk of IDDM among breastfed children. *Diabetes*. 37, 1625–32.

McKeown-Eyssen GE, Ruedy J, Neims A (1983). Methyl mercury exposure in northern Quebec. II. Neurological finding in children. *Am J Epidemiol*. 118, 470–9.

McTiernan A, Thomas DB (1986). Evidence for a protective effect of lactation on risk of breast cancer in young women: Results from a case-control study. *Am J Epidemiol*. 124, 353–8.

Needleman H, Bellinger D, Leviton A et al. (1983). Umbilical cord blood lead levels and neuropsychological performance at 12 months of age. *Pediatr Res*. 17, 179A.

Newcomb PA, Storer BF, Longnecker MP et al. (1994). Lactation and reduced risk of premenopausal breast cancer. *N Engl J Med*. 330, 81–7.

Newman J (1993). Would breastfeeding decrease risks of lead intoxication? *Pediatrics*. 90, 131.

Neville MC, Walsh CT (1995). Effects of xenobiotics on milk secretion and composition. *Am J Clin Nutr*. 61, 687S–94S.

New Zealand Government (2015). Medicines use in lactation. *Prescriber Update* 36, 22–5.

Oxtoby MJ (1988). Human immunodeficiency virus and other viruses in human milk: Placing the issues in broader perspective. *Pediatr Infect Dis J*. 7, 825–35.

Peters HA, Gocmen A, Gripps DJ et al. (1982). Epidemiology of hexachlorobenzene induced porphyria in Turkey. *Arch Neurol*. 39, 744–9.

Rabinowitz M, Leviton A, Needleman H (1985). Lead in milk and infant blood: A dose-response mode. *Arch Environ Health*. 40, 283–6.

Redel CA, Shulman RG (1994). Controversies in the composition of infant formulas. *Pediatr Clin N A*. 41, 909–24.

Rogan WJ, Gladen BC, McKinney JD et al. (1986). Neonatal effects of transplacental exposure to PCBs and DDE. *J Pediatr*. 109, 335–41.

Schaefer C, Peters P, Miller RK (2007). *Drugs During Pregnancy and Lactation*. 2nd Ed., Amsterdam: Academic Press, Elsevier.

Schreiber JS (1997). Transport of organic chemicals to breast milk: Tetra-chlorothene case study. In: Kacew S, Lambert GH, eds. *Environmental Toxicology and Pharmacology of Human Development*. Washington, DC: Taylor & Francis.

Semple JL, Lugowski SJ, Baines CJ et al. (1998). Breast milk contamination and silicone implants: Preliminary results using silicon as a proxy measurement for silicone. *Plast Reconstr Surg*. 102, 528–33.

Sigurs N, Hattevig G, Kjellman B (1992). Maternal avoidance of eggs, cow's milk and fish during lactation: Effect on allergic manifestation, skin-prick test, specific 1gE antibodies in children at age 4 years. *Pediatrics*. 89, 735–9.

Stuebe AM, Michels KB, Willett WC et al. (2009). Duration of lactation and incidence of myocardial infarction in middle to late adulthood. *Am J Obstet Gynecol*. 200, 138. e1–138.e8.

Stürtz N, Evangelista de Duffard AM, Duffard R (2000). Detection of 2,4-dichlorophenoxyacetic acid (2,4-D) residues in neonates breastfed by 2,4-D exposed dams. *Neurotoxicology*. 21, 147–54.

U.S. FDA (2015). Pregnancy, Lactation, and Reproductive potential: Labeling for Human Prescription Drug and Biological Products-Content and Format.

Takeuchi T (1968). Pathology of Minamata disease. In: Kutsune M, ed. *Minamata Disease*. Japan: Kunamoto University.

Wang RY, Needham LL (2007). Environmental chemicals: From the environment to food, to breast milk, to the infant. *J Toxicol Environ Health B*. 10, 597–609.
WHO (2002). Breastfeeding and Maternal medication: Recommendations for Drugs in the Eleventh WHO Model List of Essential Drugs.
Yamaguchi A, Yoshimura T, Kuratsune M (1971). A survey of pregnant women having consumed rice oil contaminated with chlorobiphenyls and their babies. *Fukuoka Acta Med*. 62, 117–22.

*section three*

# *Target organs and systems*

# chapter twelve

# Toxicology of the liver

**Young-Suk Jung and Byung-Mu Lee**

## Contents



## Introduction

The liver is the largest (1.4–1.6 kg in an adult person) and metabolically the most complex organ in the body, involved in the metabolism of nutrients as well as most drugs and toxicants. The latter types of substances are usually detoxified, but many of them may be bioactivated and become more toxic. Hepatocytes (hepatic parenchymal cells) comprise the bulk of the organ. These cells are responsible for the liver's central role in metabolism, and lie between blood-filled sinusoids and the biliary passages. Kupffer cells line the hepatic sinusoids and constitute an important part of the reticuloendothelial system of the body. The blood is supplied through the portal vein and hepatic artery, and it is drained through the central veins, followed by the hepatic vein into the vena cava. The biliary passages begin as tiny bile canaliculi, formed by adjacent parenchymal cells, which coalesce into ductules, interlobular bile ducts, and larger hepatic ducts (Figure 12.1). The main hepatic duct joins the cystic duct from the gall bladder to form the common bile duct, which drains into the duodenum.

Toxicity of the liver (also termed hepatic toxicity or hepatotoxicity) is often encountered during new drug development and thus, substantial numbers of new drug candidates have been withdrawn because of discovery of drug-induced liver injury (DILI) (Watkins, 2011; Chen et al., 2013). Approximately 50% of candidate compounds have produced hepatic effects at supra-therapeutic dose (Amacher, 1998). During the 1990–1998 period, 458 deaths were estimated annually from overdoses of acetaminophen (APAP), a well-known hepatotoxic drug in the United States (Nourjah et al., 2006). Hepatotoxicity is therefore considered one of the most life-threatening drug induced adverse outcomes. A website, LiverTox (available at: https://livertox.nih.gov/), provides up-to-date and comprehensive information about DILI produced by prescription and nonprescription drugs, herbal and dietary supplements (LiverTox, 2016).

The toxicology of the liver is complicated by a variety of liver injuries and by different mechanisms through which the injuries are induced. The

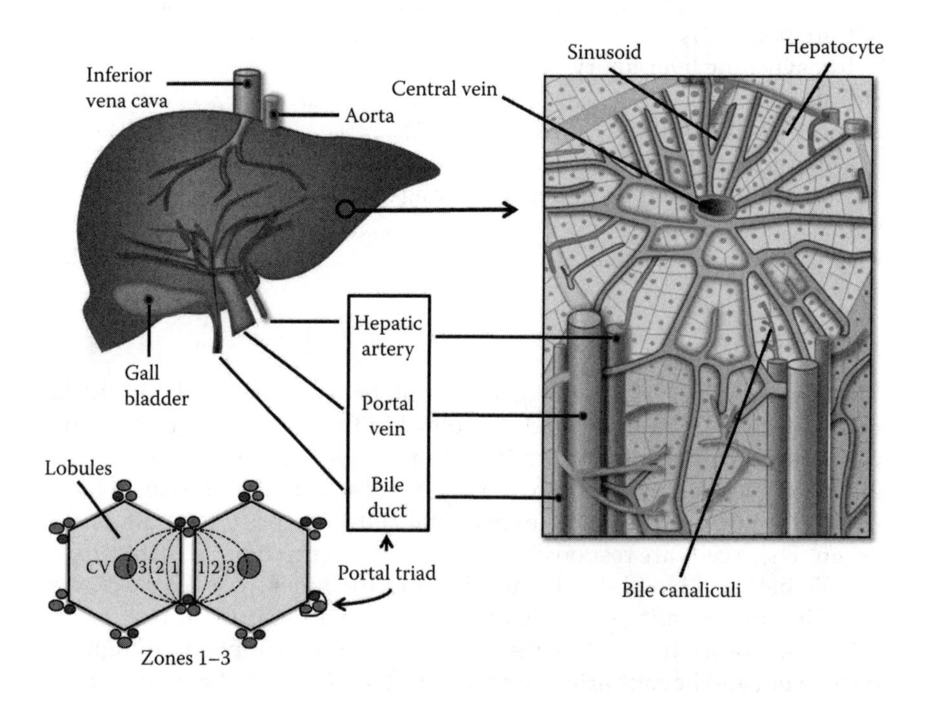


*Figure 12.1* Schematic structure of the liver showing zonation and vascular systems. (Courtesy of Dr. Byung-Mu Lee.)

types of injury, the underlying mechanisms, and morphologic and biochemical changes are described in the following sections.

## *Liver zonation and hepatotoxicity*

Zonation in the liver is categorized into zones 1, 2, and 3 based upon their position and oxygenation of hepatic lobules (50,000~100,000) as summarized in Table 12.1. Zone 1 is histologically located in the area where the oxygenated blood from hepatic arteries enters and $O_2$ levels are high (Katz et al., 1977; Jungermann and Kietzmann, 1996) (Figure 12.1). On the other hand, zone 3 is located around central veins, low in $O_2$ level, and highly susceptible to hypoxic agents leading to ischemic injury. Zone 2 is the area in between zones 1 and 3, where $O_2$ levels are intermediate. In addition, differential expression of metabolic enzymes and proteins occurs in each zone and may contribute to the incidence of differential liver injury. Zonal necrosis (zone 1 or zone 3) for example is a type of liver injury that produces a severe liver dysfunction leading to acute liver failure (Singh et al., 2011; Sacré et al., 2016).

The liver is often the target organ for a number of reasons. Most toxicants enter the body via the gastrointestinal (GI) tract, and after absorption are transported by the hepatic portal vein to the liver. The liver has a high concentration of binding sites. It also has a high concentration of xenobiotic-metabolizing enzymes (mainly cytochrome P-450), which

***Table 12.1*** Acinar zonation and characteristics in the liver

| Site | Characteristics |
|---|---|
| Zone 1 (afferent) | • High $O_2$ levels for $O_2$-dependent bioactivation<br>• Less ischemic injury<br>• Rich in enzymes and located in periportal area<br>• Rich in hormone, nutrients, and glutathione<br>• Gluconeogenesis, glycogen synthesis, and bile salt formation |
| Zone 2 | • Intermediate $O_2$ levels<br>• Intermediate zone between periportal and pericentral |
| Zone 3 (efferent) | • Low $O_2$ levels, susceptible to hypoxic toxicants, and lowest regenerative capacity due to least oxygenated blood supply<br>• More ischemic injury and less in glutathione<br>• Rich in microsomal enzymes (e.g., CYP450)<br>• Located around central veins (pericentral)<br>• Glycolysis and lipolysis |

*Source:* Bouwens L, Baekeland M, De Zanger R, Wisse E, *Hepatology*, 6, 718–22, 1986; Lough J, Rosenthall L, Arzoumanian A, Goresky CA, *J Hepatol*, 5, 190–8, 1987; Colnot S, Perret C, *Molecular Pathology of Liver Diseases*, Springer, New York, 2011.

render most toxicants less toxic and more water soluble, and thus more readily excretable. However, in some cases toxicants are activated and consequently induce lesions. The fact that hepatic lesions are often centrilobular has been attributed to the higher concentration of cytochrome P-450 in this region. In addition, the relatively lower concentration of glutathione, the antioxidant, at this site compared with that in other parts of the liver, may also play a role (Smith et al., 1979).

## *Types of liver injury*

Toxicants induce a variety of adverse effects on different organelles in liver cells (as shown in Table 12.2), exhibiting different types of tissue injury as described subsequently. These liver injuries are mediated through a number of biochemical reactions, such as oxidative stress, covalent binding, inhibition of protein synthesis, disturbance of biliary production and/or flow, immunological disorder, and perturbation of calcium homeostasis.

### *Fatty liver (steatosis)*

A fatty liver, a condition also known as fatty liver disease (FLD) or hepatic steatosis, is one that contains more than 5% lipid by weight. The presence of an excess stainable fat in such a liver is demonstrable histochemically. The lesion may be acute, such as that induced by ethionine, phosphorus,

***Table 12.2*** Effects of toxicants on subcellular organelles in liver cells

| Organelle | Effect | Examples of toxicants |
|---|---|---|
| Plasma membrane | Enzyme leakage | APAP, $CCl_4$, phalloidin |
| Nucleus | Neoplasia | Aflatoxin, Be, cycasin, tannic acid, dimethylnitrosamine (DMN) |
| Mitochondria | Swelling | $CCl_4$, cycasin, diquat, DMN, ethionine, phosphorus |
| Lysosomes | Accumulation | Be, $CCl_4$, ethionine, phosphorus |
| Peroxisomes | Proliferation | Clofibrate, TCE, high-fat diet |
| Endoplasmic reticulum | Degranulation; proliferation | $CCl_4$, DMN, ethionine, phosphorus |
| Cytoskeleton | Derangement | Cytochalasin B, phalloidin |
| Bile canaliculi | Dilatation | Lithocholate, taurocholate |

*Source:* de la Iglesia F, Sturgess JM, Feuer G, *Toxicology of the Liver*, Raven Press, New York, 1982; Stott WT, *Reg Toxicol Pharmacol.*, 8, 125–159, 1988; Plaa GL, *Casarett and Doull's Toxicology*, 4th ed, McGraw-Hill, New York, 334–353, (1993).

or tetracycline. Ethanol and methotrexate may produce either acute or chronic lesions. FLD can be classified into:

1. *Microvescular FLD*: Some toxicants, such as tetracycline and valproic acid, produce many small fat droplets in a cell (called microvescular FLD), which lead to high mortality rates.
2. *Macrovescular FLD*: On the other hand, ethanol and malnutrition induce large fat droplets in a cell (called macrovescular FLD), which displace the nucleus and may produce a low frequency of mortality. Metabolic syndrome (e.g., diabetes, hypertension, obesity, etc.) also initiates FLD.
3. *Alcoholic fatty liver disease (AFLD) and non-alcoholic fatty liver disease (NAFLD)*: NAFLD is considered the most common of all liver disorders and the most frequent cause of chronic liver disease (Youssef and McCullough, 2002).

Although lipid accumulation in the liver is the common endpoint of these toxicants, the underlying mechanisms vary. One of the mechanisms is an increased synthesis of triglyceride and other lipid moieties. However, the most common mechanism is the impairment of the release of hepatic triglycerides into plasma. Since hepatic triglycerides are secreted only when it is combined with lipoprotein (forming very low density lipoprotein), accumulation of hepatic lipid occurs as a result of a number of mechanisms:

1. Inhibition of synthesis of the protein moiety of lipoproteins
2. Reduced conjugation of triglycerides with lipoproteins
3. Loss of potassium from hepatocytes, resulting in an interference of transfer of the very low-density lipoprotein across the cell membrane (Plaa, 1993)

## *Liver necrosis*

Liver necrosis involves the death of hepatocytes. The necrosis may be focal (central, mid-zonal, and peripheral) or excessive. It is usually an acute injury. A number of chemicals have been demonstrated or reported to produce liver necrosis, which is a serious adverse manifestation but not necessarily critical because of the remarkable regenerating capacity of the liver.

Cell death occurs along with rupture of the plasma membrane. No ultrastructural changes of the membrane per se have been detected prior to its rupture. There are, however, a number of changes that precede cell death. Early morphologic changes include cytoplasmic edema, dilatation of endoplasmic reticulum, and disaggregation of polysomes. There is an accumulation of triglycerides as fat droplets in the cells. Late changes are progressive swelling of mitochondria with cristae disruption, cytoplasmic swelling, dissolution of organelles and nucleus, and rupture of plasma membrane (Bridges et al., 1983). Cyanobacterial blooms are known to produce a variety of toxins including microcystins, which subsequently attack the liver. Microcystins were reported to produce severe deformations such as plasma membrane bleb formation and loss of microvilli. In addition, microcystins produce severe hypoglycemia attributed to the failure of hepatic gluconeogenesis (Zurawell et al., 2005).

The biochemical changes are complex, and various hepatotoxicants apparently act through different mechanisms. Carbon tetrachloride ($CCl_4$) has been shown to act primarily through its reactive metabolite, the trichloromethyl radical $CCl_3$ (Recknagel and Glende, 1973), which covalently binds to proteins and unsaturated lipids and induces lipid peroxidation. Subcellular membranes are rich in such lipids and are, therefore, susceptible (Table 12.1). Recknagel et al. (1982), however, suggested that microsomal lipid peroxidation might lead to a depression of microsomal $Ca^{2+}$ pump resulting in an early disturbance of $Ca^{2+}$ homeostasis in the liver, which might then induce cell death. In addition, Shah et al. (1979) suggested that the toxicity of $CCl_4$ might be mediated through another metabolite, namely, phosgene. It is noteworthy that other drugs may act in a synergistic fashion. Chan et al. (2005) demonstrated that ketamine, an anesthetic, when administered to animals using $CCl_4$ as a model drug to study liver functions, showed that hepatotoxicity was more severe and occurred earlier (a synergistic response).

A number of chemically related compounds, such as chloroform, tetrachloroethane, and carbon tetrabromide, as well as phosphorus, appear to act in similar ways. Acetaminophen also induces liver necrosis but apparently not through lipid peroxidation (Kamiyama et al., 1993). At low doses, acetaminophen reactive metabolites conjugate with sulfate and glutathione. With increasing doses, the level of glutathione reduces, and the covalent binding of the chemical to the proteins rises. Bromobenzene is also bioactivated in the liver. Its 3,4-epoxide covalently binds to proteins and lipids and produces necrosis (see also Chapter 3). Other examples include isoniazid and iproniazid, both of which undergo bioactivation and form metabolites that bind to macromolecules and produce necrosis (Mitchell et al., 1976).

Disturbance of $Ca^{2+}$ homeostasis may also play an important role through an activation of molecular oxygen resulting in an oxidative stress, as discussed in Chapter 4 (Thomas and Reed, 1989).

Other biochemical changes include depletion of adenosine triphosphate (ATP), shifts of the $Na^+$ and $K^+$ balance between hepatocytes and blood, depletion of glutathione, damage to cytochrome P-450, and loss of nicotinamide adenine dinucleotide (NAD) and nicotinamide adenine dinucleotide phosphate (NADP) (Kulkarni and Hodgson, 1980).

## *Cholestasis*

Cholestasis is a hepatic disorder where normal flow of bile and/or secretion of bile in liver cells is reduced or impaired, which results in intrahepatic accumulation of bile acids. This type of liver damage, usually acute, is less common than fatty liver and necrosis, and more difficult to induce in animals with the possible exception of the steroids. The cholestatic agents appear to act through several mechanisms. For example, α-naphthylisocyanate (ANIT) induces cholestasis, hyperbilirubinemia, and inhibition of microsomal mixed-function oxygenases. Reduction of biliary excretory activity of the canalicular membrane appears to be the predominant mechanism for cholestasis. Further, ANIT seems to alter ductular cell permeability. Bailie et al. (1994) found that platelets seem to contribute to ANIT-induced liver injury. In addition, cholestasis is associated with complex transcriptional and post-transcriptional alterations of hepatobiliary transporters (e.g., ATP-binding cassette transporters) and enzymes participating in bile formation (Wagner et al., 2009).

A number of anabolic and contraceptive steroids as well as taurocholate, chlorpromazine, and erythromycin lactobionate were found to produce cholestasis and hyperbilirubinemia associated with canalicular bile plugs. Ethinyl estradiol and chlorpromazine seem to impair the permeability of the biliary tract, thus reducing bile salt-independent bile flow (Plaa, 1976, 1993). Ampicillin, rifampin, imipramin, and tetracycline produce cholestasis, but this type of drug-induced cholestasis is reversible shortly after medications are discontinued. Other types of cholestasis include hereditary cholestasis, extra hepatic cholestasis, intrahepatic cholestasis of pregnancy, and inflammatory cholestasis (Zollner and Trauner, 2008).

## *Cirrhosis*

Cirrhosis is characterized by the presence of septae of collagen distributed throughout most of the liver. Separated by these fibrous sheaths, clusters of hepatocytes appear as nodules. The pathogenesis is not fully understood, but in a majority of cases, cirrhosis seems to originate from single-cell necrosis associated with a deficiency in the repair mechanism. This condition then leads to fibroblastic activity and scar formation. Inadequate blood flow in the liver may be a contributing factor.

Several chemical carcinogens and long-term administration of $CCl_4$ induce cirrhosis in animals. The most important cause of human cirrhosis is chronic ingestion of alcoholic beverages. The mechanism is not fully understood, but ethanol may damage mitochondria and increase local production of reactive oxygen species (ROS). These may lead to steatosis, necrosis, and cirrhosis. This pathologic condition may be induced in animals with ethanol in combination with diets deficient in choline, proteins, methionine, vitamin $B_{12}$, and folic acid. Because this type of nutritional deficiency is common in alcoholism, Hartroft (1975) suggested the nutritional deficiency as the primary cause. Lieber and DeCarli (1976) were able to induce cirrhosis in baboons with ethanol alone and claimed, therefore, that alcohol was directly hepatotoxicity.

For the etiology of cirrhosis, (1) alcohol contributes about 60–70%, (2) viral hepatitis 10%, (3) biliary disease 5–10%, (4) autoimmune and genetic causes ~7%, (5) primary hemochromatosis 5%, and (6) other risk factors include obesity, diabetes, and iron overload. Of importance, the deficiency of vitamin D has been reported in chronic liver disease and lower levels of vitamin D are detected in alcoholic cirrhosis than in primary biliary cirrhosis, which might increase the risk of bone disease as a complication (Malham et al., 2011).

One of the mechanisms underlying hepatic cirrhosis includes ROS generation, which leads to oxidative stress (Cao et al., 2003; Kirmaz et al., 2004; Marra, 2007; Sikorska et al., 2016). Oxidative products such as ROS and lipid peroxidation products generated in injured hepatocytes initiate hepatic stellate cells (HSCs) activation. One of the central events in HSC activation is the excessive formation of extracellular matrix proteins induced mainly by TGF-β1. Kupffer cells can also release ROS and proinflammatory cytokines during the phagocytosis of cell debris or apoptotic bodies, thereby recruiting more inflammatory cells and enhancing the injury and oxidative stress. In addition, increased expression and release of the tissue inhibitor of metalloproteinase (TIMP)-1 from HSC and Kupffer cells lead to the reduced degradation of collagen.

Among mechanisms mentioned above, efforts have been made for drug discovery, in the search of HSC inactivators and antioxidants, for the treatment of liver fibrosis (Bataller and Brenner, 2005).

For diagnosis of liver fibrosis and cirrhosis, serum hyaluronic acid and alpha 2 macroglobulin (A2MG) have been suggested as biomarkers although other hepatic biomarkers (prothrombin time, platelet count, AST, ALT, albumin) have also been used (Soresi et al., 2014; Neuman et al., 2016).

## *Viral-like hepatitis*

A clinical syndrome indistinguishable from viral hepatitis has been known to be associated with various drugs. In general, it has the following characteristics (Plaa, 1993):

1. Such liver injuries are not demonstrable in animals
2. Effects in humans do not seem to be related to the dose
3. Latent period varies greatly
4. Toxicity is manifest in only a few susceptible individuals
5. Histologic picture is more variable
6. Patients usually show other signs of hypersensitivity and sometimes respond to a challenge dose
7. Fever, rash, and eosinophilia are present in many cases

The clinical picture may vary from patient to patient. For example, among those with halothane-induced hepatotoxicity, 50% of the patients displayed signs of typical immunologic reaction: fever, eosinophilia, and prior exposure to this anesthetic. Others did not exhibit these signs, and livers of fatal cases exhibited lesions similar to those induced by $CCl_4$ (Lewis and Zimmerman, 1989).

Halothane may induce a mild hepatotoxicity, which is reproducible in animals. In addition, it may act through an immune-mediated mechanism to produce the viral-like liver toxicity, which is more severe and delayed in onset (Hubbard et al., 1988).

## *Carcinogenesis*

Hepatocellular carcinoma and cholangiocarcinoma are the most common types of primary malignant neoplasms of the liver. Others include angiosarcoma, glandular carcinoma, trabecular carcinoma, and undifferentiated liver cell carcinoma. The significance of adenoma, focal basophilic hyperplasia, and hyperplastic nodule is as yet uncertain, whereas bile duct hyperplasia is likely to be a physiologic response to toxicant exposure (Newberne, 1982).

Dieldrin induces hepatocarcinogenesis via a nongenotoxic mechanism only in mice but not in rats (Kamendulis et al., 2001). Although the precise mechanisms are not known, fumonisin B, in addition to producing hepatotoxicity, induces hepatocellular adenoma and carcinoma (Li et al., 2000). On the other hand, the role of vinyl chloride in inducing angiosarcoma in humans is beyond doubt.

As discussed in Chapter 7, a large number of toxicants are known to induce liver cancers in animals. However, the carcinogenicity of these chemicals in humans, with respect to the liver, has not been well established (Wogan, 1976).

### Idiosyncratic liver injury

DILI can be classified into intrinsic and idiosyncratic liver injury, and the latter is further divided into immune-mediated and nonimmune-mediated idiosyncratic hepatotoxicity.

Idiosyncrasy is known as genetically determined abnormal reactivity to chemicals such as drugs, herbal, and food supplements (Li, 2002; Kaplowitz, 2005; Stickel et al., 2011). As it is not related to the *dose, route,* or *period of exposure,* idiosyncratic hepatotoxicity is an unusual and unpredictable injury. Although it occurs rarely and has a varying spectrum in clinical, histological, and laboratory features, idiosyncratic liver injury is a leading cause for the limited use or withdrawal of a drug from the market. Drugs with known idiosyncratic hepatotoxicity are listed in Table 12.3. The toxic mechanism is largely discriminated by an immune-mediated or nonimmune-mediated response. While halothane, nitrofurantoin, and phenytoin are considered immune idiosyncratic hepatotoxins, isoniazid, disulfiram, valproic acid, or troglitazone are thought to produce toxicity by nonimmune mechanisms. In the case of diclofenac, idiosyncratic hepatotoxicity can be induced by both immune and nonimmune responses. Immune-mediated (allergic) idiosyncratic hepatotoxicity shows characteristic symptoms and signs of an adaptive immune system reaction, including fever, skin reactions, eosinophilia, formation of autoantibodies, and a short latency time (1–6 weeks) particularly after re-exposure (Khoury et al., 2015).

## Hepatotoxicants

Some of the liver injuries described have a number of common features, namely, steatosis, necrosis, cirrhosis, and neoplasia. (1) These injuries are relatively easily produced in experimental animals. (2) Many toxicants induce several types of such injuries. For example, steatosis, necrosis, and cirrhosis result from exposure to $CCl_4$ (and related chemicals such as chloroform), aflatoxins, and phosphorus. Aflatoxins and dioxins induce necrosis, cirrhosis, and neoplasm. Steatosis and cirrhosis are seen after exposure to ethanol; bromobenzene is known to induce necrosis and cirrhosis. Chloroform was shown to produce liver cell death by depletion of glutathione and an oxidative phase characterized by mitochondrial permeability transition and protein nitration (Burke et al., 2007). Comfrey, an herbal medicine containing pyrrolizidine alkaloids, produces hepatotoxicity in

*Table 12.3* Examples of drugs with known idiosyncratic hepatotoxicity

| Type of injury | Drug (use) |
|---|---|
| **A. Immune-mediated (allergic) idiosyncratic hepatotoxicity (latency period 1–6 wks)** | |
| *Hepatocellular injury* | Diclofenac (analgesic) |
| | Dihydralazine (antihypertensive) |
| | Halothane (anaesthetic) |
| | Methyldopa (antihypertensive) |
| | Minocycline (antibiotic) |
| | Nitrofurantoin (antibiotic) |
| | Phenytoin (anticonvulsant) |
| | Propylthiouracil (antithyroid) |
| | Trovafloxacin (antibiotic) (withdrawn EU, U.S. 1999–2001) |
| *Cholestatic injury* | Amoxicillin-clavulanic acid (antibiotic) |
| | Chlorpromazine (antipsychotic) |
| | Erythromycins (antibiotic) |
| | Phenobarbital (sedative) |
| | Phenothiazines (antipsychotic) |
| | Sulfonamides (antibiotic) |
| | Sulindac (analgesic) |
| | Tricyclic antidepressants |
| **B. Nonimmune-mediated (nonallergic) idiosyncratic hepatotoxicity (latency 30 d–1 yr)** | |
| *Hepatocellular injury* | Amiodarone (anti-arrhythmic) |
| | Diclofenac (analgesic) |
| | Disulfiram (alcoholism) |
| | Isoniazid (antituberculosis) |
| | Isotretinoin (acne) |
| | Ketoconazole (antifungal) |
| | Niacin (cholesterol-lowering) |
| | Pemoline (CNS stimulant) (withdrawn, Canada 1997, U.S. 2005) |
| | Rifampin (antituberculosis) |
| | Statins (lipid-lowering) |
| | Tacrine (Alzheimer's disease) |
| | Tolcapone (Parkinson's disease) |
| | Troglitazone (diabetes) (withdrawn, Germany, U.S. 2000) |

(*Continued*)

*Table 12.3 (Continued)* Examples of drugs with known idiosyncratic hepatotoxicity

| Type of injury | Drug (use) |
|---|---|
| | Valproic acid (anticonvulsant) |
| *Cholestatic injury* | Anabolic steroids |
| | Azathioprine (immunosuppressant) |
| | Cyclosporine (immunosuppressant) |
| | Estrogens |
| | Oral contraceptives |
| | Terbinafine (antifungal) |

*Source:* Adapted from Kaplowitz N, *Nat Rev Drug Discov.*, 4, 489–499, 2005; Lucena MI et al., *Fundam Clin Pharmacol.*, 22(2), 141–58, 2008; Verma S, Kaplowitz N, *Gut.*, 58(11), 1555–64, 2009; Khoury T et al., *J Clin Transl Hepatol.*, 3(2), 99–108, 2015.

humans and livestock, and carcinogenicity by interacting with DNA in hepatocytes (Mei et al., 2010).

Mainly certain bile salts, α-naphthylisocyanate, certain anabolic and contraceptive steroids, manganese, and a number of drugs induce cholestasis. Some of these drugs and other substances are also known to induce viral-like hepatitis. For example, *p*-aminosalicylic acid, chlorpromazine, erythromycin, and phenytoin (diphenylhydantoin) appear to produce viral-like hepatitis through a type of hypersensitivity reaction. On the other hand, iproniazid, isoniazid, and hydrazine derivatives induce this effect perhaps through a metabolic abnormality.

Examples of the various types of hepatotoxicants are listed in Appendix 12.1.

## Clinical biochemical tests

A number of serum enzymes have been used as indicators of hepatic injuries. These enzymes are released to the blood from the cytosol and subcellular organelles as summarized below:

1. Serum alanine aminotransferase (ALT) or aspartate aminotransferase (AST) is increased in reliable correlation with the severity of hepatic necrosis. It is, therefore, the choice test in liver necrosis.
2. Ornithine carbamoyl transferase (OCT) and sorbitol dehydrogenase (SDH) are more sensitive, but less specific, than ALT. They are therefore often used in conjunction with ALT when testing new toxicants. The enzyme levels in blood are often used as biomarkers among humans exposed to hepatotoxicants.
3. ALT and alkaline phosphatase (AP) are greatly elevated in cholestatic lesions. On the other hand, serum cholinesterase may be reduced in

certain cases of liver diseases. For additional details, see Plaa and Charbonneau (1994).

Glutamate dehydrogenase, paraoxonase, malate dehydrogenase, and purine nucleoside phosphorylase can be used for biomarkers of hepatotoxicity by photometric methods (Ozer et al., 2008). In addition, other biomarkers such as serum F protein, arginase I, and glutathione-S-transferase alpha (GST-$\alpha$) may be applicable, but have limitations due to antibody availability and high cost.

## *Other tests*

The liver is involved in the metabolism of carbohydrate, fat, and protein as well as in the formation of prothrombin and the excretion of bilirubin and certain foreign chemicals. It is also the major site of biotransformation of toxicants. Tests have thus been devised to determine these hepatic functions.

The liver excretes for example, bilirubin, hence its level in the blood is an index of liver function, but it is relatively insensitive. The rate of excretion of bromosulfophthalein is a more sensitive indicator of liver damage. Clinically, the prolongation of prothrombin time, after excluding vitamin K deficiency, has been used in detecting acute hepatic lesions. A chemical may either potentiate or inhibit the pharmacologic and toxicologic actions of another by stimulating the hepatic microsomal enzymes. Measurements of barbiturate-induced sleeping time and the duration of zoxazolamine-induced paralysis have been used as indications of hepatic effects.

In addition, a number of biochemical tests can be performed on the liver tissue:

1. Level of triglycerides
2. Activity of glucose 6-phosphatase
3. Level of microsomal conjugated dienes, resulting from the peroxidation of microsomal lipids
4. Covalent binding of reactive metabolites to tissue macromolecules
5. Arylation or alkylation of purine and pyrimidine components of DNA and RNA (carcinogenicity)
6. Arylation or alkylation of other macromolecules (necrosis)

Because of the importance of lipid peroxidation in liver lesions, the extent of this reaction is often determined by using thiobarbituric acid. It combines with malonaldehyde (MDA), a degradation product of the lipid, to form a colored complex which can be measured quantitatively.

# *Appendix 12.1 Examples of hepatotoxic agents and associated liver injury*

**Necrosis and fatty liver**

| | |
|---|---|
| APAP[a] | Ethanol[b] |
| Aflatoxin | Ethionine[b] |
| Allyl alcohol[a] | Fumonisin B |
| | Furosemide[a] |
| Azaserine | Galactosamine |
| Beryllium[a] | Phosphorus |
| Bromobenzene[a] | Puromycin[b] |
| Carbon disulfide | Pyrrolizidine alkaloids |
| $CCl_4$ | Tannic acid[a] |
| Chloroform | Tetrachloroethane |
| Corticosteroid | Tetracycline[b] |
| Cycloheximide[b] | Thioacetamide[a] |
| Dichlorobenzene | Trichloroethylene |
| Dimethylnitrosamine | Valproic acid[b] |
| Diquat | |

**Cholestasis (drug-induced)**

| | |
|---|---|
| *p*-Aminosalicylic acid[c] | Mestranol |
| Amitriptyline | Methandrolone |
| Carbamazepine[c] | Methimazole |
| Carbarsone | Oxyphenisatin[c] |
| Chlorpromazine[c] | Perphenazine |
| Chlorthiazide | Phenindione[c] |
| Diazepam | Promazine |
| Erythromycin estolate[c] | Steroids, androgenic, and anabolic |
| Estradiol | Sulfanilamide |
| Ethacrynic acid[c] | Thiabendazole |
| Imipramine[c] | Thioridazine |
| Mepazine | |

**Viral-like hepatitis (drug induced)**

| | |
|---|---|
| Colchicine | Methoxyflurane |
| Halothane | α-Methyldopa |
| Imipramine | Papaverine |
| Indomethacin | Phenylbutazone |
| Iproniazid | Phenytoin |

(*Continued*)

| | |
|---|---|
| Isoniazid | Sulfonamides |
| 6-Mercaptopurine | Zoxazolamine |
| **Carcinogenesis (in experimental animals)** | |
| Acetylaminofluorene | Polychlorinated biphenyls |
| Aflatoxin $B_1$[d] | Pyrrolizidine alkaloids |
| Cycasin | Safrole |
| Dialkyl nitrosamines | Urethane |
| N(nitrosomethyl)urea[d] | Vinyl chloride[d] |

[a] Primary effect is necrosis.
[b] Primary effect is fatty liver.
[c] Also induces viral-like hepatitis.
[d] In humans also.

# References


Amacher DE (1998). Serum transaminase elevations as indicators of hepatic injury following the administration of drugs. *Regul Toxicol Pharmacol.* 27, 119–30.

Bailie MB, Pearson JM, Lappin PB et al. (1994). Platelets and α-naphthylisothiocyanate-induced liver injury. *Toxicol Appl Pharmacol.* 129, 207–13.

Bataller R, Brenner DA (2005). Liver fibrosis. *J Clin Invest.* 115(2), 209–18.

Bouwens L, Baekeland M, De Zanger R, Wisse E (1986). Quantitation, tissue distribution and proliferation kinetics of Kupffer cells in normal rat liver. *Hepatology.* 6, 718–22.

Bridges JW, Benford DJ, Hubbard SA (1983). Mechanisms of toxic injury. *Ann N Y Acad Sci.* 407, 42–63.

Burke AS, Redeker K, Kurten RC et al. (2007). Mechanisms of chloroform-induced hepatotoxicity: Oxidative stress and mitochondrial permeability transition in freshly isolated mouse hepatocytes. *J Toxicol Environ Health A.* 70, 1936–45.

Cao Q, Mak KM, Ren C, Lieber CS (2003). Leptin stimulates tissue inhibitor of metalloproteinase-1 in human hepatic stellate cells: Respective roles of the JAK/STAT and JAK-mediated $H_2O_2$-dependant MAPK pathways. *J Biol Chem.* 279, 4292–304.

Chan W-H, Sun W-Z, Ueng T-H (2005). Induction of rat hepatic cytochrome P450 by ketamine and its toxicological implications. *J Toxicol Environ Health A.* 68, 1581–97.

Chen M, Zhang J, Wang Y, Liu Z, Kelly R, Zhou G et al. (2013). Liver Toxicity Knowledge Base (LTKB)—A systems approach to a complex endpoint. *Clin Pharmacol Ther.* 95, 409–12.

Colnot S, Perret C (2011). Liver zonation. In: Monga SPS ed. *Molecular Pathology of Liver Diseases.* New York: Springer, pp. 7–16.

de la Iglesia F, Sturgess JM, Feuer G (1982). New approaches for assessment of hepatotoxicity by means of quantitative functional–morphological interrelationship. In: Plaa GL, Hewitt WR, eds. *Toxicology of the Liver.* New York: Raven Press.

Hartroft WS (1975). On the etiology of alcoholic liver cirrhosis. In: Khanna JM, Israel Y, Kalant H, eds. *Alcoholic Liver Pathology.* Toronto, Canada: Addiction Research Foundation.

Hubbard AK, Gandolfi AJ, Brown RR (1988). Immunological basis of anesthetic-induced hepatotoxicity. *Anesthesiol.* 69, 814–7.

Jungermann K, Kietzmann T (1996). Zonation of parenchymal and nonparenchymal metabolism in liver. *Annu Rev Nutr.* 16, 179–203.

Kamendulis LM, Kolaja KL, Stevenson DE et al. (2001). Comparative effects of dieldrin on hepatic ploidy, cell proliferation, and apoptosis. *J Toxicol Environ Health A.* 62, 127–41.

Kamiyama T, Sato C, Liu J et al. (1993). Role of peroxidation in acetaminophen-induced hepatotoxicity: Comparison with carbon tetrachloride. *Toxicol Lett.* 66, 7–12.

Kaplowitz N (2005). Idiosyncratic drug hepatotoxicity. *Nat Rev Drug Discov.* 4, 489–99.

Katz N, Teutsch HF, Jungermann K, Sasse D (1977). Heterogeneous reciprocal localization of fructose-1, 6-bisphosphatase and of glucokinase in microdissected periportal and perivenous rat liver tissue. *FEBS Lett.* 83(2), 272–6.

Khoury T, Rmeileh AA, Yosha L et al. (2015). Drug induced liver injury: Review with a focus on genetic factors, tissue diagnosis, and treatment options. *J Clin Transl Hepatol.* 3(2), 99–108.

Kirmaz C, Terzioglu E, Topalak O et al. (2004). Serum transforming growth factor beta1 (TGF-beta1) in patients with cirrhosis, chronic hepatitis B and chronic hepatitis C [corrected]. *Eur Cytokine Netw.* 15, 112–6.

Kulkarni AP, Hodgson E (1980). Hepatoxicity. In: Hodgson E, Guthrie FE, eds. *Introduction to Biochemical Toxicology.* New York: Elsevier.

Lewis JH, Zimmerman HJ (1989). Drug-induced liver disease. *Med Clin North Am.* 73, 775–92.

Li AP (2002). A review of the common properties of drugs with idiosyncratic hepatotoxicity and the "multiple determinant hypothesis" for the manifestation of idiosyncratic drug toxicity. *Chem Biol Interact.* 142, 7–23A.

Li W, Riley RT, Voss KA et al. (2000). Role of proliferation in the toxicity of fumonisin B: Enhanced hepatoxic response in the partially hepatectomized rat. *J Toxicol Environ Health A.* 60, 441–57.

Lieber CS, DeCarli LM (1976). Animal models of ethanol dependence of liver injury in rats and baboons. *Fed Proc.* 35, 1232–6.

LiverTox. Available online: http://livertox.nlm.nih.gov (accessed on 16 December 2016).

Lough J, Rosenthall L, Arzoumanian A, Goresky CA (1987). Kupffer cell depletion associated with capillarization of liver sinusoids in carbon tetrachloride-induced rat liver cirrhosis. *J Hepatol.* 5, 190–8.

Lucena MI, García-Cortés M et al. (2008). Assessment of drug-induced liver injury in clinical practice. *Fundam Clin Pharmacol.* 22(2), 141–58.

Malham M, Jørgensen SP, Ott P et al. (2011). Vitamin D deficiency in cirrhosis relates to liver dysfunction rather than aetiology. *World J Gastroenterol.* 17, 922–5.

Marra F (2007). Cellular and molecular mechanisms of hepatic fibrogenesis. *Gastroenterol Hepatol.* 30(Supl 1), 99–105.

Mei N, Guo P, Fu PP et al. (2010). Metabolism, genotoxicity and carcinogenicity of comfrey. *J Toxicol Environ Health B.* 13, 509–26.

Mitchell JR, Snodgrass WR, Gillette JR (1976). The role of biotransformation in chemical-induced liver injury. *Environ Health Persp.* 15, 27–38.

Neuman MG, Cohen LB, Nanau RM (2016). Hyaluronic acid as a non-invasive biomarker of liver fibrosis. *Clin Biochem*. 49(3), 302–15.

Newberne PM (1982). Assessment of the hepatocarcinogenic potential of chemicals: Response of the liver. In: Plaa GL, Hewitt WR, eds. *Toxicology of the Liver.* New York: Raven Press.

Nourjah P, Ahmad SR, Karwoski C, Willy M (2006). Estimates of Acetaminophen (Paracetomal)-associated overdoses in the United States, *Pharmacoepidemiol Drug Saf.* 15(6), 398–405.

Ozer J, Ratner M, Shaw M et al. (2008). The current state of serum biomarkers of hepatotoxicity. *Toxicology*. 245, 194–205.

Plaa GL (1976). Quantitative aspects in the assessment of liver injury. *Environ Health Persp*. 15, 39–46.

Plaa GL (1993). Toxic responses of the liver. In: Amdur MO, Doull J, Klaassen CD, eds. *Casarett and Doull's Toxicology*, 4th edn. New York: McGraw-Hill, pp. 334–53.

Plaa GL, Charbonneau M (1994). Detection and evaluation of chemically induced liver injury. In: Hayes AW, ed. *Principles and Methods of Toxicology*. New York: Raven Press, pp. 839–70.

Recknagel RO, Glende EA Jr (1973). Carbon tetrachloride hepatotoxicity: An example of lethal cleavage. *CRC Crit Rev Toxicol*. 2, 263–97.

Recknagel RO, Glende EA, Waller RL et al. (1982). Lipid peroxidation: Biochemistry, measurement, and significance in liver cell injury. In: Plaa GL, Hewitt WR, eds. *Toxicology of the Liver.* New York: Raven Press.

Sacré A, Lanthier N, Dano H, Aydin et al. (2016). Regorafenib induced severe toxic hepatitis: Characterization and discussion. *Liver Int*. 36(11), 1590–4.

Shah H, Martman SP, Weinhouse S (1979). Formation of carbonyl chloride in carbon tetrachloride metabolism by rat liver in vitro. *Cancer Res*. 39, 3942–7.

Sikorska K, Bernat A, Wroblewska A (2016). Molecular pathogenesis and clinical consequences of iron overload in liver cirrhosis. *Hepatobiliary Pancreat Dis Int*. 15(5), 461–79.

Singh A, Bhat T K, and Sharma OP (2011). Clinical biochemistry of hepatotoxicity. *J Clinic Toxicol*. S4, 001.

Smith ML, Loveridge N, Wills ED et al. (1979). The distribution of glutathione in rat liver lobule. *Biochem J*. 182, 103–8.

Soresi M, Giannitrapani L, Cervello M, Licata A, Montalto G (2014). Non invasive tools for the diagnosis of liver cirrhosis. *World J Gastroenterol*. 20(48), 18131–50.

Stickel F, Kessebohm K, Weimann R et al. (2011). Review of liver injury associated with dietary supplements. *Liver Int*. 31, 595–605.

Stott WT (1988). Chemically induced proliferation of peroxisomes: Implications for risk assessment. *Reg Toxicol Pharmacol*. 8, 125–59.

Thomas CE, Reed DJ (1989). Current status of calcium in hepatocellular injury. Hepatology 10, 375–84.

Verma S, Kaplowitz N (2009). Diagnosis, management and prevention of drug-induced liver injury. *Gut*. 58(11), 1555–64.

Wagner M, Zollner G, Trauner, M (2009). New molecular insights into the mechanisms of cholestasis. *J Hepatol*. 51, 565–80.

Watkins PB (2011). Drug safety sciences and the bottleneck in drug development. *Clin Pharmacol Ther*. 89, 788–90.

Wogan CN (1976). The induction of liver cell cancer by chemicals. In: Cameron HM, Linsell DA, Warwick GP, eds. *Liver Cell Cancer.* Amsterdam, The Netherlands: Elsevier.

Youssef WI, McCullough AJ (2002). Steatohepatitis in obese individuals. *Best Pract and Res in Clinical Gastroenterol.* 16, 733–47.

Zollner G, Trauner M (2008). Mechanisms of cholestasis. *Clin Liver Dis.* 12, 1–26.

Zurawell RW, Chen H, Burke JM et al. (2005). Hepatotoxic cyanobacteria: A review of the biological importance of microcystins in freshwater environments. *J Toxicol Environ Health B.* 8, 1–37.

# *chapter thirteen*

# *Toxicology of the kidney*

***Young-Suk Jung and Hyung Sik Kim***

*Contents*

## *Introduction*

The kidneys are pair of organs located toward the lower back with each kidney on each side of the spine. Kidney filters blood and excretes various toxicants from our body through urine where most toxicants are excreted. The kidney is the second major target for drug-induced target organ toxicity. Kidneys receive nearly 25% of cardiac output resulting in high volume of blood flow, and concentrated toxicants which are transported across tubular cells, where they are bioactivated or detoxified depending on the toxicants. Kidneys are one of the major organs of excretion, and thus exposed to a greater proportion of circulating drugs and chemicals. It is therefore a major target organ for adverse effects. To facilitate discussions on these effects, the renal structure and functions are briefly reviewed. Nephrotoxicity is one of the most common kidney problems and occurs when our body is exposed to a drug or toxin that produces damage to this tissue. When kidney damage occurs, it is not possible to remove excess urine, and wastes. Blood electrolytes (such as potassium and magnesium) become consequently elevated.

### *The structure*

The kidney is a complex organ whose predominant structures are the nephrons, numbering approximately $1.3 \times 10^6$. The nephrons of two normal kidneys are collectively responsible for filtering approximately 150–180 L of plasma per day, processing the filtrate to regulate fluid, electrolyte, and acid–base balance while eliminating waste products. Each nephron consists of a glomerulus and a series of tubules (Figure 13.1). The glomerulus is supplied with a high-pressure capillary system that produces an ultrafiltrate from the plasma.

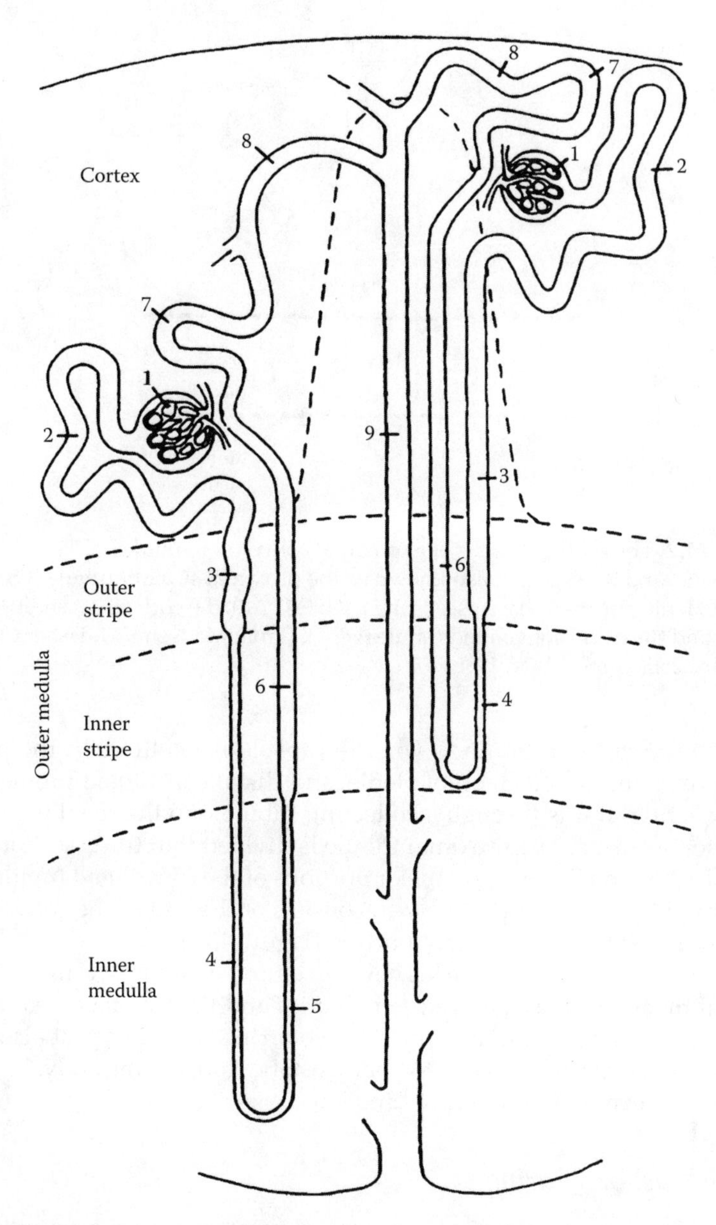


***Figure 13.1*** Schematic presentation of a cortical (short-looped) and a juxtamedullary (long-looped) nephron together with the collecting system. 1, Glomerulus with Bowman's capsule; 2, Proximal tubule (*convoluted portion*); 3, Proximal tubule (*straight portion*); 4, Descending thin limb (loop of Henle); 5, Ascending limb (loop of Henle); 6, Thick ascending limb; 7, Distal convoluted tubule; 8, Connecting tubule; 9, Collecting tubule. (From Kriz W, Bankir L, *Am J Physiol.*, 254, F1–F8, 1988.)

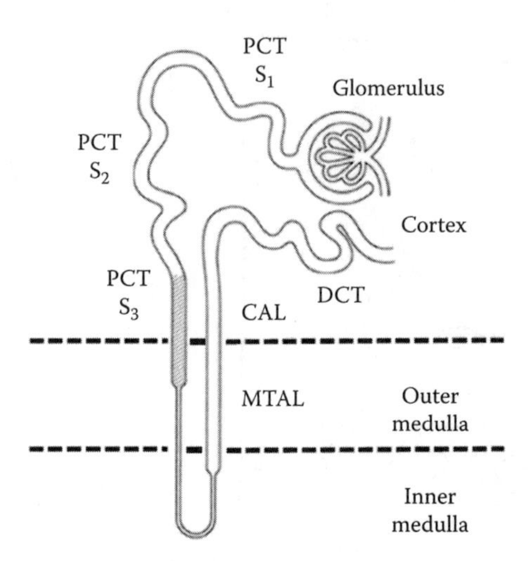


***Figure 13.2*** The tubule consists of a proximal convoluted tubule (PCT), composed of an $S_1$, $S_2$, and $S_3$ segment, also known as the proximal straight tubule (PST), the loop of Henle, the medullary ascending limb (MTAL), the cortical ascending limb (CAL), and the distal convoluted tubule (DCT). (From Madsen KM, Tisher CC, *Am J Physiol.*, 250(6 Pt 3), F1–15, 1986.)

The filtrate collected in Bowman's capsule flows through the proximal convoluted tubule, loop of Henle, and distal convoluted tubule, and subsequently drains through a collecting tubule into the renal pelvis for excretion as urine. The proximal tubule is divided into three sections ($S_1$, $S_2$, and $S_3$). $S_1$ and $S_3$ consist of major portions of the convoluted tubule and the straight portion, respectively. $S_2$ consists of the end of the convoluted portion and start of the straight portion (Figure 13.2).

The major function of the kidney is to eliminate wastes resulting from normal metabolism and excrete xenobiotics and their metabolites. These functions occur through the production of urine, a process that also contributes to the maintenance of the homeostatic status of the body. In addition, it has several nonexcretory functions.

## *The production of urine*

The production of urine is a complex process, which begins with filtration in the glomeruli. In humans, approximately 180 L of filtrate is formed per day. As only 500–2500 ml of urine is excreted, 99% of the filtered water is reabsorbed. The reabsorption of water, through diffusion, takes place first at the proximal tubules, where $Na^+$ is actively reabsorbed. Further diffusion of water takes place at the descending limb of the loop of Henle to the hyperosmolar interstitium. The hyperosmolarity is produced by the active reabsorption of $Cl^-$ (along with $Na^+$) at the ascending limb of the loop. The spatial arrangement of the loops and the vasa recta provides an effective countercurrent multiplier mechanism.

Additional water is removed from the filtrate in the distal and collecting tubules, as $Na^+$ is actively reabsorbed. The extent of removal of water from these tubules depends upon the activity of antidiuretic hormone (ADH). ADH reduces the urine volume by increasing the permeability of these structures to water.

## *Tubular resorption and secretion*

As the glomerular capillaries contain large pores (70 nm), substances with molecular weights under 60,000 Da are filtered into Bowman's capsules. Some of the filtered substances such as glucose and amino acids, which are vital to the body, are reabsorbed by the tubules. On the other hand, ammonia ($NH_3$), a metabolic waste of amino acids, diffuses through the cells to the filtrate, where it reacts with $H^+$ to form $NH_4^+$, which is nondiffusible, hence excreted.

To facilitate the passive reabsorption of water and maintain homeostasis, various electrolytes in the glomerular filtrate are nearly completely reabsorbed. The reabsorption of $Na^+$ at the distal and collecting tubules is regulated by mineralocorticoids, that of phosphorus by parathyroid hormone (PAH), and that of bicarbonate ($HCO_3^-$) by the acid–base balance. In addition, $K^+$ and $H^+$ are secreted by the tubules.

## *Nonexcretory functions*

The kidney possesses other functions such as the regulation of blood pressure and volume. This is mediated through the renin–angiotensin–aldosterone system. Renin, a proteolytic enzyme, is formed in the cells of the juxtaglomerular apparatus and catalyzes the conversion of a plasma angiotensin prohormone to angiotensin I. The latter, a decapeptide, is converted in the lungs to angiotensin II by an enzyme that removes a dipeptide from the C-terminal end.

A renal erythropoietic factor also acts on a plasma protein to form erythropoietin, which increases production of normoblasts and synthesis of hemoglobin. Renal prostaglandins are produced in the interstitial cells in the medulla and appear to have the capability of regulating renal blood flow and the excretion of $Na^+$ and urine. The kidney is also involved in the conversion of the relatively inactive 25-hydroxy-vitamin $D_3$ to the active 1,25-dihydroxy-vitamin $D_3$.

## Nephrotoxicants: Mechanism and site of action

### Classification of nephrotoxicants

The major groups of nephrotoxicants are heavy metals, antibiotics, analgesics, fungal toxins, and certain halogenated hydrocarbons (Table 13.1). All parts of the nephron are potentially subject to the detrimental effects of toxicants. However, most toxicants preferentially affect specific parts of the kidney. The mechanisms of action of nephrotoxicants include interaction with receptors, inhibition of oxidative phosphorylation, disturbance of $Ca^{2+}$ homeostasis, and disruption of plasma and subcellular membrane functions. Certain chemicals may affect one area predominantly, but the entire nephron is subject to damage.

#### *Analgesics*

Analgesics induce a nephropathy with decease in renal volume, but histologically there is thickening of the basement membrane of the loop of Henle, isolated necrosis of interstitial and papillary tubular cells followed by fibrosis and cortical interstitial nephritis (Schnellmann, 1998). For example, acetaminophen-induced renal toxicity has been attributed to cytochrome P-450 mixed function oxidase isoenzymes, prostaglandin synthetase, and *N*-deacetylase enzymes present in the kidney (Mazer and Perrone, 2008). GSH is also considered an important detoxifying element of acetaminophen and its metabolites. Acetaminophen-induced renal failure becomes evident after hepatotoxicity in most cases, but may be differentiated from hepatorenal syndrome, which may complicate fulminant hepatic failure (Mazer and Perrone, 2008; Kadowaki et al., 2012).

#### *Antibiotics*

Antibiotics used in septic patients also tend to produce acute kidney injury (AKI) including gentamicin, amikacin, vancomycin, and amphotericin-B (Eyler and Mueller, 2011). This is due to accumulation of aminoglycosides, which are taken up by PTC by the megalin/cubilin endocytotic receptor complex, to levels exceeding serum concentrations. This in turn results in problems with protein synthesis and folding, disrupted protein sorting, increased lysosomal permeability, proteolysis and mitochondrial dysfunction, and probably other damage resulting in cell death (González de Molina and Ferrer, 2011). Nephrotoxicity due to aminoglycoside mediates non-oliguric renal failure and a fall in glomerular filtration rate (GFR), generally occurring 7 days after treatment. Amphotericin-B induces renal vasoconstriction and reduces GFR by more than half (Bates et al., 2001; Harbarth et al., 2001).

***Table 13.1*** Major groups of nephrotoxicants

| Toxicants | Site of action |
|---|---|
| | **Heavy metals** |
| Cadmium | Proximal tubules |
| Chromium | Proximal tubules |
| Gold | Glomeruli |
| Lead | Proximal tubules and blood vessels |
| Mercury, inorganic | Proximal tubules and glomeruli |
| | **Antibiotics** |
| Aminoglycosides | Glomeruli and proximal tubules |
| Amphotericin-B | Glomerular blood vessels and distal tubules |
| Cephaloridine | Proximal tubules |
| Gentamicin | Glomeruli and proximal tubules |
| Puromycin | Glomeruli |
| Tetracycline | Interstitial tissues in medulla |
| | **Halogenated hydrocarbons** |
| Bromobenzene | Proximal tubules |
| Carbon tetrachloride | Proximal tubules |
| Chloroform | Proximal tubules |
| Decalin | Proximal tubules |
| Hexachlorobutadiene | Pars recta |
| Hydroquinone | Proximal tubules |
| | **Analgesics/anesthetics** |
| Acetaminophen | Various parts of a nephron and blood vessel |
| Ibuprofen | Glomeruli and proximal tubules |
| Methoxyflurane | Various parts of a nephron |
| | **Antineoplastics** |
| Adriamycin | Glomeruli |
| Cisplatin | Pars recta and other parts of a nephron proximal tubules |
| Methotrexate | Proximal tubules |
| | **Immunosuppressants** |
| Cyclosporin | Blood vessels and interstitial tissue, proximal tubules and distal tubules |
| Tacrolimus | Proximal tubular injury |

(*Continued*)

***Table 13.1 (Continued)*** Major groups of nephrotoxicants

| Toxicants | Site of action |
|---|---|
| | **Miscellaneous** |
| Glycol | Tubular blockade |
| Sulfapyridine | Tubular blockade |

*Antiviral drugs*

Ritonavir is a substrate for MRP2 and it was suggested that it might potentiate the toxicity of tenofovir disoproxil fumarate (TDF) by inhibiting exit from proximal tubule cells and increasing intracellular concentration (Vidal et al., 2006). The mechanism of this inhibition is unclear because TDF is not believed to exit through MRP2 (Cihlar et al., 2007). However, ritonavir slows TDF renal clearance in humans and increased TDF plasma concentration is associated with development of tubular toxicity. Renal function improved in both patients after discontinuing TDF. Thus, TDF-associated renal toxicity needs to be monitored during TDF therapy (Cho et al., 2016).

*Anticancer drugs*

Although the exact mechanism of doxorubicin (DXR)-induced nephrotoxicity remains unknown, it is believed that the toxicity may be mediated through free radical formation, iron-dependent oxidative damage of biological macromolecules, membrane LPO, and protein oxidation. DXR-induced changes in the kidneys of rats include increased glomerular capillary permeability and tubular atrophy (Ayla et al., 2011).

The etiology of methotrexate (MTX)-induced renal dysfunction is believed to be mediated by precipitation of MTX and its metabolites in renal tubules (Smeland et al., 1996; Widemann and Adamson, 2006) or via a direct toxic effect of MTX on renal tubules (Messmann et al., 2001). More than 90% of MTX is cleared by the kidneys. MTX is poorly soluble at acidic pH, and its metabolites, 7-OH-MTX and DAMPA, are 6–10 times less soluble than MTX, respectively (Jacobs et al., 1976; Donehower et al., 1979).

Platinum-derived chemotherapeutic agents, including the parent compound cis-diamminedichloroplatinum (II) (cisplatin, CDDP), are the principal therapeutic agents to treat various cancers, including ovarian, testicular, and bladder cancer. However, the therapeutic use of CDDP is limited by its irreversible side effects, including nephrotoxicity, neurotoxicity, and ototoxicity. Evidence of CDDP-induced kidney damage in animal models is displayed as characteristic morphological changes in the renal tubules (Won et al., 2016). It is estimated that 30% of patients treated with CDDP exhibit elevated serum Cr levels and reduced glomerular filtration rate, reflecting development of nephrotoxicity. The pathophysiological mechanisms purported to underlie CDDP-induced nephrotoxicity have been extensively examined including oxidative stress, inflammation, and apoptosis pathways (Miller et al., 2010).

### *Other chemicals*

High molecular weight organic compounds such as humic or fulvic acid, which occur naturally in lignite beds, induce a nephropathy that resembles Balkan endemic nephropathy (BEN). Ochratoxin A, a naturally occurring mycotoxin, also produced BEN as well as renal tumors (Clark and Snedeker, 2006). This is an irreversible disease and results in end-stage renal failure (Bunnell et al., 2007). The *n*-arylsuccinimides produce a chronic interstitial nephritis characterized by polyuric renal failure (Rankin, 2004). Details of these are provided in a review article by Commandeur and Vermeulen (1990). In general, men are more susceptible to chemical-induced nephrotoxicity. This is especially true among geriatric patients (Kacew et al., 1995).

Tacrolimus (FK506) is one of the principal immunosuppressive agents used after solid organ transplantations to prevent allograft rejection. Tacrolimus-induced chronic kidney injury (CKI) is characterized by fibrosis in the medullary rays, but the early morphologic findings of tacrolimus-induced AKI are not well characterized. Kidney injury molecule-1 (KIM-1) is a specific injury biomarker that was found to be useful in the diagnosis of mild to severe acute tubular injury on renal biopsies. A patient with AKI associated with elevated serum tacrolimus levels in which KIM-1 staining was present only in proximal tubules located in the medullary rays in the setting of otherwise normal light, immunofluorescent, and electron microscopy (Cosner et al., 2015). Therefore, tacrolimus-induced nephrotoxicity preferentially affects proximal tubules in medullary rays and this targeted injury is a precursor lesion for the linear fibrosis seen in CKI.

## *Major sites of nephrotoxicity*

### *Glomeruli*

The antibiotic puromycin increases permeability of the glomerulus to proteins such as albumin. This has been attributed to an alteration in the electrical charge of glomerular basement membrane (Brenner et al., 1977). On the other hand, the aminoglycoside antibiotics, such as gentamicin and kanamycin, decrease glomerular filtration, in addition to their effects on renal tubules (Humes and O'Connor, 1988). Certain toxicants, for example, gold, mercury, and penicillamine, may induce membranous glomerulonephritis by deposition of antigen–antibody conjugates in the glomerular basement membrane. Deoxynivalenol, a mycotoxin commonly found in cereal-based foods, produces deposition of immunoglobin A in the kidney, which resembles human glomerulonephritis nephropathy (Pestka and Smolinski, 2005). Ibuprofen decreases the renal blood flow and glomerular filtration rate (GFR) (Kent et al., 2007).

*Proximal tubules*

Because of their active absorptive and secretory activities, the proximal tubules often have higher concentrations of toxicants. Furthermore, proximal tubules have higher levels of cytochrome P-450 to detoxify or activate toxicants and are thus often the site of adverse effects. Heavy metals, such as mercury, chromium, cadmium, and lead alter the functions of the tubules, characterized by glycosuria, aminoaciduria, and polyuria. However, one needs to be cautious with respect to concentration or dose in terms of exposure. Diamond et al. (2003) clearly showed that exposure to cadmium produced renal toxicity as evidenced by proteinuria, but the source of cadmium inducing this effect was not derived from the diet. After higher doses, metals produce tubular cell death, elevated blood urea nitrogen (BUN), and anuria. The straight portion (pars recta) of the proximal tubules appears more susceptible than the convoluted portion to the toxicity of mercury (Phillips et al., 1977). The nephrotoxicity may result from a combination of direct cellular toxicity and ischemia secondary to vasoconstriction. Additional information on renal toxicity of metals is given in Chapter 25.

As noted above, certain antibiotics affect GFR. In addition, many antibiotics are also secreted by proximal tubules and induce alterations in the tubular functions. Various aminoglycoside antibiotics (streptomycin, neomycin, kanamycin, gentamicin, and amphotericin B) have been reported to affect proximal tubules. These drugs alter membrane phospholipid compositions, permeability, $Na^+$–$K^+$–ATPase activity, adenylate cyclase activity, and transport of $K^+$, $Ca^{2+}$, and $Mg^{2+}$ (Kaloyanides, 1984; Mingeot-Leclercq et al., 1995). Cephaloridine, unlike the antibiotics named above, is not secreted from the proximal tubules but is accumulated in these cells, thereby producing damage.

Halogenated hydrocarbons such as carbon tetrachloride and chloroform are mainly hepatotoxic, but in certain animal species they may also exert toxic effects on the kidney, especially on the proximal tubules, as reflected in functional changes. At higher doses, however, morphological changes may be produced in other parts of the nephron. Hexachlorobutadiene damage mainly the pars recta of the proximal tubules, resulting in a decreased urinary concentrating ability. Bromobenzene, similarly to hexachlorobutadiene, is also nephrotoxic, acting on the proximal tubules; while the former is bioactivated in the liver, the latter is bioactivated in the kidney, via a renal enzyme (C-S lyase) after biotransformation in the liver (Hook et al., 1982).

*Other sites*

Tetracycline, especially outdated products, may affect the renal medulla and induce interstitial nephritis. Amphotericin-B induces renal toxicity in a majority of the patients, affecting various renal structures.

Methoxyflurane, an anesthetic, is known to be nephrotoxic in humans and certain animals, producing *high-output* renal failure. This chemical was shown to be biotransformed to inorganic fluoride and oxalate. Experimental data suggest that the $F^-$ acts on several parts of the nephron to reduce reabsorption of water. First, it interferes with the capability of the proximal tubules to reabsorb water. Second, methoxyflurane inhibits the enzymes involved in the transport of ions at the ascending limb of the loop of Henle, thus reducing the interstitial osmolarity, thereby decreasing water reabsorption. This chemical also damages collecting tubules, rendering them insensitive to ADH (Mazze, 1976).

Analgesic mixtures containing aspirin and phenacetin, a derivative of acetaminophen, produce chronic renal failure, with adverse effects located predominantly in the medulla, that is the loop of Henle, vasa recta, interstitial cells, and collecting tubules (Schnellmann, 1998). The effects might be a result of vasoconstriction of the vasa recta (the blood vessels surrounding the loop of Henle) due to an inhibition of the synthesis of vasodilator prostaglandin (Nanra, 1974). Cisplatin affects many parts of the tubules in patients taking this chemotherapeutic agent (Tanaka et al., 1986). Cyclosporin produces acute thrombotic microangiopathy and chronic nephropathy with interstitial fibrosis (Racusen and Solez, 1988).

Other types of toxicity include renal carcinogenicity of DMN (dimethyl nitrosamine), and tubular blockade induced by the metabolites of sulfapyridine (acetylsulfapyridine) and glycols (oxalic acid). Penicillins and sulfonamides were reported to produce inflammatory interstitial nephritis in humans. An immunological mechanism was suggested as responsible for this toxicity (Appel and Neu, 1977). High concentrations of calcium may lead to calcification in the kidney and subsequent renal failure (Hwang et al., 2003).

## Testing procedures

Functional and morphological examinations of the kidney are routinely carried out as an integral part of short-term and long-term toxicity studies. The types of examinations involved are described in Chapter 6 and are further elaborated here.

Dogs, rabbits, and rats are the most commonly used animals in studies designed specifically for nephrotoxicity. Examinations of kidney function may be done in a number of ways.

## *Urinalysis*

### *Proteinuria*

Because of the size of their molecules, only a small amount of proteins of low molecular weight pass through the glomerular filter. The low molecular weight proteins are readily reabsorbed by the proximal tubules. The occurrence of large amounts of such proteins in the urine is thus an indication of a loss of tubular reabsorptive function, as in cadmium poisoning (Diamond et al., 2003). On the other hand, excretion of high molecular weight protein indicates a loss of integrity of glomeruli. It is to be noted that normal rat urine may contain some protein. A critical comparison of the treated animals with the controls is therefore important.

### *Glycosuria*

Glucose in the glomerular filtrate is completely reabsorbed in the tubules, provided the amount of glucose to be reabsorbed does not exceed the *transport maximum* (Tm). Glycosuria in the absence of hyperglycemia thus indicates tubular dysfunction.

### *Urine volume and osmolarity*

These two values are usually inversely related and are useful indicators of renal function in a *concentration test,* wherein water is withheld from the animal, and also in a *dilution test,* wherein a large amount of water is given to the animal. The osmolarity can be estimated from the specific gravity, but the freezing point of urine provides a more accurate measurement. A toxicant may produce high-output renal failure as noted above. On the other hand, it may induce oliguria or even anuria, resulting from tubular injury, with concomitant interstitial edema and intraluminal sediment or debris, which blocks urine flow.

### *Acidifying capacity*

This can be assessed from urine pH, titratable acids, and $NH_4^+$. This capacity is reduced when there is distal tubular dysfunction.

### *Enzymes*

Enzymes such as maltase and acid phosphatase in urine may indicate destruction of proximal tubules. Urine alkaline phosphatase, on the other hand, may be renal or hepatic in origin. Plummer (1981) suggested that the urinary enzymes are not only useful indicators of renal damage but also indicate the subcellular site of origin. For example, alkaline phosphatase is located in the endoplasmic reticulum, glutamate dehydrogenase in the mitochondria, and lactate dehydrogenase in the cytoplasm.

In general, urinary enzymes are more useful measures in acute nephrotoxic conditions.

## *New biomarkers*

The next generation of biomarkers for detecting nephrotoxicity have been widely investigated (Bonventre et al., 2010; Waring and Moonie, 2011). Potential renal biomarkers include urinary kidney injury molecule-1 (KIM-1), neutrophil gelatinase-associated lipocalin (NGAL), interleukin-18, cystatin C, clusterin, and fatty acid binding protein-liver type (Table 13.2). The site-specific biomarkers are listed in Figure 13.3. However, these new biomarkers require validation for their clinically successful application. Basic biological understanding of AKI will improve with high-throughput methodologies such as proteomics and metabolomics, and will lead to the identification and usage of novel biomarkers. Ultimately, a combination of biomarkers indicating kidney dysfunction and damage will likely be required.

### N-*acetyl-β-glucosaminidase (NAG)*

NAG; a proximal tubule lysosomal enzyme of 140 kDa with two isoforms, is widely used in screening for nephrotoxicity in human and in other species. NAG is found in both the $S_3$ segment of proximal tubular

***Table 13.2*** Major sites of nephrotoxicity and its specific biomarkers

| Site | Drugs inducing nephrotoxicity | Biomarkers |
|---|---|---|
| Glomerular | ACE inhibitors, ARB, NSAIDs, Mitomycin-C | Collagen IV, Cystatin C, Total protein |
| | Antiplatelet agents, Cyclosporin, Quinone | Cytokines (Interferons, Interleukins, TNF, CSFs) |
| Proximal tubule | Aminoglycoside antibiotics<br>Amphotericin B, Adefovir<br>Cisplatin, Foscarnet<br>Contrast stain, Cocaine, Heroin, Methadone<br>Methamphetamine | α-GST, α1-microglobulin, $β_2$-microglobulin, Clusterin, Cystatin C, HGF, KIM-1, L-FABP, Microalbumin, NAG, Netrin1, NHE3, NGAL, Osteopontin, RBP |
| Loop of Henle | | NHE3, Osteopontin |
| Distal tubule | Amphotericin B, Lithium<br>Acyclovir, Indinavir, Sulfonamides | Clusterin, H-FABP, NGAL, Osteopontin, π-GST |

*Source:* Reprinted from *Comprehensive Toxicology*, Vaidya VS, Bonventre JV, Ferguson MA, *vol. 7*, Elsevier, Oxford, pp. 197–211, Copyright 2010, with permission from Elsevier.

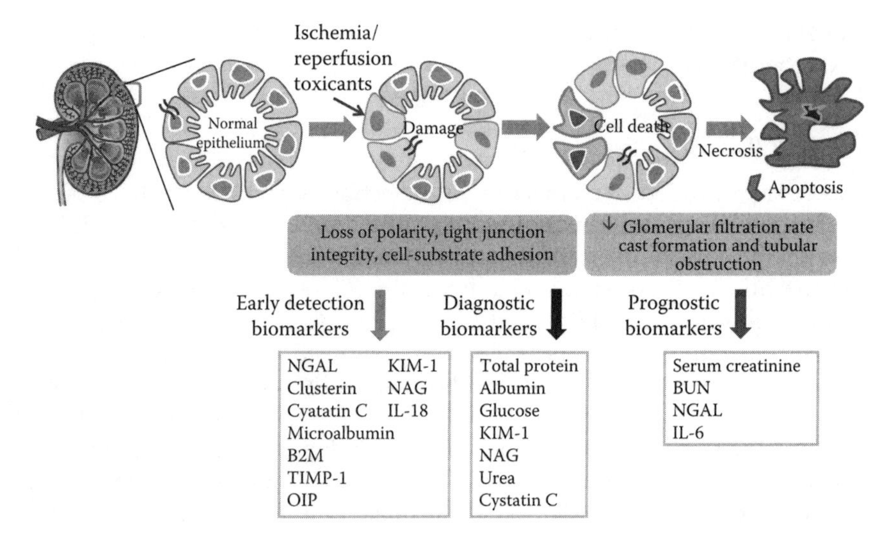


***Figure 13.3*** The cellular mechanisms involved in acute kidney injury and its urinary biomarkers. Biomarkers are renal or nonrenal derived molecules that report the functional status of kidney filtration and tubule injury. Markers may be nonrenal molecules that are filtered, secreted or reabsorbed, molecules that are constitutively expressed, or molecules that are upregulated by inflammation-mediated immune cells. (From Cheon JH et al. *Toxicol Res,* 32, 47–56, 2016.)

cells and the distal nephron. It has the highest activity in the straight ($S_3$) location of the proximal tubule (Ali et al., 2014). It is normally retarded by the passage through the glomerulus, and elevated urinary levels are an indication of proximal tubule injuries (Drake et al., 2002). Previous experiments showed that NAG is a sensitive marker of acute ischemic and oxidative stress within the kidney. A significant elevation in the urinary concentration of NAG was observed in animals exposed to gentamicin, cisplatin, or lithium (Vaidya et al., 2010b.)

*Neutrophil gelatinase-associated lipocalin (NGAL)*

NGAL is synthesized during the maturation process of granulocytes, which are involved in innate immunity (Borregaard et al., 1995). NGAL is highly upregulated following renal injury, and might be detected in serum and urine within 2 hours of injury, prior to functional changes in the kidney (Bennett et al., 2008). In AKI, NGAL is expressed in proximal tubule cells and then readily secreted into the urine without reabsorption; this occurs before SCr levels rise. Therefore, NGAL is a useful biomarker for the early diagnosis of AKI. In clinical studies, normal serum NGAL levels were approximately 80 ng/ml in healthy individuals, but increased to > 10-fold in serum and > 100-fold in urine following AKI (Mishra et al., 2005). Further, the role of NGAL as an AKI biomarker has been established after cardiac surgery (Xin et al., 2008).

*Glutathione S-transferase (GST)*

GSTs are a family of cytosolic, microsomal, and membrane-bound enzymes. The GST alpha isoform is localized to the proximal tubular cells, whereas the GST pi isoform is confined to distal tubular cells (Branten et al., 2000). The secretion level of GST is increased in response to cisplatin, cadmium, fluoride, and aristolochic acid (Usuda et al., 1998; Won et al., 2016). The highest urinary levels are detected with selective straight $S_3$ segment toxicants in rats (Frazier et al., 2012). Increased urinary pi GST ($\pi$-GST), a distal tubule cytosolic enzyme, was found in male patients following amphotericin B administration (Pai et al., 2005).

*Kidney injury molecule-1 (KIM-1)*

KIM-1 is a type-1 transmembrane glycoprotein with unknown function. KIM-1 is not expressed in normal kidney tissue but is expressed in proximal tubular cells after ischemic or nephrotoxic injury (Ichimura et al., 1998; Han et al., 2002). KIM-1 is a sensitive biomarker of kidney injury and better able to predict proximal tubule injury than SCr in a rat model (van Timmeren et al., 2007). Urinary KIM-1 levels were detected within 24 hours of acute tubular necrosis, even when SCr concentrations did not increase. A strong correlation between immunohistochemical KIM-1 expression and tubular cell injury was shown in renal allograft biopsies of patients with active antibody-mediated transplant rejection (Solez et al., 2008). Urinary excretion of KIM-1 was significantly elevated in rats treated with cisplatin at the early time points (Lee et al., 2014). Urinary KIM-1 is also associated with inflammation and renal function and reflects tissue KIM-1 levels, indicating that it can be used as a noninvasive biomarker for renal disease.

*Cystatin C*

Cystatin C is a low molecular weight protein (approximately 13.3 kDa) that is removed from the bloodstream by glomerular filtration. Cystatin C is a protease inhibitor that is normally expressed in nucleated cells and solely excreted by the kidney without muscle catabolism (de Boer et al., 2009; Beringer et al., 2009). Cystatin C is not normally detected in urine, but was found in urine of patients with tubular damage. Urinary levels of cystatin C were significantly elevated in AKI after elective cardiac surgery (Koyner et al., 2008). Compared with SCr, it is less dependent on age, gender, race and muscle mass when measured in the serum after kidney damage (Beringer et al., 2009). A reduction in kidney function and

GFR are positively correlated with blood levels of cystatin C. In patients with AKI, serum cystatin C rose by more than 50% 14 hours earlier than an observable increase in SCr (Herget-Rosenthal et al., 2004; Villa et al., 2005). Thus, this study concluded that serum cystatin C levels are useful in detection of AKI and may allow for the detection of AKI 1 to 2 days earlier than Cr.

*Osteopontin*

Osteopontin is a glycoprotein that is highly expressed in bone and epithelial tissues (Oldberg et al., 1986) and secreted in both phosphorylated and nonphosphorylated forms. It is expressed in various cell types, including macrophages, activated T cells, smooth muscle cells, and endothelial cells (Brown et al., 1992). Osteopontin is abundant in the bone matrix and present in kidney and epithelial cells as well as in other organs and body fluids (Chen et al., 1993). Osteopontin may be detected at high levels in human urine when the kidneys are markedly damaged by various nephrotoxicants, such as gentamicin, cisplatin, and cyclosporin (Beringer et al., 2009). Therefore, pharmacological inhibition of osteopontin expression may provide a novel approach for the treatment of type 2 diabetes-mediated nephrotoxicity.

*Interleukin-18 (IL-18)*

IL-18 is a proinflammatory cytokine that is activated in proximal tubule cells and excreted in the urine following kidney injury (Okamura et al., 1995). Previously, Boros and Bromberg (2006) reported that IL-18 exacerbated tubular necrosis and neutralizing antibodies against IL-18 to reduce renal injury in mice. Further, urinary excretion of IL-18 significantly rose 6 hours after pediatric cardiac surgery, whereas SCr levels did not change until 48–72 hours after surgery (Parikh et al., 2006). Therefore, the proinflammatory cytokine IL-18 is both a mediator and a biomarker of AKI in mice and humans.

*Pyruvate kinase M2 (PKM2)*

PKM2 catalyzes the final rate-limiting reaction in the glycolytic process, which is transfer of a high-energy phosphate group from phosphoenolpyruvate (PEP) to ADP, producing ATP and pyruvate (Mazurek et al., 2007; Christofk et al., 2008). In the PK subfamily, the M2 isoform (PKM2) is subjected to a complex regulation by both oncogenes and tumor suppressors, which allows for fine-tuning of PKM2 activity (Muirhead, 1990). The less active form of PKM2 directs glucose to aerobic glycolysis, while active PKM2 directs glucose towards oxidative metabolism. PKM2 was detected in the urine of rats injected with cisplatin (10 mg/kg) at 1 and 3 days after treatment (Kim et al., 2014).

## *Blood analysis*

### *Blood urea nitrogen (BUN)*

BUN is derived from normal metabolism of protein and is excreted in the urine. Elevated BUN usually indicates glomerular damage and decreased kidney function. However, its level might also be affected by poor nutrition and hepatotoxicity, which are common effects of many toxicants.

### *Creatinine*

Creatinine is a metabolite of creatine and is excreted completely in the urine via glomerular filtration. An elevation of its level in the blood is thus an indication of impaired kidney function. Further, data on its level in blood and in urine are used to estimate GFR. One drawback with this procedure is the fact that the tubules secrete some creatinine as well.

### *3-Indoxyl sulfate (3-IS)*

3-IS is a renal toxin that accumulates in the blood of uremic animals or patients as a consequence of decreased or absent urinary excretion of 3-IS, and is believed to be indicative of renal tubular injury. A marked elevation in serum 3-IS was observed following cisplatin treatment (Won et al., 2016). This is especially important for identifying biomarkers, as an increase in blood 3-IS preceded any evidence of apparent histopathological kidney damage. 3-IS is predominantly excreted via active secretion through the organic anion transporter (OAT) in proximal tubules and not via glomerular filtration, as 3-IS binding to albumin prevents it from entering the glomerulus. Thus, higher levels of 3-IS noted in blood may be indicative of renal tubular damage, as demonstrated in human studies. Thus, urinary 3-IS might be useful as a marker in clinical trials allowing therapy to be initiated at an early stage in the course of AKI (Figure 13.4).

## *Special tests*

### *Glomerular filtration rate (GFR)*

GFR can be more accurately determined by the clearance of inulin, a polysaccharide. It is diffused into the glomerular filtrate and is neither reabsorbed nor secreted by the tubules. Reduced GFR indicates impairment of glomerular filtration.

### *Renal clearance*

This is the volume of plasma of a substance that is completely cleared in a unit of time. The renal clearance of *p*-aminohippuric acid (PAH) exceeds that of inulin because it is not only filtered through the glomeruli but also secreted by the tubules. A reduction of PAH elimination without a

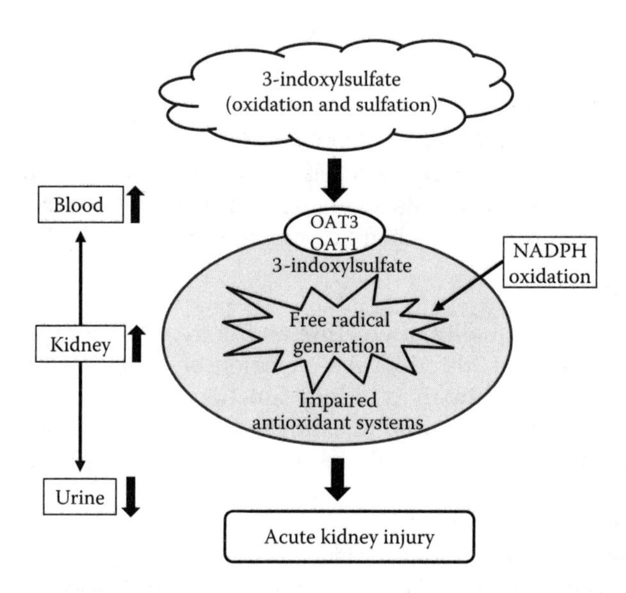


***Figure 13.4*** The molecular mechanism underlying the nephrotoxicity of 3-indoxyl sulfate. 3-Indoxyl sulfate accumulated in the blood and kidney of patient with acute kidney injury and then accelerates tubular cell injury. (From Won AJ et al., *Mol Biosyst.*, 12, 133–144, 2016.)

concomitant decrease of GFR indicates tubular dysfunction. PAH is nearly completely (up to 90%) removed from the blood in one passage. The rate of its clearance is therefore useful in determining the effective renal plasma flow. The renal blood flow is determined by the use of radiolabeled microspheres or an electromagnetic flow meter.

*Phenol sulfonphthalein excretion test*

The rate of excretion of phenol sulfonphthalein is related to renal blood flow. It is, therefore, often used in the assessment of renal function. However, a reduced secretion rate can also result from cardiovascular diseases.

## *Nature of nephrotoxicity*

The kidney has a remarkable compensatory capability. Even after appreciable changes in renal functions and morphology, the kidney may compensate and regain normal functions. Therefore, it is important to perform tests at repeated and appropriate time intervals.

Nephrotoxicants exert adverse effects on various parts of the kidney, resulting in alterations of different functions. A variety of tests therefore need to be performed. The most sensitive and reliable tests appear to vary depending on the nature of the nephrotoxicants as well as the experimental conditions (e.g., animal species, duration of exposure). Kluwe (1981) concluded from his studies that invitro accumulation of organic ions (e.g., PAH, TEA etc.), urinary concentrating ability, and kidney weight were the most sensitive and consistent indicators of nephrotoxicity. Standard urinalysis, serum analyses, qualitative enzymuria, and histopathological changes were less sensitive and less consistent. It was noted that urine osmolarity was the most sensitive indicator of the nephrotoxicity of a platinum complex, whereas GFR and effective renal plasma flow were affected only later and at higher doses.

In assessing the renal effects of a toxicant, extrarenal factors that might affect the blood volume or blood pressure need to be taken into account, since these may indirectly impair renal functions. Further, kidney diseases, such as those associated with aging, may be prevalent and also need to be considered.

## References

Appel GB, Neu HC (1977). The nephrotoxicity of antimicrobial agents (parts 1 and 2). *N Engl J Med.* 296, 663–670, 722–8.

Ayla S, Seckin I, Tanriverdi G et al. (2011). Doxorubicin induced nephrotoxicity: Protective effect of nicotinamide. *Int J Cell Biol.* 2011, 39023–8.

Ali RJ, Al-Obaidi FH, Arif HS (2014). The role of urinary *N*-acetyl beta-D-glucosaminidase in children with urological problems. *Oman Med J.* 29, 285–8.

Bates DW, Su L, Yu DT et al. (2001). Correlates of acute renal failure in patients receiving parenteral amphotericin B. *Kidney Int.* 60, 1452–9.

Borregaard N, Sehested M, Nielsen BS, Sengelov H, Kjeldsen L (1995). Biosynthesis of granule proteins in normal human bone marrow cells. Gelatinase is a marker of terminal neutrophil differentiation. *Blood,* 85, 812–7.

Bennett M, Dent CL, Ma Q et al. (2008). Urine NGAL predicts severity of acute kidney injury after cardiac surgery: A prospective study. *Clin J Am Soc Nephrol.* 3, 665–73.

Boros P, Bromberg JS (2006). New cellular and molecular immune pathways in ischemia/reperfusion injury. *Am J Transplant.* 6, 652–8.

Bonventre JV, Vaidya VS, Schmouder R, Feig P, Dieterle F. (2010). Next-generation biomarkers for detecting kidney toxicity. *Nat Biotechnol.* 28, 436–40.

Brenner BM, Bohrer MP, Baglis C et al. (1977). Determinants of glomerular permselectivity: Insights derived from observations in vivo. *Kidney Int.* 12, 229–57.

Bunnell JE, Tatu CA, Lerch HE et al. (2007). Evaluating nephrotoxicity of high-molecular weight organic compounds in drinking water from lignite aquifiers. *J Toxicol Environ Health A.* 70, 2089–91.

Brown LF, Berse B, Van de Water L et al. (1992). Expression and distribution of osteopontin in human tissues: Widespread association with luminal epithelial surfaces. *Mol Biol Cell.* 3, 1169–80.

Branten AJ, Mulder TP, Peters WH et al. (2000). Urinary excretion of glutathione S transferases alpha and pi in patients with proteinuria: Reflection of the site of tubular injury. *Nephron*. 85, 120–6.
Beringer PM, Hidayat L, Heed A et al. (2009). GFR estimates using cystatin C are superior to serum creatinine in adult patients with cystic fibrosis. *J Cystic Fibrosis*. 8, 19–25.
Chen J, Singh K, Mukherjee BB, Sodek J (1993). Developmental expression of osteopontin (OPN) mRNA in rat tissues: Evidence for a role for OPN in bone formation and resorption. *Matrix*. 13, 113–23.
Cheon JH, Kim SY, Son JY et al. (2016). Pyruvate kinase M2: A novel biomarker for the early detection of acute kidney injury. *Toxicol Res*. 32, 47–56.
Cho H, Cho Y, Cho EJ et al. (2016). Tenofovir-associated nephrotoxicity in patients with chronic hepatitis B: Two cases. *Clin Mol Hepatol*. 22, 286–91.
Christofk HR, Vander Heiden MG, Harris MH et al. (2008). The M2 splice isoform of pyruvate kinase is important for cancer metabolism and tumour growth. *Nature*. 452, 230–3.
Cihlar T, Ray AS, Laflamme G et al. (2007). Molecular assessment of the potential for renal drug interactions between tenofovir and HIV protease inhibitors. *Antivir Ther*. 12, 267–72.
Clark HA, Snedeker SM, (2006). Ochratoxin A: Its cancer risk and potentiation for exposure. *J Toxicol Environ Health B*. 9, 265–96.
Commandeur JNM, Vermeulen NPE (1990). Molecular and biochemical mechanisms of chemically induced nephrotoxicity: A review. *Chem Res Toxicol*. 3, 171–94.
Cosner D, Zeng X, Zhang PL (2015). Proximal tubular injury in medullary rays is an early sign of acute tacrolimus nephrotoxicity. *J Transplant*. 1–13.
de Boer IH, Katz R, Cao JJ et al. (2009). Cystatin C, albuminuria, and mortality among older adults with diabetes. *Diabetes Care*. 32, 1833–8.
Diamond GL, Thayer WC, Choudhury H (2003). Pharmacokinetics/pharmacodynamics (PK/PD) modeling of risks of kidney toxicity from exposure to cadmium: Estimates of dietary risks in the US population. *J Toxicol Environ Health A*. 66, 2141–64.
Donehower RC, Hande KR, Drake JC et al. (1979). Presence of 2,4-diamino-N10-methylpteroic acid after high-dose methotrexate. *Clin Pharmacol Ther*. 26, 63–72.
Drake PL, Krieg E, Teass AW, Vallyathan V (2002). Two assays for urinary *N*-acetyl-β-D-glucosaminidase compared. *Clin Chem*. 48, 1604–5.
Eyler RF, Mueller BA (2011). Medscape. Antibiotic dosing in critically ill patients with acute kidney injury. *Nat Rev Nephrol*. 7, 226–35.
Frazier KS, Seely JC, Hard GC et al. (2012). Proliferative and nonproliferative lesions of the rat and mouse urinary system. *Toxicol Pathol*. 40, 14S–86S.
González de Molina FJ, Ferrer R (2011). Appropriate antibiotic dosing in severe sepsis and acute renal failure: Factors to consider. *Crit Care*. 15, 175.
Han WK, Bailly V, Abichandani R et al. (2002). Kidney Injury Molecule-1 (KIM-1): A novel biomarker for human renal proximal tubule injury. *Kidney Int*. 62, 237–44.
Harbarth S, Pestotnik SL, Lloyd JF, Burke JP, Samore MH (2001). The epidemiology of nephrotoxicity associated with conventional amphotericin B therapy. *Am J Med*. 111, 528–34.

Herget-Rosenthal S, Marggraf G, Husing J et al. (2004). Early detection of acute renal failure by serum cystatin C. *Kidney Int.* 66, 1115–22.

Hook JB, Rose MS, Lock EA (1982). The nephrotoxicity of hexachloro–1:3-butadiene in the rat: Studies of organic anion and cation transport in renal slices and the effects of monoxygenase inducers. *Toxicol Appl Pharmacol.* 65, 373–82.

Humes HD, O'Connor RP (1988). Aminoglycoside nephrotoxicity. In: Shrier RW, Gottschalk CW, eds. *Diseases of the Kidney*, 4th ed. *vol. 2*. Boston Little, Brown.

Hwang S-J, Lai Y-H, Chiu H-F et al. (2003). Association of death from renal failure with calcium levels in drinking water. *J Toxicol Environ Health A.* 66, 2327–35.

Ichimura T, Bonventre JV, Bailly V et al. (1998). Kidney Injury Molecule-1 (KIM-1), a putative epithelial cell adhesion molecule containing a novel immunoglobulin domain, is up-regulated in renal cells after injury. *J Biol Chem.* 273, 4135–42.

Jacobs SA, Stoller RG, Chabner BA et al. (1976). 7-Hydroxymethotrexate as a urinary metabolite in human subjects and rhesus monkeys receiving high dose methotrexate. *J Clin Invest.* 57, 534–8.

Kacew S, Ruben Z, McConnell RF (1995). Strain as a determinant factor in the differential responsiveness of rats to chemicals. *Toxicol Pathol.* 23, 701–14.

Kadowaki D, Sumikawa S, Arimizu K et al. (2012). Effect of acetaminophen on the progression of renal damage in adenine induced renal failure model rats. *Life Sci.* 91, 1304–8.

Kaloyanides GJ (1984). Aminoglycoside-induced functional and biochemical defects in the renal cortex. *Fundam Appl Toxicol.* 4, 930–43.

Kent AL, Maxwell LE, Koina ME et al. (2007). Renal glomeruli and tubular injury following indomethacin, ibuprofen, and gentamicin exposure in a neonatal rat model. *Pediatr Res.* 62, 307–12.

Kim SY, Sohn SJ, Won AJ, Kim HS, Moon A. (2014). Identification of noninvasive biomarkers for nephrotoxicity using HK-2 human kidney epithelial cells. *Toxicol Sci.* 140, 247–58.

Kluwe WM (1981). Renal function tests as indicators of kidney injury in subacute toxicity studies. *Toxicol Appl Pharmacol.* 57, 414–24.

Kriz W, Bankir L (1988). A standard nomenclature for structures of the kidney. *Am J Physiol.* 254, F1–F8.

Koyner JL, Bennett MR, Worcester EM et al. (2008). Urinary cystatin C as an early biomarker of acute kidney injury following adult cardiothoracic surgery. *Kidney Int.* 74, 1059–69.

Lee YK, Park EY, Kim S et al. (2014). Evaluation of cadmiuminduced nephrotoxicity using urinary metabolomic profiles in sprague-dawley male rats. *J Toxicol Environ Health Part A.* 77, 1384–98.

Mazer M, Perrone J (2008). Acetaminophen-induced nephrotoxicity: Pathophysiology, clinical manifestations, and management. *J Med Toxicol.* 4, 2–6.

Madsen KM, Tisher CC (1986). Structural-functional relationship along the distal nephron. *Am J Physiol.* 250(6 Pt 3), F1–15.

Mazze RI (1976). Methoxyflurane nephropathy. Environ Health Perspect 15, 111–120.

Messmann R, Allegra C (2001). Antifolates. In: Chabner B, Longo D eds. *Cancer Chemotherapy and Biotherapy*. Philadelphia: Lippincott Williams & Wilkins, pp. 139–84.

Mazurek S, Drexler HC, Troppmair J et al. (2007). Regulation of pyruvate kinase type M2 by A-Raf: A possible glycolytic stop or go mechanism. *Anticancer Res.* 27, 3963–71.

Mishra J, Dent C, Tarabishi R et al. (2005). Neutrophil gelatinase-associated lipocalin (NGAL) as a biomarker for acute renal injury after cardiac surgery. *Lancet.* 365, 1231–8.

Miller RP, Tadagavadi RK, Ramesh G, Reeves WB (2010). Mechanisms of cisplatin nephrotoxicity. *Toxins* (Basel). 2, 2490–518.

Mingeot-Leclercq MP, Brasseur R, Schank A (1995). Molecular parameters involved in aminoglycoside nephrotoxicity. *J Toxicol Environ Health.* 44, 263–300.

Muirhead H. (1990). Isoenzymes of pyruvate kinase. *Biochem Soc Trans.* 18, 193–6.

Nanra RS (1974). Pathology, etiology and pathogenesis of analgesic nephropathy. *Aust NZJ Med.* 4, 602–3.

Oldberg A, Franzen A, Heinegard D (1986). Cloning and sequence analysis of rat bone sialoprotein (osteopontin) cDNA reveals an Arg-Gly-Asp cell-binding sequence. *Proc Natl Acad Sci USA.* 83, 8819–23.

Okamura H, Tsutsi H, Komatsu T et al. (1995). Cloning of a new cytokine thatinduces IFN-gamma production by T cells. *Nature.* 378, 88–91.

Pai MP, Norenberg JP, Telepak RA, Sidney DS, Yang S (2005). Assessment of effective renal plasma flow, enzymuria, and cytokine release in healthy volunteers receiving a single dose of Amphotericin B desoxycholate. *Antimicrob Agents Chemother.* 49, 3784–9.

Pestka JJ, Smolinski AT (2005). Deoxynivalenol: Toxicology and potential effects on humans. *J Toxicol Environ Health B.* 8, 39–69.

Phillips R, Yamaguchi M, Cote MG et al. (1977). Assessment of mercuric chloride-induced nephrotoxicity by *p*-aminohippuric acid uptake and the activity of four gluconeogenic enzymes in rat renal cortex. *Toxicol Appl Pharmacol.* 41, 407–22.

Parikh CR, Mishra J, Thiessen-Philbrook H et al. (2006). Urinary IL-18 is an early predictive biomarker of acute kidney injury after cardiac surgery. *Kidney Int.* 70, 199–203.

Plummer DT (1981). Urinary enzyme in drug toxicity. In: Gorrod JW, ed. *Testing for Toxicity.* London: Taylor & Francis.

Racusen LC, Solez K (1988). Cyclosporine nephrotoxicity. *Int Rev Expo Pathol.* 30, 107–57.

Rankin GO (2004). Nephrotoxicity induced by *C*- and *N*-arylsuccinimides. *J Toxicol Environ Health B.* 7, 399–416.

Solez K, Colvin RB, Racusen LC et al. (2008). Banff 07 classification of renal allograft pathology: Updates and future directions. *Am J Transplant.* 8, 753–60.

Schnellmann RG (1998). Analgesic nephropathy in rodents. *J Toxicol Environ Health B.* 1, 81–90.

Smeland E, Fuskevag OM, Nymann K et al. (1996). High-dose 7-hydroxymethotrexate: Acute toxicity and lethality in a rat model. *Cancer Chemother Pharmacol.* 37, 415–22.

Tanaka H, Ishikawa E, Teshima S et al. (1986). Histopathological study of human cisplatin nephrotoxicity. *Toxicol Pathol.* 14, 247–57.

Usuda K, Kono K, Dote T et al. (1998). Urinary biomarkers monitoring for experimental fluoride nephrotoxicity. *Arch Toxicol.* 72, 104–9.

Vaidya VS, Bonventre JV, Ferguson MA (2010a). Biomarkers of acute kidney injury. In: McQeen CA, Schnellmann RG, eds. *Comprehensive Toxicology, vol. 7.* Oxford, UK: Elsevier, 197–211.
Vaidya VS, Ozer JS, Dieterle F et al. (2010b). Kidney injury molecule-1 outperforms traditional biomarkers of kidney injury in preclinical biomarker qualification studies. *Nat Biotechnol.* 28, 478–85.
van Timmeren MM, van den Heuvel MC, Bailly V et al. (2007). Tubular kidney injury molecule-1 (KIM-1) in human renal disease. *J Pathol.* 212, 209–17.
Vidal F, Domingo JC, Guallar J et al. (2006). In vitro cytotoxicity and mitochondrial toxicity of tenofovir alone and in combination with other antiretrovirals in human renal proximal tubule cells. *Antimicrob Agents Chemother.* 50, 3824–32.
Villa P, Jimenez M, Soriano MC et al. (2005). Serum cystatin C concentration as a marker of acute renal dysfunction in critically ill patients. *Crit Care.* 9, R139–43.
Waring WS, Moonie A (2011). Earlier recognition of nephrotoxicity using novel biomarkers of acute kidney injury. *Clin Toxicol.* 49, 720–8.
Widemann BC, Adamson PC (2006). Understanding and managing methotrexate nephrotoxicity. *Oncologist.* 11, 694–703.
Won AJ, Kim S, Kim YG et al. (2016). Discovery of urinary metabolomic biomarkers for early detection of acute kidney injury. *Mol Biosyst.* 12, 133–44.
Xin C, Yulong X, Yu C et al. (2008). Urine neutrophil gelatinase-associated lipocalin and interleukin-18 predict acute kidney injury after cardiac surgery. *Renal Failure.* 30, 904–13.

# chapter fourteen

# Toxicology of the immune system

**Tae Cheon Jeong**

Contents



## General considerations

The function of the immune system is to protect the host against foreign organisms (viruses, bacteria, fungi), tumor cells, and other foreign substances such as xenobiotics. The importance of the immune system is evidenced by the consequences of immunodeficiency: patients with this disorder are prone to be susceptible to infections and develop tumors. Immunodeficiency can be congenital or acquired; the latter is also known as acquired immunodeficiency syndrome (AIDS).

The immune system is composed of several types of organs, cells, and noncellular components. The functions of the individual components are, in general, interrelated. Thus, upon encountering a foreign substance, a cascade of reactions usually appears between different types of cellular and humoral components. These reactions involve recognition, memory, and response to foreign substances, and are designed for their elimination or control.

Because of its complex cellular and molecular components, which include highly coordinated networks and rapidly dividing properties of immune cells, the immune system is one of the most sensitive targets for toxic compounds, as it can control either networks or cell division.

A variety of toxicants are known to suppress immune functions. This effect leads to lowered host resistance to bacterial, parasitic infestation, or viral infections, as well as diminished control of cancer cells formed. In addition, certain toxicants may provoke exaggerated immune reactions leading to local or systemic reactions. Furthermore, the toxicants sometimes lead to "autoimmune reactions." Therefore, the toxicity of the immune system is not only indicated by immunosuppression, but immunoenhancement as well wherein the immune function is abnormally triggered or stimulated.

This chapter briefly describes the components of the immune system and their functions and the major immunotoxicants.

## Components of the immune system

The immune system consists of a network of organs including bone marrow, thymus, spleen, and lymph nodes. From these organs, various lymphocytes and other cells with different immune functions are derived.

Some of the components are involved in specific immune responses and others in nonspecific responses. Both types of cells are derived from the pluripotent stem cells in the bone marrow. The lymphoid stem cells are generated from these cells. Some of these cells are processed through the thymus and become T cells (T lymphocytes); others go through the "bursal equivalent" tissues (including bone marrow, lymph nodes, and lymphoid tissues in the gut such as the appendix, cecum, and Peyer patches) to become B cells (B lymphocytes). Still others are released from the bone marrow without further processing. These are known as natural killer (NK) cells. Unlike T cells and B cells, NK cells are also involved in nonspecific defense against neoplasms, and certain other foreign substances (Table 14.1). Other pluripotent stem cells give rise to myeloid stem cells, from which monocytes, mast cells, and polymorphonuclear (PMN) cells are derived. Monocytes then become macrophages, which are involved in specific (acquired) and nonspecific (innate) immune reactions. In addition,

***Table 14.1*** Cells and primary soluble mediators: Innate vs. acquired immunity

| Characteristic | Innate immunity | Acquired immunity |
|---|---|---|
| Cells involved | Polymorphonuclear cells | T cells |
| | | B cells |
| | Monocyte/macrophage | Macrophages |
| | NK cells | NK cells |
| Primary soluble mediators | Complement | Antibody |
| | Lysozyme | Cytokines |
| | Acute phase proteins | |
| | Interferon α/β | |
| | Cytokines | |
| Specificity of response | None | Yes |
| Response enhanced by repeated antigen challenge | No | Yes |

*Source:* Burns LA et al., *Casarett and Doull's Toxicology*, McGraw-Hill, New York, pp. 335–402, 1996.

there are three types of PMN cells, namely, neutrophils, eosinophils, and basophils. These cells are involved in nonspecific defense mechanisms.

## *T cells*

As noted above, T cells, after passing through the thymus, enter the blood and constitute 70% of the circulating lymphocytes. Some settle in thymus-dependent areas of the spleen and lymph nodes. On contact with antigens processed by antigen-presenting cells (APCs; such as macrophages and B cells), T cells undergo proliferation and differentiation. Some of these cells become "activated" and are responsible for mediating cellular immunity. Others become memory T cells, which can be activated by combining with antigens while others become *helper* cells. Once activated, helper T cells proliferate and secrete lymphokines which induce B cells to become plasma cells secreting antigen-specific antibodies.

The activated T cells react either directly with cell membrane-associated antigens or by releasing various soluble factors known as lymphokines. There are a large number of lymphokines (see the section "Other Types of Cells").

## *B cells*

Other stem cells undergo changes in certain tissues, as noted above, to become B cells (B lymphocytes). They enter the blood to constitute 30%

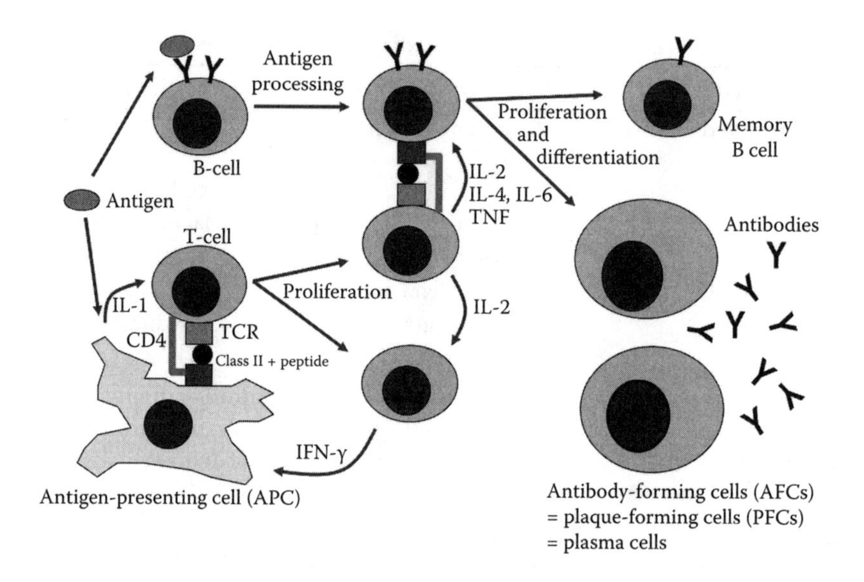


***Figure 14.1*** Cellular interactions in antibody responses.

of the lymphocytes. The primary immune response is initiated by contact of antigen with B cells, which then differentiate and proliferate. Some of these become *memory* cells, which retain the surface immunoglobulin receptors, whereas others become *plasma* cells. The latter type bears IgM and IgD immunoglobulins on the cell surface. Exposure of the memory cells to the same antigen at a later time results in the secondary immune response. Figure 14.1 briefly illustrates the cellular interactions in antibody responses.

## Other types of cells

*Other lymphocytes* lack the characteristic surface markers of T and B cells, but participate in nonspecific immune system functions and are known as the null cells. Some of these, the *natural killer* cells, display spontaneous (without prior sensitization) cytolytic activity against other cells, especially leukemia and carcinoma cells.

*Macrophages* are also derived from the stem cell pool in the bone marrow. After their release, they appear in the bloodstream as monocytes and in the tissues as histiocytes. On contact with a foreign body, they engulf the foreign body and become activated macrophages. These cells are rich in cytoplasmic hydrolytic enzymes and these enzymes readily digest most bacterial cells. Macrophages can also be activated to become APCs.

*Langerhans cells,* located in the skin, are also derived from bone marrow and act as APCs. They serve to process dermal antigens and initiate contact allergy and rejection of skin graft.

Among the *PMN cells,* neutrophil PMNs exert phagocytic activity. The eosinophils possess cytotoxic function, and basophils (which become mast cells in tissues) release histamine and other substances, thereby initiating local reactions to a foreign substance inducing immediate hypersensitivity.

## Soluble mediators

*Immunoglobins* (*Ig family*) are proteins produced by plasma cells derived from B cells with specific antibody activities. Their specificity is determined by the amino acid sequence and tertiary surface configuration. Numerous types of antibodies against specific antigens are produced by the combinatorial expression of gene fragments, which yield the specificity of acquired immunity. There are five major types of immunoglobins. Their characteristics and functions are outlined in Table 14.2.

*Interleukins* (cytokines) are proteins produced by activated T cells (lymphokines) or monocytes/macrophages (monokines) in response to antigenic or mitogenic stimulation. They promote the proliferation of T, B, and hematopoietic stem cells.

*The complement system* consists of more than 30 plasma and body fluid proteins. These proteins complement a variety of immune functions, such

***Table 14.2*** Characteristics of immunoglobulins

| Class | Mol. weight (Dalton) | Mean survival, $t_{1/2}$ (days) | Mean serum concentration (mg/dL) | Major function |
|---|---|---|---|---|
| IgG | 150,000 | 20 | 720–1500 | Most prevalent; major antibody for toxins, viruses, and bacteria |
| IgA | 170,000 | 6 | 90–325 | In secretions from mucosa; for early antibacterial and antiviral defense |
| IgM | 900,000 | 10 | 45–150 | Major antibody after exposure to most antigens |
| IgD | 180,000 | 3 | 3 | Present on B cell surface, function as an antigen receptor |
| IgE | 200,000 | 2 | 0.03 | Fixed on mast cells, responsible for immediate type hypersensitivity |

as adherence of antibody-coated bacteria to macrophages, modulation of immune response, and lysis of cells. Immunotoxicants activate or inhibit the complements. Macrophages and certain lymphocytes are capable of synthesizing certain important cytokines, such as tumor necrosis factor (Ruddle, 1994), and growth factors; the latter play a central role in the fibrotic lung lesions in humans exposed to asbestos and silica (see Chapter 12).

## Immunotoxicants

### Major immunotoxicants

A variety of substances have been found to affect the immune system. Exposure to foreign substances suppresses or enhances immune response depending upon dose, duration, and route of administration (Kreitinger et al., 2016). Some parent chemicals affect immune functions directly or may require metabolic activation. The compounds may be categorized as follows:

1. *Medicinal products*: Among these, the antineoplastic drugs cyclophosphamide, nitrogen mustards, 6-mercaptopurine, azathioprine, methotrexate, 5-fluorouracil, actinomycin, doxorubicin, and diazepam are more frequently implicated (a number of other drugs that induced autoimmune reactions are listed in Table 14.3)
2. *Heavy metals, organometals*: Beryllium, nickel, chromium, lead, gold, methylmercury, platinum, organic tin compounds, sodium arsenite and arsenate, and arsenic trioxide
3. *Pesticides*: Pyrethroids, chlordane, DDT, dieldrin, methyl parathion, carbofuran, maneb, hexachlorobenzene, carbaryl, 2,4-D, paraquat, and diquat

**Table 14.3** Examples of drugs that induce autoimmune syndromes

| Autoimmune syndrome | Examples of drugs |
|---|---|
| Hepatitis | Erythromycin, floxacillin, halothane, methyldopa |
| Hemolytic anemia | Amoxicillin, nomifensine, probenecid, tolbutamide |
| Lupus erythematosus | Hydralazine, procainamide |
| Nephritis | Captopril |
| Neutropenia | Methyldopa, penicillamine |
| Oculocutaneous syndrome | Practolol |
| Thrombocytopenia | Acetaminophen, quinine |

*Source:* Pohl LR et al., *Annu Rev Pharmacol.*, 28, 367–387, 1988; Behan PO et al., *Lancer.*, ii, 984–987, 1976.

4. *Halogenated hydrocarbons*: 2,3,7,8-tetrachlorodibenzo-*p*-dioxin, polychlorinated biphenyls, polybrominated biphenyls, trichloroethylene, chloroform, carbon tetrachloride, pentachlorophenol, perfluorooctanoic acid, and perfluorooctane sulfonate
5. *Air pollutants*: Diesel exhaust particles, ambient particulate matter, asbestos fibers, and nanoparticles
6. *Miscellaneous compounds*: Aflatoxins, benzo(*a*)pyrene, methylcholanthrene, diethylstilbestrol, 2-methoxyethanol, benzene, corticosteroids, deoxynivalenol, 12-*O*-tetradecanoylphorbol-13-*O*-acetate, ochratoxin, penicillin, sulfites, subtilisin, formaldehyde, drug of abuse including cocaine, and toluene diisocyanates

The effects of toxicants on the immune system are complex; some suppress cell-mediated immunity, others humoral immunity, and others may even stimulate certain immune functions (Table 14.4). Therefore, the adverse effects of chemicals on immune functions need to be determined via the tiered testing approach (Dean et al., 1982).

***Table 14.4*** Effects of *in vivo* exposure to chemicals on immune functions and host resistance

| Parameters | DES | BaP | TPA |
|---|---|---|---|
| Resistance to *Listeria* challenge | D | NE | I |
| Resistance to tumor challenge | D | NE | D |
| *Trichinella* expulsion | D | D | NE |
| Thymus weight | D | NE | D |
| Delayed hypersensitivity | D | NE | NE |
| Lymphocyte responses[a] | D | D[b] | D |
| T-cell quantification | D | – | D |
| Spontaneous lymphocyte cytotoxicity | NE | NE | D |
| Antibody plaque response | D | D | D |
| Immunoglobulins, M, G, and A levels | NE | NE | D |
| Macrophage phagocytosis | I | NE | I |
| Macrophage cytostasis | I | NE | I |
| RES clearance time | I | NE | I |
| Bone marrow cellularity[c] | D | D | NE |

*Source:* Dean et al., *Pharmacol Rev.*, 34, 137–148, 1982.

*Abbreviations:* BaP, benzo[*a*]pyrene; D, decreased; DES, diethylstilbesterol; I, increased; NE, no effect; –, not tested; TPA, 12-*O*-tetradecanoylphorbol-13-*O*-acetate.

[a] Lymphocyte responses to phytohemagglutinin, concanavalin A, lipopolysaccharide, and mixed lymphocyte culture.

[b] Decreased, except the response to mixed lymphocyte culture.

[c] Colony-forming units, multipotent cells, and granulocyte/macrophage progenitors.

## *Effects on immune functions*

The function of the immune system is, as noted earlier, to protect the host against foreign organisms (viruses, bacteria, etc.), tumor cells, and other foreign substances. When the system functions properly, foreign agents are eliminated promptly and efficiently. However, with certain agents and in some individuals, the immune system may respond in adverse manners manifested as (1) hypersensitivity and/or allergy; (2) autoimmunity; and (3) immunosuppression and/or immunodeficiency. These are outlined next.

### *Hypersensitivity and allergy*

There are four types of such reactions. With Type I, the reactions are immediate (usually within 15 min), resulting from a second or subsequent exposure to an antigen. The first exposure to that antigen induces production of IgE antibodies while the subsequent exposure to the same antigen triggers the release of existing histamine, heparin, serotonin, prostaglandins, chemokines, and so forth. These substances induce a variety of clinical manifestations, such as asthma, rhinitis, urticaria, and anaphylaxis. Allergenic agents are diverse in nature and notable examples of these are metals (nickel, beryllium, platinum compounds), therapeutic agents (penicillin), food additives (sulfites, monosodium glutamate, tartrazine, and benzoates), food (chocolate, peanuts), pesticides (pyrethrum), and industrial chemicals such as toluene diisocyanate (TDI).

Type II and Type III hypersensitivity reactions are less common. Type II is characterized by cytolysis through IgG and/or IgM. The targets are usually erythrocytes, leucocytes, platelets, and their progenitors. The result of the cytolysis is hemolytic anemia, leukopenia, or thrombocytopenia. The offending agents include gold salts, chlorpromazine, phenytoin, sulfonamides, and TDI. Type III, also known as Arthus reaction, is mediated mainly by IgG. The antigen–antibody complexes are deposited in the vascular endothelium. Depending upon the site, the damaged blood vessels may produce lupus erythematosus (e.g., procainamide) and glomerular nephritis (e.g., gold).

Type IV is a delayed hypersensitivity reaction whose latent period is usually between 12 and 48 hours. The reaction is mediated by T cells (rather than antibodies) and characterized by perivascular infiltration of monocytes, lymphocytes, and lymphoblasts (resulting from local transformation of lymphocytes). Clinically, this is seen in association with contact dermatitis and granulomatous reactions. A commonly encountered hypersensitivity inducer is nickel, which also induces immediate immune reaction. Others include beryllium, chromium, formaldehyde, thimerosal (a mercurial compound that was widely used as a preservative for vaccine), and TDI.

### *Autoimmunity*

In autoimmune diseases, the immune system produces antibodies to endogenous antigens, thus damaging normal tissues. Hemolytic anemia is an example of such disorders with phagocytosis of antibody-sensitized erythrocytes leading to hemolysis and anemia. Certain chemicals and metals have been reported to induce such diseases. For example, the pesticide dieldrin was found to produce hemolytic anemia. Exposure to gold and mercury has been associated with a type of glomerular nephritis that is considered an autoimmune disease (Dean et al., 1982). Trichloroethene, an industrial solvent, was shown to induce an autoimmune disorder resembling systemic lupus erythematosus (Wang et al., 2007).

In addition, a number of drugs are known to exert toxicity through their effects on the cellular or humoral immunity, inducing autoimmune diseases. Clinically these conditions are manifested as hepatitis, nephritis, hemolytic anemia, neutropenia, thrombocytopenia, and so forth. Table 14.3 is a compilation of such drugs.

The mode of action of these drugs appears to be mediated through covalent binding of the drug or its metabolite to tissue macromolecules. The target specificity may be related to differences in tissue distribution of the conjugates. In general, the incidence of these side effects is low, perhaps due to a complex genetic makeup, which determines the levels of activating and detoxicating enzymes (Pohl et al., 1988; Park and Kiteringham, 1990).

### *Immunosuppression and immunodeficiencies*

Many immunotoxicants suppress immune functions (Bondy and Pestka, 2000; Dhouib et al., 2016). An extensively studied immunotoxicant is 2,3,7,8-tetrachlorodibenzo-*p*-dioxin (TCDD) which acts on the immune system. TCDD suppresses all the specific immune functions tested, while sparing nonspecific functions, such as the NK-cell activity and macrophage functions. Its immunotoxicity is apparently mediated through binding to the *Ah* receptors in lymphoid cells (Luster et al., 1989; Esser, 2016). Cigarette smoke components are also effective immunosuppressants. Alcohol depresses immune system functions, resulting in a depletion and loss of function of $CD4^{(+)}$ T lymphocytes, and subsequent suppression of IL-2 production, which regulates both innate and adaptive immunity (Ghare et al., 2011). When the immune system is suppressed, individuals are more susceptible to infections and many diseases such as cancers, aging, diabetes, and so forth, develop.

Other immunosuppressants have more restricted activities. For example, antineoplastic drugs such as cyclosporin adversely affect B cells; T cells that have undergone antigenic differentiation may also be affected. Metals such as lead and mercury impair both humoral and cell-mediated host resistance (Luebke et al. 2006). In addition, gold may also induce glomerular nephritis through an autoimmune mechanism resulting in deposits in the glomeruli. Nickel may suppress immune functions through a variety of mechanisms; however, its major clinical effect is hypersensitivity. Organochlorine pesticides impair immune functions mainly in neonatal animals (Loose, 1982). Carbaryl depresses antibody response and phagocytosis by granulocytes. Corticosteroids depress immune functions as well as inflammatory responses.

## *Immunotoxicity*

As noted above, the immune system is composed of a variety of cellular and humoral components and exerts numerous activities. An immunotoxicant affects any one or more of these components and activities.

### *Immunocompetence tests in intact animals*

These tests are designed to study the effects of chemicals on host resistance/susceptibility to bacterial, viral, and parasitic diseases as well as to bacterial endotoxins and tumor cells. In general, mice are used because of the large number of animals required.

The test chemical is given to the animals by an appropriate route, preferably mimicking human exposure. Usually three dose groups and a control group are included in the test. The duration of the dosing is generally 14 or 90 days. After this pretreatment, animals are given a suitable quantity of the challenging agent. The quantity of the agent is selected on the basis that 10–20% of the mortality or morbidity is induced in control animals. Increased mortality or morbidity indicates decreased host resistance. A list of various infectious agents has been compiled by Bradley and Morahan (1982).

### *Cell-mediated immunity*

This can be studied in intact animals or with cells *in vitro*. In intact animals, usually mice, the most commonly used procedure is to determine the *delayed hypersensitivity* response to a specific antigen. The antigen, such as sheep erythrocytes or keyhole limpet hemocyanin, is injected into a footpad or an ear of the animal. Four days later, a challenging dose of the antigen is administered at the sensitized site. The extent of the swelling or amount of localized radioactivity is measured from a radiolabeled substance, such as $^{125}$I-labeled human serum albumin or tritiated thymidine (Luster et al., 1982; Munson et al., 1982; Sanders et al., 1982).

*In vitro* tests are conducted on cells collected from animals pretreated with the test chemical. Such tests include lymphocyte proliferation and lymphocyte subpopulation. The *lymphocyte proliferation* assay is conducted by culturing, in the presence of mitogens, lymphocytes collected from the spleen of pretreated animals. Mitogens such as phytohemagglutinin and concanavalin A are capable of inducing proliferation of normal T lymphocytes, whereas lipopolysaccharides, such as the cell membrane of Gram-negative bacteria, affect B lymphocytes. Immunosuppressive agents inhibit lymphocyte proliferation. The extent of proliferation can be determined by the incorporation of tritiated thymidine into DNA (Luster et al., 1982).

Lymphocytes, as noted above, consist of T cells, B cells, and null cells; the T-cell population is composed of T-memory, T-helper, and T-killer cells. Techniques for their enumeration include the use of immunofluorescence, rosette formation, histochemistry, cell electrophoresis, cytolysis, and fluorescence-activated cell sorting (Norbury, 1982).

## *Humoral immunity*

A commonly used procedure, the plaque assay, involves quantitative determination of plaque-forming cells of the IgM class: 4 days after the mouse has been sensitized to an antigen (e.g., sheep erythrocytes), the spleen is removed and a cell suspension is made. A quantity of the antigen, along with a suitable complement, is added to the suspension. The mixture is then spread on a slide and the number of plaque counted, representing the primary humoral immune response. A brief procedure for determining the number of plaque-forming cells is depicted in Figure 14.2. To determine the secondary immune response, the mouse is administered on day 10 a second dose of the antigen. On day 15 the spleen is removed and the above procedure is repeated with an additional step of incubation with rabbit anti mouse IgG to develop the IgG-producing plaque. Reduced plaque indicates immunosuppression (Spyker-Cranmer et al., 1982). Instead of sheep erythrocytes, which are T-dependent antigens, lipopolysaccharides that are T-independent antigens may be used.

The levels of various immunoglobulins (IgG, IgM, and IgA) in the serum may be directly measured. The techniques for their measurement have been reviewed by Davis and Ho (1976). The number of B cells in the spleen also provides information on the status of humoral immunity (Dean et al., 1982). Vos et al. (1982) have elaborated the procedures and advantages of the enzyme-linked immunosorbent assay (ELISA) in testing chemicals for immunotoxicity.

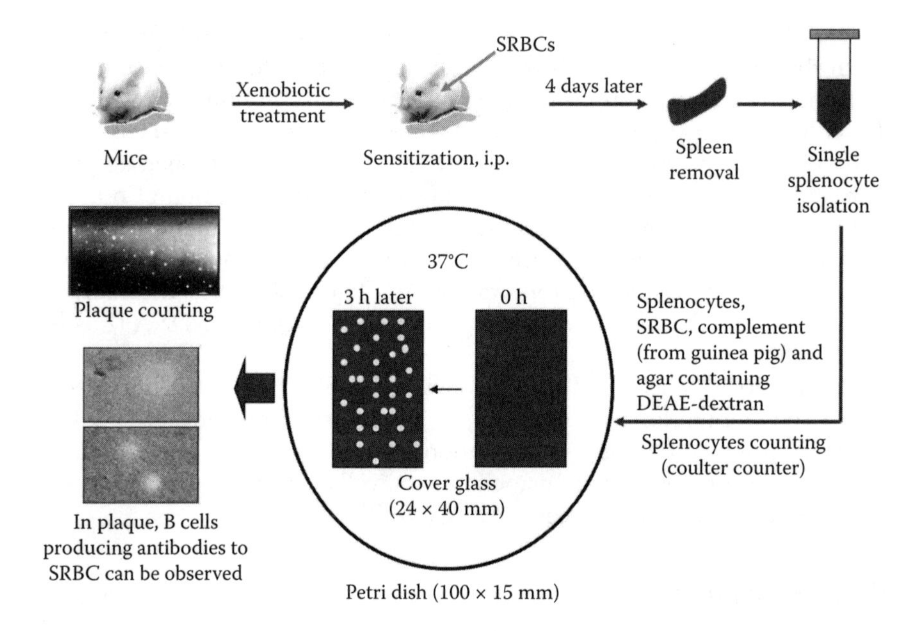


***Figure 14.2*** A procedure for determining the number of plaque-forming cells.

### *Macrophage and bone marrow*

The functions of macrophages can be tested in a number of ways: (1) number of resident peritoneal cells, (2) phagocytosis, (3) lysosomal enzymes, (4) cytostasis of tumor target cells, and (5) reticuloendothelial system uptake of $^{132}$I-triolein. Parameters of bone marrow activity include (1) cellularity, (2) colony-forming units of pluripotent cells, (3) colony-forming units of granulocyte/macrophage progenitors, and (4) iron incorporation in the bone marrow and spleen (Dean et al., 1982).

### *Others*

A variety of pathotoxicological data are also useful indicators of immune function; (1) hematology profile: erythrocyte count, leukocyte count, and differential cell count; (2) serum proteins: albumin, globulin, and albumin/globulin ratio; (3) weights: body, spleen, thymus, and adrenals; and (4) histology: thymus, adrenals, lung, kidneys, heart, spleen, and cellularity of spleen and bone marrow. For example, thymic atrophy appears to be a sensitive indicator of immunotoxicity. A paucity of lymphoid follicles and germinal centers in the spleen is indicative of B-cell deficiency, whereas T-cell deficiency is characterized by lymphoid hypoplasia in the paracortical areas (Dean et al., 1982).

In addition to the immunotoxicity testings used for conventional chemicals, new testing tools are required to better predict the immunotoxic potential of unique types of drugs, such as nanomedicinal products and nucleic acid sequences for designing nontoxic siRNAs and RNA-based vaccine adjuvants (Chaudhary et al., 2016; Giannakou et al., 2016).

## Further reading

Descates J (1999). *An Introduction to Immunotoxicology*. Philadelphia, PA: Taylor & Francis.

WHO. (1996). Principles and methods for assessing direct immunotoxicity associated with exposure to chemicals. Environ Health Criteria 180. Geneva, Switzerland: World Health Organization.

## References

Behan PO, Behan WMH, Zacharias FJ et al. (1976). Immunological abnormalities in patients who had the oculomueocutaneous syndrome associated with practol therapy. *Lancer.* ii, 984–7.

Bondy GS, Pestka JJ (2000). Immunomodulation by fungal toxins. *J Toxicol Environ Health.* B 3, 109–43.

Bradley SG, Morahan PS (1982). Approaches to assessing host resistance. *Environ Health Persp.* 43, 65–71.

Burns LA, Meade BJ, Munson AE (1996). Toxic responses of the immune system. In: Klaassen CD, ed. *Casarett and Doull's Toxicology.* New York: McGraw-Hill, pp. 335–402.

Chaudhary K, Nagpal G, Dhanda SK et al. (2016). Prediction of immunmodulaltory potential of an RNA sequence for designing non-toxic siRNAs and RNA-based vaccine adjuvants. *Sci Rep.* 6, 20678.

Davis NC, Ho M (1976). Quantitation of immunoglobulins. In: Rose NR, Friedman H, eds. *Manual of Clinical Immunology.* Washington, DC: American Society of Microbiology.

Dean JH, Luster MI, Boorman GA et al. (1982). Procedure available to examine the immuno toxicity of chemicals and drugs. *Pharmacol Rev.* 34, 137–48.

Dhouib I, Jallouli M, Annabi A et al. (2016). From immunotoxicity to carcinogenicity: The effects of carbamate pesticides on the immune system. *Environ Sci Pollut Res Int.* 23 (10), 9448–58.

Esser C (2016). The aryl hydrocarbon receptor in immunity: Tools and potential. *Methods Mol Biol.* 1371, 239–57.

Ghare S, Patil M, Hote P et al. (2011). Ethanol inhibits lipid raft-mediated TCR signaling and IL-2 expression: Potential mechanism of alcohol-induced immune suppression. *Alcohol Clin Exp Res.* 35, 1435–44.

Giannakou C, Park MV, de Jong WH et al. (2016). A comparison of immunotoxic effects of nanomedicinal products with regulatory immunotoxicity testing requirements. *Int J Nanomedicine.* 11, 2935–52.

Kreitinger JM, Beamer CA, Shepherd DM (2016). Environmental immunology: Lessons learned from exposure to a select panel of immunotoxicants. *J Immunol.* 196 (8), 3217–225.

Loose LD (1982). Macrophage induction of T-suppressor cells in pesticide exposed and protozoan-infected mice. *Environ Health Persp.* 43, 89–97.

Luster MI, Ackermann MF, Germolec DR et al. (1989). Perturbations of the immune system by xenobiotics. *Environ Health Persp.* 81, 157–62.

Luster MI, Dean JH, Boorman GA (1982). Cell-mediated immunity and its application in toxicology. *Environ Health Persp.* 43, 31–6.

Luebke RW, Chen DH, Dietert R et al. (2006). The comparative immunotoxicity of five selected compounds following developmental or adult exposure. *J Toxicol Environ Health B.* 9, 1–26.

Munson AE, Sanders VM, Douglas KA et al. (1982). In vivo assessment of immunotoxicity. *Environ Health Persp.* 43, 41–52.

Norbury KC (1982). Immunotoxicology in the pharmaceutical industry. *Environ Health Persp.* 43, 53–9.

Park BK, Kiteringham N (1990). Drug–protein conjugation and its immunological consequences. *Drug Metab Rev.* 22, 87–144.

Pohl LR, Satoh H, Christ DD et al. (1988). The immunologic and metabolic basis of drug hypersensitivities. *Annu Rev Pharmacol.* 28, 367–87.

Ruddle NH (1994). Tumor necrosis factor (TNFα) and lymphotoxin (TNFβ). *Curr Opin Immunol.* 4, 327–32.

Sanders VM, Tucker AN, White KL Jr et al. (1982). Humoral and cell-mediated immune status in mice exposed to trichloroethylene in the drinking water. *Toxicol Appl Pharmacol.* 62, 358–68.

Spyker-Cranmer JM, Barnett JB, Avery DL et al. (1982). Immunoteratology of chlor-dane: Cell-mediated and humoral immune responses in adult mice exposed in utero. *Toxicol Appl Pharmacol.* 62, 402–8.

Vos JG, Krajnac EI, Beekhof P (1982). Use of the enzyme-linked immunosorbent assay (ELISA) in immunotoxicity testing. *Environ Health Persp.* 43, 115–21.

Wang G, Ansari GAS, Khan MF (2007). Involvement of lipid peroxidation-derived aldehyde–protein adducts in autoimmunity mediated by trichloroethene. *J Toxicol Environ Health A.* 70, 1977–85.

# *chapter fifteen*

# *Respiratory system toxicology*

***Kyuhong Lee***

*Contents*



## *Introduction*

The respiratory system of humans is increasingly exposed through the inhalation route to airborne toxicants such as cigarette smoke, fine particles, heavy metals, automobile exhaust gases, volatile organic compounds (VOCs), and microorganisms. Inhalation toxicities refer to toxic responses produced in the respiratory tract via exposure to these toxicants. Air pollution episodes that caused human deaths include the Meuse Valley air pollution episode (Belgium in 1930), the Donora episode (Pennsylvania in 1948),

| Structure | Diameter (μm) | Cilia | Cartilage | Goblet cell (mucus) |
|---|---|---|---|---|
| Larynx | 35–45 | +++ | +++ | +++ |
| Trachea | 20–25 | +++ | +++ (C-shaped) | +++ |
| Main bronchi | 12–16 | +++ | +++ (rings) | ++ |
| Lobar bronchi | 10–12 | +++ | +++ (plates) | ++ |
| Segmental bronchi | 8–10 | +++ | +++ (plates) | ++ |
| Small bronchi | 1–8 | +++ | +++ (plates) | + |
| Bronchiole | 0.5–1 | ++ | 0 | + |
| Terminal bronchiole | <0.5 | ++ | 0 | 0 |

***Figure 15.1*** Anatomical diameter and respiratory system.

and the London smog episode (England in 1952). These episodes have provided the basis for present-day regulations to reduce toxic substances from emissions and to improve air quality (ambient, indoor). We now know that pulmonary toxicity is highly dependent upon physicochemical properties (e.g., diameter, size) of particles inhaled into the lungs (Figure 15.1).

# *Respiratory defense system*

## *Structure*

The respiratory tract is a complex system, both in structure and function. It consists of the nasopharynx, the tracheal and bronchial tract, and the pulmonary acini, which are composed of respiratory bronchioles, alveolar ducts, and alveoli (Figure 15.2). The nasopharynx serves to remove large particles from the inhaled air, add moisture, and moderate the temperature. The tracheal and bronchial tract serves as the conducting airway to the alveoli (McClellan and Henderson, 2009).

## *Functions*

The pulmonary acini are the sites where oxygen and carbon dioxide are exchanged between the blood and the air, and are the main sites of absorption of toxicants that exist in the form of gases and vapors. The alveoli are lined with epithelial cells, especially those of type I. These cells have a very thin cytoplasm (0.1–0.2 μm), but each covers a relatively large surface (2290 $\mu m^2$). The cuboidal (63 $\mu m^2$) type II cells can undergo mitosis and, in time, mature to type I cells. In addition, there are endothelial cells, macrophages, and fibroblasts.

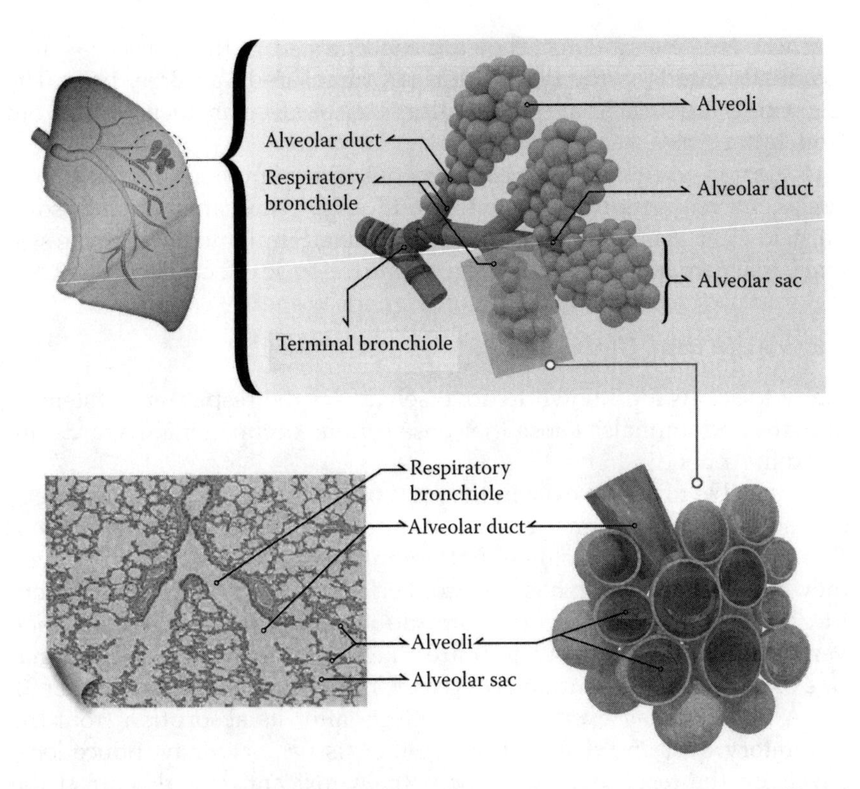


*Figure 15.2* Structure of the lungs: trachea, bronchi, bronchioles, terminal bronchioles, respiratory bronchioles, alveolar duct, and alveoli.

Apart from its vital function in the exchange of oxygen and carbon dioxide, the respiratory system also regulates the blood concentrations of angiotensins, biogenic amines, and prostaglandins. Furthermore, it can excrete toxicants that have been absorbed from the lungs or via other routes. Although the liver is the primary site of blood detoxification, pulmonary tissue possesses cytochrome P-450 (CYP-450) enzymes involved in xenobiotic detoxication.

## Defense mechanisms

The trachea and bronchi are lined with ciliated epithelium and covered with a thin layer of mucus secreted by certain cells in the epithelial lining. This lining, with the cilia and mucus, can move particles deposited on the surface up to the mouth. The particle-containing mucus can then be eliminated from the respiratory tract by spitting or swallowing.

The respiratory tract has various CYP-450 enzyme systems, which may detoxify certain toxicants. However, many toxicants may be activated by these enzyme systems. They are concentrated in the Clara cells and, to a lesser extent, in the type II cells (Dormans and Van Bree, 1995). The Clara cells are located at the boundary where alveolar ducts branch out from bronchioles.

Apart from clearance and detoxication, the respiratory tract also possesses mechanisms to phagocytize and engulf toxicants, notably solid particles. The main effector is the macrophage. Similar to the enzyme systems, the macrophage may also aggravate the toxic effects (Brain, 1992).

## *Toxicants and their effects*

Many toxicants are known to adversely affect the respiratory system in humans and animals. Those that pose serious occupational hazards are listed in Appendix 15.1.

Inhalable toxicants exist in the form of gases, vapors, liquid droplets, and solid particulate matters. Gases and vapors are readily absorbed. The droplets and particulate matters may also be absorbed, however, they vary in size, which has a marked effect on the extent of absorption. In general, large particles (>10 μm) do not enter the respiratory tract. Very small particles (<0.01 μm) are likely to be exhaled. The optimal size of particle for retention is between 1 and 3 μm (see also Chapter 2).

A toxicant may exert systemic effects after its absorption from the respiratory tract and distribution to other tissues or it may induce local effects on the respiratory tract, or both. A toxicant may also affect the respiratory tract after exposure from other routes.

### *Systemic effects*

Many chemicals can be absorbed from the inspired air. After absorption, they are carried by the circulating blood to various parts of the body and exert their effects, such as in a general anesthesia.

Toxic gases can be absorbed from various parts of the respiratory tract including the nasopharynx. The main site of absorption, however, is the alveoli, and the principal mechanism of absorption is simple diffusion. In addition, liquid aerosols and solid particulate matter can also be absorbed via different mechanisms. Further details regarding the uptake of toxicants are provided in Chapter 2.

### *Pulmonary effects*

A variety of pulmonary effects have been observed. These are briefly described under five categories. Additional details and references have been provided by Gordon and Amdur (1994).

### *Local irritation*

Ammonia and chlorine are classic examples of irritant gases. They produce bronchial constriction and edema, which result in dyspnea, but chronic effects are rare. Arsenicals induce irritation on acute exposure; after prolonged exposure they might induce development of lung cancer. Similarly, chronic exposure to cigarette smoke results in irritation in lung airways and ultimately in lung cancer. Residing in highly industrialized cities or in the vicinity of traffic has been shown to produce lung dysfunction and subsequently development of diseases such as asthma due to ambient particulate matter or diesel exhaust particles. Dust generated during storms was reported to produce lung irritation and leads to an increase in the frequency of respiratory distress cases.

### *Cellular damage and edema*

Toxic *gases*, such as ozone and oxides of nitrogen, produce cellular damage, perhaps through generation of reactive oxygen species and reactive nitrogen species followed by peroxidation of cellular membranes. Edema ensues as a result of the increased permeability through the damaged membrane. The edematous fluid, however, accumulates in the airway instead of in the interstitial space, as is the case with other tissues. Such effects are also observed after inhalation of toxicants that exist in small particles, such as diesel exhaust, nickel carbonyl, and certain beryllium and boron compounds.

Cellular damage usually affects type I cells in the alveoli. Death of these cells leads to proliferation of type II cells, which then flatten and become type I cells. However, more extensive damage will result in the exudation of fibrin-rich protein, neutrophils, and debris into the alveoli. These eventually become fibrous tissue. Asbestos fibers are known to produce fibrotic reactions and mesothelioma.

Certain organic *solvents*, such as perchloroethylene and xylene, are rapidly absorbed after inhalation and distributed to various parts of the body including the liver, which is the major site of biotransformation. Part of the solvent reenters the lungs through circulation and may form reactive metabolites, leading to covalent binding to macromolecules there. This process, in turn, produces pulmonary cellular damage and edema. It is also noteworthy that the lungs serve as a conduit for chemicals into the circulation followed by activation in other tissues and development of diseases in different organs. An example is benzene that enters via the lungs and forms reactive intermediates in the liver, which subsequently react with bone macromolecules, resulting in leukemia.

*Ipomeanol* is a toxin produced by the mold *Fusarium solani*, which grows on sweet potatoes. This toxin is interesting in that it produces necrosis of one type of cell only, namely, the Clara cells. These cells bioactivate the toxin to a reactive metabolite, which binds to the macromolecules and produces cellular necrosis. This is followed by edema, congestion, and hemorrhage in the lungs. Death may ensue (Timbrell, 1991).

Glucans are polyglucose compounds, which are constituents of fungi and bacteria that produce inflammatory lung diseases characterized by hypersensitivity and pneumonitis (Schuyler et al., 1998). Monocrotaline, a pyrrolizidine alkaloid, was reported to produce lung injury and pulmonary hypertension. In fact, monocrotaline is used as a model to study causes of pulmonary hypertension in humans (Schultze and Roth, 1998).

*Fibrosis (Pneumoconiosis)*

Pulmonary fibrosis is a serious, debilitating lung disease that results from the inhalation of "inorganic dust." *Silicosis*, with a history that goes back to thousands of years, is produced by crystalline forms of silica (silicon dioxide). Of the crystalline forms, quartz is the most stable. On heating, such as in volcanic eruption and mining, quartz may become tridymite or cristobalite. Both of these forms are more fibrogenic than quartz. The toxic effect stems from the rupture of the lysosomal membrane in a macrophage. The released lysosomal enzymes digest the macrophage and this process, in turn, releases the silica from the lysed macrophage in a continuous process. It was suggested that the damaged macrophage releases factors that stimulate the fibroblasts and the formation of collagen (Brain, 1980). Other cells, such as fibroblasts and epithelial cells, in response to macrophage inflammatory proteins, may also play a role in the fibrotic changes (Driscoll et al., 1993). Kuhn et al. (1995) suggest that cytokine is involved in the fibrosis and its increase precedes deterioration of pulmonary function, hence may serve as a biomarker for initiating intervention in exposed workers.

Another major cause of pulmonary fibrosis is *asbestos*. Asbestos refers to a large number of fibrous hydrated silicates of magnesium, calcium, and others. In addition, some of these mineral fibers, such as blue asbestos (crocidolites), produce bronchogenic carcinoma and mesothelioma. The white variety (chrysotile) appears to have no effect on the incidence of mesothelioma. The potency of asbestos seems related to its chemical and physical properties. Fibers measuring 5 μm in length and 0.3 μm in diameter appear to be most potent. Various types of man-made refractory ceramic fibers have been used in the place of asbestos. In the rat, they also induce fibrosis and carcinoma, but appear to be less carcinogenic than asbestos (Mast et al., 1995). However, the incidence of carcinoma is markedly increased in smokers exposed to asbestos indicating that the presence of asbestos creates a more susceptible individual to lung cancer development.

Other fibrogenic substances include coal dust, kaolin, talc, aluminum, beryllium, and carbides of tungsten, titanium, and tantalum (Appendix 15.1).

Coal worker's pneumoconiosis (also known as black lung disease) is produced by long exposure to coal dust, graphite, or man-made carbon.

*Emphysema* is also a debilitating disease. It may be induced by cigarette smoking or exposure to aluminum, cadmium oxide, or oxides of nitrogen, ozone, and others. It was suggested that the elastic fibers surrounding and supporting the alveoli and bronchi may be damaged by the elastase released from polymorphonuclear granulocytes under certain conditions (Spitznagel et al., 1980).

#### *Allergic response*

This type of response is usually induced by pollens, spores of molds, bacterial contaminants, cotton dust, cement dust, and so on. Detergents containing enzymes derived from *Bacillus subtilis* were reported to produce asthma among workers. A common chemical used in the plastic industry, toluene diisocyanate, as other isocyanates, also produces hypersensitivity reactions. It is probable that this reactive chemical binds to proteins in the blood or lungs to form antigens, which stimulate antibody formation. The major response is bronchoconstriction triggered by the reaction between the antigens and circulating or fixed antibodies (Karol and Jin, 1991). Long-term exposure may result in other pulmonary effects such as chronic bronchitis and fibrosis.

#### *Lung cancer*

Cigarette smoke contains a number of carcinogens, co-carcinogens, and irritants (Hoffmann and Hoffmann, 1997). These substances initiate and promote carcinogenesis. Furthermore, many other substances may induce oxidative stress, thereby adversely affecting health (Appendix 15.2). Some details on this topic have been outlined by Halliwell and Cross (1994). It is well established that cigarette smoking is the leading cause of lung cancer in many countries and that it greatly increases the incidence of lung cancers among asbestos workers (Chapter 5). Other causes of lung cancer include arsenic, chromate, nickel, uranium, and coke oven emissions.

Asbestos has been well known for its carcinogenicity in the respiratory tract in humans and animals. Man-made refractory ceramic fibers also appear to be carcinogenic, but only at maximum tolerated doses. Much investigation is in progress to determine their health hazards, if any, in humans. One important approach is to assess their persistence, which is a determinant of their toxicity (Bignon et al., 1994).

## *Effects on upper respiratory tract*

Large airborne particles in the inhaled air are mainly deposited in the nasal passages. They may produce hyperemia, squamous- or transitional-cell metaplasia, hyperplasia, ulceration, and, in certain cases, carcinoma.

For example, nickel sub-sulfide, nickel oxide, and nickel usually exist in large particles during their production and mining; therefore, their effects are mainly on the nasal passage (NAS, 1975). Inhalation of diesel exhaust particles was found to produce immediate nasal hyperresponsiveness, antioxidant responses, marked epithelial inflammation, and specific humoral responses (Nikasinovic et al., 2004). The larynx is also a site of chemical carcinogenesis, for example, with asbestos and chromium (Salem and Katz, 1998). Inhalation of gases and vapors such as sulfur dioxide and toluene may produce irritation of the trachea and bronchi. Other toxic effects include deciliation, goblet-cell hyperplasia, and squamous metaplasia.

## *Effects of exposure from routes other than inhalation*

*Paraquat*, a herbicide, produces lung damage not only after exposure by inhalation but also after ingestion (Clark et al., 1966). Its storage in the lungs and its inherent toxicity are apparently the reasons for its pulmonary effects after noninhalation routes. It is of interest that ingestion of paraquat was used as a means of suicide. The mechanism of paraquat toxicity is the generation of reactive oxygen species, which is dependent on the mitochondrial inner transmembrane potential (Castello et al., 2007). In contrast, a closely related herbicide, diquat, although also toxic to cultured lung cells, is not toxic to the lungs either after inhalation or after ingestion, and interestingly is not retained by the lungs.

A number of drugs are known to induce pulmonary fibrosis in humans. These include bleomycin, busulfan, cyclophosphamide, gold salts, melphalan, methotrexate, BCNU, chlorambucil, and mitomycin. In these cases, there is an increase in interstitial collagen and in the number of type II cells. Methotrexate and streptomycin were found to induce pulmonary eosinophilia. Phenylbutazone, oxyphenylbutazone, aspirin, retinoic acid, and sulfonamides may produce pulmonary edema.

In addition, a number of amphiphilic drugs, such as chlorphentermine, chloroquine, amiodarone, and triparanol, are known to interact with the phospholipids in certain cells to form myeloid bodies and pulmonary foam cells in humans and animals. These bodies and cells were suggested to lead to alterations in cell activities and later to impairment of respiratory functions (Hruban, 1984). However, there is no evidence that drug-induced pulmonary phospholipidosis results in any functional changes in lung activity. It would seem that this is a morphological alteration, but not a functional disturbance, and can be considered adaptive. This adaptive change disappears upon drug cessation and pulmonary function remains normal.

## *Outbreak of pulmonary fibrosis by humidifier disinfectants*

Recently, there was a case report in South Korea that the use of biocide products to sterilize humidifiers injured and in some cases caused death in humans (KCDC, 2011). PHMG-phosphate (polyhexamethylene guanidine phosphate) and PGH (oligo(2-(2-ethoxy)ethoxyethyl guanidine chloride) formed aerosols of approximately 100 nanometer in size through humidifiers, and several months of exposure to these compounds resulted in serious lung injury, presenting clinical features such as pulmonary inflammation and fibrosis (Hong et al., 2014; Kim et al., 2014). Inhalation toxicity studies using animals and cells showed that exposure to PHMG-phosphate produced lung damage, as evidenced by inflammation and fibrosis reported in human patients (Park et al., 2014; Song et al., 2014; Kim et al., 2015, 2016; Lee et al., 2016). Currently, the toxicological mechanisms underlying pulmonary injury remain to be elucidated.

*Appendix 15.1 Site of action and pulmonary disease produced by selected occupationally inhaled toxicants*

| Toxicant | Common name of the disease | Acute effect | Chronic effect |
|---|---|---|---|
| Aluminum dust | Aluminosis | Cough, shortness of breath | Interstitial fibrosis |
| Aluminum abrasives | Shaver's disease, corundum smelter's lung, bauxite lung | Alveolar edema | Fibrotic thickening of alveolar walls, interstitial fibrosis, emphysema |
| Ammonia | | Immediate upper and lower respiratory tract irritation, edema | Chronic bronchitis |
| Arsenic | | Bronchitis | Lung cancer, bronchitis, laryngitis |
| Asbestos | Asbestosis | | Pulmonary fibrosis, pleural calcification, lung cancer, pleural mesothelioma |
| Beryllium | Berylliosis | Edema, pneumonia | Pulmonary fibrosis, progressive dyspnea, interstitial granulomatosis, cor pulmonale |
| Cadmium oxide | | Cough, pneumonia | Emphysema, cor pulmonale |
| Carbides of tungsten, titanium, tantalum | Hard metal disease | Hyperplasia and metaplasia of bronchial epithelium | Fibrosis, peribronchial, and perivascular fibrosis |

(*Continued*)

| Toxicant | Common name of the disease | Acute effect | Chronic effect |
|---|---|---|---|
| Chlorine | | Cough, hemoptysis, dyspnea, tracheobronchitis, bronchopneumonia | |
| Chromium (VI) | | Nasal irritation, bronchitis | Lung tumors and cancers |
| Coal dust | Pneumoconiosis (coal workers pneumoconiosis, anthracosis) | | Pulmonary fibrosis |
| Coke oven emissions | | | Tracheobronchial cancers |
| Cotton dust | Byssinosis | Tightness in chest, wheezing, dyspnea | Reduced pulmonary function, chronic bronchitis |
| Hydrogen fluoride | | Respiratory irritation, hemorrhagic pulmonary edema | |
| Iron oxides | Siderotic lung disease<br>Silver finisher's lung | Cough | Subpleural and perivascular aggregations of macrophages |
| | Hematite miner's lung | | Diffuse fibrosis-like pneumoconiosis |
| | Welder's lung | | Bronchitis |
| Isocyanates | | Cough, dyspnea | Asthma, reduced pulmonary function |
| Kaolin | Kaolinosis | | Pulmonary fibrosis |
| Nickel | | Pulmonary edema, delayed by 2 days (NiCO) | Squamous-cell carcinoma of nasal cavity and lungs |

*(Continued)*

| Toxicant | Common name of the disease | Acute effect | Chronic effect |
|---|---|---|---|
| Oxides of nitrogen | | Pulmonary congestion and edema | Emphysema |
| Ozone | | Pulmonary edema | Emphysema |
| Phosgene | | Edema | Bronchitis |
| Perchloroethylene | | Pulmonary edema | |
| Silica | Silicosis, pneumoconiosis | | Pulmonary fibrosis |
| Sulfur dioxide | | Bronchoconstriction, cough, tightness in chest | |
| Talc | Talcosis | | Pulmonary fibrosis |
| Tin | Stenosis | | Widespread mottling of x-ray without clinical signs |
| Vanadium | | Upper airway irritation and mucus production | Chronic bronchitis |

## Appendix 15.2 Mechanisms underlying the oxidative stress induced by cigarette smoke

1. Smoke contains many free radicals, especially peroxyl radicals that might attack biological molecules and deplete antioxidants, such as vitamin C and a-tocopherol.
2. Smoke contains oxides of nitrogen, including the unpleasant nitrogen dioxide ($NO_2$–).
3. The tar phase of smoke contains hydroquinones. These are lipid soluble and can redox cycle to form $O_2$– and $H_2O_2$. They can enter cells and may even reach the nucleus to cause oxidative DNA damage. Some hydroquinones may release iron from the iron-storage protein ferritin in lung cells and respiratory tract lining fluids.
4. Smoking may irritate lung macrophages, activating them to make $O_2$–.[a]
5. Smokers' lungs contain more neutrophils than the lungs of nonsmokers, and smoke might activate these cells to make $O_2$–.[a]
6. Smokers often eat poorly and drink more alcohol than nonsmokers and have a low intake of nutrient antioxidants.
7. Cigarette smoke contains large amounts of fine nanoparticles <50 nm, which generate reactive oxygen species.

[a] Superoxide anion.

## References

Bignon J, Saracci R, Touray JC (1994). Biopersistence of respirable synthetic fibers and minerals. *Environ Health Persp.* 102(Suppl 5), 3–5.

Brain JD (1980). Macrophage damage in relation to the pathogenesis of lung diseases. *Environ Health Persp.* 35, 21–8.

Brain JD (1992). Mechanisms, measurement and significance of lung macrophage function. *Environ Health Persp.* 97, 5–10.

Castello PR, Drechsel DA, Patel M (2007). Mitochondria are a major source of paraquatinduced reactive oxygen species production in the brain. *J Biol Chem.* 282, 14186–93.

Clark DG, McElligott TF, Hurst EW (1966). The toxicity of paraquat. *Br J Ind Med.* 23, 126–32.

Dormans JAMA, Van Bree L (1995). Function and response of type II cells to inhaled toxicants. *Inhal Toxicol.* 7, 319–42.

Driscoll KE, Hassenbein DG, Carter J et al. (1993). Macrophage inflammatory proteins 1 and 2: Expression by rat alveolar macrophages, fibroblasts, and epithelial cells and in rat lung after minimal dust exposure. *Am J Respir Cell Mol Biol.* 8, 311–8.

Gordon T, Amdur MO (1994). Responses of the respiratory system to toxic agents. In: Amdur MO, Doull J, Klaassen CD, eds. *Casarett and Doull's Toxicology: The Basic Science of Poisons,* 4th edn. New York, McGraw-Hill, 443–62.

Halliwell B, Cross CE (1994). Oxygen-derived species: Their relation to human disease and environmental stress. *Environ Health Persp.* 102(Suppl 10), 5–12.

Hoffmann D, Hoffmann I (1997). The changing cigarette, 1950–1995. *J Toxicol Environ Health.* 50, 307–64.

Hong SB, Kim HJ, Huh JW, Do KH, Jang SJ Song JS, Choi SJ et al. (2014). A cluster of lung injury associated with home humidifier use: Clinical, radiological and pathological description of a new syndrome. *Thorax.* 69(8), 694–702.

Hruban Z (1984). Pulmonary and generalized lysosomal storage induced by amphiphilic drugs. *Environ Health Persp.* 55, 53–76.

Karol MH, Jin R (1991). Mechanism of immunotoxicity to isocyanates. *Chem Res Toxicol.* 4, 503–9.

Kim HJ, Lee MS, Hong SB et al. (2014). Cluster of lung injury cases associated with home humidifier use an epidemiological investigation. *Thorax.* 69(8), 703–8.

Kim HR, Shin DY, Chung KH (2015). The role of NF-kB signaling pathway in polyhexamethylene guanidine phosphate induced inflammatory response in mouse macrophage RAW264.7 cells. *Tox Lett.* 233, 148–55.

Kim HR, Lee KH, Park CW et al. (2016). Polyhexamethylene guanidine phosphate aerosol particles induce pulmonary inflammatory and fibrotic responses. *Arch. Toxicol.* 90 (3), 617–32.

Kim KW, Ahn K, Yang HJ et al. (2014). Humidifier disinfectant-associated children's interstitial lung disease. *Am J Respir Crit Care Med.* 189(1), 48–56.

KCDC (Korea Centers for Disease Control and Prevention). (2011). In-depth investigation on the cases of lung injury with unknown cause. *Public Health Wkly.* 4 (45), 829–32.

Kuhn DC, Stauffer JL, Gaydos LJ et al. (1995). Inflammatory and fibrotic mediator release by alveoli macrophages from coal miners. *J Toxicol Environ Health.* 45, 9–21.

Lee SJ, Park JH, Lee JY et al. (2016). Establishment of a mouse model for pulmonary inflammation and fibrosis by intratracheal instillation of polyhexamethyleneguanidine phosphate. *J Toxicol Pathol.* 29(2), 95–102.

Mast RW, McConnell EE, Anderson R et al. (1995). Studies on the chronic toxicity (inhalation) of four types of refractory ceramic fiber in male Fischer 344 rats. *Inhal Toxicol.* 7, 425–67.

McClellan RO, Henderson RF (2009). *Concepts in Inhalation Toxicology*, 2nd ed. New York,: Informa Healthcare.

National Academy of Sciences (NAS) (1975). *Nickel.* Washington, DC: National Academy of Sciences.

Nikasinovic L, Momas I, Just J (2004). A review of experimental studies on diesel exhaust particles and nasal epithelium alterations. *J Toxicol Environ Health B.* 7(2), 81–104.

Park S, Lee K, Lee EJ et al. (2014). Humidifier disinfectant-associated interstitial lung disease in an animal model induced by polyhexamethylene guanidine aerosol. *Am J Respir Crit Care Med.* 190(6), 706–8.

Salem H, Katz SA (1998). *Inhalation Toxicology*, 2nd ed. Boca Raton, FL: Taylor & Francis.

Schultze AE, Roth RA (1998). Chronic pulmonary hypertension—The monocrotaline model and involvement of the hemostatic system. *J Toxicol Environ Health B.* 1, 271–346.

Schuyler M, Gott K, Cherne A (1998). Effect of glucan on murine lungs. *J Toxicol Environ Health A*. 53, 493–505.
Song JA, Park HJ, Yang MJ et al. (2014). Polyhexamethyleneguanidine phosphate induces severe lung inflammation, fibrosis, and thymic atrophy. *Food Chem. Toxicol*. 69, 267–75.
Spitznagel JK, Moderzakowski MC, Pryzwansky KB et al. (1980). Neutral proteases of human polymorphonuclear granulocytes: Putative mediators of pulmonary damage. *Environ Health Persp*. 35, 29–38.
Timbrell JA (1991). *Principles of Biochemical Toxicology*. London: Taylor & Francis.

# chapter sixteen

# Toxicology of the skin

**Ok-Nam Bae**

Contents



## General considerations

The human body, as well as that of other animals, is almost entirely covered by skin. As a result, it is exposed to a variety of chemicals such as ingredients in cosmetics, household products, topical medications, and environmental contaminants including heavy metals and industrial pollutants, especially in certain workplaces. Dermal exposure to chemicals might result in various types of lesions. Ultraviolet (UV) irradiation is also one of the common stimuli which directly induce skin damage, and chemicals exposed to skin can be photoactivated by UV irradiation leading to chemical-phototoxicity. Further, skin lesions may occur following systemic exposure to chemicals and subsequent distribution of chemicals via dermal microcirculation.

The skin consists of the epidermis and dermis, which rests over the subcutaneous tissue (Figure 16.1). The epidermis is relatively thin, averaging 0.1–0.2 mm in thickness, whereas the dermis is approximately 2 mm thick. These two layers are separated by a basement membrane.

The living layer of epidermis consists of a basal cell layer (stratum germinativum), which provides the other layers with new cells. These new cells become prickle cells (stratum spinosum) and later, the granular cells (stratum granulosum) whose nuclei disintegrate and dissolve. In addition, these cells produce keratohydrin, which subsequently becomes keratin in the outermost stratum corneum, the horny layer which is gradually shed. This development process takes about 4 weeks. The epidermis also contains melanocytes, which produce pigments; Langerhans cells, which act as macrophages; and lymphocytes. The latter two types of cells are involved in immune responses. The epidermis thus forms an important protective cover for the body.

The dermis is mainly composed of collagen and elastin, which are important components for the support of the skin. This layer consists of several types of cells, the most abundant being the fibroblasts, which are involved in the biosynthesis of the fibrous proteins and ground substances

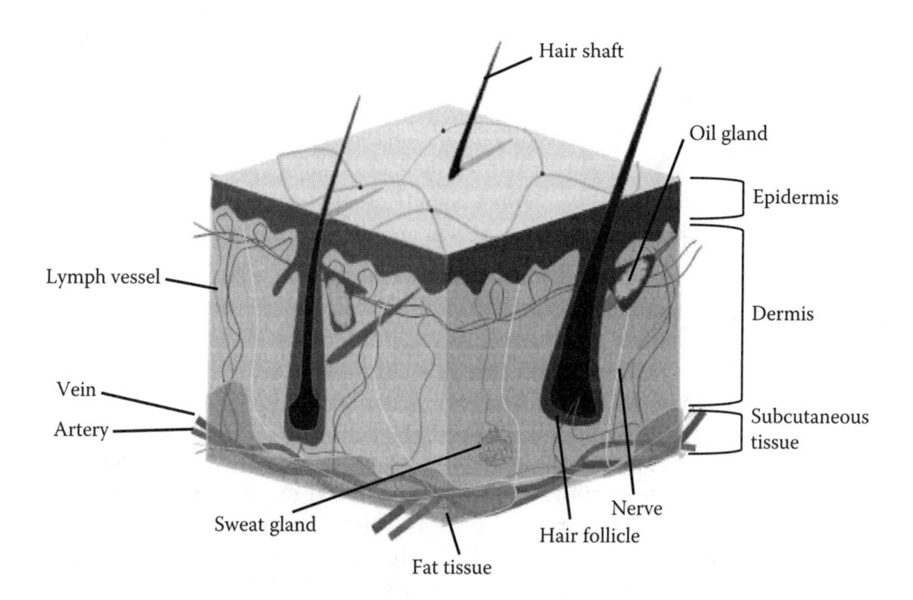


*Figure 16.1* Skin structure. Cross section of the skin showing the two major layers of the epidermis and dermis, and the various structures in the dermis.

such as hyaluronic acid, chondroitin sulfates, and mucopolysaccharides. The other types of cells include fat cells, macrophages, histiocytes, and mast cells. Beneath the dermis lies the subcutaneous tissue.

There are, in addition, a number of other structures, such as hair follicles, sweat glands (the exocrine glands), sebaceous glands, small blood vessels, and neural elements.

The possibility of systemic toxicity following dermal exposure to toxicants is discussed in Chapter 2. In addition, dermal reactions may appear following systemic administration of toxicants. Various types of toxicity attributed to pesticides, industrial chemicals, heavy metals, and industrial chemicals from dermal exposure are discussed in Chapters regarding these chemicals.

## Types of toxic effects and dermatotoxicants

A variety of effects result from dermal exposures to toxicants. Most of the effects involve the skin itself, but some of them affect its appendages including hair, sebaceous glands, and sweat glands.

### Primary irritation

Irritation is a reaction of the skin to chemicals such as strong alkalis, acids, solvents, and detergents. Irritation ranges in severity from hyperemia, edema, and vesiculation to ulceration (corrosion). Primary irritations occur at the site of contact and, in general, on the first contact. Irritation is thus different from sensitization.

### Sensitization reaction

The skin may show little or no reaction on the first contact with a chemical. However, a reaction or a more severe reaction occurs after a subsequent exposure to the chemical. The induction period ranges from a few days to years. A subsequent exposure to the specific toxicant elicits a reaction after a delay of 12–48 hours. It is therefore known as "delayed type IV hypersensitivity." A complex immune mechanism is involved in this reaction. Briefly, the toxicant, upon entering the skin, becomes bonded to the surface of certain cells (the antigen presenting cells), which process it for reaction with T lymphocytes. After such reaction, sensitized T lymphocytes may release a variety of substances upon re-exposure to the same toxicant and result in hyperemia and edema.

Interestingly, the skin sensitization reaction has recently been explained as a representative toxicity model of Adverse Outcome Pathway (AOP). AOP, a pathway-based toxicological concept that provides a framework for organizing knowledge regarding the progression of toxicity events, has attracted significant attention as a paradigm shift for chemical safety from descriptive to mechanism-based and predictive toxicology (Ankley et al., 2010; Groh and Tollefsen, 2015). AOP encompasses all processes of a complicated toxicity from a molecular initiating event (MIE), which indicates a direct interaction of chemical with its biological target molecule, to subsequent responses at cellular, tissue, organ and individual level. Molecular initiating events provide a foundation for alternative approaches to assess or predict potential hazards, ultimately contributing to regulatory applications (Perkins et al., 2010). Defining key events (KEs) and their relationship (KER) may be very important steps to understand the orchestrated adverse outcome in this pathway-based approach.

In an attempt to apply the AOP concept to regulatory toxicity testing and assessment, the OECD published a document where the state of knowledge of AOP for skin sensitization has been well described (2012; Figure 16.2). Four KE in skin sensitization are used to explain the coordination between keratinocytes, dendritic cells, and T cells (Leist et al., 2014). Skin sensitization is a complicated biological process where diverse cell types orchestrate the final toxicity following exposure to chemicals,

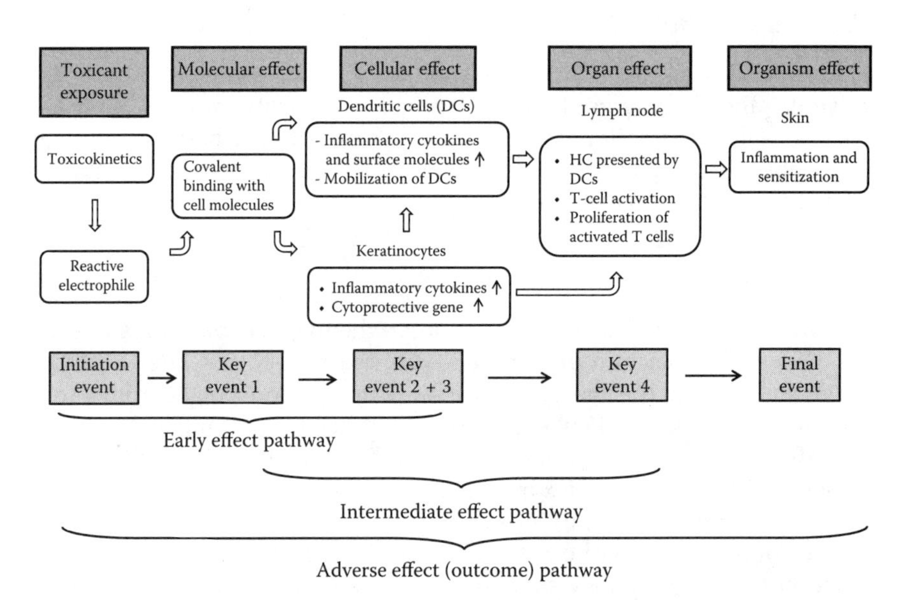


*Figure 16.2* Skin sensitization adverse outcome pathway (AOP). Skin sensitization is a toxicological event resulting from complicated relationship between KEs in keratinocytes, dendritic cells, and T cells in skin tissue. Histocompatibility complexes (HC). (Modified from Leist et al., *ALTEX*, 31, 341–356, 2014.)

**Table 16.1** Selected dermal sensitizers

| | |
|---|---|
| Antibiotics | Neomycin |
| Hair dye ingredient | *p*-Phenylenediamine |
| Local anesthetics | Benzocaine |
| Metals | Nickel and nickel salts, beryllium, chromium salts, organomercurials (thimerosal) |
| Pesticides | Captan, ethylenediamine |
| Poisonous plants | Poison ivy, poison oak |

and the representative approach of skin sensitization AOP is currently providing an important toxicological insight into understanding of pathway-based toxicity and development of future toxicity testing methods to evaluate or predict chemical toxicity.

A variety of chemicals, including topical medications, induce sensitization reactions. Table 16.1 lists a number of them. The chemicals produce a positive response in human patch test with a frequency of 5–11% (Nethercott et al., 1994).

Toluene diisocyanate (TDI), is an allergenic agent, producing asthma and other effects in the respiratory tract. In addition, it may induce skin sensitization after inhalation (Ebino et al., 2001). TDI is used in the pharmaceutical industry for development of anti-asthmatic medications.

## *Phototoxicity and photoallergy*

These two types of skin reaction are similar in that both are light (i.e., UV irradiation) -induced and may follow either systemic administration or topical application of the offending chemical. However, photoallergy involves immune reactions, whereas *phototoxicity* does not. This and other differences are summarized in Table 16.2. The term *photoirritation* is often used to refer to phototoxicity (Thong and Maibach, 2008), however, here the term *phototoxicity* is used to represent chemical-induced nonimmunologic toxicity following photo-activation of the chemical.

Phototoxicity is more common than photoallergy. The most commonly reported phototoxic chemicals in humans, according to Harber et al. (1987), are aminobenzoic acid derivatives, anthraquinone dyes, chlorpromazine, chlorothiazides, phenothiazines, sulfanilamide, and coal tar derivatives (e.g., anthracene, pyridine, acridine, and phenanthrene). Two different mechanisms are known to initiate phototoxicity. One is photodynamic reaction as seen in cases of most of the drugs or coal tar derivatives, and this reaction requires oxygen as exemplified in photodynamic therapy (PDT)

*Table 16.2* Comparison of phototoxic and photoallergic reactions

| Reaction | Phototoxic | Photoallergic |
|---|---|---|
| Reaction possible on first exposure | Yes | No |
| Incubation period necessary after first exposure | No | Yes |
| Chemical alteration of photosensitizer | No | Yes |
| Covalent binding with carrier | No | Yes |
| Clinical changes | Usually like sunburn; Erythema, edema, vesicles, and bullae | Varied morphology; Eczematous lesions, and pruritic |
| Flares at distant previously involved sites possible | No | Yes |
| Persistent light reactions can develop | No | Yes |
| Crossreactions to structurally related agents | Infrequent | Frequent |
| Concentration of drug necessary for reaction | High | Low |
| Incidence | Usually relatively high | Usually very low |
| Action spectrum | Usually similar to absorption | Usually higher wavelength than absorption |
| Passive transfer | No | Possible |
| Lymphocyte stimulation test | No | Possible |
| Macrophage migration inhibition test | No | Possible |
| Diagnosis | | |
| Topical agent | Clinical | Photopatch tests |
| Systemic agent | Clinical + phototests | Clinical + phototests; possibly photopatch tests |

*Source:* Harber LC, Baer RL, *J Invest Dermatol.*, 58, 327–342, 1972; Thong HY, Maibach HI, *Dermal Absorption and Toxicity Assessment*, Boca Raton, FL: Taylor & Francis, 2008.

in treatment of certain types of cancer and acne (Sakamoto et al., 2010; Agostinis et al., 2011). The other mechanism is nonphotodynamic which does not require oxygen, and this is the main mechanism for phototoxicity of psoralens (Thong and Maibach, 2008). A phototoxic skin reaction

***Table 16.3*** Examples of phototoxic photoallergic chemicals

| Chemicals | Phototoxicity | Photoallergy |
|---|---|---|
| Aminobenzoic acid derivatives | + | + |
| Chlorpromazine | + | + |
| Chlorothiazide | + | + |
| Methoxy psoralens | + | – |
| Psoralens | + | – |
| Sulfonamides | + | + |
| Tetracyclines | + | – |
| Coal tar derivatives | + | – |
| Nonsteroidal anti-inflammatory drugs | + | – |

consists of a delayed erythema, followed by hyperpigmentation and desquamation.

The most commonly reported photoallergic chemicals include aminobenzoic acids, chlorpromazine, chlorpropamide, 2,2-thiobis(4-chlorophenol) (Fentichlor), halogenated salicylanilides, promethazine, sulfanilamide, and thiazides (Harber et al., 1987) (Table 16.3). Many compounds are, therefore, both phototoxic and photoallergic. Clinically, photoallergy usually manifests as delayed papules and eczema, but it may also appear as immediate urticarial reaction. Histologically, it is characterized by a dense perivascular round cell infiltrate in the dermis. The delayed reactions are Type IV T-cell-mediated immune response, whereas the immediate reaction is probably antibody mediated.

The most biologically active rays that produce erythema and pigmentation are in the shorter ultraviolet range, that is, wavelengths below 320 nm. The sunlight ranges from 290 nm upward, but the UV rays emitted by artificial light sources may be shorter. However, the longer UV rays (UVA; 320–400 nm) per se are less erythrogenic, but are responsible for both phototoxic and photoallergic reactions to chemicals (see the section "Testing Procedures for Skin Toxicities"). While UVA may reach capillary blood in dermis, UVB (290–320 nm) mostly acts on epidermis due to its limited penetration. Therefore, UVA is considered to be important to activate topically or systemically exposed chemicals, and UVB irradiation is considered to be relevant for topically applied chemicals (ICHEWG, 2013).

## *Contact urticaria/urticarial reactions*

These skin reactions, in the form of urticaria or eczema, appear within minutes to an hour after contact with the offending substance. Hence, these are different from the sensitization reaction described above.

The mechanism may be nonimmunological, such as the case with aspirin and methyl nicotinate. In other cases, for example, latex rubber and penicillin, an immunologic mechanism, is involved. However, unlike the sensitization reaction described earlier, an antibody (IgE), rather than T cell is involved. In both immunological and nonimmunological cases, vasoactive substances elicit dermal reactions, for example, histamine along with prostaglandins, leukotrienes, and kinins. A great variety of substances have been reported to induce these reactions, including metals (copper and platinum), medications (antibiotics and local anesthetics), and biogenic polymers released from arthropods (jellyfish). Amin et al. (1995) provided extensive lists of agents that induce immunological and nonimmunological immediate contact reactions. Urticarial actions may also follow ingested or parenterally administered agents.

## *Cutaneous cancer*

It has been known for over two centuries that soot produces skin cancer. More recent studies confirm that soot and related substances, such as coal tars, creosote oils, shale oils, and cutting oil, induce cancers of the skin and other sites in animals and humans. In addition, arsenic and certain arsenic compounds have been reported to be associated with skin cancer in humans.

A number of polycyclic aromatic hydrocarbons (e.g., benzo[*a*]pyrene) and heterocyclic compounds (e.g., benz[*c*]acridine) are known to induce skin cancer after topical applications on animals (IARC, 1973). UV radiation is an important cause of skin cancer in humans, and a number of chemicals influence the effect of UV light and vice versa (Forbes, 1995; Brozyna and Chwirot, 2006). Other risk factors for skin cancer include chronic wounds, inflammation, irritation, acute trauma, and a history of sunburns early in life (Kasper et al., 2011).

## *Effects on epidermal adnexa*

### *Hair*

Loss of hair may result from various antimitotic agents used in cancer chemotherapy. These agents affect the anagen phase of hair growth. The affected hair starts to shed after about 2 weeks of therapy, but hair growth resumes about 2 months after the suspension of therapy.

A number of other medications are known to cause hair loss by converting hair follicles in the anagen phase to telogen phase. In such cases, hair shedding generally starts 24 months after therapy. The medications involved in this type of hair loss include oral contraceptives, anticoagulants, propranolol, and triparanol.

*Sebaceous glands*

These glands secrete lipid through expulsion of their lipid-laden cells and are therefore known as *holocrine*. Their activity is hormone dependent. For example, androgens stimulate and estrogens inhibit excretion. Adrenocortical steroids and thyroid hormones also have some stimulatory activity. Acne may be formed as a result of proliferation of the follicular epithelium of the sebaceous gland. Topically applied substances such as greases and oils, and systemically administered substances such as iodides and bromides, may increase the formation of acnes.

A number of chlorinated aromatic hydrocarbons produce various skin lesions, including *chloracne*, which is characterized by small straw-colored cysts and comedones in which the sebaceous gland is replaced by a keratinous cyst. The severity of chloracne varies, but it has been noted among occupational workers. However, it was more notable in the outbreaks in Japan among individuals after their consumption of a batch of rice oil contaminated with polychlorinated biphenyls (WHO, 1976), and in Seveso, Italy, among residents near a factory that accidentally released a large amount of 2,3,7,8-tetrachlorodibenzo-*p*-dioxin (Pocchiari, 1980).

*Sweat glands*

Sweating serves useful physiological functions such as regulation of body temperature, and chemical-induced hyper- or hypohidrosis might increase the risk of embarrassment or heat exhaustion (Cheshire and Fealey, 2008). Blockage of the sweat ducts, a disorder known as miliaria, may occur after topical application of 95% phenol and chloroform (Shelley and Horvath, 1950).

## Testing procedures for skin toxicities

### Primary irritation

This effect is in general measured by a patch test on the skin of rabbits (Draize, 1959). A small amount (0.5 g or 0.5 ml) of the chemical to be tested is introduced under a 1-inch$^2$ gauze pad that is placed over a shaved part of the skin. The pad is suitably fastened over the animal for 24 hours. At the end of this period, the pad is removed and the skin reaction is graded according to the extent of *(i)* erythema and eschar formation and *(ii)* edema formation. The skin reaction is read again at the end of 72 hours. The same test is done on other rabbits, except that the skin has been abraded. The 24- and 72-hour readings from both groups are added to obtain the *primary irritation index* (PII).

There are a number of modified skin irritation tests based on the Draize procedure. The modifications involve the animal species and the

**Table 16.4** *In vitro* OECD test guidelines for skin toxicity

| TG No. | Title | Date |
|---|---|---|
| TG 439 | *In Vitro* Skin Irritation: Reconstructed Human Epidermis Test Method | July 25, 2015 |
| TG 442C | *In Chemico* Skin Sensitisation Direct Peptide Reactivity Assay (DPRA) | February 5, 2015 |
| TG 442D | *In Vitro* Skin Sensitisation ARE-Nrf2 Luciferase Test Method | February 5, 2015 |
| TG 442E | *In Vitro* Skin Sensitisation Human Cell Line Activation Test (h-CLAT) | July 29, 2016 |
| TG 432 | *In Vitro* 3T3 NRU Phototoxicity Test | November 23, 2004 |

number of animals used, quantity of the test material applied, repetitive applications, and types of examinations.

While evaluation of skin irritation is an important issue for safety regulation of topically applied drugs or chemicals, the movement against the cruelty of animal testing has led to two bans concerning animal testing for cosmetic ingredients/products in the European Union in 2009. The first ban was about animal testing itself to evaluate the safety of cosmetic ingredients, and the second ban, which has been in place since 2013, prohibits the sale of cosmetic products that contain ingredients tested on animals (Mehling et al., 2012). Based upon the efforts to develop and validate the *in vitro* alternative tests to replace the rabbit Draize test, several *in vitro* skin irritation tests using 3D reconstructed human epidermis (RhE), such as EpiSkin, EpiDerm, and SkinEthic were developed and approved as OECD test guidelines (Macfarlane et al., 2009; OECD, 2015). The *in vitro* test system of RhE was found to mimic the physiological/biochemical properties of epidermis, and these test guidelines measure chemical-induced skin irritation using cell viability as readout (OECD, 2015; Table 16.4).

### *Sensitization reaction*

The procedure described by Draize (1959) calls for the use of guinea pigs that are given the chemical by 10 repeated intradermal injections on one flank and a challenging dose on the other flank after a 10- to 14-day resting period. A greater reaction after the challenging dose, in comparison with that after the sensitizing doses, indicates sensitization.

The Draize test is generally considered insufficiently sensitive to identify allergic potential. Magnusson and Kligman (1969), therefore, recommended the use of the *maximization test* in which the guinea pigs are given the test substance intradermally on day 0 with and without Freund's complete adjuvant. On day 7, the substance is applied at the same site occlusively. Two weeks later, the test substance is applied topically over the pretreated areas in these animals. Different concentrations of the agent are used in the challenge. OECD (1992) has adopted this and the Buehler test which requires the application of the chemical under closed patches.

Similar to the evaluation of skin irritation, there has been continuing efforts to apply the 3R concept, *Replacement, Reduction and Refinement* of animal experiments, the basic principle for development of animal alternatives (Rusche, 2003), to test methods for skin sensitization. Local lymph node assay (LLNA; TG No. 429) in mouse was developed to reduce the pain in experimental animals compared to the Buehler test (OECD, 2010), and the advanced modified tests for LLNA were also developed and approved. Nonanimal test methods to evaluate and predict skin sensitizing potential of chemicals have been actively developed based on the complicated interactions between sensitizing chemicals and different cellular parts of skin (Mehling et al., 2012). Recently approved OECD TGs for skin sensitization are presented in Table 16.4.

Human experience is obtained either in patch tests or in a controlled population. In the latter case, the substance is widely distributed to the target population for use as directed. Their skin reactions are examined and evaluated. A patch test usually involves 100 men and 100 women, covering a wide age range. The test material (0.5 ml or 0.5 g) is applied by patch to an area on the arm or back. The skin reaction is examined on the following day after the removal of the patch.

## *Phototoxicity and photoallergy*

Phototoxicity appears to be more readily demonstrable in the hairless mouse, the rabbit, and the guinea pig. The substance to be tested may be administered topically or by a systemic route. The reaction of the skin to nonerythrogenic light (wavelength greater than 320 nm) is then determined. Significant erythema, compared with controls, indicates phototoxicity.

For the detection of photoallergy, albino guinea pigs are especially useful. The procedure involves, in principle, an induction of photosensitization by repeatedly applying a small amount of the chemical on a shaved and depilated area of the skin and exposing that area to appropriate UV rays. After a 3-week interval, the guinea pigs are exposed to the chemical and the UV rays to elicit photoallergy.

An *in vitro* assay to evaluate phototoxicity was developed as 3T3 neutral red uptake (NRU) phototoxicity assay (3T3 NRU PT) using mouse fibroblast (OECD, 2004; Table 16.4). This test method is the most widely used phototoxicity assay and included in ICH S10 guideline for photosafety evaluation of pharmaceuticals (ICHEWG, 2013). Due to the high percentage of false positive results, a positive outcome in this method should not be regarded to indicate a clinical phototoxic potential. However, in case a chemical compound is negative in this test, the compound has a very low probability of being phototoxic in humans, based on the high sensitivity of 3T3 NRU PT. This method is not appropriate to predict the potential of photoallergy.

### *Contact urticaria*

A number of animal models have been proposed based on the procedure devised by Jacobs (1940). These generally involve a patch test on the flank and nipples of guinea pigs. A test using guinea pig ears has been found to be satisfactory in screening human contact with urticarigenic substances (Lahti and Maibach, 1984).

The open patch test can be applied to human volunteers or to patients suspected of being susceptible to the chemical. In the latter case, all necessary resuscitation equipment and qualified personnel should be available to respond to anaphylactoid reaction.

Any immunological involvement can be demonstrated by the passive transfer test in which 0.1 ml fresh serum from the patient is injected intradermally into the forearm of a volunteer and challenged 24 hours later by applying the suspected chemical to the injection site.

### *Cutaneous cancer*

The procedure involves topical application of the substance on a shaved area of the skin. The substance per se, in case of a liquid, is applied directly. Otherwise, it is dissolved or suspended in a suitable vehicle. The skin painting is usually done once a week or more frequently. The most commonly used animal is the mouse. It is advisable to include a vehicle control group as well as a positive control group, which is treated with a known skin carcinogen such as benzo(*a*)pyrene.

## *References*

Agostinis P, Berg K, Cengel KA, Foster TH, Girotti AW, Gollnick SO, Hahn SM et al. (2011). Photodynamic therapy of cancer: An update. *CA Cancer J Clin.* 61, 250–81.

Amin S, Lahti A, Maibach HI (1995). Immediate contact reactions: Contact urticaria and the contact urticaria syndrome. In: Marzulli FN, Maibach HI, eds. *Dermatotoxicology*, 5th ed. Washington, DC: Taylor & Francis.

Ankley GT, Bennett RS, Erickson RJ, Hoff DJ, Hornung MW, Johnson RD, Mount DR, Nichols JW et al. (2010). Adverse outcome pathways: A conceptual framework to support ecotoxicology research and risk assessment. *Toxicol Sci*. 148, 14–25.

Brozyna A, Chwirot BW (2006). Porcine skin as a model system for studies of ultraviolet effects in human skin. *J Toxicol Environ Health A*. 69, 1155–65.

Cheshire WP, Fealey RD (2008). Drug-induced hyperhidrosis and hypohidrosis: Incidence, prevention and management. *Drug Saf*. 31, 109–26.

Draize JH (1959). Dermal toxicity. In: Editorial Committee of the Association of Food and Drug Officials of the United States, eds. Appraisal of the Safety of Chemicals in Foods, Drugs and Cosmetics. Association of Food & Drug Officials of the United States.

Ebino K, Ueda H, Kawakatsu H et al. (2001). Isolated airway exposure to toluene diisocyate results skin sensitization. *Toxicol Lett*. 121, 79–85.

Forbes PD (1995). Carcinogenesis and photocarcinogenesis test methods. In: Marzull FN, Maibach HI, eds. *Dermatotoxicology*. Washington, DC: Taylor & Francis.

Groh KJ, Tollefsen KE (2015). The Challenge: Adverse outcome pathways in research and regulation—Current status and future perspectives. *Environ Toxicol Chem*. 34, 1935.

Harber LC, Baer RL (1972). Pathogenic mechanisms of drug-induced photosensitivity. *J Invest Dermatol*. 58, 327–42.

Harber LS, Shalita AR, Armstrong RB (1987). Immunologically mediated contact photosensitivity in guinea pigs. In: Marzulli FN, Maibach HI, eds. *Dermatotoxicology*. Washington, DC: Hemisphere, 413–30.

ICH Expert Working Group (2013). International Conference on Harmonisation of Technical Requirements for Registration of Pharmaceuticals for Human Use; S10 Photosafety Evaluation of Pharmaceuticals.

IARC (1973). Certain polycyclic aromatic hydrocarbons and heterocyclic compounds. IARC Monographs on the Evaluation of Carcinogenic Risk of the Chemical to Man, Vol. 3. Lyon, France: International Agency for Research on Cancer.

Jacobs JL (1940). Immediate generalized skin reactions in hypersensitive guinea pigs. *Proc Soc Exp Biol Med*. 43, 641–3.

Kasper M, Jaks V, Are A et al. (2011). Wounding enhances epidermal tumorigenesis by recruiting hair follicle keratinocytes. *Proc Natl Acad Sci*. 108, 4099–104.

Lahti A, Maibach HI (1984). An animal model for nonimmunologic contact urticaria. *Toxicol Appl Pharmacol*. 76, 219–24.

Leist M, Hasiwa N, Rovida C, Daneshian M, Basketter D, Kimber I, Clewell H et al. (2014). Consensus report on the future of animal-free systemic toxicity testing. *ALTEX*. 31, 341–56.

Macfarlane M, Jones P, Goebel C, Dufour E, Rowland J, Araki D, Costabel-Farkas M et al. (2009). A tiered approach to the use of alternatives to animal testing for the safety assessment of cosmetics: Skin irritation. *Regul Toxicol Pharmacol*. 54, 188–96.

Magnusson B, Kligman AM (1969). The identification of contact allergens by animal assay. The guinea pig maximization test. *J Invest Dermatol*. 52, 268–76.

Mehling A, Eriksson T, Eltze T, Kolle S, Ramirez T, Teubner W, van Ravenzwaay B et al. (2012). Non-animal test methods for predicting skin sensitization potentials. *Arch Toxicol.* 86, 1273–95.

Nethercott JR, Holness DL, Adams RM et al. (1994). Multivariate analysis of the effect of selected factors on the elicitation of patch test response to 28 common environmental contactants in North America. *Am J Contact Dermatitis.* 5, 13–8.

OECD. (1992). OECD Guidelines for Testing Chemicals. Test No. 406: Skin Sensitisation. Paris: Organization for Economic Cooperation and Development.

OECD. (2004). OECD Guidelines for Testing Chemicals. Test No. 432: In Vitro 3T3 NRU Phototoxicity Test. Paris: Organization for Economic Cooperation and Development.

OECD. (2010). OECD Guidelines for Testing Chemicals. Test No. 429: Skin Sensitisation: Local Lymph Node Assay. Paris: Organization for Economic Cooperation and Development.

OECD. (2012). The Adverse Outcome Pathway for Skin Sensitisation Initiated by Covalent Binding to Proteins. Part 2: Use of the AOP to Develop Chemical Categories and Integrated Assessment and Testing Approaches. Series on Testing and Assessment. No. 168. ENV/JM/MONO(2012)/PART2.

OECD. (2015). OECD Guidelines for Testing Chemicals. Test No. 439: In Vitro Skin Irritation: Reconstructed Human Epidermis Test Method. Paris: Organization for Economic Cooperation and Development.

Perkins EJ, Antczak P, Burgoon L, Falciani F, Garcia-Reyero N, Gutsell S, Hodges G et al. (2010). Adverse outcome pathways for regulatory applications: Examination of four case studies with different degrees of completeness and scientific confidence. *Environ Toxicol Chem.* 29, 730–41.

Pocchiari F (1980). Accidental release of 2,3,7,8-tetrachlorodibenzo-*p*-dioxin (TCDD) at Seveso, Italy. *Ecotoxicol Environ Saf.* 4, 282.

Rusche B (2003). The 3Rs and animal welfare—Conflict or the way forward? *ALTEX.* 20, 63–76.

Sakamoto FH, Torezan L, Anderson RR (2010). Photodynamic therapy for acne vulgaris: A critical review from basics to clinical practice: Part II. Understanding parameters for acne treatment with photodynamic therapy. *J Am Acad Dermatol.* 63, 195–211.

Shelley WB, Horvath PN (1950). Experimental miliaria in man. II. Production of sweat retention anhidrosis and *Miliaria crystallina* by various kinds of injury. *J Invest Dermatol.* 1, 9–20.

Thong HY, Maibach HI (2008). Photosensitivity induced by exogenous agents; Phototoxicity and photoallergy. In: Roberts MS, Walters KA, eds. *Dermal Absorption and Toxicity Assessment.* Boca Raton, FL: Taylor & Francis.

WHO. (1976). Polychlorinated biphenyls and terphenyls. *Environ Health Criteria,* 2nd ed. Geneva, Switzerland: World Health Organization.

# *chapter seventeen*

# *Toxicology of the eye*

**Sam Kacew**

*Contents*



## *General considerations*

Although the eyes are relatively small, they are important to one's well-being and are complex in structure.

The eye is a spherical body that is covered mainly by three coats of tissues: The sclera, choroids, and retina. These coats mainly consist of, respectively, fibrous tissues; pigments and blood vessels; and nerve fibers, cells, and special receptors. They are nontransparent. However, light is admitted through the front of the eye, where the three coats are replaced by a number of tissues, notably the cornea and the lens (Figure 17.1a).

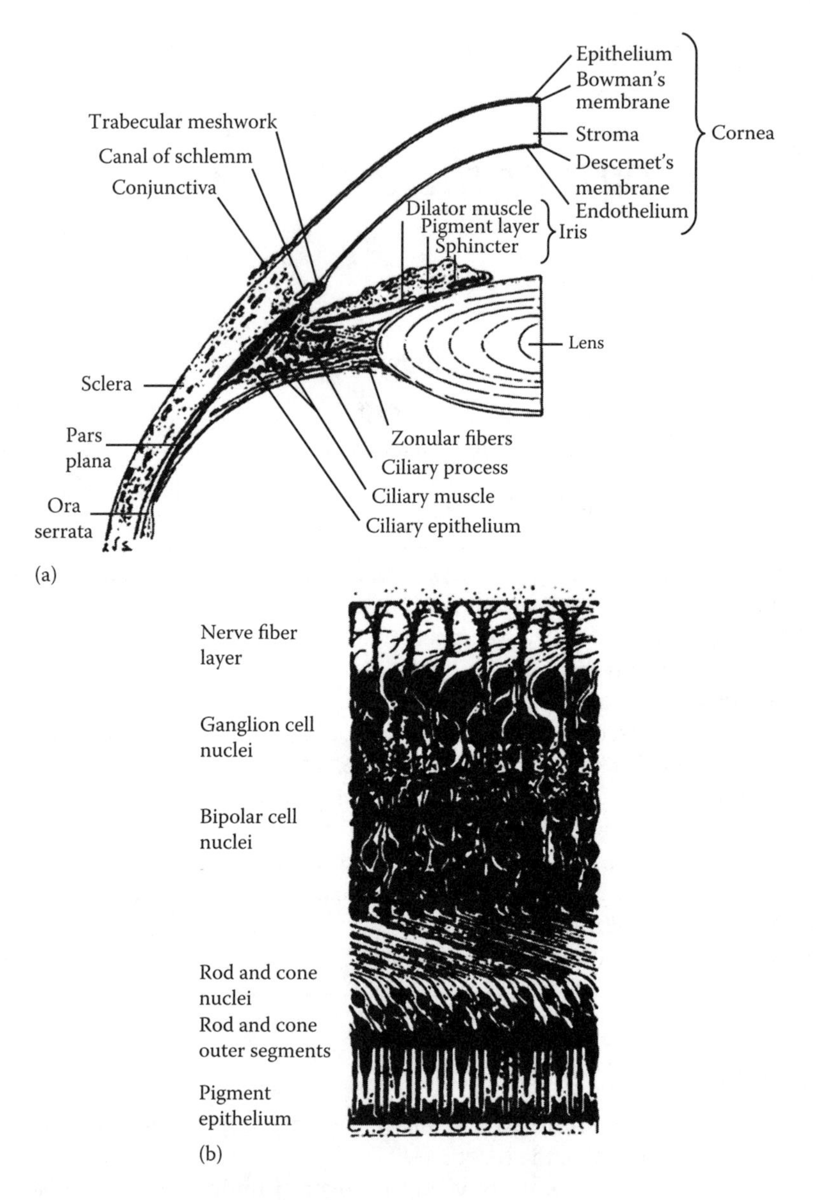


***Figure 17.1*** (a) Cross section of the anterior chamber angle and surrounding structures. (b) Cross section of the retina. (From Vaughan D, Ashbury T, *General Ophthalmology*, 10th ed., Lange Medical Publications, Los Altos CA, 1983; Polyak S, *The Retina*, University of Chicago Press, Chicago IL, 1940.)

The cornea is a continuum of the sclera and it consists of a relatively thick stroma which is covered in the front by an epithelium, consisting of several layers of cells and Bowman's membranes, and behind by Descemet's membrane and an endothelium. The cornea and the front portion of the sclera, as well as the inside of the eyelids, are covered by a thin layer of conjunctiva.

The lens consists of transparent fibers enclosed in the lens capsule. It is suspended by the ciliary zonule to the ciliary body and its curvature is adjustable by the contraction and relaxation of the ciliary muscle. The space between the lens and the cornea is filled with the aqueous humor. Also in this space, and immediately in front of the lens, is the iris. It is rich in blood vessels and heavily pigmented. The iris has a central opening, the pupil. Filling the space between the lens and retina is the vitreous humor.

The retina is the ocular structure that responds to light stimuli. It consists of several layers (Figure 17.1b). The outermost is a pigmented epithelium. Next to it are the retinal rods and cones, which are the light-responsive neural structures. They are connected via the bipolar cells to the ganglion cells. The axons from the latter cells converge and exit from the eye at the optic papilla as the optic nerve. Because of their diverse physiological nature and spatial relations, these various ocular structures may exhibit a variety of effects as a result of exposure to toxicants.

## *Toxicants and ocular sites affected*

### *Cornea*

The cornea is a delicate structure and is subject to toxic effects of chemicals, mainly from external exposure. Chemicals that affect the cornea include acids, alkali, detergents, organic solvents, and smog. Acids and alkali can readily damage the cornea. The extent of damage ranges from minor, superficial destruction of the tissue which heals completely, to opacity of the cornea or even perforation. Acid burns are related to the low pH as well as the affinity of the anion for the corneal tissue. The effects of alkali usually have slower onset than those induced by acids and are essentially pH-dependent. However, the ammonium ion, which is present in many household products, penetrates the cornea more readily and thereby affects the iris (Potts, 1996).

Detergents are useful household and industrial products which may damage the cornea. In general, nonionic detergents are less damaging than ionic agents, while cationic agents are more damaging than anionic ones (Draize and Kelley, 1952). Organic solvents, such as acetone, hexane, and toluene, may enter the eye as a result of industrial or lab accidents. These substances dissolve fat and damage the corneal epithelial cells.

Smog is a mixture of industrial smoke and fog. However, it now refers more often to the photochemical reaction products of automobile exhaust which accumulate under certain meteorological conditions (see Chapter 23). They mainly affect the respiratory tract, but even at low concentrations they irritate the corneal sensory nerve endings and cause reflex lacrimation.

Other chemicals affect the cornea following *systemic administration*. These include quinacrine, chloroquine, and chlorpromazine. Potts (1996) reviewed the corneal effects of these drugs and other chemicals. They affect the cornea via tears and/or after passing through the blood–aqueous barrier. However, they affect humans rarely and only after large doses.

## *Iris, aqueous humor, and ciliary body*

Because of its proximity to the cornea, the iris is susceptible to physical trauma and chemical irritation. The effects of such irritation consist of leakage of serum proteins and fibrin, as well as leukocytes, from the blood vessels. These may be followed by fibroblast metaplasia. Severe damage to the iris initiates liberation of melanin granules from the posterior epithelium of the iris.

The iris is innervated by sympathetic nerves (for the dilator muscles) and parasympathetic nerves (for the constrictor muscles). Therefore, the pupil can be dilated by chemicals that are sympathomimetic or parasympatholytic, and it can be constricted by parasympathomimetic and sympatholytic chemicals. Further, the size of the pupil can be altered via the central nervous system by chemicals such as morphine and general anesthetics.

The aqueous humor is secreted by the epithelium of the ciliary body into the posterior chamber. It flows through the pupil into the anterior chamber and drains through the canal of Schlemm at the angle of the anterior chamber. Inflammatory changes of the iris block the drainage of the fluid through the canal of Schlemm and raise the intraocular pressure, thereby inducing glaucoma. Atropine and other mydriatics may also precipitate glaucoma by dilating the pupil, thus blocking the drainage. Corticosteroids, applied topically or systemically, also increase the intraocular pressure and produce glaucoma.

The ciliary muscle lies in the ciliary body. The contraction of the ciliary muscle allows relaxation of the ciliary zonule, which in turn allows the lens capsule to assume a more spherical form. This muscle is parasympathetically innervated; therefore, acetylcholinesterase inhibitors and parasympatholytic agents such as atropine cause the lens to be fixed in different states of visual accommodation.

## *Lens*

A number of chemicals are known to alter the lenticular transparency, resulting in the formation of cataracts. Examples are 2,4-dinitrophenol, corticosteroids, busulfan, triparanol, and thallium. Their cataractogenic property has been noted in humans as well as in animals, such as the rabbit, rat, and young fowl. The effects generally follow systemic exposure, but with certain chemicals (e.g., corticosteroids and anticholinesterases), they may occur after topical application (Woods et al., 1967; Axelsson, 1968).

Diabetic patients are more likely to have cataracts, which can also be produced in rats and rabbits rendered diabetic with alloxan or streptozotocin (Heywood, 1982). In addition, rats fed large amounts of galactose develop cataracts (Sippel, 1966). This condition may be comparable to the cataracts observed in infants with galactosemia. Such galactosemia results from a metabolic inability, inherited as an autosomal recessive trait, to convert galactose to glucose, because of the absence of the enzyme galactose-1-phosphate uridylyl transferase (Kinosita, 1965). On the other hand, deficiencies of certain nutrients may also induce cataracts. These nutrients include tryptophan, proteins, vitamin E, riboflavin, and folic acid (Gehring, 1971).

The mechanism underlying the formation of cataracts is not fully understood. It is likely that it varies with the nature of the toxicant. For example, corticosteroid cataracts may be mediated through an inhibition of protein synthesis in the lens (Ono, 1972). Busulfan may act through an interference of mitosis of the lenticular epithelial cells (Grimes and von Sallmann, 1966). Triparanol may interfere with the $Na^+$ pump, resulting in an increase of $Na^+$ and water in the lens (Harris and Gruber, 1972). The effect of dinitrophenol is likely to be mediated through the uncoupling of oxidative phosphorylation (see also Chapter 4).

An extensive review of cataractogenic chemicals has been prepared by Gehring (1971). The cataractogenic chemicals are listed in Appendix 17.1.

Apart from cataractogenic effects, which are permanent, transient lens opacity has been noted in young beagle dogs following administration of some tranquilizers, some diuretics, and diisophenol. In addition, the transparency and refraction of the lens may also be altered by dimethyl sulfoxide and *p*-chlorophenylalanine (Heywood, 1982).

Ultraviolet (UV)-A or UV-B radiation can induce cataracts, and lead to impaired vision and transient or permanent blindness (Roberts, 2011). Increased risks for cataracts, even at low to moderate radiation doses, were observed among Japanese A-bomb survivors and Chernobyl clean-up workers (Shore et al., 2010). Other risk factors include aging, women, smoking, heavy drinking, myopia, and long-term exposure to heavy metals (e.g., lead, gold, and copper).

## Retina

Certain polycyclic compounds, such as chloroquine, hydroxychloroquine, and thioridazine, induce retinopathy in humans and animals. They affect the visual acuity, dark adaptation, and retinal pigment pattern. Hyperoxia and iodate may also induce retinal changes. Different mechanisms are involved in these retinal effects. Inhibition of protein metabolism in the pigment epithelium has been suggested as the primary toxic effect of chloroquine and hydroxychloroquine, which have strong affinity for melanin (Meier-Ruge, 1972). Increased oxygen supply to the retina induces vasoconstriction, which is associated with a decrease in the supply of nutrients. The latter effect is probably responsible for the hyperoxia-induced retinal changes. Iodate apparently affects the pigment epithelium, the derangement of which results in the degeneration of the rod layer. Various modes of action have been provided by Heywood (1982). These include the early formation of membranous cytoplasmic bodies (myeloid bodies), degenerative changes in the cell body of the rods and cones, derangement of the intracytoplasmic rods, and appearance of vacuoles around these rods in the tapetum.

Leong et al. (1987) reported that an important chemical intermediate, 4,4-methylenedianiline, a well-known hepatotoxicant, induces degeneration of the inner and outer segments of the photoreceptor cells in albino and pigmented guinea pigs. Other retinal effects include hemorrhage from the rupture of blood vessels or disturbance of blood clotting mechanism and exudates, which may cause partial detachment of the retina.

Hayasaka et al. (2011) reported that supplementation of long-term (exceeding a few years) ornithine and high blood concentrations (exceeding 600 μmol/L) of ornithine can induce retinal toxicity in gyrate atrophy of the choroid and retina (GA). Therefore, patients with GA were recommended to avoid taking ornithine; amino acid supplementation should be administered carefully for patients with the hyperornithinemia–hyperammonemia–homocitrullinuria syndrome.

## Optic nerve

As noted above, the retina contains among other structures, the ganglion cells, the axons of which form the optic nerve. Toxicants can affect either the ganglion cells or the optic nerve. Damage to one of them often results in the degeneration of the other.

Some toxicants affect mainly the central vision. The most notable example is methanol. Others include carbon disulfide, disulfiram, ethambutol, and thallium. On the other hand, quinine, chloroquine, pentavalent arsenic, and carbon monoxide cause constriction of the visual field by damaging the structures responsible for peripheral vision. Interestingly, nitrobenzol affects both the central and peripheral vision (Harrington, 1976). While methylmercury also constricts the visual field, its toxic effect is on the visual cortex instead of the optic nerve (Chapter 21).

These toxicants can also be classified according to their effects on other peripheral nerves. For example, quinine, ethambutol, and methanol generally do not affect other peripheral nerves, while carbon disulfide, disulfiram, and thallium produce both optic and peripheral neuropathies. It is worthy to note that certain organic solvents induce peripheral neuropathy but spare the visual system. These include tri-*o*-cresyl phosphate, acrylamide, *n*-hexane, and methyl *n*-butyl ketone (Grant, 1980).

Clioquinol (also known as Vioform and Entero-Vioform) was widely used for the prevention and treatment of "traveler's diarrhea." It has reportedly induced more than 10,000 cases of subacute myelo-opticoneuropathy, a disease affecting the optic nerves, spinal tracts, and peripheral nerves (Potts, 1996).

## *Testing procedures for eye toxicities*

Effects on the eye can be examined after topical application of the toxicants. In addition, systemic administration can also result in ocular alterations. Several types of examinations are available. Albino rabbits are commonly used to determine the ocular irritancy of ophthalmic medications and other chemicals that might come in contact with the eye. Dogs and non-human primates (rhesus monkeys) have also been used. For studying the effects of toxicants on the lens, retina, and optical nerve, many species of animals are used such as rat, rabbit, cat, dog, monkey, and pig.

### *Gross examination*

The test described by Draize and Kelley (1952) has been a standard procedure for testing ocular irritancy. It specifies the use of nine rabbits. Into one eye of each rabbit, 0.1 ml of the test material is instilled. In three of nine rabbits, the test material is washed with 20 ml lukewarm water 2 seconds after the instillation, and in three others, the washing is done with a 4-second delay. In the three remaining rabbits, the material is left in the eye. The ocular reactions are read with the unaided eye or with the aid of a slit-lamp at 24, 48, and 72 hours and at 4 and 7 days after treatment. The reactions on the conjunctiva (redness, chemosis, and discharge), cornea (the degree and extent of opacity), and iris (congestion, swelling, and circumcorneal injection) are scored according to a specified scale. A series of colored pictures, originally provided by the U.S. Food and Drug Administration in 1965 as a guide for grading eye irritation, are available from the U.S. Consumer Product Safety Commission, Washington, DC Samples were reproduced in Hackett and McDonald (1995).

Several modified versions of the Draize and Kelley test have been proposed. Griffith et al. (1980) reported on their results of assessing eye irritancy of a large number of substances. The irritancy ranged from nil to corrosive. The authors recommend that the following points should be taken into account in conducting eye irritation tests:

1. A 0.01 ml dose, or its weight equivalent for solids and powders, should be applied directly to the central corneal surface of at least six eyes without subsequent rinsing or manipulation of the eyelids.
2. Evaluation of the irritancy should be based on the median duration for the eyes to return to normal, instead of using a scoring system based on the type and extent of the effects.

The latest U.S. federal agency regulation (CPSC, 1988) requires the use of six albino rabbits for each test substance. For test liquids, 0.1 ml of the test material is used, and for solids and pastes, 100 mg of the test material is used. The test material is instilled into one eye of each rabbit without washing. Ocular examinations are done after 24, 48, and 72 hours. A rabbit is considered as having positive reaction if the eye shows, on any examination, ulceration or opacity of the cornea, inflammation of the iris, or swelling of the conjunctiva with partial eversion of the eyelids.

Another variation of the Draize procedure calls for the use of three rabbits whose eyes are examined at 1, 24, 48, and 72 hours. However, only one albino rabbit should be used first, if marked effects are expected. Further, if it is thought that the substance may cause unreasonable pain, a local anesthetic should be used. The grading of the eye irritation is as shown in Appendix 17.2 (OECD, 1987).

## *Instrumental examinations*

### *Ophthalmoscopy*

The ophthalmoscope is used in assessing effects of toxicants on various parts of the retina. The examination is generally intended to discover the existence of edema, hyperemia, or pallor; atrophy of the optic disk, pigmentation, or the state of the blood vessels. Changes in the vitreous humor, lens, aqueous humor, iris, and cornea can also be observed.

### *Visual perimetry*

Effect on the visual field can be readily determined in humans, but not in lab animals, except nonhuman primates. Merigan (1979) described a procedure using macaque monkeys to demonstrate the loss of peripheral vision resulting from exposure to methylmercury.

#### *Other procedures*

Visual acuity and color vision are sensitive and useful indicators of effects on the visual system in humans. Procedures involving instrumentation, such as electrooculography, and visual-evoked responses are also useful and can be incorporated in animal experimentation (Grant, 1980).

### *Histological and biochemical examinations*

Light microscopy can usually pinpoint the site of action of toxicants, electron microscopy can demonstrate ultrastructural changes, and biochemical studies can reveal the mechanism of toxic effects. For example, with light microscopy, chloroquine has been observed to initiate a thickening of the pigment epithelium, followed by migration of the pigment to the outer nuclear layer, and finally total atrophy of the photoreceptors (Meier-Ruge, 1968). Electron microscopy showed mitochondrial swelling and disorganization of the endoplasmic reticulum in the photoreceptor inner segment (Solze and McConnell, 1970). Biochemical studies revealed inhibition of many enzymatic reactions, especially those related to protein metabolism of the pigment epithelium.

#### In vitro *tests*

Owing to humane concerns about the use of animals in eye irritation tests, a number of *in vitro* tests have been developed. These involve the use of cells from isolated cornea and chorioallantoic membrane and measuring their uptake of dyes, such as neutral red, as an indicator of toxicity. Other proposed procedures include isolated rabbit eye and isolated chicken eye (Green, 1998). However, these tests apparently require refinement and extensive validation.

## *Evaluation*

Eye irritation tests are widely used to assess the ocular irritancy of chemicals. In general, the albino rabbit is the animal of choice. Some intra-lab and inter-lab variations in the scores were noted in a collaborative study (Marzulli and Ruggles, 1973). Nevertheless, periodic collaborative studies tend to improve the reliability of the scores. The various modifications made on the Draize test also tend to reduce the variability of the results.

A large number of animal experimentations and clinical studies indicate that there is a fair correlation between humans and animals in their reactions to toxicants with respect to cataract formation and retinopathy (Grant, 1980; Potts, 1996).

## *Appendix 17.1 Cataractogenic chemicals*

| | |
|---|---|
| Sugars (glucose, galactose, xylose) | Tyrosine |
| Streptozotocin | 2,4-Dinitrophenol and related compounds |
| Corticosteroids | |
| Naphthalene | Alkylating agents |
| Mimosine (leucenol) | Anticholinesterases |
| Methoxsalen | Chlorpromazine |
| Methionine sulfoximine | Triparanol |
| Polyriboinosinic acid | Dimethyl sulfoxide |
| Polyribocytidylic acid | 2,4,6-Trinitrotoluene |
| Quietidine (1,4-bis(phenylisopropyl)-piperazine·2HCl) | Sympathomimetic drugs and morphine-like drugs |
| *N*-phenyl-â-hydrazinopropionitriles and related compounds | 2,6-Dichloro-4-nitroaniline |
| | Iodoacetic acid |
| 4 [3(7-Chloro-5,11-dihydrodibenz [*b*,*e*] [1,4]-oxyazepin-5-YL)propyl]-1-piperazine ethanol dichloride | Mephenytoin |
| | Diquat |
| | Oral contraceptives |
| | Sulfaethoxypyridazine |
| | Thallium |
| | Paradichlorobenzene |
| | Heptachlor |
| | Desferal |
| | Thioacetamide |

## Appendix 17.2 Grading of eye irritation

| Cornea | |
|---|---|
| No ulceration or opacity | 0 |
| Scattered or diffuse areas of opacity (other than slight dulling of normal luster), details of iris clearly visible | 1 |
| Easily discernible translucent area, details of iris slightly obscured | 2 |
| Necrotic area, no details of iris visible, size of pupil barely discernible | 3 |
| Opaque cornea, iris not discernible through the opacity | 4 |
| **Iris** | |
| Normal | 0 |
| Markedly deepened rugae, congestion, swelling, moderate circumcorneal heperemia, or injection; any of these or combination of any thereof, iris still reacting to light (sluggish reaction is positive) | 1 |
| No reaction to light, hemorrhage, gross destruction (any or all of these) | 2 |
| **Conjunctiva redness (refers to palpebral and bulbar conjunctiva, cornea, and iris)** | |
| Blood vessels normal | 0 |
| Some blood vessels definitely hyperemic (injected) | 1 |
| Diffuse, crimson color, individual vessels not easily discernible | 2 |
| Diffuse beefy red | 3 |
| **Chemosis: Lids and/or nictitating membranes** | |
| No swelling | 0 |
| Any swelling above normal (includes nictating membranes) | 1 |
| Obvious swelling with partial eversion of lids | 2 |
| Swelling with lids about half-closed | 3 |
| Swelling with lids more than half-closed | 4 |

*Source:* OECD., *OECD Guidelines for Testing of Chemicals*, Organization for Economic Cooperation and Development, Paris, 1987; OECD., *OECD guidelines for the testing of chemicals test no. 405. Acute Eye irritation/corrosion*, available online, 2002.

## References

Axelsson U (1968). Glaucoma, miotic therapy and cataract III. Visual loss due to lens changes in glaucoma eyes treated with paraoxon (Mintacol), echothiophate or pilocarpine. *Acta Ophthalmol.* 46, 831.

CPSC (1988). Consumer product safety commission. Test for eye irritants. Code of federal regulations, Title 16. Federal Hazardous Substances Act Regulation, Part 1500.42.

Draize JH, Kelley EA (1952). Toxicity to eye mucosa of certain cosmetic preparations containing surface-active agents. *Proc Sci Sect Toilet Goods Assoc.* 17, 1–4.

Gehring PJ (1971). The cataractogenic activity of chemical agents. *CRC Crit Rev Toxicol.* 1, 93–118.

Grant WM (1980). The peripheral visual system as a target. In: Spencer BS, Schaumburg HH, eds. *Experimental and Clinical Neurotoxicology*. Baltimore, MD: Williams & Wilkins.

Green S (1998). Update on agency initiatives in alternative methods. In: Margulli FN, Maribach HI, eds. *Dermatology Methods: The Laboratory Worker's Vade McCum*. Philadelphia, PA: Taylor & Francis, 377–82.

Griffith JF, Nixon GA, Bruce RD et al. (1980). Dose–response studies with chemical irritants in the albino rabbit eye as a basis for selecting optimum testing conditions for predicting hazard to the human eye. *Toxicol Appl Pharmacol.* 55, 501–13.

Grimes P, Von Sallmann L (1966). Interference with cell proliferation and induction of polyploidy in rat lens epithelium during prolonged Myleran treatment. *Exp Cell Res.* 62, 265–73.

Hackett RB, McDonald TO (1995). Assessing ocular irritation. In: Marzulli FN, Maibach HI, eds. Dermatotoxicology. Washington, DC: Taylor & Francis.

Harrington DO (1976). *The Visual Fields*. St. Louis, MI: Mosby.

Harris JE, Gruber L (1972). Reversal of triparanol-induced cataracts in the rat. II. Exchange of 22Na, 42K, 86Rb in cataractous and clearing lenses. *Invest Ophthalmol Vis Sci.* 11, 608–16.

Hayasaka S, Kodama T, Ohira A (2011). Retinal risks of high-dose ornithine supplements: A review. *Br J Nutr.* 106, 801–11.

Heywood R (1982). Histopathological and laboratory assessment of visual dysfunction. *Environ Health Perspect.* 44, 35–45.

Kinosita JH (1965). Cataracts in galactosemia. *Invest Ophthalmol Vis Sci.* 4, 786–99.

Leong BKJ, Lund JE, Groehn JA et al. (1987). Retinopathy from inhaling 4,4′-methylenedianiline aerosols. *Fundam Appl Toxicol.* 9, 645–58.

Marzulli FN, Ruggles DI (1973). Rabbit eye irritation test: Collaborative study. *J Am Assoc Anal Chem.* 56, 905–14.

Meier-Ruge M (1968). The pathophysiological morphology of the pigment epithelium and its importance for retinal structure and function. *Med Prob Ophthalmol.* 8, 32–48.

Meier-Ruge W (1972). Drug-induced retinopathy. *CRC Crit Rev Toxicol.* 1, 325–60.

Merigan WH (1979). Effects of toxicants on visual systems. *Neurobehav Toxicol.* 1(Suppl. 1), 1522.

OECD. (1987). OECD Guidelines for Testing of Chemicals. Paris: Organization for Economic Cooperation and Development.

OECD. (2002). OECD guidelines for the testing of chemicals test no. 405. Acute Eye irritation/corrosion. Available from: http://www.oecd-ilibrary.org/environment/testno-405-acute-eye-irritation-corrosion_9789264070646-en.

Ono S (1972). Presence of corticol-binding protein in the lens. *Ophthalmic Res.* 3, 233–40.

Polyak S (1940). *The Retina*. Chicago, IL: University of Chicago Press.

Potts AM (1996). Toxic responses of the eye. In: Klaassen CD, ed. *Casarett and Doull's Toxicology*. New York, NY: McGraw-Hill.

Roberts JE (2011). Ultraviolet radiation as a risk factor for cataract and macular degeneration. *Eye Contact Lens.* 37, 246–9.

Shore RE, Neriishi K, Nakashima E (2010). Epidemiological studies of cataract risk at low to moderate radiation doses: (Not) seeing is believing. *Radiat Res.* 174, 889–94.

Sippel TO (1966). Changes in water, protein and glutathione contents of the lens in the course of galactose cataract development in rats. *Invest Ophthalmol Vis Sci.* 5, 568–75.

Solze DA, McConnell DG (1970). Ultrastructural changes in the rat photoreceptor inner segment during experimental chloroquine retinopathy. *Ophthal Res.* 1, 140–8.

Vaughan D, Ashbury T (1983). *General Ophthalmology,* 10th ed. Los Altos, CA: Lange Medical Publications.

Woods DC, Contaxis I, Sweet D et al. (1967). Response of rabbits to corticosteroids. I. Influence on growth, intraocular pressure and lens transparency. *Am J Ophthalmol.* 63, 841–9.

# *chapter eighteen*

# *Toxicology of the nervous system*

***Ok-Nam Bae***

*Contents*

## Introduction

As a vital part of the body, the nervous system is shielded from toxicants in the blood by a unique protective mechanism, namely, the blood–brain barrier (BBB) and blood–nerve barrier (BNB). Nonetheless, it is susceptible to a variety of toxicants. For example, methylmercury (MeHg) mainly affects the nervous system, although its concentration in the brain is comparable to that in most other tissues, and in fact it is much lower than that in the liver and kidneys.

The greater susceptibility may be attributed partly to the fact that neurons have a high metabolic rate, with little capacity for anaerobic metabolism. Further, being electrically excitable, neurons tend to lose cell membrane integrity more readily. The great length of the axons is another reason for the nervous system being susceptible to adverse effects, because the cell body must supply its axon structurally and metabolically. To facilitate the description of the various types of toxic effects and the procedures for their testing, in the following, the various parts of the nervous system are described.

### Central and peripheral nervous system

The nervous system consists of two major parts: the central nervous system (CNS) and the peripheral nervous system (PNS). The CNS is comprised of the brain and the spinal cord, and the PNS covers the cranial and spinal nerves, which are either motor or sensory. The neurons of the sensory spinal nerves are located in the ganglia in the dorsal roots. In addition, the PNS also includes the sympathetic nerve system, which arises from neurons in the thoracic and lumbar region of the spinal cord, and the parasympathetic system, which stems from nerve fibers leaving the CNS via the cranial nerves and the sacral spinal roots.

### Cells and appendages

The principal cells in the nervous system are neurons, composed of perikarya, along with their dendrites and axons. These structures are responsible for the conduction of nerve impulses. The main supporting structure consists of various types of glial cells. Apart from a lack of conductivity, glial cells differ from neurons in that the former, as most other types of cells, do reproduce, whereas the latter do not.

In the CNS, the glial cells include astrocytes, oligodendrocytes (oligodendroglia), and microglia. Astrocytes help to maintain a proper microenvironment around the neurons and support the BBB. Oligodendroglia surrounds the axons in the CNS with a lipid-rich material, the myelin sheath, which provides electrical insulation. Microglia are basically macrophages that are located in the CNS. In the PNS, the Schwann cells provide the myelin sheath, which wraps around the axon and is interrupted by the nodes of Ranvier.

## *Neurotransmitters*

Neurons are connected, via their axons, to other neurons at their dendrites, or to the receptors in the glands or muscles. At nerve terminals, on excitation by an action potential, chemical neurotransmitters are released. The most common transmitters are acetylcholine and norepinephrine. However, there are several amine neurotransmitters in addition to norepinephrine, such as dopamine, serotonin, and histamine. Further, the following amino acids also act as neurotransmitters: 7-aminobutyric acid (GABA), glycine, glutamate, and aspartate. These transmitters are small molecules and act rapidly. They are synthesized in the presynaptic terminals. These neurotransmitters are presynthesized, stored in synaptic vesicles, and released upon excitation. Nitric oxide (NO), a recently discovered neurotransmitter, is different from the others in that, as a labile free radical, it is not presynthesized for storage in synaptic vesicles. It is synthesized, on demand, from l-arginine by NO synthase (Zhang and Snyder, 1995).

In addition to these small-molecule neurotransmitters, a large number of neuropeptides are slow-acting neurotransmitters/modulators. Some are released by the pituitary gland: ACTH, β-endorphin, growth hormone, thyrotropin, oxytocin, and vasopressin. A number of peptide transmitters act on the gut and brain, for example, leucine enkephalin and methionine enkephalin.

## *Blood–brain and blood–nerve barriers*

These barriers protect the nervous system from certain neurotoxicants. Differences in neurotoxicity sometimes might be explained on the basis of these barriers.

### *Blood–brain barrier*

The endothelium in the brain is impermeable to substances of medium molecular weight, such as horseradish peroxidase (molecular weight:

40,000 Da; diameter: 5–6 nm), because the adjacent cells are tightly joined. Further, these cells have few micropinocytotic vesicles, which in capillaries of other tissues serve as an important transport mechanism across endothelial cells. Four major cellular elements such as endothelial cells (ECs), astrocyte end-feet, microglial cells, and pericytes play an important role in structural integrity and genesis of the blood–brain barrier (BBB) (Correale and Villa, 2009). However, highly lipid-soluble substances and the nonionized fraction of a chemical are more permeable across the BBB. It is, therefore, similar to intact cell membranes in permeability.

The BBB is absent where the cells produce hormones or act as hormonal or chemoreceptors. Glutamate and a number of related compounds were shown to affect areas in the brain not protected by the BBB, such as the arcuate nucleus of the hypothalamus and the *area postrema* in various lab animals. These effects, while not observed in humans, are of interest because they may be used as tools in the study of such clinical conditions as Huntington's disease, drug-induced Parkinsonism, tardive dyskinesia, and sulfur amino acidopathies.

The BBB is effective in excluding many neurotoxicants, such as diphtheria, staphylococcus, and tetanus toxins. This is also the case with doxorubicin, which affects the dorsal root ganglia but not CNS. Mercuric chloride is a small molecule but is hydrophilic and exists mainly in ionic form. Its concentration in the brain is minimal and so are its CNS effects. On the other hand, MeHg is lipophilic and thus readily crosses the BBB, thereby damaging the brain.

The recent concept of *neurovascular unit* (Figure 18.1), a modular structure emphasizing the interaction between cells composing the microenvironment in the brain, provides a new insight into understanding neurobiology and toxicology (Xing et al., 2012; Kim et al., 2013). The toxicity of neurons, or brain endothelial cells, is not independent or separated events, but brain damage is a matter of the complex of neurons, vascular cells, and the supportive system including astrocytes. The effects of opioids, amphetamine, alcohol, and nicotine on the neurovascular unit have been reviewed by Egleton and Abbruscato (2014).

#### *Blood–nerve barrier*

Peripheral nerves are enclosed by two connective tissue sheaths, the perineurium and epineurium, and interlaced with the endoneurium. The blood–nerve barrier (BNB), also known as the blood–nerve interface, is nourished by the blood vessels in the endoneurium and supplemented by the lamellated cells of the perineural sheath. The BNB is not as effective as the BBB; therefore, the dorsal root ganglia are generally more susceptible than neurons in the CNS to neurotoxicants. For example, doxorubicin

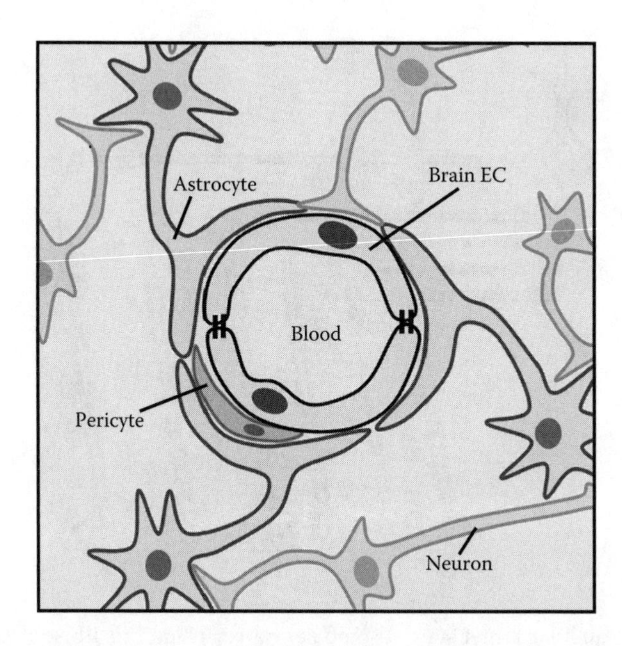


***Figure 18.1*** Neurovascular unit. An integrated functional framework where BBB endothelial cells, neurons, and supportive cells including astrocytes interact to maintain a normal microenvironment in the brain. (From Kim JH *Toxicol Res.*, 29, 157–164, 2013.)

affects neurons in the dorsal root ganglia but not those in the brain. Lead (Pb) intoxication produces endothelial damage, increases permeability of blood–nerve interface, and produces demyelination as a primary pathological event (Mizisin and Weerasuriya, 2011).

## Neurotoxic effects and neurotoxicants

The effects may be classified according to the site of action. These include the neurons, axons, glial cells, and vascular system. A toxicant, however, may affect more than one site. The following is a brief description of certain neurotoxic effects, along with the putative mode of action, grouped according to the site of action.

Figure 18.2 depicts damage to neurons, axons, and the myelin sheath. *Neuronopathy* is represented by the damage to a second-order sensory neuron (4), which innervates corpuscle A, and a neuron in the dorsal root ganglion (3), which innervates corpuscle B. *Axonopathy* is represented by the damaged central axonal process of a sensory neuron, which innervates corpuscle C, and the axons of the lower motor neurons (2), which

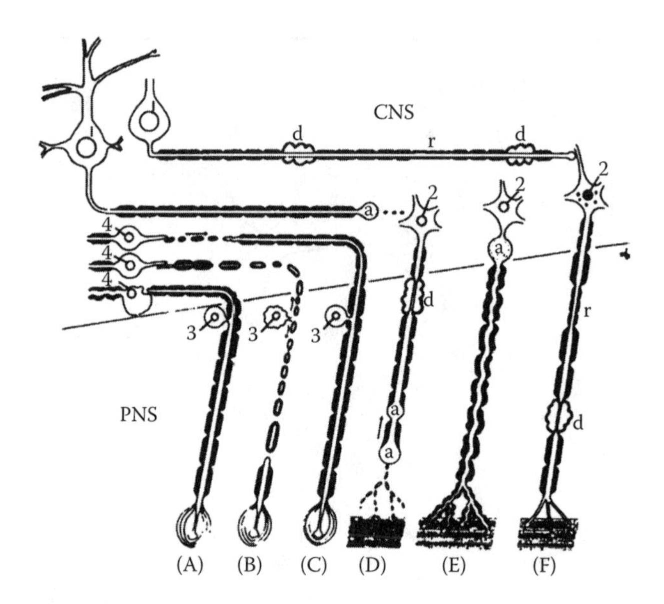


***Figure 18.2*** Cellular target sites of some neurotoxic chemicals illustrated by upper (1) and lower (2) motor neurons, dorsal root ganglion cells (3), and second-order sensory neurons (4) in the gracile nucleus of the medulla oblongata. The central nervous system (CNS) is represented above the sloping horizontal line and the peripheral nervous system (PNS) below. The peripheral receptors on fibers (A–C) are pacinian corpuscles. Fibers (D–F) innervate extrafusal muscle fibers: a, axonal degeneration; d, demyelination; r, remyelination of ventral root, and medulla oblongata. (From Spencer PS et al., *Experimental and Clinical Neurotoxicology*, Williams & Wilkins, Baltimore, MD, 743–757, 1980.)

innervates muscle fibers D and E. *Myelinopathy* is shown along the axons of upper (1) and lower (2) motor neurons which innervates muscle fiber F.

Some neurotoxicants that induce these and other damage are listed in Table 18.1 and described in further detail.

## *Neuronopathy*

Neurons, being dependent mainly on glucose as an energy source, are susceptible to anoxic and hypoglycemic conditions. A number of chemicals are well known for their anoxygenic effects in the brain. Barbiturates induce anoxia in the brain, especially in the hippocampus and cerebellum. Permanent CNS damage even after a barbiturate coma, however, is rare, possibly because of reduced cell metabolism. On the other hand, prolonged exposure to carbon monoxide may induce permanent changes in the brain, arising from the development of a diffuse sclerosis of the white

***Table 18.1*** Representative neurotoxicants and their mode of action

| | |
|---|---|
| Acrylamide—A | *n*-hexane—A |
| Actinomycin—M | IDPN—A |
| AETT—M | Kainic acid—N |
| Alcohol—N, T | Lead—MS |
| Alanosine—N | Leptophos—A |
| Aluminum—N | Lysolecithin—M |
| 6-Aminonicotinamide—BV | Methyl *n*-butyl ketone—A |
| Anatoxin—C | Methylmercury—N, BV |
| Arseni—BV | Nicotine—C |
| Azide—N | Organic solvents—A |
| Barbiturate—N | Organotin—N |
| Botulinum toxin—C | Pyrethroids—C |
| Carbon monoxide—N | Saxitoxin—C |
| Clioquinol—A | Tellurium—BV, M |
| Cyanide—N, BV | Tetanoplasmin—C |
| DDT—C | Tetrodotoxin—C |
| Diphtheria toxin—M | Thallium—A |
| Doxorubicin—N | TOCP—A |
| EPN—A | Triethyltin—M, BV |
| Ethidium bromide—M | Triparanol—M |
| Glutamate—N | Vincristine—A |
| Hexachlorophene—M, BV | |

*Abbreviations:* A, axonopathy; AETT, acetyl ethyl tetramethyl tetralin; BV, blood vessel and edema; C, conduction and transmission; M, myelinopathy; MS, multiple sites; N, neuropathy; T, teratogenicity.

matter (leukoencephalopathy). Cyanide and azide inhibit cytochrome oxidase, thereby producing cytotoxic anoxia. Contamination of food products with tricresyl phosphate was shown to produce a delayed neuropathy related to the inhibition of "neuropathy target esterase" whereby there is damage to spinal nerves, the spinal cord, brain, and other tissues (Craig and Barth, 1999). This type of neuropathy also occurs following exposure to organophosphorus (OP) insecticides (Pope, 1999; see below).

The cell body of neurons may be affected directly by toxicants. Methylmercury first produces focal loss of ribosomes and then disintegration and disappearance of the Nissl substances, especially in the small cells. These are followed by nuclear and perinuclear changes and finally by the loss of the entire neuron including its axon (Jacobs et al., 1977). The herbicide paraquat produces destruction of dopaminergic neurons via oxidative stress (Yang and Tiffany-Castiglioni, 2008). Paraquat-induced neuronal effects resemble the manifestations in Parkinson's disease.

Doxorubicin (Adriamycin) affects neurons by intercalating with DNA, leading to a breakdown of the helical structures (Cho et al., 1980). This derangement inhibits synthesis of RNA and neuronal protein. Since this drug does not cross the BBB, it might affect the neurons in the dorsal root ganglia (Figure 18.2B) and autonomic ganglia, but not those in the CNS. On the other hand, MeHg penetrates the BBB and thus damages neurons in the CNS as well as those in the dorsal root ganglia.

Organotins are used as pesticides and as plasticizers. Upon entering the nervous system, these compounds accumulate in the Golgi-like structures in the cell body. The cells then undergo swelling and necrosis (Bouldin et al., 1981).

Aluminum (Al) also penetrates the BBB and induces encephalopathy with neurofibrillar degeneration in cats and rabbits (DeBoni et al., 1976). Reviews in toxicology conclude that the use of Al cooking utensils and the use of various Al-containing food additives are safe (Soni et al., 2001; Krewski et al., 2007). Aluminum increases the permeability of BBB by changing its ultrastructure and expression of occludin and F-actin, but zinc protects the integrity of BBB and inhibits decrease of tight junction protein occludin and F-actin expression in BBB in rats exposed to Al (Song et al., 2008).

Glutamate and related chemicals, in very large doses, are known to affect areas of the CNS devoid of BBB (see the section "Blood–Brain Barrier") and are considered as exerting neuroexcitatory and neurotoxic effects. The dendrites are the primary site of action. The perikarya are then affected, but the axons are spared (Figure 18.2A). The toxicity may be mediated through NO (Dawson et al., 1991). Kainic acid derived from a particular seaweed has been used in ascariasis; it is similar to glutamate but much more potent (Olney et al., 1974).

Alcohol in pregnant women may induce nervous system abnormalities in their offspring including abnormal neuronal migration and abnormal development of dendritic spines (Abel et al., 1983).

## *Axonopathy*

Some axons are very long (up to 1 m), and the elements in the axons, such as neurofibrils, are synthesized not locally but in the cell body, and transported along the axon. The axon may therefore be attacked either directly by toxicants or indirectly through damage to the cell body. Lesions may occur either in the proximal or in the distal sections of axons.

### *Proximal axonopathy*

β,β-Iminodiproprionitrile (IDPN) produces typical lesions of this type. IDPN has therefore been used as a model to study motor neuron diseases such as amyotrophic lateral sclerosis. The primary effect of IDPN is the impairment of slow axonal transport of neurofilaments, probably through aberrant phosphorylation of neurofilaments (Gold and Austin, 1991), while their synthesis is continued in the cell body. Accumulation of neurofilaments in the proximal axon leads to enlargement and atrophy of the distal axon (Figure 18.2E). The enlarged proximal axon in turn elicits local proliferation of the subpial astrocytic processes and extension of the processes filled with glial filaments along the proximal ventral root. The proximal swelling also stimulates splitting of myelin at the intraperiod line, formation of intramyelinic vacuoles, and ultimate demyelination. The Schwann cells in the demyelinated segment divide and remyelinate, and repeated demyelination and remyelination yield "onion-bulb" formation (Griffin and Price, 1980).

*Distal axonopathy*

Axons contain three types of neurofibrillary structures, namely, neurotubules, neurofilaments, and microfilaments as well as mitochondria and smooth endoplasmic reticulum. These structures are especially susceptible to a variety of neurotoxicants. For example, thallium induces mitochondrial swelling and degeneration, and certain OP compounds and organic solvents produce derangement of neurofibrillary structures, resulting in distal axonopathy.

An important type of distal axonopathy is produced by certain OP compounds such as tri-*o*-cresyl phosphate (TOCP), ethyl-4nitrophenyl phenylphosphonothioate (EPN), and leptophos. These compounds, besides inhibiting acetylcholinesterase (AChE), produce *delayed neuropathy*, which is manifested mainly as muscle paralysis. This affects especially long and large nerve fibers, hence the hindlimbs are paralyzed before the forelimbs. TOCP induced delayed neuropathy in 10,000 humans. Although a number of other animals may also be affected, especially after repeated exposures, this toxicity is readily reproduced in hens, usually with a delay of 8–10 days after exposure. Because of the severity of delayed neurotoxicity, new OP chemicals are routinely tested for this potential hazard. OECD (1984) and EPA (1994) published guidelines for such tests both after a single dose and after repeated administrations, using domestic hens. The condition is unrelated to (AChE) inhibition because potent inhibitors such as malathion, parathion, and carbaryl do not possess this toxic property. It is apparently associated with phosphorylation of the enzyme neuropathy target esterase (NTE; formerly known as neurotoxic esterase) (Abou-Donia, 1981; Johnson, 1990; Pope, 1999).

A different type of distal axonopathy is known to be produced by hexacarbons such as *n*-hexane and methyl *n*-butyl ketone. These solvents, such as acrylamide, produced toxic polyneuropathy among industrial workers

(Exon, 2006). Both produce marked neurofilament proliferation in axons, probably as a result of altered phosphorylation of certain proteins (Berti-Mattera et al., 1990). However, giant axonal swellings are common with hexacarbons (Figure 18.2D), but are rare with acrylamide. Further, sensory nerves are involved early with acrylamide but later with hexacarbons, which affect certain motor nerves first. Vincristine may produce accumulation of neurofibrils in the perikarya and axons. Vincristine disrupts the axonal neurotubules and neurofilaments, and blocks axoplasmic transport of these ultrastructures.

Clioquinol, a popular remedy and preventive drug for "travelers' diarrhea" in the 1960s and 1970s, induced disorders of the nervous system known as subacute myelo-optico-neuropathy in thousands of individuals (Appendix 1.2). In humans and experimental animals, this compound produces central axonal degeneration of the dorsal root ganglion (Figure 18.2C), as well as of the optic nerves (Worden et al., 1978).

Distal axonopathy has also been postulated as resulting from impairment of glycolytic enzyme activities in the axon (Spencer et al., 1979). These enzymes are responsible for the transport of neurofilaments, which are synthesized in the perikaryon and transported along the axon. Impairment of the activities of these enzymes would thus first affect the distal portion of the axon as well as the large, long nerve fibers, which have a greater energy demand on the perikarya. A second hypothesis postulates that the neurofilaments are directly affected by toxicants such as hexacarbons and acrylamide (Savolainen, 1977). Neurofilaments exposed to the toxicant for the longest period, namely, those located distally in long fibers, are affected first.

*Conduction and transmission*

Rapid neuronal communications are mediated by electrical or chemical signals through conduction and transmission. Toxicants affecting these pathways may alter intracellular or intercellular signal transfer.

*Interference with impulse conduction*

A number of toxicants act mainly on nerve membranes. These membranes normally maintain a negative resting potential. When stimulated, an action potential is generated. The resting and action potentials result from differences in the $Na^+$ and $K^+$ concentrations across the membrane, and the $Na^+$ channels maintain their concentrations. Tetrodotoxin, the toxic principle of puffer fish, was shown to block the action potential by blocking the $Na^+$ channels. Saxitoxin, the toxic principle produced by the dinoflagellate *Gonyaulax* and taken up by the clam *Saxidomas giganteus*, also acts by blocking the $Na^+$ channels. Consumption of improperly cleaned puffer fish or contaminated clams may result in death by respiratory failure. DDT and pyrethroids are markedly different in chemical structure. However, their effects on the nervous systems are similar. They prolong the opening of the $Na^+$ channel, thereby initiating repetitive activity at the synapses and neuromuscular junctions (Narahashi, 1992).

### *Interference with synaptic transmission*

Botulinum toxin, the most potent biologic toxin, is produced by *Clostridium botulinum*. Botulinum toxin induces the paralysis of muscles by impairing the release of acetylcholine (ACh) from motor nerve endings. Black widow spider venom, on the other hand, induces an excessive release of ACh and results in cramps and paralysis.

Tetanoplasmin, from the microbe *Clostridium tetani*, produces tetanus through its effect on the CNS. Tetanoplasmin blocks release of the inhibitory amino acid transmitters GABA and glycine, thereby producing spastic paralysis. The molecular weight of this proteinaceous dimer is about 150,000, and therefore, it is too large to cross the BBB; however, it reaches the CNS by retrograde axonal transport (Schield et al., 1977).

Certain neurotoxins (e.g., anatoxin-S) may be produced by cyanobacteria in eutrophic lakes and ponds. These toxins interfere with the transmission of impulses from nerve terminals to muscles, thereby inducing muscle paralysis (Carmicheal, 1994).

Acrylamide produces neurotoxicity by interfering with kinesin-related motor proteins in neurofilaments that are involved in fast antegrade transport of nerve signals between axons. Inhibition of these motor proteins, and transaxonal transport of nerve growth factors, result in impaired molecular transport from the cell body to distal axon, leading to the death of the nerve body. This is manifested as hindlimb splay, ataxia, and skeletal muscle weakness (Exon, 2006).

## *Glial cells and myelin*

### *Myelinating cells*

Demyelination may result from injuries to myelinating cells (oligodendrocytes and Schwann cells). Neurotoxins of this type include Pb, which affects Schwann cells possibly by interfering with their $Ca^{2+}$ transport. Hypocholesterolemic agents such as triparanol, as expected, disrupt the myelin sheath because of the high (70%) lipid content of myelin. However, these drugs produce ultrastructural changes in oligodendrocytes before demyelination occurs. Diphtheria toxin demyelinates, possibly by affecting both myelin and myelinating cells. Triethyltin, ethidium bromide, and actinomycin are other examples of demyelinating toxins that act on the myelinating cells. The pesticide rotenone produces degeneration of the ganglion cell layer resulting in a neurodegenerative disorder associated with the destruction of the mitochondria (Zhang et al., 2006). This phenomenon is found in Leber's optic neuropathy and Parkinson's disease.

#### *Myelin sheath*

Demyelination may also occur from impacts on the myelin sheath. This type of effect generally involves a disruption of the membrane structure. Other modes of action include (1) inhibition of carbonic anhydrase or other enzymes involved in ion and water transport, (2) inhibition of enzymes involved in oxidative phosphorylation, and (3) chelation of metals. Neurotoxicants that act directly on the myelin sheath include triethyltin, lysolecithin, isoniazid, cyanate, hexachlorophene, and Pb. Acetyl ethyl tetramethyl tetralin also produces myelinopathy through a complex mechanism (Figure 18.2F).

Lead has been known for centuries as a neurotoxicant. Lead affects various parts of the nervous system, including the myelin sheath. The PNS is affected before the CNS. In addition, Pb affects motor nerves before the sensory ones, resulting in "wrist-drop" and "foot-drop." Its effects on the blood vessels are discussed next.

### *Blood vessels and edema*

The permeability of the vascular system in the CNS and PNS may be increased by higher blood pressure or lower plasma osmolarity. It may also result from exposure to certain toxins. The greater permeability generally leads to an accumulation of fluids in the extracellular space. In addition, a number of neurotoxicants are known to induce cellular edema.

#### *Extracellular edema*

Lead damages the endothelial cells and produces extravasation of plasma in the brain, especially in the white matter, which has a greater compliance than gray matter. The fact that suckling rats are more susceptible to Pb has been attributed to the immaturity of the vascular system (Press, 1977). Lead has similar effects on the endoneurium, leading to increased endoneural fluid pressure and demyelination. Organic Pb, such as tetraethyl lead, more readily penetrates the barriers and is therefore more toxic in this respect.

Mercury (Hg) compounds damage the endothelial cells and increase their permeability. Organic arsenicals produce edema and focal hemorrhages in the brain. Tellurium produces edema in the endoneurium. Chronic alcoholism is associated with endoneural edema.

Endoneural edema might also result from intramyelinic edema in hexachlorophene intoxication. Endoneural edema may also be associated with Wallerian degeneration due to mechanical injury.

### Cellular edema

Various parts of neurons may become edematous following exposure to toxicants. For example, 6-aminonicotinamide affects the perikaryon; cyanide and carbon monoxide affect the axon; and ouabain and methyl sulfoxime affect the presynaptic nerve endings.

Edema of astrocytes and oligodendrocytes may be produced by 6-aminonicotinamide. Ouabain may also affect astrocytes. Edema of Schwann cells may be induced by Pb, which, as noted above, may also produce extracellular edema.

Triethyltin and isoniazid also produce edema of the myelin sheaths in the CNS. Hexachlorophene induces edema of myelin sheaths both in white matter of the brain and in peripheral nerves.

## Testing procedures for neurotoxicities

### Functional observational battery

A battery of observations, namely the functional observational battery (FOB), was devised to assess neurotoxic effects (EPA, 1994; Kallman and Fowler, 1994). This is done in intact animals, usually rats or mice. These animals are exposed to the toxicant at two or three doses by an appropriate route. The duration of treatment and observation period vary from days to months according to the nature of the toxicant. The animals are observed for the following abnormalities:

(a) Unusual body position, activity level, gait, etc.
(b) Unusual behavior such as compulsive biting, self-mutilation, circling, and walking backward
(c) The presence of convulsions, tremors, lacrimation, red-colored tears, salivation, diarrhea, vocalization, etc.
(d) Changes in sensory and motor functions (for details, see the following sections)

### Neurologic examinations

These examinations often provide an indication of the site of neurotoxicity. Most of these examinations can be performed in humans as well as in animals. The exceptions relate to the determination of *mental state* and many *sensory functions*, which can be more readily assessed in humans.

*Cranial nerves* I through XII have different functions, and their tests therefore vary. For example, tests of the acoustic and optic nerves involve the evaluation of responses to sound and light stimuli.

*Motor examination* includes inspection of muscles for weakness, atrophy, and fasciculation, which indicate dysfunction of the lower motor neuron, that is, the anterior horn cells, motor roots, and peripheral nerves. Spasticity is a sign of dysfunction of the upper motor neurons in the brain and their axons down to the spinal cord. Resting tremor is often associated with lesions in the basal ganglia or cerebellum. Intention tremor occurs during voluntary movement and is a manifestation of cerebellar disease.

*Reflex examination* includes deep tendon reflexes, the functioning of which involves the intrafusal receptors, dorsal root ganglia, anterior horn cells and their axons, neuromuscular junction, and muscle. Damage to any of these structures will cause these reflexes to be absent or hypoactive. On the other hand, when there is upper motor neuron dysfunction, these reflexes will be exaggerated. The Babinski reflex is the most important superficial cutaneous reflex. Abnormal response is an indication of corticospinal dysfunction.

*Gait abnormalities* may also aid in locating the site of toxicity. For example, lower motor neuron disease causes a high-stepping gait. A scissoring, or stiff, gait indicates upper motor neuron lesion. Cerebellar dysfunction results in an ataxic or reeling gait.

## Morphologic examinations

Neurotoxicants may act on the CNS, PNS, or both. Neurotoxicants may induce lesions in the neuronal perikaryon or its axon, either proximally or distally, myelinating cells or myelin sheath itself, astrocytes, or endothelial cells. Morphologic examinations are, therefore, important in establishing the precise site of toxic lesions on an anatomic level. Examinations on cellular and ultrastructural levels often facilitate the differential diagnosis of the neuropathy.

Some of the commonly used techniques, along with a list of references, have been provided by Spencer et al. (1980). It is worth noting, however, that damage to endothelial cells may be demonstrated not only by signs of edema (fewer cells and nerve fiber per unit area), but also by increases in the pressure of the intracranial and endoneural fluids as well as by the penetration of tracer substances, such as horseradish peroxidase, through the endothelium.

## Electrophysiological examinations

### Peripheral nerves

A frequently used examination involves the measurement of *motor nerve* conduction velocity. This can be done on intact animals subjected to short-term or chronic exposure to neurotoxicants or on exposed nerves after local application of the toxicants. *Sensory nerve* conduction velocity and action potentials have also been measured in the study of neurotoxicity.

#### *Electromyography*

This procedure calls for the examination of the electrical activities of a muscle, at rest and when contracted, recorded with the aid of a needle electrode inserted into the muscle. Neurotoxicity may manifest as (1) abnormal insertional activity, (2) occurrence of spontaneous electrical activity of a resting muscle, and (3) interference pattern of electrical activity of motor units during voluntary muscle contraction (Goodgold and Eberstein, 1977).

## *Behavioral studies: Testing procedures*

There is a large body of information on behavioral toxicology, resulting from a widespread feeling that behavior is a subtle and sensitive indicator of toxicity. However, this view has been questioned by Norton for example (1980), who stated: "Scientific data supporting this view are not only scanty but the available evidence often flatly contradicts this assumption." It is the hope that improved testing procedures will increase the sensitivity and utility of this approach in neurotoxicology. A few highlights of this subject are presented here.

The tests involve two types of responses: (1) unconditioned responses, which are either emitted (spontaneous) or elicited (reflex); (2) conditioned responses, which may be considered as either "classic conditioning" (Pavlov) or operant conditioning (Skinner). The extent of the training required of the experimental animals and the neurobehavioral function to be assessed is also a useful criterion for the classification of the tests.

### *Simple tests*

Tilson et al. (1980) listed tests that require little or no prior training of the experimental animals (rats and mice) (Table 18.2).

### *More involved tests*

The tests listed in Table 18.3 require extended or special training, frequent evaluation, and/or manipulation of motivational factors.

### *Procedures to enhance sensitivity*

Because of the large functional reserve of the brain, focal damage may not result in any overt brain dysfunction. Such damage, however, may be

*Table 18.2* Examples of primary level neurobehavioral tests for rats or mice

| Neurobehavioral function | Behavioral test |
|---|---|
| | **Sensory** |
| Visual, olfactory, somatosensory, auditory | Localization |
| Pain | Tail flick |
| Orientation in space | Negative geotaxis |
| | **Motor** |
| Spontaneous activity | Activity in Automex |
| Muscular weakness | Forelimb grip; hindlimb extensor |
| Fatigability | Swim endurance |
| Tremor | Frequency of occurrence |
| | **Cognitive: Associative** |
| Learning and retention | One-way avoidance; step-through passive avoidance |
| | **Affective: Emotional** |
| Responsiveness | Startle to air puff; emergence in a novel environment |
| | **Physiological: Consummatory** |
| Thermoregulation | Body weight; food and water ingestion; core temperature |

*Source:* Tilson HA et al., *Experimental and Clinical Neurotoxicology*, Williams & Wilkins, Baltimore, MD, pp. 758–766, 1980.

*Note:* EPA (1994) has provided some guidelines on schedule-controlled operant behavior.

demonstrated clinically with the use of *provocative* tests. These involve administering sodium amobarbital, raising body temperature, or lowering blood pH with the intravenous infusion of ammonium chloride (Lehrer, 1974).

### *Animal models other than rats and mice*

Apart from rats and mice, other animals such as pigeons, cats, dogs, and monkeys are also commonly used, with testing procedures similar to those listed earlier.

## *Evaluation*

In view of the wide range of toxic effects on the nervous system, as outlined above, there is clearly a need for a battery of tests for the evaluation

***Table 18.3*** Examples of secondary level neurobehavioral tests for rats or mice

| Neurobehavioral function | Behavioral test |
|---|---|
| | **Sensory** |
| Visual, auditory, olfactory | Operant psychophysics |
| Gustatory | Taste discrimination |
| Somatosensory | T-maze discrimination |
| Orientation in space | T-maze discrimination |
| Pain | Operant titration |
| | **Motor** |
| Spontaneous activity | Diurnal cyclicity; patterning |
| Muscular strength | Operant response force |
| Tremor | Spectral analysis |
| | **Cognitive: Associative** |
| Learning and retention | Autoshaping; temporal discriminating; repeated acquisition |
| | **Affective: Emotional** |
| CNS excitability | Brain self-stimulation; aversion thresholds |
| | **Physiologic: Consummatory** |
| Thermoregulation | Diurnal patterning; cyclicity; preference |

*Source:* Tilson HA et al., *Experimental and Clinical Neurotoxicology*, Williams & Wilkins, Baltimore, MD, pp. 758–766, 1980.

of neurotoxicants. It is also worth noting that the choice of animal species is critical in eliciting certain types of toxicity, such as delayed neurotoxicity. Further, the nature of the toxicity on the nervous system, as on other organs, varies according to duration of exposure. For example, *n*-hexane and TOCP produce, after acute exposure, narcosis, but induce axonopathy after repeated exposures.

The significance of a neurotoxic effect depends on its reversibility. In general, irreversible effects are more serious than reversible ones. The site of the effect also plays an important role. There are areas in the nervous system more critical to physiologic function than others. In addition, focal damage in areas with abundant functional reserve is likely to be less serious.

The behavioral effects are especially susceptible to endogenous and environmental variations. Norton (1980) reported data to indicate a large variability of results both between animals of the same species and within the same animal at different times. It is therefore important to adhere to proper experimental procedures, such as sufficiently large number of animals, rigorously controlled experimental environments, and proper statistical analysis of results. The need for randomization and blind outcome has also been emphasized to reduce bias in neurobehavioral scores in animal studies (Hirst et al., 2014).

## References


Abel EJ, Jacobson S, Sherwin BJ (1983). In utero ethanol exposure: Functional and structural brain damage. *Neurobehav Toxicol Teratol* 5, 139–46.

Abou-Donia MB (1981). Organophosphorus ester-induced delayed neurotoxicity. *Annu Rev Pharmacol Toxicol* 21, 511–48.

Berti-Mattera LN, Eichberg J, Schrama L et al. (1990). Acrylamide administration alters protein phosphorylation and phospholipid metabolism in rat sciatic nerve. *Toxicol Appl Pharmacol.* 103, 502–11.

Bouldin TW, Gaines ND, Bagvell CR et al. (1981). Pathogenesis of trimethyltin neuronal toxicity. *Am J Pathol.* 104, 237–49.

Carmicheal WW (1994). The toxins of cyanobacteria. *Sci Am.* 270, 78–86.

Cho ES, Spencer PS, Jortner BS (1980). Doxorubicin. In: Spencer PS, Schaumberg HH, eds. *Experimental and Clinical Neurotoxicology.* Baltimore, MD: Williams & Wilkins, pp. 440–55.

Correale J, Villa A (2009). Cellular elements of the blood-brain barrier. *Neurochem Res.* 34, 2067–77.

Craig PH, Barth ML (1999). Evaluation of the hazards of industrial exposure to tricresyl phosphate: A review and interpretation of the literature. *J Toxicol Environ Health B.* 2, 281–300.

Dawson VL, Dawson TM, London ED et al. (1991). Nitric oxide mediates glutamate neurotoxicity in primary cortical culture. *Proc Natl Acad Sci USA.* 88, 6368–71.

DeBoni U, Otros A, Scott JW et al. (1976). Neurofibrillary degeneration induced by systemic aluminum. *Acta Neuropathol.* 35, 285–94.

EPA (1994). Health Effects Testing Guidelines. Code Federal Refutations, Title 40, Part 798.

Egleton RD, Abbruscato T (2014). Drug abuse and the neurovascular unit. *Adv Pharmacol.* 71, 451–80.

Exon JH (2006). A review of the toxicology of acrylamide. *J Toxicol Environ Health B.* 9, 397–412.

Gold GB, Austin DR (1991). Regulation of aberrant neurofilament phosphorylation in neuronal perikarya. *Brain Res.* 563, 151–62.

Goodgold J, Eberstein A (1977). *Electrodiagnosis of Neuromuscular Diseases.* Baltimore, MD: Williams & Wilkins.

Griffin JW, Price DL (1980). Proximal axonopathies induced by toxic chemicals. In: Spencer PS, Schaumberg HH, eds. *Experimental and Clinical Neurotoxicology.* Baltimore, MD: Williams & Wilkins, pp. 161–78.

Hirst JA, Howick J, Aronson JK, Roberts N, Perera R, Koshiaris C, Heneghan C (2014). The need for randomization in animal trials: An overview of systematic reviews. *PLoS One.* 9, e98856.

Jacobs JM, Carmichael N, Cavanagh JB (1977). Ultrastructural studies in the nervous system of rabbits poisoned with methyl mercury. *Toxicol Appl Pharmacol.* 39, 249–61.

Johnson MK (1990). Contemporary issues in toxicology, organophosphates and delayed neuropathy—Is NTE alive and well? *Toxicol Appl Pharmacol.* 103, 385–99.

Kallman MJ, Fowler SC (1994). Assessment of chemically induced alterations in motor functions. In: Chang LW, ed. *Principles of Neurotoxicology.* New York: Marcel Dekker, 373–96.

Kim JH, Byun HM, Chung EC, Chung HY, Bae ON (2013). Loss of integrity: Impairment of the blood-brain barrier in heavy metal-associated ischemic stroke. *Toxicol Res.* 29, 157–64.

Krewski D, Yokel RA, Nieboer E et al. (2007). Human health risk assessment for aluminium, aluminium oxide, and aluminium hydroxide. *J Toxicol Environ Health B.* 10(Suppl. 1), 1–269.

Lehrer GM (1974). Measurement of minimal brain dysfunction. In: Xintaras C, Johnson BL, de Groot I, eds. *Behavior Toxicology.* Washington, DC: National Institute for Occupational Safety and Health.

Mizisin AP, Weerasuriya A (2011). Homeostatic regulation of the endoneurial micro-environment during development, aging and in response to trauma, disease and toxic insult. *Acta Neuropathol.* 121, 291–312.

Narahashi T (1992). Nerve membrane $Na^+$ channels as targets of insecticides. *Trends Pharmacol Sci.* 13, 236–41.

Norton S (1980). Behavioral toxicology: A critical appraisal. In: Witschi HR, ed. *The Scientific Basis of Toxicity Assessment.* Amsterdam, The Netherlands: Elsevier/North Holland, pp. 91–107.

OECD. (1984). Delayed neurotoxicity of organophosphorus substances. In: Guidelines for Testing Chemicals. Paris, France: Organization for Economic Cooperation and Development.

Olney JW, Rhee V, Ho OL (1974). Kainic acid: A powerful neurotoxic analogue of glutamate. *Brain Res.* 77, 507–12.

Pope CN (1999). Organophosphorous pesticides: Do they all have the same mechanism of toxicity? *J Toxicol Environ Health B.* 2, 161–81.

Press MF (1977). Lead encephalopathy in neonatal Long-Evans rats: Morphologic studies. *J Neuropathol Exp Neurol.* 36, 169–93.

Savolainen J (1977). Some aspects of the mechanism by which industrial solvents produce neurotoxic effects. *Chem Biol Interact.* 18, 1–10.

Schield LK, Griffin JW, Drachman DB et al. (1977). Retrograde axonal transport: A direct method for measurement of rate. *Neurology.* 27, 393.

Song Y, Xue Y, Liu X et al. (2008). Effects of acute exposure to aluminum on blood-brain barrier and the protection of zinc. *Neurosci Lett.* 445, 42–6.

Soni MG, White SM, Flamm WG et al. (2001). Safety evaluation of dietary aluminum. *Reg Toxicol Pharmacol.* 33, 66–79.

Spencer PS, Bischoff MC, Schaumberg HH (1980). Neuropathological methods for the detection of neurotoxic disease. In: Spencer PS, Schaumberg HH, eds. *Experimental and Clinical Neurotoxicology.* Baltimore, MD: Williams & Wilkins, pp. 743–57.

Spencer PS, Sabri MI, Schaumberg HH et al. (1979). Does a defect in energy metabolism in the nerve fiber cause axonal degeneration in polyneuropathies? *Ann Neurol.* 5, 501–7.

Tilson HA, Cabe PA, Burne TA (1980). Behavioral procedures for the assessment of neurotoxicity. In: Spencer PC, Schaumberg HH, eds. *Experimental and Clinical Neurotoxicology.* Baltimore, MD: Williams & Wilkins, pp. 758–66.

Worden AN, Heywood R, Prentice DE et al. (1978). Clioquinol toxicity in the dog. *Toxicology.* 9, 227.

Xing C, Hayakawa K, Lok J, Arai K, Lo EH (2012). Injury and repair in the neurovascular unit. *Neurol Res.* 34, 325–30.

Yang W, Tiffany-Castiglioni E (2008). Paraquat-induced apoptosis in human neuroblastoma SH-SY5Y cells: Involvement of p53 and mitochondria. *J Toxicol Environ Health A.* 71, 289–99.

Zhang J, Snyder SH (1995). Nitric oxide in the nervous system. *Am Rev Pharmacol Toxicol.* 35, 213–33.

Zhang X, Jones D, Gonzalez-Lima F (2006). Neurodegeneration produced by rotenone in the mouse retina: A potential model to investigate environmental pesticide contributions to neurodegenerative diseases. *J Toxicol Environ Health A.* 69, 1681–97.

*chapter nineteen*

# *Toxicology of the cardiovascular systems*

**Ok-Nam Bae**

*Contents*



## *General considerations*

The cardiovascular system is composed of two parts: the heart and the blood vessels. The heart is a vital organ in the body, providing essential energy sources to each organ. Although the heart is not a common target organ for xenobiotic-associated toxicity, it can be damaged by a variety of chemicals. These compounds act either directly on the myocardium or indirectly through the nervous system or blood vessels. In terms of blood vessels, smooth muscle cells and endothelial cells may be major target cells for chemical-mediated toxicity, since they are continuously exposed to absorbed xenobiotics by the systemic circulation. A list of chemicals showing cardiotoxicity is presented in Table 19.1. Table 19.2 provides a list of chemicals with vascular toxic potential.

***Table 19.1*** Cardiotoxic drugs and chemicals

| | |
|---|---|
| **Cardiomyopathy** | |
| Allylamine | Adrenergic agonists |
| Furazolidone | Methysergide |
| Ethanol | Vasodilators |
| Cobalt | |
| **Mitochondrial dysfunction** | |
| Doxorubicin | Anticancer drugs |
| Rosiglitazone | Antidiabetic drugs |
| Alcohol | |
| **Interference with nucleic acid metabolism and protein synthesis** | |
| Antineoplastic drugs | |
| **Electrophysiological mechanisms** | |
| Cardiotonic drugs | Local anesthetics |
| Phenytoin (diphenylhydantoin) | Emetine |
| Tricyclic antidepressants | Chlordimeform |
| Clofibrate | Contrast media |
| Lithium | Antimalarial drugs |
| Propylene glycol | Calcium antagonists |
| **Nonspecific myocardial depression** | |
| Lipid-soluble, organic compounds | Antimicrobial antibiotics |
| Myocardial depressant factor | Carbromide, carbromal |
| **Involvement with lipid metabolism** | |
| High cholesterol diet | Brominated vegetable oils |
| Rapeseed oil | |
| **Miscellaneous** | |
| Phenothiazines | |

*Source:* Van Stee EW, *The Scientific Basis of Toxicity Assessment*, Elsevier/North Holland, New York, 1980; Varga ZV et al., *Am J Physiol Heart Circ Physiol.*, 309, H1453–H1467, 2015.

**Table 19.2** Vasculotoxic drugs and chemicals

| | |
|---|---|
| **Endothelial impairment** | |
| VEGF inhibitors | Anticancer drugs |
| Cisplatin | Anticancer drugs |
| Bleomycin | Anticancer drugs |
| Rofecoxib | Anti-inflammatory drugs |
| Arsenic | Heavy metal |
| Monocrotaline | Plant toxin |
| **Smooth muscle dysfunction** | |
| Arsenic | Heavy metal |
| 5-Fluorouracil | Anticancer drugs |
| Sorafenib | Anticancer drugs |
| **Miscellaneous** | |
| Allylamines | |

## Toxic effects on the heart

The heart is mainly composed of myocardial cells, each measuring about 15 × 80 μm. Unlike skeletal muscle cells, each of which is innervated, only some of the heart muscle cells are innervated. However, these cells are joined, at their ends, to each other by the nexus which has low resistance and thus allows a rapid transmission of electrical stimulus from one cell to the next. These characteristics are essential to the programmed sequence of contraction of different parts of the heart. The myocardium is also different from skeletal muscles in that there is less contractile material (50% vs. 80%) but greater mitochondrial matter (35% vs. 2%). Mitochondria thus play an important role in cardiac contractility and serve as a common subcellular target of cardiotoxicity.

Myocardial contraction involves the liberation of energy from oxidative metabolism, conservation of the energy by adenosine triphosphate and creatine phosphate, and utilization of energy by contractile proteins. The most vulnerable mechanisms include the utilization of energy and intracellular movement of calcium ions, which is involved in the contractility of the myocardium as well as regulating enzyme activities, and transduction of hormonal information. Since the regulation of myocardial cell contraction and myocardial systolic function is regulated by delicate signaling pathways in cellular and organ levels, alterations of these pathways consequently results in cardiotoxicity. There is an emerging concern for drug-induced cardiotoxicity, as exemplified in chemotherapy-related

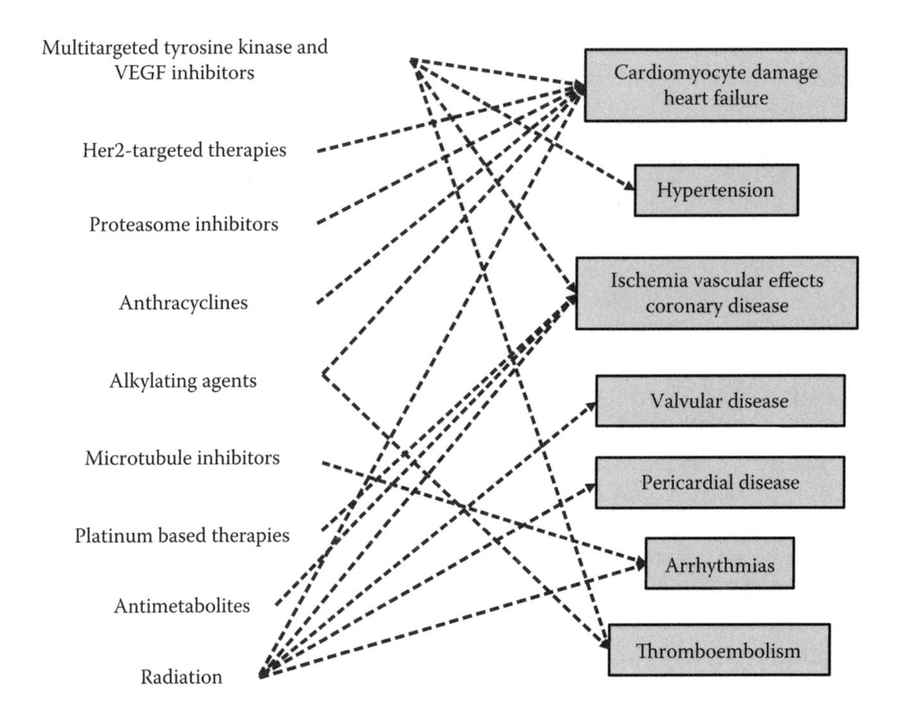


***Figure 19.1*** Cardiotoxocity of chemotherapy. (Modified from Lenneman CG and Sawyer DB, *Circ Res.*, 118, 1008–1020, 2016.)

cardiac dysfunction (Figure 19.1), and therefore a closer monitoring and understanding of the mode of action is needed to prevent chemical-associated cardiotoxicity.

## *Cardiomyopathy*

The main mechanisms of cardiomyopathy induced by drugs and chemicals are summarized as dysregulation of intracellular calcium, mitochondrial impairments, and oxidative stress. Cobalt is known to produce a number of serious and fatal cases of cardiomyopathy, and studies suggested that intramitochondrial accumulation of calcium may mediate cobalt-associated cardiotoxicity. The toxicity of cobalt on the heart was markedly enhanced by malnutrition, especially deficiency of certain amino acids. Grice (1972) noted that cobalt ions reduced oxygen uptake and interfered with cardiac energy metabolism in the tricarboxylic acid cycle, as thiamine deficiency increased. Cobalt may reduce the available myocardial $Ca^{2+}$ by complexing with macromolecules and could also be antagonistic to endogenous $Ca^{2+}$.

Adrenergic β-receptor agonists, isoproterenol in particular, and vasodilating antihypertensive drugs, such as hydralazine, are capable of inducing myocardial necrosis. The former chemicals have direct adrenergic effects, whereas the antihypertensive drugs exert adrenergic effects via the induced hypotension. These effects produce an augmented transmembrane calcium influx, which subsequently induce an increase in the rate and force of contraction. This, along with the concomitant hypotension, results in cardiac hypoxia. Hypoxia and calcium deposits in the mitochondria produce disintegration of organelles and sarcolemma (Balazs et al., 1981).

The anthracycline antibiotics, including doxorubicin, are known to be associated with acute adverse effects of hypotension, tachycardia, and arrhythmias. More prolonged administration of these drugs produce degeneration and atrophy of cardiac muscle cells and interstitial edema and fibrosis. Anthracycline antibiotics are known to generate reactive oxygen species (ROS) in cardiac myocytes, and consequently induced oxidative damage in protein, nucleic acids, and lipid. These modifications of key macromolecules in cardiomyocytes ultimately lead to dysregulation in contractile function and cell death such as apoptosis or necrosis (Zhang et al., 2012). The mechanism of doxorubicin-induced cardiotoxicity is particularly involved in apoptosis mediated by calcium overload and iron-catalyzed formation of free radicals while the anticancer mode of action is due to the inhibition of topoisomerase II (Bernard et al., 2011). Doxorubicin, containing quinones in its chemical structure, enhances ROS generation in primary cultures of cardiomyocytes in a time- and concentration-dependent manner (Fu et al., 2010).

## *Interference with nucleic acid synthesis and DNA damage*

As described above, the generation of oxidative stress is suggested as one of the main mechanism of cardiotoxicity of anthracycline antibiotics, doxorubicin, and daunorubicin. In addition, the binding of these antibiotics to mitochondrial and nuclear DNA, which subsequently interferes with the synthesis of RNA and protein, may be a potential mechanism. This effect on the heart is important because the half-life of the contractile proteins is relatively short (12 weeks). Other possible mechanisms of action include peroxidation of membrane lipids and hypotension resulting from release of cytokines (Van Stee, 1980).

Of note, mitochondrial DNA is known to be highly susceptible to oxidative stress compared to nuclear DNA, since the mitochondria is one of the main cellular location of ROS generation, and protective mechanisms against DNA damage such as histones or a DNA repair system are limited in mitochondria (Marzetti et al., 2013). The oxidative mitochondrial DNA may be one of the mechanisms for cardiotoxicity as observed in alcoholic cardiomyopathy (Piano and Phillips, 2014).

## *Arrhythmias*

A number of fluorocarbons are capable of producing cardiac arrhythmias. This effect is mediated by a sensitization of the heart to epinephrine, depression of contractility, reduction of coronary blood flow, and reflex rise in sympathetic and vagal impulses to the heart following irritation of mucosa in the respiratory tract (Aviado, 1978).

Tricyclic antidepressants also induce cardiac arrhythmias. These effects are likely the result of imbalances within the autonomic regulatory system of the heart. Propylene glycol, a common solvent, converts ventricular tachycardia induced by deslanoside into ventricular fibrillation (Keller et al., 1992).

Arrhythmias are also suggested as one of the most common toxicities mediated by taxanes, antineoplatic chemotherapeutic agents (Lenneman and Sawyer, 2016). Paclitaxel decreased calcium increase and contraction in cardiomyocytes, and reduced the time from the maximum contracted state to relaxation (Howarth et al., 1999). Different types of arrhythmias were enhanced by taxane, as bradyarrhythmias, spraventricular arrhythmias including atrial fibrillation, atrial flutter, and atrial tachycardias were observed following taxane exposure.

## *Myocardial depression*

A number of lipid-soluble organic compounds, such as general anesthetics, depress cardiac contractility. The probable mechanism of action is a nonspecific expansion of various cellular membranes by the insertion of chemically indifferent molecules in the hydrophobic regions of integral proteins and membrane phospholipids.

Antibiotics, such as amphotericin B, chloramphenicol, streptomycin, and tetracycline, produce hypotension through depression of cardiac contractility. The mechanism of action appears to be related to an inhibition of $Ca^{2+}$ bound to superficial membrane sites (Keller et al., 1992).

## *Miscellaneous*

Rapeseed oil, a common cooking oil in many parts of the world, produces accumulation of lipid globules in heart muscles of rats. This effect was attributed to the high content of erucic acid in rapeseed oil. Brominated vegetable oils, used in adjusting the density of flavoring oils and in enhancing cloudy stability in beverages, induce biochemical and morphological changes in cardiac myofibrils. The coloring Brown FK also produces severe morphological changes in the heart muscles.

## Toxic effects on blood vessels

The vascular system consists of arteries, arterioles, capillaries, venules, and veins. A toxicant may affect any of these vessels; the seriousness of the effect depends upon the physiological role of the organ that is supplied by the affected blood vessels (Herrmann et al., 2016). The representative adverse symptoms associated with vascular toxicity are illustrated in Figure 19.2. Vascular smooth muscle cells and endothelial cells are known to be affected by several vasotoxicants and the mechanism of vascular

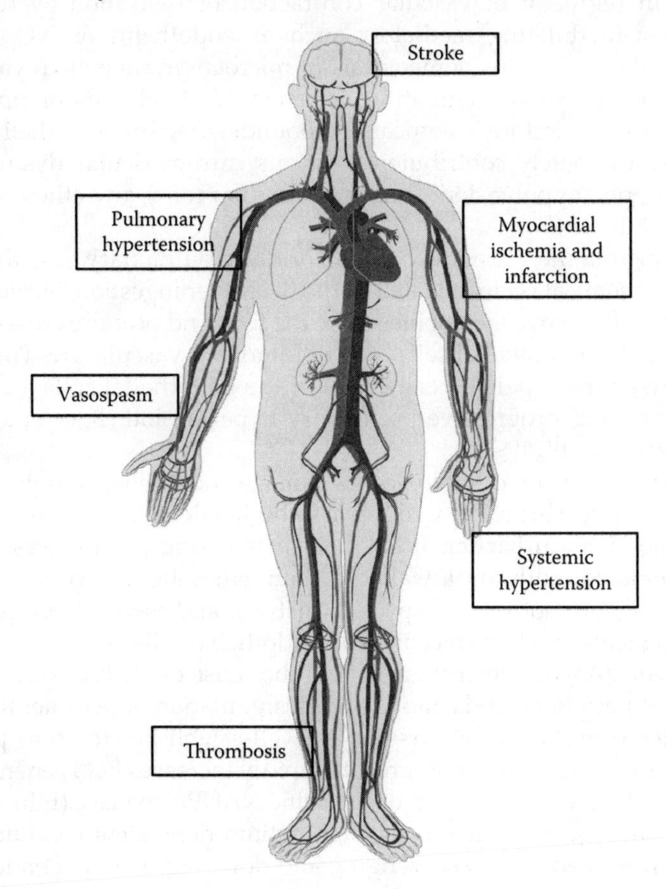


***Figure 19.2*** Vascular toxocity and related symptoms. (Modified from Herrmann J et al., *Circulation*, 133, 1272–1289, 2016.)

toxicity varies according to the target molecules affected by the toxicants. Representative mechanisms are enhancement of ROS generation, disruption of cGMP/NO/NOS pathway, or DNA damage for endothelial toxicity, and interruption of contractile machinery, such as Rho kinase pathway or phosphorylation of myosin light chain, or calcium dysregulation for smooth muscle toxicity.

## *Endothelial damage and increased capillary permeability*

Endothelium, the lining of endothelial cells, is a critical interface between blood and vessels which can be a primary target for toxicants. Endothelium is a main regulator of vascular contraction or relaxation by releasing vasomotor-modulating mediators such as endothelin or NO, respectively. It also maintains homeostasis in microenvironments in vascular/hemostatic system by regulating adhesion of blood cells or uptake of lipoproteins. Therefore, chemical compounds affecting endothelial function may ultimately contribute to various cardiovascular dysfunctions such as hyper/hypotension (abnormal vascular tone), and atherosclerosis (Mason, 2016).

Monocrotaline, a plant toxin, may produce pulmonary vascular damage. This chemical is bioactivated in the liver after ingestion, but sufficient amounts of the active metabolites leave the liver and produce cross-linking of DNA in the endothelial cells of the pulmonary vasculature. This effect can damage the repairing capability of the endothelial cells leading to thrombosis and progressive pulmonary hypertension (Boor et al., 1995; Schultze and Roth, 1998).

Lead and several other toxicants damage endothelial cells of capillaries in the brain. This effect will result in brain edema and an impairment of the blood–brain barrier. Inhalation of irritating gas induces pulmonary edema. Recently, multiwalled carbon nanotubes (MWCNT) used in electronics, automotive, aerospace industries, and medical devices were found to increase cell permeability in endothelial cells.

Arsenic (As) has been suggested as the cause of the *black-foot* disease, a result of peripheral endarteritis and dysregulation of peripheral microcirculation (Lin et al., 1998). Arsenic is a well-established toxicant, producing endothelial damage. Inorganic As rapidly increases ROS generation in endothelial cells via activation of a specific NADPH oxidase (Ellinsworth, 2015). It subsequently attenuates endothelium-dependent conduit artery dilation mediated by NO scavenging and downregulation of endothelial NO synthase. This mechanism is suggested to contribute to As-associated cardiovascular diseases in populations exposed to As-contaminated drinking water (Lee et al., 2003; Bae et al., 2008).

## Vasoconstriction and vasodilatation

Ingestion of ergot alkaloids (fungal contaminants in certain foods) may produce gangrene resulting from vasoconstriction. Exposure to pure oxygen over a prolonged period may result in blindness, especially among premature infants, evidently because of the associated vasoconstriction in the eye. Arsenic is also known to induce calcium sensitization, resulting in increased vasoconstriction in smooth muscle cells (Lee et al., 2005). An anticancer agent sorafenib induces impaired regulation of Rho kinase, contributing to potential vasospasm (Arima et al., 2009).

Occupational workers exposed to nitroglycerin were reported to suffer sudden mortality due to heart attack on their days off. Apparently, the continued exposure to a coronary dilator rendered the workers accustomed to a low level of coronary flow, and sudden cessation of exposure to the coronary dilator precipitated coronary insufficiency.

The musculature of the coronary artery may be damaged by large doses of certain hypotensive drugs such as minoxidil and hydralazine. The lesion may be a result of exaggerated pharmacodynamic changes (Boor et al., 1995).

## Atherosclerosis

Atherosclerosis is a complex degenerative disease mainly affecting large blood vessels such as the coronary and carotid arteries. Narrowing of these arteries may result in heart attacks and strokes, respectively. While the etiology of atherosclerosis is complex, certain toxicants may aggravate the pathological condition. Carbon monoxide may increase the permeability of capillaries surrounding these arteries and promote degenerative processes (Yang et al., 1998). Exposure to air pollutants resulted in an increased frequency of hospital admissions for cardiovascular disease, congestive heart failure, and higher mortality (Chung et al., 2005; Dominic et al., 2005; Yang, 2008). Carbon disulfide ($CS_2$) produces damage to the endothelium. Ramos et al. (1994) observed that certain allylamines and aromatic hydrocarbons might contribute to the development of atherosclerosis. These toxicants may act through NO and endothelin on the smooth muscle and endothelium of arteries, and induce vascular lesions, which could contribute to the development of atherosclerosis.

## Fibrosis

Cadmium and lead may affect blood vessels in kidneys producing renal fibrosis. The impairment of blood supply may interfere with the "nonexcretory functions" of the kidneys, and indirectly produce hypertension.

### *Hypersensitivity reaction*

Gold salts, penicillin, sulfonamides, and a number of other toxicants may induce vasculitis or exacerbate preexisting polyarteritis. The condition usually affects small vessels and is associated with the infiltration of eosinophils and mononuclear cells, indicating an involvement of the immune system.

### *Tumors*

Tumors of blood vessels may result from certain toxicants. For example, vinyl chloride was reported to produce hemangiosarcoma in the liver of humans and animals; hemangioendothelioma was shown to result from exposure to thorium dioxide.

## *Testing procedures for cardiovascular toxicities*

Cardiovascular toxicity can be studied in intact normal animals, in animals with specific pathological conditions, such as hypertension or diabetes mellitus, or in isolated hearts and blood vessels.

### *Normal animals*

Various examinations for cardiovascular toxicity can be performed on animals in conventional toxicity studies. These include blood pressure, heart rate, and electrocardiography. The rate of blood flow is a useful indicator of the functions of the cardiovascular systems and is measured using, among others, pulsed Doppler flow meter (Haywood et al., 1981). The status of the arterioles, capillaries, and venules can be studied either at a specific site of organism (e.g., conjunctiva and retina) or through microvascular chamber which can be chronically placed on a lab animal (Smith et al., 1994). Functional tests, such as swimming until exhaustion, have been suggested. At necropsy, the organ weight is often determined. Gross, light, and in particular, electron microscopic examinations are valuable. Biochemical studies of the myocardium and of the blood are also useful.

### *Animals with pathological conditions*

The hearts of rabbits fed a diet containing 2% cholesterol become atherosclerotic. These hearts are more susceptible to myocardial ischemia (Lee et al., 1978). Other models, such as infarcted myocardium, cardiomyopathic hamster, obesity, and drug interaction models have been described and referenced by Van Stee (1980).

### *Isolated heart or cultured cardiomyocytes*

The isolated, perfused heart is a common model for studying the effects of drugs on the strength and rate of heart contractions and rate of coronary flow. It is also used to detect the cardiac effects produced by toxicants. Toy et al. (1976) showed that certain halogenated alkanes depressed the peak left ventricular pressure as well as the rate of rise of that pressure. The isolated atrium and cultured heart cells have also been used in the study of cardiotoxicity (Adams et al., 1978; Sperelakis, 1978).

*In vitro* assays using cultured myocytes are relevant models to study functional alterations of excitation or contraction, however, the replicating integrated cardiovascular physiology along with achieving the efficiency and reproducibility has been challenged. Recently, stem cell-derived cardiomyocytes were thought to develop *in vitro* cardiovascular functions (Peters et al., 2015), and these cells, which beat spontaneously, are getting attention for toxicity screening.

### *Isolated vessels or cultured vascular cells*

The isolated aortic rings can be applied to study vascular contraction or relaxation in an organ bath system. Primary isolated or cultured smooth muscle cells have been used to evaluate the effects of chemicals on essential signaling pathways in contractile machinery. Primary or cultured endothelial cells, which have intact NO signaling pathway, are also useful to evaluate vascular toxicity. Recent progress using endothelial progenitor cells contribute to study xenobiotic-associated endothelial damage.

### *Evaluation*

The cardiovascular toxicity of chemicals is not readily detected in conventional toxicity studies. For example, the toxic effects of cobalt and anthracycline antibiotics on the heart were reproduced in animal experiments only after they were detected in humans first. Negative results, therefore, do not necessarily exclude potential cardiotoxicity.

To demonstrate such toxicity, specific testing procedures may be required. These procedures usually mimic the clinical conditions. For example, intermittent administration of the anthracycline antibiotics was necessary to elicit cardiotoxicity; presumably continuous treatment caused the animals to die from other toxic effects before heart lesions developed.

The toxicity of adrenergic β-receptor agonists is best detected in acute studies; the effects of prolonged treatment may be masked by tolerance development (Balazs and Ferrans, 1978).

## *References*

Adams HR, Parker JL, Durrett LR (1978). Cardiac toxicities of antibiotics. *Environ Health Perspect*. 26, 217–31.

Arima Y, Oshima S, Noda K, Fukushima H, Taniguchi I, Nakamura S, Shono M et al. (2009). Sorafenib-induced acute myocardial infarction due to coronary artery spasm. *J Cardiol*. 54, 512–5.

Aviado DM (1978). Effects of fluorocarbons, chlorinated solvents, and inosine on the cardiopulmonary system. *Environ Health Perspect*. 26, 207–16.

Bae ON, Lim KM, Han JY, Jung BI, Lee JY, Noh JY, Chung SM et al. (2008). U-shaped dose response in vasomotor tone: A mixed result of heterogenic response of multiple cells to xenobiotics. *Toxicol Sci*. 103, 181–90.

Balazs T, Ferrans VJ (1978). Cardiac lesions induced by chemicals. *Environ Health Perspect*. 26, 181–91.

Balazs T, Ferrans VJ, El-Hage A et al. (1981). Study of the mechanism of hydralazine-induced myocardial necrosis in the rat. *Toxicol Appl Pharmacol*. 59, 524–34.

Bernard Y, Ribeiro N, Thuaud F et al. (2011). Flavaglines alleviate doxorubicin cardiotoxicity: Implication of Hsp27. *PLoS One*. 6, e25302.

Boor PJ, Gotlieb AI, Joseph EC et al. (1995). Chemical-induced vasculature injury. *Toxicol Appl Pharmacol*. 132, 177–95.

Chung CC, Tsai SS, Ho SC et al. (2005). Air pollution and hospital admissions for cardiovascular disease in Taipei. *Environ Res*. 98, 130–9.

Dominic F, McDermott A, Daniels M et al. (2005). Revised analysis of the national morbidity, mortality and air pollution study: Mortality among residents of 90 cities. *J Toxicol Environ Health A*. 68, 1071–92.

Ellinsworth DC (2015). Arsenic, reactive oxygen, and endothelial dysfunction. *J Pharmacol Exp Ther*. 353, 458–64.

Fu Z, Guo J, Jing L et al. (2010). Enhanced toxicity and ROS generation by doxorubicin in primary cultures of cardiomyocytes from neonatal metallothionein-I/II null mice. *Toxicol In Vitro*. 24, 1584–91.

Grice HC (1972). The changing role of pathology in modern safety evaluation. *CRC Crit Rev Toxicol*. 1, 119–52.

Haywood JR, Shaffer RA, Fink GD et al. (1981). Regional blood flow measurements with pulsed Doppler flowmeter in conscious rat. *Am J Physiol*. 241, 14273–8.

Herrmann J, Yang EH, Iliescu CA, Cilingiroglu M, Charitakis K, Hakeem A, Toutouzas K et al. (2016). Vascular toxicities of cancer therapies: The old and the new—An evolving avenue. *Circulation*. 133, 1272–89.

Howarth FC, Calaghan SC, Boyett MR, White E (1999). Effect of the microtubule polymerizing agent taxol on contraction, Ca2+ transient and L-type Ca2+ current in rat ventricular myocytes. *J Physiol*. 516, 409–19.

Keller RS, Parker JL, Adams HR (1992). Cardiovascular toxicity of antibacterial antibiotics. In: Costa D, ed. *Cardiovascular Toxicology*. New York: Raven Press, pp. 165–95.

Lee MY, Jung BI, Chung SM, Bae ON, Lee JY, Park JD, Yang JS et al. (2003). Arsenic-induced dysfunction in relaxation of blood vessels. *Environ Health Perspect.* 111, 513–7.

Lee MY, Lee YH, Lim KM, Chung SM, Bae ON, Kim H, Lee CR et al. (2005). Inorganic arsenite potentiates vasoconstriction through calcium sensitization in vascular smooth muscle. *Environ Health Perspect.* 113, 1330–5.

Lee RJ, Zaidi IH, Baky SH (1978). Pathophysiology of the atherosclerotic rabbit. *Environ Health Perspect.* 26, 225–31.

Lenneman CG, Sawyer DB (2016). Cardio-oncology; An update on cardiotoxicity of cancer-related treatment. *Circ Res.* 118, 1008–20.

Lin TH, Huang YL, Wang MY (1998). Arsenic species in drinking water, hair, fingernails and urine of patient's with blackfoot disease. *J Toxicol Environ Health A.* 53, 85–93.

Marzetti E, Csiszar A, Dutta D, Balagopal G, Calvani R, Leeuwenburgh C (2013). Role of mitochondrial dysfunction and altered autophagy in cardiovascular aging and disease: From mechanisms to therapeutics. *Am J Physiol Heart Circ Physiol.* 305, H459–76.

Mason JC (2016). Cytoprotective pathways in the vascular endothelium. Do they represent a viable therapeutic target? *Vascul Pharmacol.* doi: 10.1016/j.vph.2016.08.002. [Epub ahead of print].

Peters EB, Liu B, Christoforou N, West JL, Truskey GA (2015). Umbilical cord blood-derived mononuclear cells exhibit pericyte-like phenotype and support network formation of endothelial progenitor cells in vitro. *Ann Biomed Eng.* 43, 2552–68.

Piano MR, Phillips SA (2014). Alcoholic cardiomyopathy: Pathophysiologic insights. *Cardiovasc Toxicol.* 14, 291–308.

Ramos KS, Bowes RC, Ou XL et al. (1994). Responses of vascular smooth cells to toxic insult: Cellular and molecular perspectives for environmental toxicants. *J Toxicol Environ Health.* 43, 419–40.

Schultze AE, Roth RA (1998). Monocrotaline pulmonary hypertension—The monocrotaline model and involvement of the hemostatic system. *J Toxicol Environ Health B.* 1, 271–346.

Smith TL, Koman LA, Mosberg AT (1994). Cardiovascular physiology and methods for toxicology. In: Hayes AW, ed. *Principles and Methods of Toxicology.* New York: Raven Press.

Sperelakis N (1978). Cultured heart cell reaggregate model for studying cardiac toxicology. *Environ Health Perspect.* 26, 243–67.

Toy PA, Van Stee EW, Harris AM et al. (1976). The effects of three halogenated alkanes on excitation and contraction in the isolated, perfused rabbit heart. *Toxicol Appl Pharmacol.* 38, 7–17.

Van Stee EW (1980). Myocardial toxicity. In: Witschi HR, ed. *The Scientific Basis of Toxicity Assessment.* New York: Elsevier/North Holland.

Varga ZV, Ferdinandy P, Liaudet L, Pacher P (2015). Drug-induced mitochondrial dysfunction and cardiotoxicity. *Am J Physiol Heart Circ Physiol.* 309, H1453–67.

Yang CY (2008). Air pollution and hospital; Admissions for congestive heart failure in a subtropical city: Taipei, Taiwan. *J Toxicol Environ Health A.* 71, 1085–90.

Yang W, Jennison BL, Omaye ST (1998). Cardiovascular disease hospitalization and ambient levels of carbon monoxide. *J Toxicol Environ Health A*. 55, 185–96.

Zhang S, Liu X, Bawa-Khalfe T, Lu LS, Lyu YL, Liu LF, Yeh ET (2012). Identification of the molecular basis of doxorubicin-induced cardiotoxicity. *Nat Med*. 18, 1639–42.

# *chapter twenty*

# *Toxicology of the reproductive systems*

***Hyung Sik Kim***

*Contents*



## *Reproductive system*

### *Reproductive process and organs*

The reproductive process starts with gametogenesis. In females, oogenesis involves the formation of primary oocytes from the primordial germ cells (oogonia) through mitosis. This development takes place during the fetal period and ceases at the time of giving birth. Primary oocytes divide by meiosis to form secondary oocytes prior to ovulation.

In males, spermatogenesis starts with gonocytes during the fetal period, after which these cells are transformed into spermatogonia after birth. Spermatogonia remain dormant until puberty, when proliferative activity begins again. Some of the spermatogonia multiply to form additional spermatogonia while others mature to spermatozoa. There are three intermediate stages of spermatogenesis; spermatogonia divide by mitosis to form primary spermatocytes, which divide by meiosis to form secondary spermatocytes, which subsequently divide to form spermatids; and finally spermatids become spermatozoa by metamorphosis. The entire process is a continuous one, and the time required for spermatogonia to become spermatozoa is about 60 days (Figure 20.1).

Fertilization requires not only functional ovum and spermatozoa but also effective delivery of the sperm and proper milieu. The conceptus and fertilized ovum is then implanted in the uterus and develops through embryonic and fetal stages. At the end of the gestational period, parturition takes place. Preparation for parturition involves coordinated changes in both mother and fetus. The mother needs to develop the ability to produce and eject milk in order to feed the newborn. The pups suckle until weaning and then grow and mature to start the reproductive process again, thus completing a reproductive cycle.

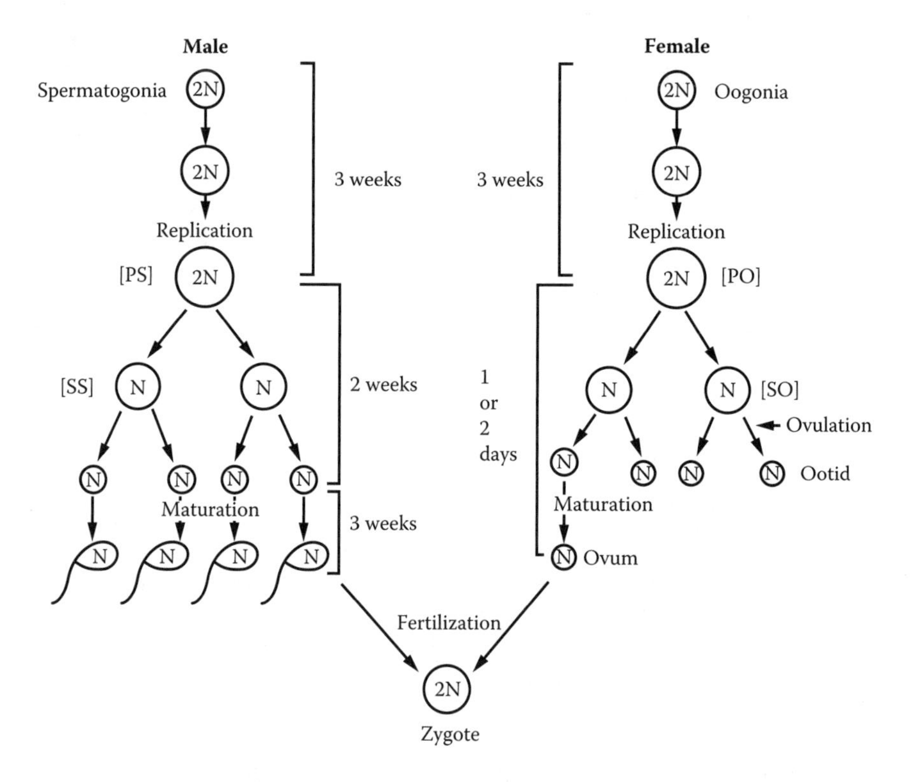


*Figure 20.1* Gametogenesis and fertilization. *Abbreviations*: 2N, diploid; N, haploid; PO, primary oocyte; PS, primary spermatocyte; SO, secondary oocyte; SS, secondary spermatocyte. (From Brusick D, *Principles of Genetic Toxicology*, 2nd ed., Plenum Press, New York, 1987.)

## Other cells and organs

While gametocytes are the essential elements of the reproductive process, other cells and organs also play important roles in reproduction. In the male reproductive system, spermatogenesis occurs in testicular seminiferous tubules. In these tubules are the Sertoli cells, extending from the basement membrane to the lumen of the seminiferous tubules, which contain androgen-binding proteins (ABPs). The ABPs facilitate movement of androgen to the spermatocytes for development. In addition, there are Leydig cells, which are located in the interstitial tissue surrounding the seminiferous tubules. These cells are the main sites of synthesis of testosterone, which is essential not only for development of the reproductive system but also for proper functioning.

After leaving the testis spermatozoa are stored in the epididymis, where they undergo changes in order to gain fertile capacity and for later delivery into the female reproductive system. In addition, the accessory organs, prostate, and seminal vesicle provide special nutrients and proper milieu for the sperm. These organs respond to the effect of testosterone, and hence their weights are indicators of the blood level of this hormone.

The external female genitals consist of numerous parts, including the vaginal opening, clitoris, urethra, labia minora, and labia. The female reproductive system is designed to carry out several functions. The female reproductive system produces egg cells necessary for reproduction, termed ova or oocytes. The system is designed to transport the ova to the site of fertilization. The ova may be affected by chemicals while they are in the ovaries. However, it is more often the fertilized ova that are affected either directly or indirectly through damage to the uterus.

## Pharmacokinetics

Throughout the reproductive cycle, toxicants may act directly on the reproductive system or the conceptus, or indirectly via certain endocrine organs. Before chemicals act directly, they need to reach the target organs in sufficiently high concentrations. This level may be higher or lower than the concentration in blood. For example, in case of DDT, the concentration is almost 80 times higher in the ovary than plasma. A number of other substances have also been shown to penetrate the oocyte, oviduct, uterine fluid, and blastocyst (Fabro, 1978).

Unlike the ovaries, the testis is protected by the blood–testis barrier (BTB) (Lee and Dixon, 1978). The BTB is a complex of a multicellular system composed of capillary endothelial cells, myoid cells, and membranes surrounding the seminiferous tubules and the tightly joined Sertoli cells in the tubules. This barrier, however, is less effective than the blood–brain barrier (BBB). The penetration rate of chemicals into the testis is governed by their molecular weights, partition coefficients, and ionic characteristics. The BTB is constituted of coexisting junctions between Sertoli cells near the basement membrane, which include tight junctions, basal ectoplasmic specializations, gap junctions, and desmosome-like junctions although the BBB and the blood–retina barrier constitute tight junctions between endothelial cells (Su et al., 2011).

The testis contains both activating and detoxicating enzyme systems. These two enzyme systems, as noted in Chapter 3, are capable of increasing and reducing toxicities of chemicals, respectively. Further, there is an efficient DNA repair mechanism in the premeiotic spermatogenic cells, but none exists in spermatids or in spermatozoa; mutations in these cells may therefore be induced by genotoxic substances.

## *Toxicants and their effects*

Reproductive toxicity includes the toxic effects of a substance on the reproductive ability of an organism and the development of its offspring. Reproductive toxicity is defined by the Globally Harmonized System as adverse effects of chemicals on sexual function and fertility in both males and females, as well as developmental toxicity in the offspring. The reproductive functions may be affected by many toxicants through their effects on the reproductive system of either gender. In the male, the formation, development, storage, and delivery of spermatozoa may be adversely affected. The oocytes, in the females, are also susceptible to certain toxicants. In addition, the implantation of the fertilized ova as well as the growth and development of the conceptus may be affected. In both genders, some of the toxic effects are mediated through hormonal or nervous system activities. For example, 2,3,7,8-tetrachlorodibenzo-*p*-dioxin (TCDD) exposure leads to altered folliculogenesis in ovary and TCDD exposure decreases the number of antral follicles without increasing in atresia. These results suggest that TCDD exerts an antiproliferative effect on the rat ovary (Karman et al., 2012). Although TCDD has been associated with alterations in ovarian function and hormones in animals, the influence of the toxicant has not been studied in humans. On July 10th, 1976, an explosion exposed residents of Seveso, Italy, to the highest levels of TCDD in their blood. Twenty years later, the Seveso Women's Health Study to study reproductive health was initiated (Warner et al., 2006).

Outcomes of reproductive toxicity were assessed to be relevant to humans using laboratory animals under study conditions. In general, adverse responses on reproductive ability or capacity or on development in humans demonstrating that a chemical classify three categories by reproductive toxicity tests. For example, two categories for positive results (clear evidence and some evidence); one category for uncertain findings (equivocal evidence); one category for no observable effects (no evidence); and one category for experiments that cannot be evaluated because of major design or performance flaws (inadequate study). It is clear that relationships exist between reproductive outcomes such as spontaneous abortions, congenital malformations, low birth weight, developmental disabilities, and infertility. In addition, multiple effects have been shown for many developmental toxicants (Table 20.1).

## *Male reproductive system*

Many chemicals adversely affect spermatogenesis and produce testicular atrophy. These include food colorings (e.g., Oil Yellow AB and Oil Yellow OB) (Allmark et al., 1955), pesticides (e.g., dibromochloropropane [DBCP]), plastics (phthalates), metals (e.g., arsenic, tin, lead, and cadmium), and organic solvents. A variety of other chemicals affect the testis, such as steroid hormones, alkylating agents, cyclohexylamine, and hexachlorophene (Schardein, 1976).

In addition to a reduced sperm count resulting from adverse effects on spermatogenesis, a toxicant may render spermatozoa defective, less mobile, or even dead. For example, both methyl methane sulfonate (MMS) and busulfan produce lethal mutations, but MMS affects spermatids and spermatozoa, whereas busulfan affects the pre-spermatogenic cells. These alkylating agents apparently attack the DNA of these cells, which undergo different repair mechanisms (Lee, 1983).

Spermatozoa may also be affected while being stored in the epididymis. For example, the male antifertility agent α-chlorohydrin inhibits the fertilizing capacity of spermatozoa. Gossypol, another such agent that was extensively employed in China (Qian and Wang, 1984), probably acts through a similar mechanism.

The testis is hormonally regulated by the hypothalamus–pituitary–testis axis: follicle-stimulating hormone (FSH) is required in the initiation of spermatogenesis through the production of ABP in Sertoli cells, whereas luteinizing hormone (LH) acts on Leydig cells to synthesize testosterone (Figure 20.2).

There are potential male reproductive toxicants among many industrial and pharmaceutical chemicals. However, no complete list exists of male reproductive hazards in the workplace. Scientists are just beginning to understand as how these hazards affect the male reproductive system. Although more than 1000 workplace chemicals have been demonstrated to possess reproductive toxicities in experimental animals, most have not been studied in humans. The potential hazards of chemicals against the male reproductive system are shown in Table 20.2.

*Table 20.1* Adverse effects of chemical exposure associated with multiple adverse reproductive outcomes

| | Adverse outcomes | | | | |
|---|---|---|---|---|---|
| Chemicals | Spontaneous abortion | Congenital malformation | Low birth weight | Developmental disabilities | Infertility |
| Alcohol | X | X | X | X | |
| Mercury | X | X | X | | X |
| Lead | X | | X | X | |
| Organic solvents | X | X | | X | |
| Smoking | X | X | X | | |
| Thalidomide | | X | | | |
| Diethylstilbestrol | | X | | X | |
| Valproic acid | | X | | | |
| Isotretinoin | | X | | | |

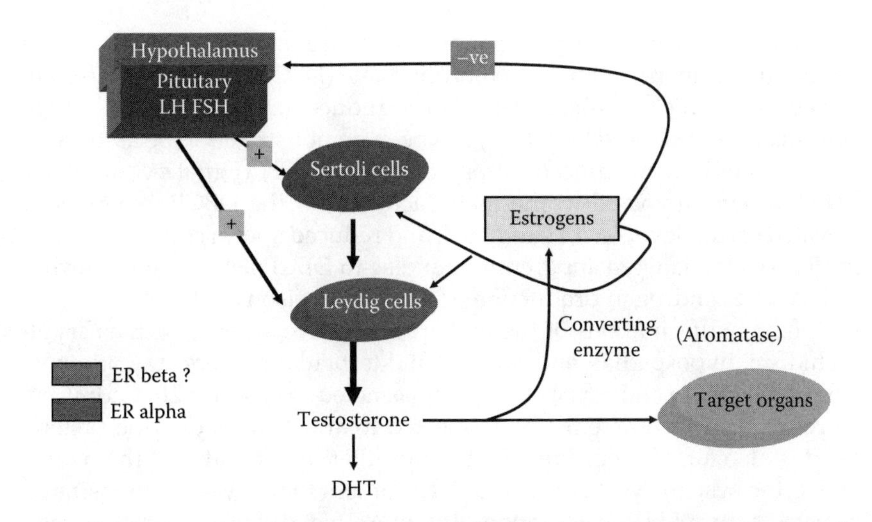


***Figure 20.2*** Possible sites of action for estrogens and androgens on the reproductive axis in male rats. (From Ferin M, *Reproductive Endocrinology, Surgery, and Technology, vol. 1*, Lippincott-Raven, Philadelphia, pp. 103–21, 1996.)

***Table 20.2*** Potential male reproductive toxicants

| Compound | Clinical manifestation | Chemical reactivity site | Mechanism/target |
|---|---|---|---|
| DBCP | | Sperm | Number of sperm |
| | | | Sperm shape |
| Lead | | Hypothalamus | Decreased FSH |
| | | Pituitary | Decreased progesterone |
| | | Ovary | |
| Mercury | | Hypothalamus | Altered gonadotrophin production and secretion |
| | | Ovary | Follicle toxicity |
| | | | Granulosa cell proliferation |
| Cadmium | | Ovary | Vascular toxicity |
| | | Pituitary | Granulosa cell cytotoxicity |
| | | Hypothalamus | Cytotoxicity |
| | | Oogenesis | Disruption of DNA/RNA synthesis |
| Phthalates | | Hypothalamus | Oestrogen agonist |
| DDT | | Pituitary | FSH, LH disruption |
| PCBs, PBBs | | | FSH, LH disruption |

Some toxicants may affect reproductive function via the action of endocrine hormones. Dibromochloropropane (DBCP), a fumigant used in agriculture, which has been reported to induce azoospermia and oligospermia in occupational workers, has been demonstrated to be associated with elevated serum concentrations of LH and FSH (Egnatz et al., 1980). Male workers involved in the manufacturing of the DBCP experienced elevated serum levels of LH and FSH, and reduced sperm count and fertility. These effects were apparently sequelae to DBCP actions upon Leydig cells to alter androgen production or action (Mattison et al., 1990).

Some malformations of the male reproductive system, such as cryptorchidism, hypospadias, and prostate and testicular cancers may originate from exposure to endocrine-disruptors (as noted in Chapter 21). Cadmium, mercury, lead, and arsenic are suspected to affect the endocrine system. Lead is also a male reproductive toxicant that directly affects the neuroendocrine system. Men exposed to lead for less than 1 year demonstrated elevated serum LH concentrations, but this effect did not progress in men exposed to the metal for more than 5 years. On the other hand, serum levels of free testosterone were significantly reduced after exposure to lead for 3 to 5 years (Rodamilans et al., 1988). In contrast, serum concentrations of LH, FSH, total testosterone, prolactin, and total neutral 17-ketosteroids were not markedly changed in workers with lower circulating levels of lead, even though the distribution frequency of sperm count was altered (Assennato et al., 1986). Cigarette smoke contains about 30 metals, of which cadmium, arsenic, and lead are present in the highest concentrations, and the cadmium body burden in smokers is about double that of nonsmokers (ATSDR). Further, excessive generation of reactive oxygen species (ROS) in the sperm results in lipid peroxidation of polyunsaturated fatty acids in their plasma membrane (Koppers et al., 2008). Several metals, including iron, copper, nickel, lead, and cadmium, may increase ROS production, decrease glutathione and other antioxidant levels, enhance lipid peroxidation of the cell membrane, initiate apoptosis, and contribute to oxidative damage of DNA (Jones et al., 1979; Liang et al., 1990; Aitken et al., 1993; Wellejus et al., 2000). Transition metals may adversely affect male reproductive system in terms of causing a disruption of spermatogenesis, a reduction in sperm count, motility, and viability, an increase in oxidative stress, an inhibition of testicular steroidogenesis, serum testosterone, libido, and a decline in fertility. Exposure to 2-ethoxyethanol has also been reported to reduce sperm count without a concurrent change in serum LH, FSH, or testosterone concentrations in shipyard painters (Welch et al., 1988).

Some compounds possess structural similarity with sex steroid hormones bind to the endocrine receptor, thus acting as agonists or antagonists, and disrupt biological responses. Chlordecone, an insecticide that binds to estrogen receptors (ER), resulted in reduced sperm count and motility. These effects result from interference induced by chlordecone on estrogen actions at the neuroendocrine or testicular level. DDT and its metabolites also exhibit steroidal properties and might be expected to alter male reproductive function by interfering with steroidal hormone functions. PCBs, polybrominated biphenyls (PBBPs), and organochlorine pesticides may also interfere with male reproductive functions by exerting estrogenic agonist/antagonist activity (Mattison et al., 1990).

Reproductive functions are also under the influence of the autonomic nervous system. Thus, the hypotensive drug losulazine, which acts by depleting norepinephrine levels, produces reversible infertility in male rats, probably through altered sexual behavior and ejaculatory disturbances (Mesfin et al., 1989). Guanethidine, another hypotensive drug, may produce or fail to induce pregnancy by interfering with seminal emission (Palmer, 1976).

Carlsen et al. (1992) reported from a meta-analysis that human sperm concentration has subsequently declined from $113 \times 10^6$/ml to $66 \times 10^6$/ml of semen during the last 50 years. Additionally, the incidence of human male hypospadias, cryptorchidism, and testicular cancer has also been markedly increased over the last 50 years (Giwercman et al., 1991). Although many investigators indicated gradual incidence of human testicular cancer, there exists no definitive evidence to prove causality that environmental chemicals induce such adverse human health effects. There is clear evidence that exposure to some chemicals increase the incidence of testicular cancer. For example, the herbicide linuron may induce Leydig cell tumors and tumorigenesis was observed to be mediated through sustained hypersecretion of LH (Cook et al., 1993). In contrast to rats, which are likely to develop Leydig cell tumors, testicular tumors are more likely to arise from germ cells in men. Cadmium exposure was found to induce prostate cancer in men (Waalkes and Rehm, 1994).

## *Female reproductive system*

Mechanisms underlying female reproductive toxicity are complex. Numerous xenobiotics have been demonstrated to be toxic to the male reproductive process compared to females. However, it is not known whether the difference is due to underlying differences in toxicity or the greater ease of studying sperm than oocytes. The potential hazards of chemicals against female reproductive system are shown in Table 20.3. Oocytes may be damaged by chemotherapeutic agents such as heavy metals, nitrogen mustard, vinblastine, and polycyclic aromatic hydrocarbons such as 3-methylcholanthrene and benzo(*a*)pyrene. Data exist, which clearly demonstrate that oocytes can be damaged by alkylating agents. These drugs destroy oocytes in humans and animals (Morgan et al., 2012). Lead,

*Table 20.3* Potential female reproductive toxicants

| Compound | Clinical manifestation | Site | Mechanism/target |
|---|---|---|---|
| | | **Chemical reactivity** | |
| Alkylating agents | Altered menses | Ovary | Granulosa cell cytotoxicity |
| | Amenorrhoea | | Oocyte cytotoxicity |
| | Ovarian atrophy | Uterus | Endometrial cell cytotoxicity |
| | Decreased fertility | | |
| | Premature menopause | | |
| Lead | Abnormal menses | Hypothalamus | Decreased FSH |
| | Ovarian atrophy | Pituitary | Decreased progesterone |
| | Decreased fertility | Ovary | |
| Mercury | Abnormal menses | Hypothalamus | Altered gonadotrophin production and secretion |
| | | Ovary | Follicle toxicity |
| | | | Granulosa cell proliferation |
| Cadmium | Follicular atresia | Ovary | Vascular toxicity |
| | Persistent diestrus | Pituitary | Granulosa cell cytotoxicity |
| | | Hypothalamus | Cytotoxicity |
| | | **Structural similarity** | |
| Azathioprine | Reduction in follicle numbers | Ovary | Purine analog |
| | | Oogenesis | Disruption of DNA/RNA synthesis |
| Chlordecone | Impaired fertility | Hypothalamus | Oestrogen agonist |
| DDT | Altered menses | Pituitary | FSH, LH disruption |
| PCBs, PBBs | Abnormal menses | | FSH, LH disruption |

*Source:* Mattison DR et al., *Environ Health Perspect* 48, 43–52, 1983; Morgan S et al., *Hum Reprod Update*. 18, 525–35, 2012; Trabert et al., *Environ Health Perspect*. 118, 1280–5, 2010; Porpora MG et al., *Environ Health Perspect*. 117, 1070–5, 2009.

*Note:* These compounds are suggested to be direct-acting reproductive toxicants based primarily on toxicity testing in experimental animals.

mercury, and cadmium also lead to ovarian damage that may be mediated through toxic effects on oocyte. The pesticide DDT isomer induces suppression of progesterone production with potencies apparently equal to that of estradiol. DDT may affect the development and growth of the conceptus and thus lower fetal weight (Fabro, 1978). Previous studies reported association between occurrence of endometriosis and elevated blood PCB levels in women, while a subsequent small clinical study found no significant correlations between disease severity in women and serum levels of halogenated aromatic hydrocarbons (Porpora et al., 2009; Trabert et al., 2010).

Prostaglandin synthetase inhibitors, for example aspirin-like drugs, may block ovulation. Oocytes are more resistant before puberty to the adverse effects of chemicals, evidently because they are dormant. Certain organochlorine pesticides such as methoxychlor, similar to estradiol, may increase the weight of the uterus (Eroschenko and Rourke, 1992). Prostaglandin synthetase inhibitors may also affect other reproductive functions. Haloperidol was shown to prevent implantation. Spironolactone may interfere with ovulation and implantation of the fertilized ovum; it may also retard the development of the sex organs of the offspring (Nagi and Virgo, 1982). Gossypol is also toxic to females as it suppresses ovarian steroid hormone secretion, interrupts regular cyclicity, and inhibits embryo implantation (Lin et al., 1994).

There is a relationship between the extent of cigarette smoking and the onset of menopause; menopause is an indication of oocyte depletion (Miller et al., 1987; Zenzes et al., 1995). The toxic effects that are specifically related to the production of congenital anomalies are dealt with in Chapter 9. Further detailed analysis of isolated granulosa cell responses to xenobiotics is needed to define the utility of this assay system.

Considering that these persistent, bioaccumulative perfluorinated compounds have been in the market for decades, it is likely that many of these studies show the effects on a second generation of exposed children. Effects in adults, especially women, are also of great concern, which range from disruption of thyroid hormones and reproductive function, to polycystic ovary syndrome, and early menopause.

## *Routine testing: Multigeneration reproduction studies*

### *Animals and doses*

In general, rats are the animals of choice for routine testing. A minimum of 20 female and 10 male rats are usually placed in each of three dose groups and a control group. OECD Guidelines (1995) recommends 10 animals of each gender. The doses are selected so that the high dose will produce some minimal toxic signs but will not result in mortality greater than 10%. The low dose will not induce any observable effect.

Prior to breeding, animals are dosed for 10 weeks prior to mating. However, because of the difference in the time required for maturation of the gametes, the males are dosed for 70 days (the period of spermatogenesis) and females for 14 days (the length of the development of the ova). Dosing of females is continued through gestation and lactation periods.

The test chemical should be administered by a route that most closely resembles that of human exposure.

To determine the potential effect of the chemical on the reproductive function of the offspring ($F_1$), a second-generation offspring ($F_2$) is bred and reared to reproductive maturity.

### *Observations and examinations*

The adult animals are observed for changes in body weight, food consumption, general appearance, estrus cycle, and mating behavior. In addition, the fertility and nesting and nursing behaviors are also noted. Half of the maternal rats are sacrificed on day 13 of gestation for examination of corpora lutea, implantation, and resorption.

The other half of the pregnant rats are allowed to deliver their pups. These are examined for litter size, number of stillborn, gender distribution, and congenital anomalies. In addition, the viability and pup weight are recorded at the time of birth, on day 4, and at weaning, and preferably also on day 12 or 14. Auditory and visual function and behavior are also examined for subtle congenital defects.

An appropriate number of males and females are randomly selected from all generations and examined by gross necropsy and histopathology, especially with respect to the reproductive organs. In males, the weight and histopathology of the testes, epididymides, seminal vesicles, prostate, and pituitary often provide useful information on the site of action of the toxicant under test. Other indicators of the effects are the sperm count, its motility and morphology, as well as the levels of certain hormones, especially testosterone, FSH, and TH. In females, the weight and histopathology of the vagina, uterus, oviduct, ovaries, and pituitary should be assessed along with the levels of the relevant hormones.

Additional details and references to the reproduction and fertility studies are provided in the EPA test guidelines (1994). The EPA may obtain data on the potential male reproductive toxicity of an agent from various sources including, but not limited to, studies carried out according to the agency's test guidelines. These may include acute, subchronic, and chronic testing as well as reproduction and fertility studies. Male-specific endpoints that may be encountered in such studies are identified in Table 20.4. A variety of measures to evaluate the integrity of the female reproductive system has been used in toxicity studies. With appropriate measures, a comprehensive evaluation of the reproductive process can be achieved, including identification of target organs and possible elucidation of the mechanisms involved in the agent's effect(s). Areas that may be examined in evaluations of the female reproductive system are listed in Table 20.5.

***Table 20.4*** Male-specific endpoints of reproductive toxicity

| | |
|---|---|
| Organ weight | Testes, epididymides, seminal vesicles, prostate, pituitary |
| Visual examination and histopathology | Testes, epididymides, seminal vesicles, prostate, pituitary |
| Sperm evaluation[a] | Sperm number (count) and quality (morphology, motility) |
| Sexual behavior[a] | Mounts, intromissions, ejaculations |
| Hormone levels[a] | Luteinizing hormone, follicle stimulating hormone, testosterone, estrogen, prolactin |
| Developmental effects | Testis descent[a], preputial separation, sperm production[a], ano-genital distance, structure of external genitalia[a] |

*Source:* EPA, *Guidelines for Reproductive Toxicity Risk Assessment*, Federal Register 61, (212), 56274–56322, 1996.

[a] Reproductive endpoints that can be obtained or estimated relatively noninvasively with humans.

***Table 20.5*** Female-specific endpoints of reproductive toxicity

| | |
|---|---|
| Organ weight | Ovary, uterus, vagina, pituitary |
| Visual examination and histopathology | Ovary, uterus, vagina, pituitary, oviduct, mammary gland |
| Estrous (menstrual[a]) cycle normality | Vaginal smear cytology |
| Sexual behavior[a] | Lordosis, time to mating, vaginal plugs, or sperm |
| Lactation[a] | Offspring growth, milk quantity and quality |
| Development | Normality of external genitalia[a], vaginal opening, vaginal smear cytology, onset of estrous behavior (menstruation[a]) |
| Senescence | Vaginal smear cytology, ovarian histology (menopause[a]) |

*Source:* EPA, *Guidelines for Reproductive Toxicity Risk Assessment*, Federal Register 61, (212), 56274–56322, 1996.

[a] Endpoints that can be obtained relatively noninvasively with humans.

## *Evaluations*

From these data, a number of disturbances of reproductive function can be deduced using the following indices:

1. *Fertility index:* The percentage of mating resulting in pregnancy
2. *Gestation index:* The percentage of pregnancies resulting in the birth of live litters
3. *Viability index:* The percentage of live pups that survive for 4 days or longer
4. *Lactation index:* The percentage of pups alive on day 4 and that survive for 21 days or longer

Other indicators of effects include (*i*) mating index (the percentage of estrus cycles that had mating), (*ii*) male fertility index (the percentage of males exposed to fertile nonpregnant females that resulted in pregnancies), (*iii*) female fertility index (the percentage of females exposed to fertile males that resulted in pregnancies), and (*iv*) 12- or 14-day survival indices.

Multigeneration reproductive study can reveal a variety of toxic effects on the reproductive function as well as on the *conceptus*. Examples are indices of gestation, viability, and survival. However, nonspecific response (e.g., nonpregnancy) is common. It may follow unusual routes of administering the chemical, such as inhalation, topical application to the eye or nose, and parenteral administration. Excessive handling may also disturb the normal reproductive function. A number of other interfering factors have been discussed by Palmer (1976).

The pathological examination may reveal suppression of spermatogenesis, advanced rates of follicle atresia, and ovulatory or meiotic failure.

## *Alternative reproductive toxicity tests*

A number of alternative test guidelines have been suggested in previous studies (Lamb, 1985; Lamb and Chapin, 1985; EPA, 1996). There is no necessity to replace the standard reproductive toxicity tests; data from these protocols may be used depending upon the nature of test chemicals. Moreover, some alternative toxicity tests may offer an expanded array of endpoints and increased flexibility (Francis and Kimmel, 1988).

Assessment of reproductive toxicity by continuous breeding has been developed by the NTP (Lamb and Chapin, 1985; Morrissey et al., 1989; Gulati et al., 1991). This protocol is a one-generation test, but dosing is extended into the $F_1$ generation to make it compatible with the EPA recommendations for a two-generation study (Francis and Kimmel, 1988). A distinctive feature of this protocol is the continuous cohabitation of male–female pairs (in the P generation) for 14 weeks.

Up to five litters can be produced after removing the pups soon after the birth. This protocol provides various information, such as the spacing, number of litters, and size over the 14-week dosing interval. In this protocol, three doses and control groups are initiated in postpubertal males and females (11 weeks of age) 7 days before cohabitation and continued throughout the test period. Offspring that are removed from the dam soon after birth are counted and examined for viability, litter and/or pup weight, sex, external abnormalities, and then discarded. The last litter may remain with the dam until weaning in order to study the effects of in utero as well as perinatal and postnatal exposures. If effects on fertility are observed in the P or F generations, additional reproductive evaluations may be conducted, including fertility studies and crossover mating, to define the affected gender and site of toxicity.

The sequential production of litters from the same adults allows observation of the timing of onset of an adverse effect on fertility. In addition, it improves the ability to detect subfertility due to the potential to produce larger numbers of pregnancies and litters than in a standard single- or multigeneration reproduction study. With continuous treatment, a cumulative effect could increase the incidence or extent of expression with subsequent litters. However, unless offspring are allowed to grow and reproduce (as they are routinely in the more recent version of the RACB protocol) (Gulati et al., 1991), it is not possible to attain useful information on postnatal development or reproductive capability of the second generation.

Sperm measures, including sperm number, morphology, motility, and vaginal smear cytology to detect changes in estrous cyclicity have been added to the RACB protocol at the end of the 12-test period, and their utility has been examined using model compounds in the mouse (Morrissey et al., 1989).

Another test method combines the use of multiple endpoints in both rat genders with initiation of treatment at weaning (Gray et al., 1988). Thus, morphologic and physiologic changes associated with puberty are included as endpoints. Both parent (P) genders are treated (at least three dose levels plus controls) continuously through breeding, pregnancy, and lactation. The $F_1$ generation is mated following a continuous breeding protocol. Vaginal smears are recorded daily throughout the test period to evaluate estrous cycle normality and confirm breeding and pregnancy (or pseudopregnancy). Pregnancy outcome is monitored in both the P and $F_1$ generations at all doses, and terminal studies on both generations include a comprehensive assessment of sperm measures (number, morphology, motility) as well as organ weight, histopathology, and serum and tissue levels of appropriate reproductive hormones. This protocol combines the advantages of a continuous breeding design with acquisition of sex-specific multiple endpoint data at all doses. In addition, identification of pubertal effects makes this protocol particularly useful for detecting compounds with hormone-mediated actions such as environmental estrogens or antiandrogens. It is possible that the effects revealed in multigeneration reproduction studies outlined above will have resulted from paternal, maternal, or fetal exposure. Thus, additional tests are often conducted to establish the cause of the effect. A few such tests are outlined here.

*Pathological examinations* are useful in identifying a variety of toxic effects of toxicants. The weight of testis is a simple but sensitive index of testicular damage. The extent and nature of such damage can often be assessed microscopically. The weight of the prostate and seminal vesicle are often correlated with levels of testosterone. Similarly, a gross and microscopic analysis of *semen* is useful in epidemiological and animal studies. The sperm count and motility, survival, and morphology of spermatozoa often provide information regarding adverse effects of toxicants on the testis (Eliasson, 1978). As noted above, certain toxicants affect reproductive function by inducing disturbances in hormones, especially testosterone, estrogen, FSH, and LH. Assays of their levels may indicate the mode of action of the toxicant.

The perfused male reproductive tracts were found to be useful models in studying the effects of chemicals on the secretion and accumulation of androgens (Bardin et al., 1978).

Certain biomarkers have been used in a variety of tests for studying disorders of the reproductive system. For example, DNA probes were employed to detect gene mutation and excessive deletions and translocations in meiotic and postmeiotic germ cells as well as Sertoli and Leydig cells in the testis (Hecht, 1987).

## References

Aitken RJ, Harkiss D, Buckingham D (1993). Relationship between iron-catalysed lipid peroxidation potential and human sperm function. *J Reprod Fertil*. 98, 257–65.

Allmark MG, Grice HC, Lu FC (1955). Chronic toxicity studies on food colors: Observations on the toxicity of FD&C Yellow No. 3 (Oil Yellow AB) and FD&C Yellow No. 4 (Oil Yellow OB) in rats. *J Pharm Pharmacol*. 7, 591–603.

Assennato GC, Paci ME, Baser R, Molinini RG, Candela BM, Giogino AG (1986). Sperm count suppression with endocrine dysfunction in lead-exposed men. *Arch Environ Health*. 41, 387–90.

Bardin CW, Baker HWG, Jefferson LS et al. (1978). Methods for perfusing male reproductive tract: Models for studying drugs and hormone metabolism. *Environ Health Perspect*. 24, 51–9.

Brusick D (1987). *Principles of Genetic Toxicology*, 2nd ed. New York: Plenum Press.

Carlsen E, Giwercman A, Keiding N, Skakkebaek NE (1992). Evidence for decreasing quality of semen during past 50 years. *BMJ*. 305, 609–12.

Cook JC, Mullin LS, Frame SR et al. (1993). Investigation of a mechanism for Leydig cell tumorigenesis by linuron. *Toxicol Appl Pharmacol*. 119, 195–204.

Egnatz DG, Ott MG, Townsend JC, Olson RD, Johns DB (1980). DBCP and testicular effects in chemical workers: An epidemiological survey in Midland, Michigan. *J Occup Med*. 22, 727–32.

Eliasson R (1978). Semen analysis. *Environ Health Perspect*. 24, 81–5.

EPA (1994). Health Effects Test Guidelines. Washington, DC: U.S. Environmental Protection Agency.

EPA (1996). Guidelines for Reproductive Toxicity Risk Assessment. Published on October 31, Federal Register 61(212), 56274–322.

Eroschenko VP, Rourke AW (1992). Stimulating influences of the technical grade methoxychlor and estradiol on protein synthesis in the uterus of the immature mouse. *J Occup Med Toxicol.* 1, 307–15.

Fabro S (1978). Penetration of chemicals into the oocyte, uterine fluid and preimplantation blastocyst. *Environ Health Persp.* 24, 25–9.

Ferin M (1996). The menstrual cycle: An integrative view. In: Adashi EY, Rock JA, Rosenwaks Z, eds. *Reproductive Endocrinology, Surgery, and Technology, vol. 1.* Philadelphia: Lippincott-Raven, pp. 103–21.

Francis EZ, Kimmel GL (1988). Proceedings of the workshop on one- vs. two-generation reproductive effects. *J Am Coll Toxicol.* 7, 911–25.

Giwercman A, Müller J, Skakkebaek NE (1991). Prevalence of carcinoma in situ and other histopathological abnormalities in testes from 399 men who died suddenly and unexpectedly. *J Urol.* 145, 77–80.

Gray LE, Ostby J, Sigmon R, Ferrell J, Linder R, Cooper R, Goldman J et al. (1988). The development of a protocol to assess reproductive effects of toxicants in the rat. *Reprod Toxicol.* 2, 281–7.

Gulati DK, Hope E, Teague J, Chapin RE (1991). Reproductive toxicity assessment by continuous breeding in Sprague-Dawley rats: A comparison of two study designs. *Fundam Appl Toxicol.* 17, 270–9.

Hecht NB (1987). Detecting the effects of toxic agents on spermatogenesis using DNA probes. *Environ Health Perspect.* 74, 31–40.

Jones R, Mann T, Sherins RJ (1979). Peroxidative breakdown of phospholipids in human spermatozoa: Spermicidal effects of fatty acid peroxides and protective action of seminal plasma. *Fertil Steril.* 31, 531–7.

Karman BN, Basavarajappa MS, Craig ZR, Flaws JA (2012). 2,3,7,8-Tetrachlorodibenzo-*p*-dioxin activates the aryl hydrocarbon receptor and alters sex steroid hormone secretion without affecting growth of mouse antral follicles in vitro. *Toxicol Appl Pharmacol.* 261, 88–96.

Koppers AJ, De Iuliis GN, Finnie JM, McLaughlin EA, Aitken RJ (2008). Significance of mitochondrial reactive oxygen species in the generation of oxidative stress in spermatozoa. *J Clin Endocrinol Metab.* 93, 3199–207.

Lamb JC (1985). Reproductive toxicity testing: Evaluating and developing new testing systems. *J Am Coll Toxicol.* 4, 163–71.

Lamb JC, Chapin RE (1985). Experimental models of male reproductive toxicology. In: Thomas JA, Korach KS, McLachlan JA, eds. *Endocrine Toxicology.* New York: Raven Press, pp. 85–115.

Lee IP (1983). Adaptive biochemical repair response toward germ cell DNA damage. *Am J Ind Med.* 4, 135–47.

Lee IP, Dixon RL (1978). Factors influencing reproduction and genetic toxic effects on male gonads. *Environ Health Perspect.* 24, 117–27.

Liang R, Senturker S, Shi X, Bal W, Dizdaroglu M, Kasprzak KS (1990). Effects of Ni(II) and Cu(II) on DNA interaction with the N-terminal sequence of human protamine P2: Enhancement of binding and mediation of oxidative DNA. *Carcinogenesis.* 20, 893–8.

Lin YC, Coskun S, Sanbuissho A (1994). Effects of gossypol on in vitro bovine oocyte maturation and steroidogenesis in bovine granulosa cells. *Theriogenology.* 41, 1601–11.

Mattison DR, Plowchalk DR, Meadows MJ, Al-Juburi AZ, Gandy J, Malek A (1990). Reproductive toxicity: Male and female reproductive systems as targets for chemical injury. *Med Clin N Am*. 74, 391–411.

Mattison DR, Plowchalk DR, Shiromizu K (1983). Effects of toxic substances on female reproduction. *Environ Health Perspect* 48, 43–52.

Mesfin GM, Morris DF, Seaman WJ et al. (1989). Testicular lesions in rats treated with a sympatholytic hypotensive agent (losulazine). *J Am Coll Toxicol*. 8, 525–38.

Miller RK, Kellogg CK, Saltzman RA (1987). Reproductive and perinatal toxicology. In: Haley TJ, Berndt WO, eds. *Handbook of Toxicology*. Washington, DC: Hemisphere, pp. 195–309.

Morgan S, Anderson RA, Gourley C, Wallace WH, Spears N (2012). How do chemotherapeutic agents damage the ovary? *Hum Reprod Update*. 18, 525–35.

Morrissey RE, Lamb JC, Morris RW, Chapin RE, Gulati DK, Heindel JJ (1989). Results and evaluations of 48 continuous breeding reproduction studies conducted in mice. *Fundam Appl Toxicol*. 13, 747–77.

Nagi S, Virgo BB (1982). The effects of spironolactone on reproductive functions in female rats and mice. *Toxicol Appl Pharmacol*. 66, 221–8.

OECD. (1995). OECD guidelines for testing of chemicals: Reproduction/developmental toxicity screening test. Paris, France: Organization of Economic Development.

Palmer AK (1976). Assessment of current test procedures. *Environ Health Perspect*. 18, 97–104.

Porpora MG, Medda E, Abballe A, Bolli S, De Angelis I, di Domenico A, Ferro A et al. (2009). Endometriosis and organochlorinated environmental pollutants: A case-control study on Italian women of reproductive age. *Environ Health Perspect*. 117, 1070–5.

Qian S, Wang Z (1984). Gossypol: A potential antifertility agent for males. *Annu Rev Pharmacol Toxicol*. 24, 329–60.

Rodamilans M, Osaba MJM, To-Figueras J, Rivera Fillat F, Marques JM, Perez P, Corbella J (1988). Lead toxicity on endocrine testicular function in an occupationally exposed population. *Hum Toxicol*. 7, 125–8.

Schardein JL (1976). *Drugs as Teratogens*. Boca Raton, FL: CRC Press.

Su L, Mruk DD, Cheng CY (2011). Drug transporters, the blood-testis barrier, and spermatogenesis. *J Endocrinol*. 208, 207–23.

Trabert B, De Roos AJ, Schwartz SM, Peters U, Scholes D, Barr DB, Holt VL (2010). Non-dioxin-like polychlorinated biphenyls and risk of endometriosis. *Environ Health Perspect*. 118, 1280–5.

Waalkes MP, Rehm S (1994). Cadmium and prostate cancer. *J Toxicol Environ Health*. 43, 251–69.

Warner M, Eskenazi B, Olive DL, Samuels S, Quick-Miles S, Vercellini P, Gerthoux PM et al. (2006). Serum dioxin concentrations and quality of ovarian function in women of Seveso. *Environ Health Perspect*. 115, 336–40.

Welch LS, Schrader SM, Turner TW, Cullen MR (1988). Effects of exposure to ethylene glycol ethers on shipyard painters: II. Male reproduction. *Am J Ind Med*. 14, 509–26.

Wellejus A, Poulsen HE, Loft S (2000). Iron-induced oxidative DNA damage in rat sperm cells *in vivo* and *in vitro*. *Free Radical Res*. 32, 75–83.

Zenzes MT, Krishnan S, Krishnan B (1995). Cadmium accumulation in follicular fluid of women in IVF is higher in smokers. *Fertil Steril*. 64, 599–603.

# *chapter twenty-one*

# *Toxicology of endocrine-disrupting chemicals*

***Hyung Sik Kim***

*Contents*

## Introduction

Endocrine-disrupting chemicals (EDCs) are considered important in the field of toxicology because of their significant impact on both the ecosystem and public health. The endocrine system is a highly complex organ that regulates numerous body functions and developments. The main function of the endocrine system is to maintain homeostasis, which it achieves using hormones synthesized and secreted from glands such as the hypothalamus, the pituitary gland (produces the luteinizing and follicle-stimulating hormones), the pineal gland (produces melatonin), the pancreas (produces insulin), and sex organs such as ovaries (produce estrogens and progestins) and testes (produce androgens), the thyroid, parathyroid, and adrenal glands (produce corticosteroids). Endocrine glands represent a collection of specialized cells that produce hormones. These hormones are generally classified as lipid derivatives (e.g., eicosanoids/steroids), peptides, and amines, which are synthesized from arachidonic acid/cholesterol, proteins, and amino acids (e.g., tyrosine, tryptophan), respectively.

The endocrine system is crucial for regulation of metabolic processes. Disruption, which involves excess or diminished hormone secretion, results in developmental and reproductive toxicity, carcinogenicity, mutagenicity, neurotoxicity, and immunotoxicity (Choi et al., 2004). Many chemicals act as endogenous estrogens and have been implicated as risk factors for cancer, cardiovascular disease, obesity, diabetes, and behavioral and learning disorders including attention deficit/hyperactivity (ADHD) disorder (Baillie-Hamilton, 2002; Thayer et al., 2012; Birnbaum, 2013). EDCs were the subjects of Rachel Carson's book *Silent Spring* published in 1962. In the intervening half-century, concern over EDCs has grown. It is beyond the scope of this chapter to describe the entire endocrine system; instead, the focus will be on the major endocrine systems that are affected by EDCs. Viewed from this general perspective, the threat posed by EDCs, with endocrine effects (either agonist or antagonistic), has been increasingly serious not only in humans, but also in ecosystems.

## Endocrine-disrupting chemicals

EDCs (also called endocrine-disrupting compounds or endocrine-disruptors) are defined as exogenous chemicals that are structurally

**Table 21.1** Preliminary list of chemicals with endocrine-disrupting effects by animal study

| Type | Chemicals | |
|---|---|---|
| Industrial chemicals | Bisphenol A, phthalate esters, *p*-nonylphenol, octylphenol, polychlorinated biphenyls, pentachlorophenol, styrene, 2,3,7,8-TCDD, tributyltin chloride | |
| Pesticides | Herbicides | Alachlor, amitrole, atrazine, 2,4-D, metribuzin, nitrofen, 2,4,5-T, trifluralin |
| | Insecticides | β-BHC, γ-BHC (lindane), carbaryl, chlordane, *p,p'*-DDD, *p,p'*-DDE, *p,p'*-DDT, dicofol, dieldrin, endosulfan, heptachlor, heptachlor epoxide, methomyl, methoxychlor, mirex, trans-nonachlor, oxychlordane, parathion, pyrethroids (synthetic), toxaphene |
| | Nematocides | Aldicarb, 1,2-dibromo-3-chloropropane |
| Heavy metals | Cadmium, lead, mercury, arsenic | |
| Pharmaceuticals | Diethylstilbestrol, tamoxifen, raloxifene, flutamide, finasteride | |
| Plant and fungal agents | Zearalenone, coumestrol, genistein, daidzein | |

*Source:* Choi and Lee, *J Toxicol Environ Health.*, 451–63, 7, 2004.

*Abbreviations:* DDT, dichlorodiphenyltrichloroethane; TCDD, tetrachlorodibenzo-*p*-dioxin.

similar to hormones, which interfere with the synthesis, secretion, transport, metabolism, and binding action of natural endogenous hormones (EPA, 1998). Initially, concern focused on chemicals with estrogen-like activities, but it has become increasingly apparent that EDCs may mimic or interfere with the actions of all endocrine hormones including androgens, thyroid, adrenal, and pituitary hormones (Colborn et al., 1993; DeRosa et al., 1998; Whitehead and Rice, 2006). Further, an EDC may exert multiple hormonal effects, including estrogenic/antiestrogenic, androgenic/antiandrogenic, or thyroid/antithyroid effects (McKinney and Waller, 1998). EDCs are present in the environment and foods, and sources include pesticides, combustion products, plasticizers, detergents, and heavy metals (Table 21.1).

## Classification of EDCs

Humans are exposed to various environmental chemicals with endocrine-disrupting properties during daily life because EDCs are found in low quantities in a variety of consumer products. EDCs commonly found in

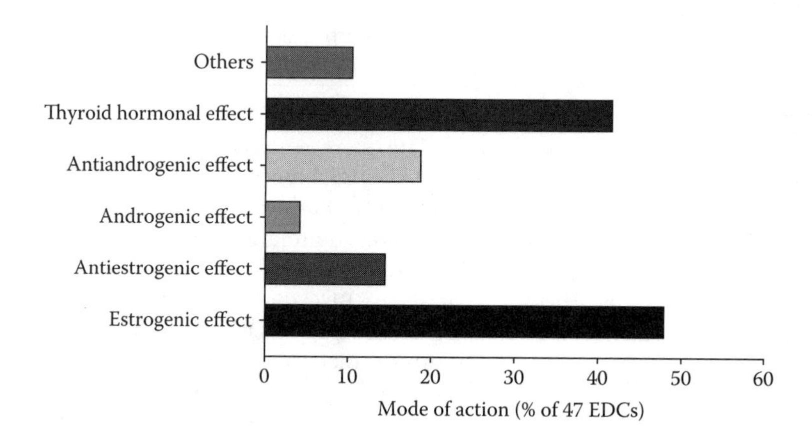


***Figure 21.1*** Hormone-modulating effects of 48 endocrine-disrupting chemicals (EDCs) classified by the Centers for Disease Control and Prevention (CDC). EDCs that have multiple hormone-modulating effects are only counted once.

the environment include herbicides, fungicides, insecticides, and industrial/commercial agents such as bisphenol A (BPA), triclosan, alkylphenol, phthalates, polychlorinated biphenyls (PCBs), and other chlorinated compounds. Accordingly, various EDCs including PCBs, 2,3,7,8-tetrachlorodibenzo-*p*-dioxin (TCDD), dichlorodiphenyl trichloroethane (DDT), BPA, polybrominated diphenyl ethers (PBDEs), and a variety of phthalate esters (PEs) are commonly detected in human blood and urine. These chemicals are classified as estrogenic/antiestrogenic, androgenic/antiandrogenic chemicals, or those that affect thyroid hormone functions (Choi et al., 2004) (Figure 21.1). It is also possible that these compounds affect other important hormones like insulin.

## *Diethylstilbestrol*

Estrogenic chemicals, such as ethinyl estradiol, mestranol, norethynodrel, and megestrol acetate, were developed as contraceptive agents. These drugs are also used in therapy for specific diseases in humans (Newburgh, 1975). In 1971, a clinical report associated diethylstilbestrol (DES) with vaginal adenocarcinoma, which was detected in a small number (<0.1%) of adolescent daughters of women who had taken the drug during the pregnancy period (Herbst et al., 1971). Subsequently, DES was also linked to more frequent benign reproductive tract problems in an estimated 95% of DES-exposed daughters; the manifestations included reproductive organ dysfunction, abnormal pregnancies, reduced fertility, and disorders of the immune system (Giusti et al., 1995). Similarly,

DES-exposed male offsprings demonstrated structural, functional, and cellular abnormalities after prenatal exposure including hypospadias, microphallus, retained testes, inflammation, and decreased fertility (Tomatis, 1994). Based on this medical catastrophe, DES may be viewed as the original EDC. Further, the possibility of second-generation effects has been reported (Newbold et al., 1998, 2000). Using developmentally exposed DES mouse models, multiple mechanisms were identified that play a role in this drug-mediated carcinogenic and toxic effects.

Recent results suggest that perinatal exposure to DES may be expected to increase the incidence of obesity in a sex-dependent manner and act as a potential chemical stressor for obesity and obesity-related disorders (Hao et al., 2012). In the study, DES induced 3T3-L1 preadipocyte differentiation and activated expression of estrogen receptor (ER) and peroxisome proliferator-activated receptor-gamma (PPAR-$\gamma$) in the target genes.

## *Alkylphenol polyethoxylates*

Alkylphenol polyethoxylates (APEs) are used as nonionic surfactants in industrial and household cleaning agents, in manufacture of paints and plastics, in pesticide formulations, and in synthesis of rubber goods (Giger et al., 1984). APEs released into sewage are metabolized by microbes in sewage sludge to alkylphenolic compounds (APs). These compounds are relatively stable and have been detected in surface water, sediments, and fish fat (Klecka et al., 2010). Several experimental studies demonstrated that APs possess some estrogenic activity (Munkittrick et al., 1998).

Nonylphenols are substances with weak estrogen receptor (ER) binding potency, which is 1000–1,000,000 lower than 17-β-estradiol (White et al., 1994; Preuss et al., 2010). Nonylphenol is also antagonistic to androgenic receptors (ARs) (Paris et al., 2002; Lee et al., 2003; Roy et al., 2004). A multigenerational study assessing the effects of 4-*n*-nonylphenol indicated only minor effects on reproductive system parameters in the offspring of tested rats at the highest doses applied (Chapin et al., 1999). A later study confirmed the observation of a possibly lower epididymal weight in male offspring at higher 4-*n*-nonylphenol dose exposure (15–75 mg 4-*n*-nonylphenol/kg/day for 8 days) (Hossaini et al., 2001). Molecular modeling of the potential interaction of nonylphenol with the estrogen receptor α shows that nonylphenol is likely to bind to the ERα (Amaro et al., 2014). However, a recent study suggested that exposure to nonylphenol may lead to thyroid dysfunction, as it may be a potential contributor to thyroid hormone disruption (Xi et al., 2013). According to the European Union (EU) risk assessment, a daily intake of NP by consumers was estimated to be in the range of 150 μg/day/person. The estimated intake included the potential intake via use of foodborne TNPP. The risk assessment clearly concluded that this low intake did not result in any adverse human risk.

Although the mechanisms are unclear, octylphenol (OP) suppresses testicular function significantly in adult male rats. In particular, it reportedly reduces testes size, lowers testosterone concentrations, and decreases spermatogenesis (Blake and Boockfor, 1997). OP was also shown to be toxic to aquatic animals and adversely affect murine splenocytes (Nair-Menon et al., 1996). Of the APs tested for estrogenicity, OP was approximately 1000 times less potent than 17β-estradiol (E2) *in vitro* (White et al., 1994).

## *Bisphenol A*

Bisphenol A (BPA) is a major component in epoxy and polycarbonate (PC) resins, which are widely used as ingredients in protective coatings on food containers and as adhesives in packaging products (Howe and Borodinsky, 1998). PC is widely used in the manufacture of plastic, and BPA accounts for about 63% of the total consumption of PC (Chemical Profile, 1999). Brotons et al. (1995) demonstrated estrogenic activity in components extracted from canned foodstuffs and identified BPA from the inner coating as an estrogenic material. Krishnan et al. (1993) reported BPA release from PC flasks and coated food cans (10–20 g/can) during autoclaving. BPA has since been detected at concentrations ranging from 4–23 g/can in both extracted foods and water from autoclaved cans (Perez et al., 1998). In addition, BPA has also been used as a sealant in dentistry and found in saliva (90–931 μg) collected from subjects 1 hour after dental therapy (Olea et al., 1996). Based on the results of studies of the migration of BPA from packing into food, the European Union (EU) initially established a specific migration limit for BPA of 3 mg/kg of food in 2002. In 2004, the limit was amended to 0.6 mg/kg in 2004. The maximal acceptable dose for BPA established by the Environmental Protection Agency (EPA) is 50 μg/kg of body weight per day (EPA, 1997).

BPA has been evaluated as a weak estrogenic agent in uterotrophic assays using immature or ovariectomized animals. The ability of BPA to induce uterotrophic activity varies among species, strains, and routes of exposure, and between immature and ovariectomized animals. Gould et al. (1998) found that BPA (150 mg/kg/day) orally administered to immature Sprague–Dawley female rats did not induce any uterotrophic response, but did find that uterine progesterone levels were significantly increased. Coldham et al. (1997) showed that a subcutaneous injection of 320 mg/kg/day BPA was inactive in immature mouse uterotrophic assays, and in a recent study, no uterotrophic response to BPA was observed in immature mice following BPA administration at 100 mg/kg/day subcutaneously, but BPA at 1000 mg/kg/day did induce a positive uterotrophic response (Mehmood et al., 2000). Although it is controversial, overall it is considered that BPA does not pose a significant health risk to humans, including newborns and babies (Willhite et al., 2008; Hengstler et al., 2011). BPA was proposed to increase the risk of obesity, brain diseases, cancer, asthma, and heart disease, as well as disrupt the hormone system/reproduction system (Rezg et al., 2014). Due to the obesogenic effects of EDCs, the term *obesogens* has been applied.

## *Phthalate esters*

Phthalate esters (PEs) are found in some soft toys, flooring, medical equipment, cosmetics, and air fresheners. Di(2-ethylhexyl) phthalate (DEHP) is the most abundant phthalate in the environment and mono-(2-ethylhexyl) phthalate is its primary metabolite, which correlates toxicokinetically with DEHP (Koo and Lee, 2007). Other important phthalates include di(n-butyl) phthalate, diethyl phthalate, butyl-benzyl phthalate, and di(*n*-octyl) phthalate. PEs are a potential health concern, because these compounds are suspected to modulate the endocrine systems of animals and have been implicated with increased male reproductive system disorders (Barlow and Foster, 2003; Kim et al., 2004; Swan, 2006). The potential detriment to the reproductive system of infants exposed to PE is of particular concern (Kaiser, 2005).

In 2002, the U.S. Food and Drug Administration (FDA) released a report that cautioned against polyvinyl chloride (PVC) devices containing DEHP. However, DEHP is widely used as a plasticizer in the manufacture of various plastics including PVC and synthesis of many medical devices. This widespread use leads to significant exposure through contaminated foods, food packaging materials, and medical products (Koo and Lee, 2004; Silva et al., 2005). California, Korea, the EU, and Japan have banned manufacturers from using some phthalates in children's toys. However, risk assessments have shown that human exposure levels to PEs generally do not exceed safe limits (Koo and Lee, 2005).

## *Polybrominated diphenyl ethers*

Polybrominated diphenyl ethers (PBDEs) are found in fire retardants, in the plastic cases of televisions and computers, and in electronic items, carpets, lighting, bedding, clothing, car components, foam cushions, and other textile materials. Commercial PBDE products are predominantly penta-, octa- and decabromodiphenyl ethers. Today, decabromodiphenyl ether (deca-BDE) accounts for over 80% of the PBDEs produced, whereas pentabromodiphenyl ether (penta-BDE) and octabromodiphenyl ether (octa-BDE) products constitute about 12 and 6%, respectively (de Wit, 2002). PBDEs have been found in indoor and outdoor air (Wilford et al., 2004), and dust samples (Stapleton et al., 2005). PBDEs are being increasingly detected in human milk, tissue, and serum samples (Mazdai et al., 2003), and the most prevalent PBDE congeners in human samples are PBDE-47 and PBDE-99 (Figure 21.2). Research suggests PBDE levels in people in North America are higher compared to levels of people in Europe or Japan (Hites, 2004). PBDEs have been found in the breast milk of U.S. women at levels 10 to 100 times higher than those found in Europe (Viberg et al., 2008; Schecter et al., 2010). Therefore, the widespread uses of PBDEs and their increasing levels in the environment have raised concerns regarding possible adverse effects on human health.

PBDEs have the potential to disrupt thyroid hormone balance and may contribute to a variety of neurological and developmental defects, including lower IQ and learning disabilities. However, no significant correlation between serum thyroxin (T4) and total PBDE concentration was reported in another study (Kim et al., 2012). PBDEs are structurally similar to PCBs and exert similar neurotoxic effects (Figure 21.3).

The adverse human health effects of PBDEs have not been definitively established. Rats and mice that ingested food with moderate amounts of PBDEs for a few days showed damage to the thyroid gland (ATSDR, 2004); those that consumed smaller amounts for weeks or months displayed adverse effects on the thyroid and liver. High concentrations of PBDEs may produce neurobehavioral alterations and affect the immune system in animals. Moreover, many differences in effects are seen between highly

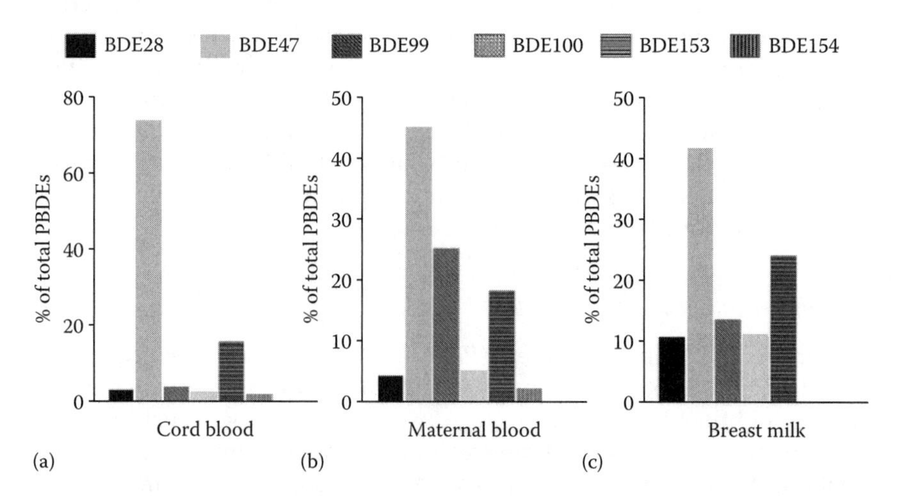


***Figure 21.2*** Distribution of polybrominated diphenyl ethers (PBDEs) congeners in paired umbilical cord blood (a), maternal blood (b), and breast milk samples (c). Congener concentrations are presented as the mean percentage of the RPBDE concentrations. (From Kim TH et al., *Chemosphere.*, 87, 97–104, 2012.)

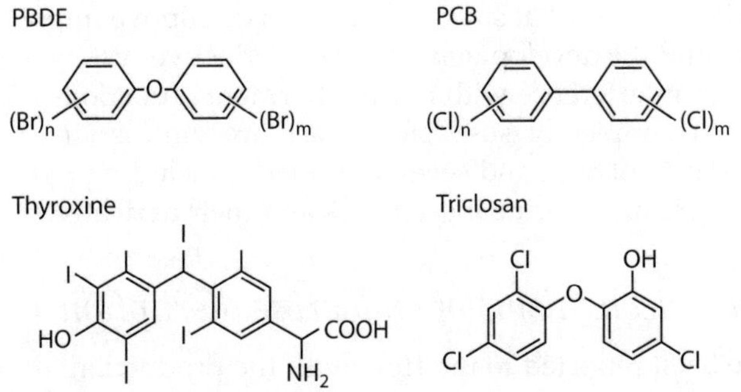

PBDE

PCB

Thyroxine

Triclosan

***Figure 21.3*** Chemical structure of PCBs, PBDEs, and thyroxine, triclosan.

brominated and less-brominated PBDEs in animal studies. Nonetheless, many of the most common PBDEs were banned in 2006 by the EU. EPA received commitments from the principal manufacturers and importers of decaBDE to initiate reductions in the manufacture, import, and sales of decaBDE starting in 2010, with all sales to cease by 2013. The proposed risk management measure was that prohibitions would apply to the manufacture, use, sale, offer for sale, and the import and export of all PBDEs (tetraBDE, pentaBDE, hexaBDE, heptaBDE, octaBDE, nonaBDE, and decaBDE) and any resin or polymer containing these substances. The Government of Canada proposed implementing regulations to extend the existing PBDE prohibition to ban use, sale, offer for sale, and import to heptaBDE, octaBDE, nonaBDE, and decaBDE. As a result, the commercial mixture DecaBDE would be banned.

## *Other suspected endocrine disruptors*

Other suspected EDCs include xenoestrogens, such as DDT and its metabolites (*o,p′*-DDT or *p,p′*-DDE), which bind to ER. The fungicide procymidone binds to the androgen receptor (AR) and acts as a competitive inhibitor of androgen (Gray et al., 1999). Environmental contaminants, such as some polycyclic aromatic hydrocarbons (PAHs) and PCBs, act as antiandrogens *in vitro*, but the mode of action of these compounds remains to be determined (Schrader and Cooke, 2003). An environmental contaminant of uncertain origin, tris-(4-chlorophenyl)-methanol, is also a potent AR antagonist. The wide use of triclosan in soaps may be causing more harm than good by promoting the emergence of strains of bacteria resistant to common antibacterial agents. In a recent statement, the U.S. FDA announced its decision to ban triclosan in soaps (FDA, 2016). Concerns about the public health impact of triclosan and related chemicals, such as triclocarban, were heightened by studies that suggested it has a disruptive impact on animal metabolism and the development of the reproductive system of young animals through interference with normal hormonal functions (DeLeo et al., 2011). Other examples of suspected EDCs are vinclozolin, zearalenone, dioxins, furans, phenols, and several pesticides including pyrethroid, carbamate, and organochlorine insecticides and their derivatives.

## *Molecular mechanisms of endocrine disruption*

EDCs have been reported to interfere with the production, release, transport, metabolism, binding, actions, and elimination of the natural hormones responsible for maintaining homeostasis and regulating body development. While the contributions of these activities to cancer risk have not been clearly defined, data from several sources collectively indicate that studies of EDC action need to take into consideration cellular environment, genetic, and possibly epigenetic changes. The effects of xenobiotics on development of several human cancers were identified several decades ago. Although the mechanisms of EDC-related cancer have not been fully elucidated, possible modes of action include alterations of metabolic activation, interactions between endogenous hormones, growth factors, and perturbations of transcription pathways.

Disruption of the endocrine system might occur in various ways. Some chemicals mimic a natural hormone, fooling the body into overresponding to the stimulus (e.g., a growth hormone that results in increased muscle mass), or responding at inappropriate times (e.g., producing insulin when it is not needed). Other endocrine disruptors block the effects of a hormone from certain receptors (e.g., growth hormones required for normal development). Still other compounds directly stimulate or inhibit the endocrine system and initiate overproduction or underproduction of hormones (e.g., an over- or underactive thyroid). Certain drugs are used to intentionally produce some of these effects, such as birth control pills. In many situations involving environmental chemicals, however, an endocrine effect is not desirable.

### *Free radical production*

As previously described (Choi et al., 2004), EDCs may exhibit a wide-ranging variety of endocrine-disrupting effects including developmental disorders, carcinogenicity, mutagenicity, immunotoxicity, and neurotoxicity. Choi and Lee (2004) demonstrated that about 94% of the 48 EDCs classified by the Centers for Disease Control and Prevention generate free radicals and that this might represent a common toxic mechanism underlying the effects of EDCs (Figure 21.4). Later, it was also postulated that oxidative stress induced by EDCs is a common mechanism of carcinogenesis (Keri et al., 2007).

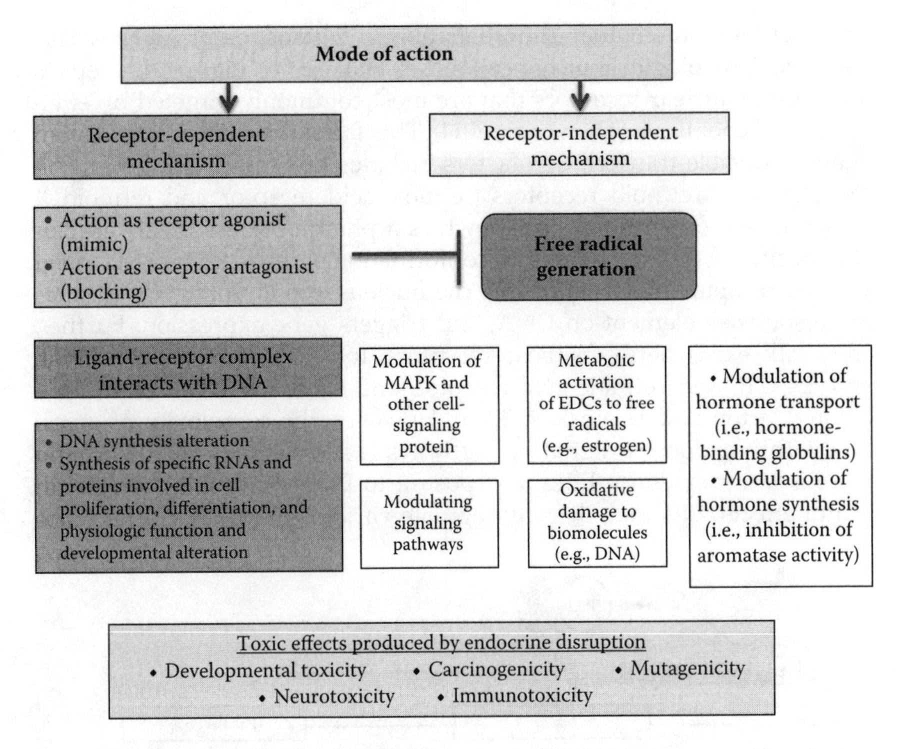


***Figure 21.4*** The mode of action and toxicities of endocrine disruptors during cancer development.

## *Nuclear receptor-mediated toxicity*

Exposure to EDCs may increase the risk of cancer in hormone-dependent organs (prostatic, breast, testicular, and endometrium). EDCs including *o,p'*-DDT, PCBs, pesticides, and heavy metals act as initiators and/or promoters of carcinogenesis (Yusof and Edwards, 1990). EDCs may also play important roles in the development of human cancer via interactions with estrogens, growth factors (and their receptors), transduction signaling pathways, oncogene activation, or tumor suppressor gene inactivation (Janosek et al., 2006). The receptor-mediated mechanism involves the activation of responsive elements on DNA, which results in an increased expression of target genes. Alternatively, interactions between compounds and receptors might negatively affect receptor binding to responsive elements on DNA, and thus suppress receptor action.

The nuclear receptor superfamily is a large group of receptors that regulate a wide range of physiological functions, including cell growth and proliferation, cellular differentiation, maintenance of homeostasis, and other toxicological outcomes (Janosek et al., 2006). Figure 21.5 depicts the various nuclear receptors that are most commonly targeted by environmental chemicals (Yoon et al., 2014). This family of structurally related ligand-inducible transcription factors includes ER, AR, thyroid hormone receptor (TR), retinoid receptors (retinoic acid receptor and retinoid X receptor), and other molecules known as orphan receptors. After binding of a specific ligand, the structural conformation of the receptor is changed and the receptor translocates into the nucleus, binds to the corresponding responsive element on DNA, and triggers gene expression. Further, cross-talk exists between these receptors, for example, between PPAR and ER, TR, and retinoic acid receptor, and this modulates gene regulation (Corton and Lapinskas, 2005). However, the complexity of cross-talk within endocrine signaling pathways is not clearly understood and there is scant evidence linking exposure to EDCs with adverse human health effects. ERs may directly regulate various genes, including those

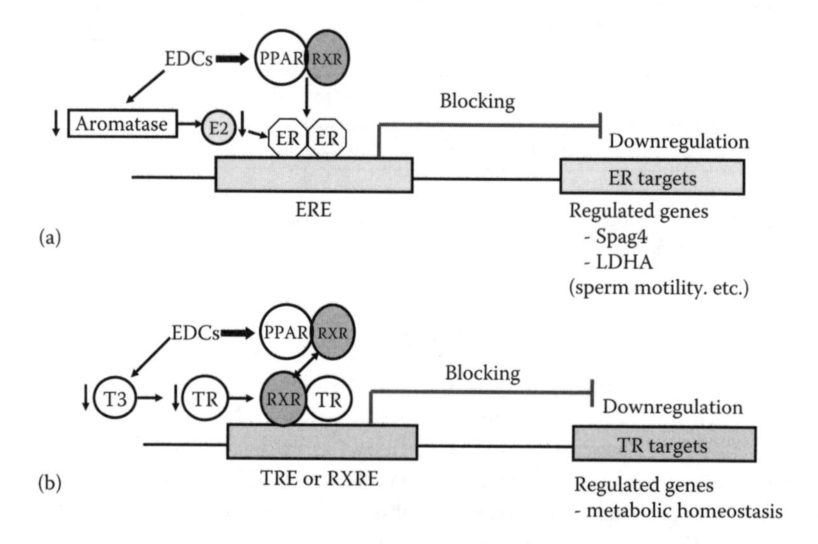


***Figure 21.5*** Mode of cross-talk between peroxisome proliferator-activated receptors (PPARs) and other nuclear receptors. (a) Cross-talk between PPAR and estrogen receptor (ER). Heterodimers for binding to an estrogen receptor element (ERE). The result is either up- or downregulation by endocring disrupting chemicals (EDCs) depending on the promoter context of the ERE. (b) Cross-talk between PPAR and thyroid hormone receptor (TR) or retinoic acid receptor (RAR). PPAR can prevent activation by thyroid hormone receptor (TR)-retinoid X receptor (RXR) heterodimers or RAR-RXR heterodimers limiting amount of RXR. This results in downregulation of genes under control of thyroid hormone response elements (TRE) or retinoic acid response elements (RARE). E2, estradiol.

encoding hormones, proteases, angiogenesis promoters (e.g., vascular endothelial growth factor), cell survival proteins (e.g., Bcl-2 and Bax) and cell proliferation proteins (e.g., cyclin D and CDKs). In addition, ERs may affect transcription without directly binding to DNA by associating with other transcription factors, such as, activator protein-1 (AP-1) or specificity protein 1 (Spl). In addition, the development of tumors in reproductive organs often depends upon the actions of sex hormones, but the mechanisms involved are unclear.

Many compounds produce adverse effects at multiple levels of thyroid signaling *in vitro* and *in vivo* (Langer, 1998). Thyroid hormone receptor-α1 (TR-α1) mRNA levels are elevated by chronic DBP exposure in rats and the TR directly affects both development of prepubertal testes and regulation of follicle-stimulating hormone receptor and luteinizing hormone receptor gene expression, which may further modulate the effects of gonadotropins on testis functions (Rao et al., 2003; Ryu et al., 2007). Further, TR-1 protein and mRNA levels are expressed at significantly higher levels in testes of DBP exposed rats, implicating TR-α1 as an essential mediator of the adverse effects of DBP and as a contributor to DBP-induced dysgenesis of testicular growth and development (Ryu et al., 2007).

## *Epigenetic regulation of transgenerational diseases*

Binding of EDCs to endogenous hormone receptors alters hormone signaling, which influences the normal endocrine system (McKinney and Waller, 1998). In particular, exposure to estrogenic chemicals during embryonic or postnatal development may produce transgenerational abnormalities in male reproductive tissues, including testes, seminal vesicles, and prostate (Anway and Skinner, 2008) as well as increase the risk of tumor development (Ho et al., 2006a). The possible involvement of epigenetic mechanisms in endocrine disruption helps explain the transgenerational effects of some EDCs. Early studies showed that treatment with DES during pregnancy resulted in vaginal adenocarcinoma in female offspring in humans (Herbst et al., 1971) and mice (McLachlan et al., 1980). It now appears that these transgenerational phenotypes are in part involved in the epigenetic reprogramming of male germline cells. Thus, epigenomic alterations seem to provide a mechanism for transgenerational changes in imprinting genes. For example, exposure to the fungicide vinclozolin during embryonic gonadal sex determination alters the epigenetic programming of the male germline to induce altered DNA methylation patterns in various genes (Birnbaum and Fenton, 2003). Ho et al. (2006b) demonstrated that exposure of rats to low doses of estradiol or BPA during the neonatal developmental period enhanced susceptibility to precancerous prostatic lesions in aged animals and sensitized the prostate gland in adult-induced hormonal carcinogenesis. These findings support the correlation between fetal exposure to EDCs and cancer development (Birnbaum and Fenton, 2003).

The epigenetic mechanism for endocrine disruption induced by EDCs involves altered DNA methylation in the germline that appears to transmit transgenerational adult-onset diseases, such as spermatogenic defects, prostate disease, kidney disease, and cancer (Anway and Skinner, 2008). These epigenetic changes occur as a consequence of mechanisms involving DNA methylation, histone modifications, and noncoding RNAs in the regulation of gene expression patterns. Epigenetic mechanisms are essential for normal development and differentiation. However, these mechanisms may be misdirected, which leads to disease, most notably cancer. Mounting evidence indicates that environmental exposure to EDCs, particularly during early development, might induce epigenetic changes that may be transmitted in subsequent generations or serve as the basis for diseases that develop later in life. Methylation profiles are used as molecular markers to distinguish subtypes of cancers and potentially as predictors of disease outcome and treatment response. The role of epigenetics in diagnosis and treatment are likely to increase as mechanisms are revealed which lead to the transcriptional silencing of genes involved in human cancer.

Emerging evidence suggests that epigenetic programming has the potential to affect protein function later in life and potentially across generations, which adds a layer of complexity to the impact of early life exposure to EDCs on endocrine homeostasis across the life span and into subsequent generations. The multifactorial nature of endocrine-related disorders also needs to be considered when designing studies and selecting appropriate animal models for mechanistic studies.

## *Adverse effects of endocrine disruptors*

It is clear from numerous investigations that EDCs pose a threat to wildlife, animals, and humans. Ever since Rachel Carson described the harmful impact of EDCs on wildlife in her book *Silent Spring*, its influences on various animals and humans has been continuously reported. The main harmful impact of EDCs is to produce abnormal conditions within the body by mimicking hormones at the molecular level.

### *Wildlife species*

Many researchers have observed the harmful impacts of EDCs on species such as shellfish, reptiles, fish, birds, and mammals.

*Shellfish*: The most representative harmful impact on a wildlife species is imposex that occurs among gastropods, such as turban shells or sea snails, whereby a female becomes a male due to the superimposition of a male sex organ on its body. This ecological phenomenon produces drastic population decreases because it affects female sterility. Imposex was first discovered in female sea snails from Plymouth, England, in 1969. This was shown to result from seawater contamination by organotin compounds like tributyltin (Birchenough et al., 2002).

*Birds*: The reproductive damage of DDT in birds is unequivocal. The mechanism responsible is a lack of eggshell calcification, which results in a failure to hatch (Rattner et al., 1984). This phenomenon mostly affects birds higher on the food chain, such as sea gulls, cormorants, herons, pelicans, falcons, and eagles. In the case of sea gulls, abnormal female–female pairing and multiple egg laying have been observed. Decreases in sexual intercourse frequency, indifference to the opposite sex, mating between the same sex, decrease in newborns, and reductions in immune function have also been reported.

*Fish*: In Japan, while confirming sexual imbalance among carp due to reduced numbers of males in some streams, it was found that the sexual imbalance was associated with relatively high levels of APEs (Diamanti-Kandarakis et al., 2009). Many reports have described the impacts of substances like APEs, which are the degradation products of synthetic detergents or nonionic surfactants. Discoveries in various parts of England of fish with ambiguous gender identities also seem to be related to APEs (Rice et al., 2003). When these APEs were injected into tanks containing rainbow trout, researchers found that testicular development was hindered. In the same experiment, it was found that vitellogenin, which is normally produced only in the liver of females, was produced in males. In addition, observations of abnormal reproductive ability and male immaturity were reported in Coho (silver) salmon inhabiting Lake Erie (Leatherland et al., 1982).

*Reptiles and Amphibians*: The representative case for reptiles was reported in Lake Apopka, Florida, where the population of alligators was reduced by 50% after accidental DDT leakage. This contamination produced male alligators to become females and male sex organ shrinkage (Semenza et al., 1997). In the case of red-eared sliders, PCB exposure was found to reduce successful egg hatching, and led the majority of eggs to become females (Moss et al., 2009). In addition, many reports on frogs showed that exposure to dioxins, heavy metals, or dibenzofurans reduced the hatching rates and increased the frequency and type of mutations (Fort et al., 2004).

## *Mammals*

Various reports have been issued on the harmful impacts attributed to EDCs on mammals. For example, marked reductions in otter counts, a high death rate among minke whale infants, population decrease among polar bears, and mass mortality of striped dolphins in the Mediterranean Sea have been reportedly related to EDCs (Sonne et al., 2009). The harmful impacts frequently reported in mammals are population decreases, male sex organ disorders, and immune system disorders, which are now also issues of concern in humans. Female rats exposed to endocrine disrupters during early development end up with fewer eggs in their ovaries and are at risk of losing their ability to reproduce at an earlier age. These findings have enhanced our knowledge of how EDCs affect the female reproductive system. These results raised concern that EDCs may also affect egg reserves in women and lead to earlier menopause.

## *Humans*

EDCs probably exert harmful effects on humans, but supporting evidence is limited. In Taiwan, growth delay, attention deficit hyperactivity disorder, and undersized penises during puberty were observed in children whose mothers used cooking oil contaminated with PCBs (Yu et al., 2000). A mother who had been exposed to synthetic estrogen was found to have a daughter with a rare type of vaginal cancer and her son possessed a malformed penis (Mericskay et al., 2005). Among women whose diets contained fish from the Great Lakes when young, the proportion of children with a small brain size at birth with developmental disabilities was relatively large (Seegal, 1999). In Danish men, sperm counts fell from 113 million/ml to 66 million/ml (Carlsen et al., 1992). In French men, counts fell from 89 million/ml in 1976 to 60 million/ml and sperm motility decreased (Auger et al., 1995). In Japan, it was found that the average sperm count of a man in his 20s living in the Tokyo suburbs was 46 million/ml, which was only half that of a man in his 40s (84 million/ml). Researchers proposed that estrogen might be a possible cause. In the United States, it was concluded that women exposed to DDT or PCBs are at the risk of developing breast cancer (Wolff and Toniolo, 1995). Taken together, reduced sperm counts, increasing numbers of (breast, prostate, and testicular) cancers, increased sterility, malformations, attention deficit hyperactivity disorders, and learning disorders in children might be related to exposure to EDCs. However, unambiguous evidence is needed.

## *Evaluation of endocrine disruptors*

The Organization for Economic Cooperation and Development (OECD) and the U.S. EPA approved various *in vitro* and *in vivo* assays for EDCs. In particular, the U.S. EPA Office of Chemical Safety and Pollution Prevention introduced EDC testing methods in Test Guideline Series 890. Detailed information on these test methods can be found at: http://www.epa.gov/endo/. OECD test guidelines for EDCs and test details are available and are briefly summarized here (OECD, 2012).

### In vitro *assays*

#### *Androgen receptor binding assay*

The AR binding assay is an *in vitro* screening assay that examines whether the test substance has the potential to interact with AR. The assay uses AR isolated from the ventral prostate of rats. This screening assay measures the receptor-binding affinity of a test substance by evaluating its ability to substitute bound reference androgen, usually 5α-dihydrotestosterone or R1881 (a synthetic androgen). The AR binding assay consists of two saturation-binding and competitive-binding experiments (EPA, 2009a).

#### *Estrogen receptor binding assay*

This competitive inhibition assay determines whether the test substance has the potential to interact with ER as a substitute for radiolabeled 17β-estradiol, an endogenous hormone. This screening assay uses ER prepared from the uterine cytosol of rats. This assay consists of two saturation binding and competitive binding experiments (EPA, 2009b).

#### *Estrogen receptor transcriptional activation assay*

The estrogen receptor transcriptional activation assay is an *in vitro* screening assay that determines whether a test substance binds to and activates ER (EPA, 2011a). After incubating a human cervical tumor from a human estrogen receptor-alpha (hERα)-HeLa-9903 cell line with a test substance, this assay is based on the measurement of luciferase activity using a luminometer after lysing cells and adding luciferin substrate.

#### *Aromatase (human recombinant) assay*

The assay determines whether the test substance inhibits the catalytic activity of cytochrome P450 enzyme aromatase (also known as CYP19) (EPA, 2011b). This assay measures aromatase activity using liquid scintillation counting of tritiated water ($^3H_2O$) released when [$^3H$] ASDN is converted into estrone.

*Steroidogenesis assay*

This assay uses human adrenocortical carcinoma H295R cell line to measure cell viability and the levels of relevant hormones (testosterone and estradiol).

## In vivo *assay*

*Amphibian metamorphosis assay*

The screening assay is used to determine whether the test substance interferes with the normal function of the hypothalamus-pituitary–thyroid axis (OECD, 2009). The assay is conducted using a negative (clean water) control after exposing Nieuwkoop–Faber stage 51 African clawed frog (*Xenopus laevis*) tadpoles to the test substance administered in at least three different concentrations for 21 days. Observational endpoints are hindlimb length, snout-to-vent length, developmental stage, body weight, thyroid histopathology, and daily observations of mortality and clinical signs. This experimental method is important because it is the only assay capable of detecting thyroid activity in animals undergoing morphological development.

*Fish short-term reproduction assay*

This screening assay is also used to determine whether the test substance interferes with the normal structure and function of the hypothalamic–pituitary–gonadal axis. The assay is conducted using a negative control by exposing sexually mature male and female fathead minnows (*Pimephales promelas*) to at least three different concentrations of the test substance for 21 days. The observational endpoints are survival (mortality), fecundity, fertilization success, gonado-somatic index, gonad histology, plasma vitellogenin, sex steroid levels, secondary sex characteristics, and other clinical signs.

*Female pubertal assay*

This screening assay is used to determine whether the test substance interacts with the endocrine system during pubertal development and affects thyroid function in juvenile/peripubertal female rats. The assay is conducted by administering the test substance daily by oral gavage to Sprague–Dawley male rats from postnatal day 22 to 42. Observational endpoints include daily body weight, vaginal opening, organ weight, histology (including colloid area and follicular cell height in thyroid), hormones [total serum thyroxine (T4), serum thyroid-stimulating hormone], estrous cyclicity, and clinical serum chemistry.

*Male pubertal assay*

This screening assay is used to measure whether the test substance interacts with the endocrine system during pubertal development and affects thyroid function in intact juvenile/peripubertal male rats. The test substance is administered daily by oral gavage to Sprague–Dawley male rats from postnatal day 23 to 53. Observational endpoints include daily body weight, preputial separation, reproductive system organ weight, histology (including colloid area and follicular cell height in thyroid), hormones (total serum testosterone, total serum thyroxine (T4), serum thyroid-stimulating hormone), and clinical serum chemistry.

*Uterotrophic assay*

This screening test is used to determine whether the test substance shows the physiological activity expected of an estrogen agonist (e.g., 17β-estradiol), as measured by an increase in uterine weight (EPA, 2009d). Test animals are young adult female rats (Sprague–Dawley and Wistar strains are preferred) after ovariectomy with adequate time for uterine tissues to regress. The test substance is administered daily for a minimum of three consecutive days. The recommended reference estrogen agonist is 17α-ethynyl estradiol (at 0.3 μg/kg/day subcutaneous or 1 μg/kg/day by oral gavage) as the positive control and distilled water as the negative control. Twenty-four hours after the last administration, test animals are autopsied and the uterus weights are measured. For test substances, it is recommended that the agonist component be administered at least at two doses (a high dose at or just below the maximum tolerated dose but not exceeding the dose limit (1000 mg/kg/day).

*Androgenic or antiandrogenic activity (Hershberger assay)*

The Hershberger assay is a short-term screening test that uses accessory tissues of the male reproductive tract to examine androgenic or antiandrogenic activity of the test substance (Hershberger et al., 1953; EPA, 2009c). The five androgen-dependent tissues examined are ventral prostate, seminal vesicle (plus fluids and coagulating glands), *levator ani* plus *bulbocavernosus,* paired Cowper's glands, and glans penis. This assay is based on the weight changes of these five androgen-dependent tissues in castrated-peripubertal male rats (Sprague–Dawley and Wistar strains are recommended, not Fischer 344). The reference androgen agonist used is testosterone propionate (at 0.2 or 0.4 mg/kg/day subcutaneous), and the reference androgen antagonist is flutamide (3 mg/kg/day) as the positive control. For test substances, it is recommended that the androgen agonist component be administered at least at two doses (a high dose at or just below the maximum tolerated dose but not exceeding the dose limit of 1000 mg/kg/day), and the androgen antagonist component be administered in at least three doses.

## *Test Guideline 407*

OECD Test Guideline 407 (TG407) originally was a repeated-dose 28-day oral toxicity study in rodents. A recent draft document proposed updated parameters on endocrine effects. The major updated contents were concerning the estrous cycle, sexual maturity, sex organ observation, and relevant hormone measure. Details of this experimental method can be found at http://www.oecd.org/dataoecd/.

### *ToxCast phase I assays*

The Endocrine Disruptor Screening Program (EDSP) began a multiyear transition to validate and more efficiently use computational toxicology methods. High-throughput screens (HTS) will enable more rapid and cost-effective assessment of potential EDC toxicity. The aims of EDSP are to prioritize and screen chemicals to determine their potential to interact with estrogen, androgen, or thyroid bioactivity by using computational or in silico models. In addition to leveraging advances in technology, the initiative also emphasizes strategic coordination and timing of chemical evaluations in the context of existing regulatory frameworks (Rotroff et al., 2013).

The U.S. EPA believes that ongoing adoption of alternative methods and technologies will continue to advance EDSP screening of chemicals for bioactivity in the estrogen, androgen, and thyroid pathways. The EPA is continuing research on the "ER Model" to determine if ToxCast™ assays can provide comparable information as that of the female rat pubertal and the fish short-term reproduction assays. In addition, research continues on the ToxCast "AR Model" for bioactivity which, if fully validated, may be considered as an alternative (alone or with the "ER Model") for the following current Tier 1 assays: AR binding, Male Rat Pubertal, Hershberger, and Fish Short-Term Reproduction. Research is also underway to develop steroidogenesis ToxCast (STR) and thyroid (THY) bioactivity models. Table 21.2 illustrates the evolution of screening in the EDSP and indicates combinations of various alternative assays and models that might overlap for evaluating potential bioactivity of chemicals.

***Table 21.2*** Preliminary list of chemicals with endocrine-disrupting activity tested by EDSP Tier 1 assay

| Current EDSP Tier 1 battery of assays | Alternative high-throughput assays and computational model for EDSP Tier 1 battery |
|---|---|
| Estrogen receptor (ER) binding | ER Model (alternative) |
| Estrogen receptor transactivation (ERTA) | ER Model (alternative) |
| Uterotrophic assay | ER Model (alternative) |
| Female rat pubertal assay | ER, STR, and Thyroid (THY) Models *(Future)* |
| Male rat pubertal assay | AR, STR, and THY Models *(Future)* |
| Androgen receptor (AR) binding | AR Model *(Future)* |
| Hershberger assay | AR Mode *(Future)* |
| Aromatase | STR Model *(Future)* |
| Steroidogenesis (STR) | STR Model *(Future)* |
| Fish short-term reproduction | ER, AR, and STR Models *(Future)* |
| Amphibian metamorphosis | THY Model *(Future)* |

# References

Agency for Toxic Substances and Disease Registry (ATSDR) (2004). Toxicological Profile for Polybrominated Biphenyls and Polybrominated Diphenyl Ethers. Atlanta, GA: U.S. Department of Health and Human Services, Public Health Service.

Amaro AA, Esposito AI, Mirisola V et al. (2014). Endocrine disruptor agent nonylphenol exerts an estrogen-like transcriptional activity on estrogen receptor positive breast cancer cells. *Curr Med Chem.* 21, 630–40.

Anway MD, Skinner MK (2008). Epigenetic programming of the germ line: Effects of endocrine disruptors on the development of transgenerational disease. *Reprod Biomed Online.* 16, 23–5.

Auger J, Kunstmann JM, Czyglik F et al. (1995). Decline in semen quality among fertile men in Paris during the past 20 years. *New Engl J Med.* 332, 281–5.

Baillie-Hamilton PF (2002). Chemical toxins: A hypothesis to explain the global obesity epidemic. *J Altern Complement Med.* 8, 185–92.

Barlow NJ, Foster PMD (2003). Pathogenesis of male reproductive tract lesions from gestation through adulthood following in utero exposure to di(n-butyl) phthalate. *Toxicol Pathol.* 31, 397–410.

Birchenough AC, Barnes N, Evans SM et al. (2002). A review and assessment of tributyltin contamination in the North Sea, based on surveys of butyltin tissue burdens and imposex/intersex in four species of neogastropods. *Mar Pollut Bull.* 44, 534–43.

Birnbaum LS, Fenton SE (2003). Cancer and developmental exposure to endocrine disruptors. *Environ Health Perspect.* 111, 389–94.

Birnbaum LS (2013). State of the Science of Endocrine Disruptors. *Environ Health Perspect.* 121(4), a107.

Blake CA, Boockfor FR (1997). Chronic administration of the environmental pollutant 4-tert-octylphenol to adult male rats interferes with the secretion of luteinizing hormone, follicle-stimulating hormone, prolactin, and testosterone. *Biol Reprod.* 57, 255–66.

Brotons JA, Olea-Serrano MF, Villalobos M et al. (1995). Xenoestrogens released from lacquer coatings in food cans. *Environ Health Perspect.* 103, 608–12.

Carlsen E, Giwercman A, Keiding N et al. (1992). Evidence for decreasing quality of semen during past 50 years [see comments]. *BMJ.* 305, 609–13.

Carson R (1962). *Silent Spring.* New York: Houghton Mifflin.

Chapin RE, Delaney J, Wang Y et al. (1999). The effects of 4-nonylphenol in rats: A multigeneration reproduction study. *Toxicol Sci.* 52, 80–91.

Chemical Profile (1999). ChemoExpo profile archives "Bisphenol-A". Available from: http://www.fobchemicals.com.

Choi SM, Lee BM (2004). An alternative mode of action of endocrine-disrupting chemicals and chemoprevention. *J Toxicol Environ Health Part B.* 7, 451–63.

Choi SM, Yoo SD, Lee BM (2004). Toxicological characteristics of endocrine-disrupting chemicals: Developmental toxicity, carcinogenicity, and mutagenicity. *J Toxicol Environ Health Part B.* 7, 1–24.

Colborn T, vom Saal FS, Soto AM (1993). Developmental effects of endocrine-disrupting chemicals in wildlife and humans. *Environ Health Perspect.* 101, 378–84.

Coldham NG, Dave M, Sivapathasundaram S et al. (1997). Elevation of a recombinant yeast cell estrogen screening assay. *Environ Health Perspect.* 105, 734–42.

Corton JC, Lapinskas PJ (2005). Peroxisome proliferator-activated receptors: Mediators of phthalate ester-induced effects in the male reproductive tract? *Toxicol Sci.* 83, 4–17.

DeLeo PS, Pawlowski S, Barton C, Fort DJ (2011). Comment on "Effects of triclocarban, triclosan, and methyl triclosan on thyroid hormone action and stress in frog and mammalian culture systems". *Environ Sci Technol.* 45, 10283–4.

DeRosa C, Richter P, Pohl H et al. (1998). Environmental exposures that affect the endocrine system: Public health implications. *J Toxicol Environ Health B.* 1, 3–26.

de Wit CA (2002). An overview of brominated flame retardants in the environment. *Chemosphere.* 46, 583–624.

Diamanti-Kandarakis E, Bourguignon JP, Giudice LC et al. (2009). Endocrine-disrupting chemicals: An Endocrine Society scientific statement. *Endocr Rev.* 30, 293–342.

EPA (1997). U.S. Environmental Protection Agency "Integrated Risk Information System" online.

EPA (1998). Research Plan for Endocrine Disruptors. EPA/600/R-98/087. Washington, DC: U.S. Environmental Protection Agency, Office of Research and Development. Available from: http://www.epa.gov/scipoly/oscpendo/docs/edstac/exesum14.pdf.

EPA (2009a). Endocrine disruptor screening program test guidelines OPPTS 890.1150: Androgen receptor binding (rat prostate cytosol). EPA 640-C-09-003. Washington, DC.

EPA (2009b). Endocrine disruptor screening program test guidelines OPPTS 890.1250: Estrogen receptor binding (rat uterine cytosol). EPA 740-C-09-005. Washington DC.

EPA (2009c). Endocrine disruptor screening program test guidelines OPPTS 890.1400: Hershberger Bioassay. EPA 740-C-09-008. Washington DC.

EPA (2009d). Endocrine disruptor screening program test guidelines OPPTS 890.1600: Uterotrophic Assay. EPA 740-C-09-0010. Washington DC.

EPA (2011a). Estrogen Receptor Transcriptional Activation (Human Cell Line – Hela-9903) Standard Evaluation Procedure (SEP). Available from: http://www.epa.gov/endo/pubs/toresources/seps/Final_890.1300_ERTA_SEP_9.15.11.pdf.

EPA (2011b). Aromatase Assay (Human Recombinant) OCSPP Guideline 890.1200 Standard Evaluation Procedure (SEP). Endocrine Disruptor Screening Program. U.S. Environmental Protection Agency Washington, DC. Available from: http://www.epa.gov/endo/pubs/toresources/seps/Final_890.1200_Aromatase_Assay_SEP_%208.1.11.pdf.

FDA News Release (2016). FDA issues final rule on safety and effectiveness of antibacterial soaps. September 2, 2016. http://beyondpesticides.org/programs/antibacterials/triclosan.

Fort DJ, Thomas JH, Rogers RL et al. (2004). Evaluation of the developmental and reproductive toxicity of methoxychlor using an anuran (Xenopus tropicalis) chronic exposure model. *Toxicol Sci.* 81, 443–53.

Giger W, Brunner PH, Schaffner C (1984). 4-Nonylphenol in sewage sludge: Accumulation of toxic metabolites from nonionic surfactants. *Science.* 225, 623–5.

Giusti RM, Iwamoto K, Hatch EE (1995). Diethylstilbestrol revisited: A review of the long-term health effects. *Ann Intern Med.* 122, 778–88.

Gould JC, Leonard LS, Maness SC et al. (1998). Bisphenol A interacts with the estrogen receptor alpha in a distinct manner from estradiol. *Mol Cell Endocrinol.* 142, 203–14.

Gray LE Jr, Wolf C, Lambright C et al. (1999). Administration of potentially antiandrogenic pesticides (procymidone, linuron, iprodione, chlozolinate, *p,p'*-DDE, and ketoconazole) and toxic substances (dibutyl- and diethylhexyl phthalate, PCB 169, and ethane dimethane sulphonate) during sexual differentiation produces diverse profiles of reproductive malformations in the male rat. *Toxicol Ind Health.* 15, 94–118.

Hao CJ, Cheng XJ, Xia HF, Ma X. (2012). The endocrine disruptor diethylstilbestrol induces adipocyte differentiation and promotes obesity in mice. *Toxicol Appl Pharmacol.* 263, 102–10.

Hengstler JG, Foth H, Gebel T et al. (2011). Critical evaluation of key evidence on the human health hazards of exposure to bisphenol A. *Crit Rev Toxicol.* 41, 263–91.

Herbst AL, Ulfelder H, Poskanzer DC (1971). Adenocarcinoma of the vagina. Association of maternal stilbstrol therapy with tumor appearance in young women. *New Eng J Med.* 284, 878–81.

Hershberger L, Shipley E, Meyer R (1953). Myotrophic activity of 19-nortestosterone and other steroids determined by modified levator ani muscle method. *Proc Soc Exp Biol Med.* 83, 175–80.

Hites R (2004). Polybrominated diphenyl ethers in the environment and in people: A meta-analysis of concentrations. *Environ Sci Technol.* 38(4), 945–56.

Ho SM, Leung YK, Chung I (2006a). Estrogens and antiestrogens as etiological factors and therapeutics for prostate cancer. *Ann New York Acad Sci.* 1089, 177–93.

Ho SM, Tang WY, Belmonte de Frausto J et al. (2006b). Developmental exposure to estradiol and bisphenol A increases susceptibility to prostate carcinogenesis and epigenetically regulates phosphodiesterase type 4 variant 4. *Cancer Res.* 66, 5624–32.

Hossaini A, Dalgaard M, Vinggaard AM et al., (2001). In utero reproductive study in rats exposed to nonylphenol. *Reprod Toxicol.* 15, 537-43.

Howe SR, Borodinsky L (1998). Potential exposure to bisphenol A from food-contact use of polycarbonate resins. *Food Addit Contam.* 15, 370–5.

Janosek J, Hilscherová K, Bláha L et al. (2006). Environmental xenobiotics and nuclear receptors—Interactions, effects and in vitro assessment. *Toxicol In Vitro.* 20, 18–37.

Kaiser J (2005). Toxicology panel finds no proof that phthalates harm infant reproductive systems. *Science.* 310, 422.

Keri RA, Ho SM, Hunt PA et al. (2007). An evaluation of evidence for the carcinogenic activity of bisphenol A. *Reprod Toxicol.* 24, 240–52.

Kim HS, Kim TS, Shin JH et al. (2004). Neonatal exposure to di(*n*-butyl) phthalate (DBP) alters male reproductive-tract development. *J Toxicol Environ Health.* 67, 2045–60.

Kim TH, Bang du Y, Lim HJ et al. (2012). Comparisons of polybrominated diphenyl ethers levels in paired South Korean cord blood, maternal blood, and breast milk samples. *Chemosphere.* 87, 97–104.

Klecka G, Persoon C, Currie R (2010). Chemicals of emerging concern in the Great Lakes Basin: An analysis of environmental exposures. *Rev Environ Contam Toxicol.* 207, 1–93.

Koo HJ, Lee BM (2004). Estimated exposure to phthalates in cosmetics and risk assessment. *J Toxicol Environ Health Part A.* 67, 1901–14.

Koo HJ, Lee BM (2005). Human monitoring of phthalates and risk assessment. *J Toxicol Environ Health.* 68, 1379–92.

Koo HJ, Lee BM (2007). Toxicokinetic relationship between di(2-ethylhexyl) phthalate (DEHP) and mono(2-ethylhexyl) phthalate in rats. *J Toxicol Environ Health Part A.* 70, 383–7.

Krishnan AV, Stathis P, Permuth SF et al. (1993). Bisphenol-A: An estrogenic substance is released from polycarbonate flasks during autoclaving. *Endocrinology.* 132, 2279–86.

Langer P (1998). Mini review: Polychlorinated biphenyls and the thyroid gland. Endocrine Regul. 32, 193–203.

Leatherland JF, Copeland P, Sumpter JP et al. (1982). Hormonal control of gonadal maturation and development of secondary sexual characteristics in coho salmon, *Oncorhynchus kisutch*, from lakes Ontario, Erie, and Michigan. *Gen Comp Endocrinol.* 48, 196–204.

Lee HJ, Chattopadhyay S, Gong EY et al. (2003). Antiandrogenic effects of bisphenol A and nonylphenol on the function of androgen receptor. *Toxicol Sci.* 75, 40–6.

Mazdai A, Dodder NG, Abernathy MP et al. (2003). Polybrominated diphenyl ethers in maternal and fetal blood samples. *Environ Health Perspect.* 111, 1249–52.

McKinney JD, Waller CL (1998). Molecular determinants of hormone mimicry: Halogenated aromatic hydrocarbon environmental agents. *J Toxicol Environ Health B.* 1, 27–58.

McLachlan JA, Newbold RR, Bullock BC (1980). Long-term effects on the female mouse genital tract associated with prenatal exposure to diethylstilbestrol. *Cancer Res.* 40, 3988–99.

Mehmood Z, Smith AG, Tucker MJ et al. (2000). The development of methods for assessing the in vivo oestrogen-like effects of xenobiotics in CD-1 mice. *Food Chem Toxicol.* 38, 493–501.

Mericskay M, Carta L, Sassoon D (2005). Diethylstilbestrol exposure in utero: A paradigm for mechanisms leading to adult disease. *Birth Defects Res Part A Clin Mol Teratol.* 73, 133–5.

Moss S, Keller JM, Richards S et al. (2009). Concentrations of persistent organic pollutants in plasma from two species of turtle from the Tennessee River Gorge. *Chemosphere.* 76, 194–204.

Munkittrick KR, McMaster ME, McCarthy LH et al. (1998). An overview of recent studies on the potential of pulp-mill effluents to alter reproductive parameters in fish. *J Toxicol Environ Health Part B.* 1, 347–71.

Nair-Menon JU, Campbell GT, Blake CA (1996). Toxic effects of octylphenol on cultured rat and murine splenocytes. *Toxicol Appl Pharm.* 139, 437–44.

Newbold RR, Hanson RB, Jefferson WN et al. (2000). Proliferative lesions and reproductive tract tumors in male descendants of mice exposed developmentally to diethylstilbestrol. *Carcinogenesis.* 21, 1355–63.

Newbold RR, Hanson RB, Jefferson WN et al. (1998). Increased tumors but uncompromised fertility in the female descendants of mice exposed developmentally to diethylstilbestrol. *Carcinogenesis.* 19, 1655–63.

Newburgh RW (1975). Toxicology of the reproductive system. In: Casarett LJ, Doull J, eds. *Toxicology The Basic Science of Poisons.* New York, NY: Macmillan. pp. 261–74.

OECD. (2009). Guideline for the Testing of Chemicals: The Amphibian Metamorphosis Assay. Test Guideline 231, Adopted 7 September 2009. Organisation for Economic Co-operation and Development: Washington Center. Available from: www.oecdwash.org.

OECD. (2012). Endocrine Disrupter Testing and Assessment. Available from: http://www.oecd.org/document/62/0,2340,en_2649_34377_2348606_1_1_1_1,00.html.

Olea N, Pulgar R, Pérez P et al. (1996). Estrogenicity of resin-based composites and sealants used in dentistry. *Environ Health Perspect.* 104, 298–305.

Paris F, Balaguer P, Terouanne B et al. (2002). Phenylphenols, biphenols, bisphenol-A and 4-tert-octylphenol exhibit alpha and beta estrogen activities and antiandrogen activity in reporter cell lines. *Mol Cell Endocrinol.* 193, 43–9.

Perez P, Pulgar R, Olea-Serrano F et al. (1998). The estrogenicity of bisphenol A-related diphenylalkanes with various substituents at the central carbon and the hydroxy groups. *Environ Health Perspect*. 106, 167–74.

Preuss TG, Gurer-Orhan H, Meerman J et al. (2010). Some nonylphenol isomers show antiestrogenic potency in the MVLN cell assay. *Toxicol In Vitro*. 24, 129–34.

Rao JN, Liang JY, Chakraborti P et al. (2003). Effect of thyroid hormone on the development and gene expression of hormone receptors in rat testes in vivo. *J Endocrinol Invest*. 26, 435–43.

Rattner BA, Eroschenko VP, Fox GA et al. (1984). Avian endocrine responses to environmental pollutants. *J Exp Zool*. 232, 683–9.

Rezg R, El-Fazaa S, Gharbi N, Mornagui B (2014). Bisphenol A and human chronic diseases: Current evidences, possible mechanisms, and future perspectives. *Environ Int*. 64, 83–90.

Rice CP, Schmitz-Afonso I, Loyo-Rosales JE et al. (2003). Alkylphenol and alkylphenolethoxylates in carp, water, and sediment from the Cuyahoga River, Ohio. *Environ Sci Technol*. 37, 3747–54.

Rotroff DM, Dix DJ, Houck KA et al. (2013). Using in vitro high throughput screening assays to identify potential endocrine-disrupting chemicals. *Environ Health Perspect*. 121, 7–14.

Roy P, Salminen H, Koskimies P et al. (2004). Screening of some anti-androgenic endocrine disruptors using a recombinant cell-based in vitro bioassay. *J Steroid Biochem Mol Biol*. 88, 157–66.

Ryu JY, Lee BM, Kacew S, Kim HS (2007). Identification of differentially expressed genes in the testis of Sprague-Dawley rats treated with di(*n*-butyl) phthalate. *Toxicology*. 234, 103–12.

Schrader TJ, Cooke GM (2003). Effects of Aroclors and individual PCB congeners on activation of the human androgen receptor in vitro. *Reprod Toxicol*. 17, 15–23.

Schecter A, Colacino J, Sjodin A et al. (2010). Partitioning of polybrominated diphenyl ethers (PBDEs) in serum and milk from the same mothers. *Chemosphere*. 78, 1279–84.

Seegal RF (1999). Are PCBs the major neurotoxicant in Great Lakes salmon? *Environ Res*. 80, S38–45.

Semenza JC, Tolbert PE, Rubin CH et al. (1997). Reproductive toxins and alligator abnormalities at Lake Apopka, Florida. *Environ Health Perspect*. 105, 1030–2.

Silva MJ, Reidy JA, Samandar E et al. (2005). Detection of phthalate metabolites in human saliva. *Arch Toxicol*. 79, 647–52.

Sonne C, Wolkers H, Leifsson PS et al. (2009). Chronic dietary exposure to environmental organochlorine contaminants induces thyroid gland lesions in Arctic foxes (Vulpes lagopus). *Environ Res*. 109, 702–11.

Stapleton HM, Dodder NG, Offenberg JH et al. (2005). Polybrominated diphenyl ethers in house dust and clothes dryer lint. *Environ Sci Technol*. 39, 925–31.

Swan SH (2006). Prenatal phthalate exposure and anogenital distance in male infants. *Environ Health Perspect*. 114, A88–9.

Thayer KA, Heindel JJ, Bucher JR et al. (2012). Role of environmental chemicals in diabetes and obesity: A national toxicology program workshop report. *Environ Health Perspect*. 120, 779–89.

Tomatis L (1994). Transgeneration carcinogenesis: A review of the experimental and epidemiological evidence. *Jpn J Cancer Res.* 85, 443–54.

Viberg H, Frederiksson A, Eriksson P (2003). Neonatal exposure to polybrominated diphenyl ether (PBDE 153) disrupts spontaneous behavior, impairs learning and memory, and decreases hippocampal cholinergic receptors in adult mice. *Toxicol Appl Pharmacol.* 192, 95–106.

Whitehead SA, Rice S (2006). Endocrine-disrupting chemicals as modulators of sex steroid synthesis. *Best Pract Res Clin Endocrinol Metabol.* 20, 45–61.

White R, Jobling S, Hoare SA et al. (1994). Environmentally persistent alkylphenolic compounds are estrogenic. *Endocrinology.* 135, 175–82.

Wilford BH, Harner T, Zhu J, Shoeib M, Jones KC (2004). Passive sampling survey of polybrominated diphenyl ether flame retardants in indoor and outdoor air in Ottawa, Canada: Implications for sources and exposure. *Environ Sci Technol.* 38, 5312–8.

Willhite CC, Ball GL, McLellan CJ (2008). Derivation of a bisphenol A oral refernce dose (RfD) and drinking water equivalent concentration. *J Toxicol Environ Health B.* 11, 69–146.

Wolff MS, Toniolo PG (1995). Environmental organochlorine exposure as a potential etiologic factor in breast cancer. *Environ Health Perspect.* 103(Suppl 7), 141–5.

Xi Y, Li D, San W (2013). Exposure to NP may lead to thyroid dysfunction. It may be a potential contributor to thyroid disruption. *Regul Pept.* 185, 52–6.

Yoon K, Kwack SJ, Kim HS, Lee BM (2014). Estrogenic endocrine-disrupting chemicals: Molecular mechanisms of actions on putative human diseases. *J Toxicol Environ Health B.* 17, 127–74.

Yu ML, Guo YL, Hsu CC et al. (2000). Menstruation and reproduction in women with polychlorinated biphenyl (PCB) poisoning: Long-term follow-up interviews of the women from the Taiwan Yucheng cohort. *Int J Epidemiol.* 29, 672–7.

Yusof YA, Edwards AM (1990). Stimulation of DNA synthesis in primary rat hepatocyte cultures by liver tumor promoters: Interactions with other growth factors. *Carcinogenesis.* 11, 761–70.

*section four*

---

# *Toxic substances and risk assessment*

# *chapter twenty-two*

# *Food additives, contaminants, and safety*

***Sam Kacew and Byung-Mu Lee***

*Contents*

# Introduction

As the global population increases, there has been a growing demand for more food. Various physical means and chemical substances have been developed and utilized to enhance food supply. However, the increased efficiency of farming has reduced the number of farmers. In addition, with industrialization and urbanization, many more individuals are residing away from farmlands. These social changes have resulted in an ever-increasing demand for processed foods, which can be transported from farms to the cities, that will retain their nutritive value and organoleptic properties. These demands have been met largely by addition of chemicals known as food additives. These chemicals serve a variety of technological functions, as described in the section "Functional Groups of Direct Food Additives."

## *Legal definition of food additives*

The following definition has been adopted by the Codex Alimentarius Commission, an intergovernmental agency consisting of more than 150 nations (FAO/WHO, 1994).

A *food additive* is "any substance not normally consumed as a food by itself and not normally used as a typical ingredient of the food, whether or not it has nutritive value. The intentional addition of this to food, for a technological (including organoleptic) purpose, in the manufacture, processing, preparation, treatment, packing, packaging, transport, or holding of such food, results or is reasonably expected to result (directly or indirectly) in it or its byproducts becoming a component of, or otherwise, affecting the characteristics of such foods." The definition does not include "contaminants" or substances added to food for maintaining or improving nutritional qualities.

The U.S. legal definition appearing in the U.S. Federal Food, Drug, and Cosmetic Act, as amended in October 1976 (1979), is different from the above in several aspects. The U.S. legislation excludes color additives and those substances that are to be added to food, but are defined as "generally recognized as safe (GRAS)." On the other hand, U.S. legislation considers nutritional supplements and irradiated foods as food additives.

## *Classification of food additives and contaminants*

### *Functional groups of direct food additives*

A number of chemicals are added to food to increase its shelf life, to render food more amenable to mass production, or to enhance its consumer appeal with respect to color, flavor, texture, and convenience. These chemicals are grouped according to their technological functions. Detailed listing of various groups of food additives and their uses is given in a Codex document (FAO/WHO, 1994). The major functional groups and some examples are listed in Appendix 22.1.

### *Indirect (unintentional) food additives*

The substances mentioned above are intentionally added to foods for specific technological purposes. Consequently, these are considered "direct" or "intentional" food additives. However, a number of substances may become part of the foods as a result of their use during the production, processing, or storage of the foods. These include antibiotics and anabolic agents used during the raising of farm animals, residue from food processing machinery, and migrants from packaging materials. In recent years, the genetic modification of crops has yielded greater production of food products, with a similar nutritive value; however, the consequences with respect to human health still remain unresolved. The genetically modified food may not be able to be metabolized by humans or may produce byproducts that individuals cannot handle and subsequently produce toxic reactions. Genetically modified foods (GMFs) play a crucial role in increasing the food supply, but one needs to be aware of the potential adverse effects.

### *Food contaminants*

These substances are present in foods as a result of environmental pollution or faulty handling of food. In other words, they serve no useful purpose either in the final food product or in its processing. Examples are mercury in fish harvested from contaminated fish farms, and mycotoxins found in improperly stored nuts and grains. Thus, they differ from both direct and indirect food additives.

## *International aspects*

Food, raw and processed, is commonly traded internationally. The additives and contaminants (and residue from pesticides) must be considered acceptable for the protection of the health of consumers. However, food that is considered acceptable by an exporting country may not be considered acceptable by the importing country. This was the case with beef from Canada after the outbreak of the "Mad Cow Disease," which was controlled by eradication of all infected animals, yet the importing countries still did not accept Canadian cattle.

In an attempt to reduce such disputes, the World Health Organization (WHO) and the Food and Agriculture Organization of the United Nations (FAO), at the request of governments, established mechanisms to provide independent toxicological evaluations. The mechanisms created were the Joint FAO/WHO Expert Committee on Food Additives and Contaminants (JECFA) and the Joint FAO/WHO Meeting of Experts on Pesticide Residues (JMPR). Members of these committees were selected from a panel of internationally known experts, acting independently.

Since their inception in the early 1960s, they have been convened annually. During these meetings, they have evaluated and reevaluated many food additives, contaminants, and pesticide residue. Acceptable daily intakes (ADIs) are allocated to those chemicals that the toxicological data so indicates. The ADIs are used by regulatory agencies in some countries.

More importantly, the ADIs are used by the Joint FAO/WHO Food Standard Program and the Codex Alimentarius Commission to establish international food standards. There are more than 150 nations that are members of the commission. Some details on the relationship among the national food regulatory agencies, national research facilities, and the Codex Alimentarius Commission are given in Chapter 30. A comprehensive review of this subject is provided in a review (Lu, 1988).

## *Toxicological testing and evaluation*

### *Categories of data required*

As these chemicals are added to foods to be consumed by large numbers of people, they are in general extensively tested and strictly evaluated. Further, because of their low toxicity, precise $LD_{50}$s are, as a rule, not required. The studies required by JECFA are categorized as follows:

1. Biochemical, including absorption, distribution, elimination (and storage), biotransformation, and effects on enzymes and other biochemical parameters
2. Acute toxicity
3. Short-term toxicity
4. Chronic toxicity
5. Reproductive toxicity
6. Mutagenicity
7. Carcinogenicity
8. Teratogenicity (developmental)
9. Clinical observations in humans

### *Extent of testing*

The JECFA considers, as a general rule, that the types of biological data listed above are required for proper evaluation of food additives.

However, for certain groups of additives, depending on their chemical nature, source, and usage, much less data are required. These include:

1. Components of food and closely related chemicals including vitamins
2. Certain enzymes used in food processing
3. Certain food colors
4. Certain metals (e.g., copper, iron, and zinc)

Detailed descriptions of the types of additives and the required data are given in several WHO reports (WHO, 1974, 1982, 1986). These descriptions are summarized in a review article (Lu, 1988).

The U.S. Food and Drug Administration (FDA) established a set of criteria to determine the "level of concern" (LOC), which in turn dictates the extent of testing required (FDA, 1982). The LOC was determined by the chemical structure of the additive and concentration in food. Additives are placed in three categories according to their chemical structure: A, B, and C. Additives of low probable toxicity are assigned to category A. This category comprises nine types of chemicals, such as simple aliphatic, noncyclic hydrocarbons with no unsaturation; sugars and polysaccharides; fats and fatty acids; and endogenous inorganic salts of alkali metals (Na and K) and alkaline earth metals (Mg and Ca). Additives with functional groups of high probable toxicity are assigned to category C. Additives of intermediate or unknown probable toxicity are assigned to category B.

## *Evaluation*

The toxicological evaluation of food additives follows the procedure of determining the adequacy of data, establishing an appropriate no-observed effect level, and selecting a proper safety factor to obtain the acceptable daily intake. This procedure is generally adopted by many national regulatory agencies, including the U.S. Food and Drug Administration, as well as the international organizations WHO and FAO. The toxicological basis for drafting the provisions for food additives in the International Food Standards is provided by the JECFA. The interrelationship between the various national and international bodies is described in a review article (Lu, 1988).

## *Generally recognized as safe*

As noted above, the U.S. legislation considers certain chemicals to be "generally recognized as safe." This was done originally in 1958, and that list included more than 600 direct additives, with a variety of technological functions, and some 2000 indirect additives. Since then, the list of direct additives has been expanded, mainly by the addition of more than 1000 flavoring ingredients proposed by the Flavor and Extract Manufacturers' Association. GRAS substances are evaluated by the Select Committee on GRAS Substances.

On the basis of new toxicological information, the safety of a number of substances on the list has since been questioned. The most notable was the suspected carcinogenicity of the artificial sweetener cyclamate. As a result, the FDA, in 1970, asked the Life Sciences Research Office of the Federation of American Societies for Experimental Biology to evaluate the safety of all the substances on the GRAS list. A Select Committee on GRAS Substances was formed and issued many reports containing its conclusion and summaries of the available information on 468 substances. A detailed account of the study by the committee is given by Carr (1987).

## *Additives of toxicological concern*

Some 600 intentional food additives are being added to a variety of our foods. The toxicity of most of these additives has been evaluated according to the prevailing procedure and considered to be "safe." However, the use of some additives has been restricted, suspended, or requires label declaration, because of toxicological concern.

### *Carcinogenicity*

The safety of *saccharin*, for example, has been questioned because of its reported carcinogenicity. In fact, the first study that revealed increased bladder tumors in rats involved the dosing of the animals with a combination of saccharin and cyclamate in a ratio of 1:9. Saccharin has been found to be excreted as such and is nonmutagenic in most test systems. However, a large-scale experiment carried out in a Canadian government laboratory showed that rats that fed on a diet with 7.5% saccharin developed bladder tumors (Arnold et al., 1977). The significance of this finding is somewhat doubtful because of the excessively high dosage and because the tumors occurred mainly among the male rats of the second generation. A recent epidemiological study suggests that artificial sweeteners including consumption of saccharin and aspartame may not be associated with cancer risk in Italy (Bosetti et al., 2009), whereas, increased cases of urinary tract tumors were observed in a case control study in Argentina (Andreatta et al., 2008).

*Cyclamates* were considered innocuous and were used widely in foods and beverages for many years. However, doubt was cast on their safety because of the discovery that they were metabolized to cyclohexylamine by intestinal flora in animals and humans, which appears to be more toxic (Classen et al., 1968). Its use as a food additive was suspended in 1969, when it was discovered that a mixture of saccharin and cyclamate increased the incidence of bladder tumors in rats (Price et al., 1970). Subsequent studies on cyclamate showed no carcinogenicity, and the short-term mutagenicity tests yielded no consistent results. This was also true of cyclohexylamine. Summaries of the reports are included in two publications (IARC, 1980; WHO, 1982). Its use has been restored in a number of countries, although it is still not permitted for use as an additive in the United States.

*Nitrates* and *nitrites* are useful preservatives and they impart a special color and flavor to treated meat such as ham and corned beef. However, they can form, with certain amines, a variety of nitrosamines, many of which are potent carcinogens. However, nitrates and nitrites are valuable in controlling toxin-forming microorganisms such as *Clostridium botulinum*. In addition, some of the epidemiological and clinical studies demonstrated that nitrates and nitrites of plant origin may play essential physiological roles in supporting cardiovascular health and gastrointestinal immune function (Hord et al., 2009). Further, nitrites occur in the body, notably in the saliva, and it has been demonstrated that nitrosation of certain amines can occur in the stomach. For these reasons, the use of these preservatives has not been suspended, but the amount used has been reduced.

On the other hand, the preservative *diethyl pyrocarbonate* (DEPC) presents a distinctly different picture. It has been used in a variety of beverages, but its use has been suspended. This decision was based on the finding that DEPC may combine with the ammonium ion in beverages to form urethane, a wide-spectrum carcinogen in all animal species tested, and on the fact that its use is not indispensable.

*Butylated hydroxyanisole* (BHA) and *butylated hydroxytoluene* (BHT) are widely used antioxidants and have been investigated in several long-term studies without revealing any serious adverse effects. However, Ito et al. (1983) reported that BHA, at very high dietary levels, induced hyperplasia and tumors in the forestomach of rats. As the tumors were only found in the forestomach, the relevance of this finding in terms of human health hazard was questioned. Additional studies using species without a forestomach were performed. The results were negative in dogs, and the increased mitotic rate in the esophagus of pigs was questionable (WHO, 1989). Olsen et al. (1983) reported an increase in hepatocellular adenoma and carcinoma. However, several other studies yielded negative results. Further, other studies on these antioxidants produced cancer-protective effects (Prochaska et al., 1985). In spite of these conflicting results, BHA and BHT are still being used.

## *Hypersensitivity reactions*

A number of food additives are known to induce hypersensitivity reactions in susceptible individuals. As they affect only a small proportion of the general population, and because their effects are usually mild and transitory, most regulatory agencies consider label declaration as a sufficient method to provide warning to these individuals. The following are the more commonly known ones.

*Tartrazine*, a widely used yellow color in a variety of processed foods, has been known to induce allergic reactions, especially among those who are allergic to aspirin (Juhlin, 1980).

*Sulfur dioxide* and related chemicals, such as bisulfites and metabisulfites, are used as preservatives in processed foods as well as salads. In the latter case, these chemicals help to preserve the freshness of the vegetables. As it is difficult to provide warning labels, such use has been discouraged.

*Monosodium glutamate* (MSG) has been used as a flavor enhancer for many decades in China and Japan. No untoward effects have been reported. However, a "Chinese restaurant syndrome" has been reported (Schaumberg et al., 1969). It usually appears after the individual has consumed a special Chinese soup, which contains relatively large amounts of MSG. The hypersensitivity reaction consists of a burning sensation, tingling in the face and neck, tightness in the chest, and so on. On account of these findings, it is now possible, in many restaurants, to order soups and other dishes specifying "no MSG." For additional details, see Kenney (1986) and Jinap and Hajeb (2010). The fact that adverse reactions to MSG have not been observed in the Far East is evidently related to the custom of consuming the soup as the last course, that is, on a full stomach, thereby delaying the absorption of this chemical and preventing a dramatic rise in blood levels.

## *Other adverse effects*

In addition to carcinogenicity and hypersensitivity reactions, the discovery of other adverse effects has prompted regulatory decisions or additional investigations. The examples are heart lesions in lab animals associated with brominated vegetable oils (BVO), a suspending agent in certain beverages, and liver lesions associated with Orange RN and Ponceau 2R, which were responsible for the suspension of their use. Other effects such as red blood cell damage (Orange RN), storage in tissues (BVO), and testicular atrophy (cyclohexylamine from cyclamate) were contributing factors to the toxicological decisions on these additives (see Lu, 1979a).

## *Indirect additives and contaminants*

Apart from direct food additives, there are a large number of indirect additives and some contaminants that pose toxicological problems and require different control measures. The problems are highlighted as follows.

### *Indirect food additives*

The most important of these chemicals are: (1) constituents of the packaging material, which may migrate into the food that is in contact with them, and (2) animal drug residues that are commonly used in raising food-producing animals.

#### *Food packaging materials*

A number of substances may migrate from food containers, wrappers, and the like, to the food that is packaged in them. Most of the chemicals that might migrate from the conventional types of packaging materials, such as paper and wood, had been considered safe and were included in the FDA's GRAS list. More recently, however, the packaging items are generally made of polymeric materials. The polymers per se are generally inert, but the components, the monomers, which are present to some extent, residual reactants, intermediates, manufacturing aids, solvents, and plastic additives, as well as the products of side reaction and chemical degradation by-products may migrate into the food that is in contact with them. Some of these chemicals have been shown to be toxic.

Vinyl chloride has been shown to be a human carcinogen at high levels of exposure, and acrylonitrile is a probable human carcinogen. Both are carcinogenic in a number of animal species (Chapter 8). Currently, bisphenol A, which is widely used in the linings of metal cans and feeding bottles, was found to be an endocrine-disrupting chemical in animals in very high quantities (Willhite et al., 2008). The release of phthalates from food packaging has raised concerns, due to the estrogenic effects of these compounds in animals. Administration of phthalates in very high concentrations is known to produce testicular dysfunction in rats (Kim et al., 2004). However, no human data showing an abnormal reproductive function in humans are available, as the concentration of phthalates or bisphenol A released is exceedingly small and not environmentally realistic. Thus, because of the exceedingly low levels of exposure from migration to food, these chemicals continue to be used and provisionally approved. The difficulty one faces is that the adverse responses reported are due to the concentration, but when there is interpolation to risk, the concentration cannot be attained by humans.

*Animal drug residue in human food*

There are essentially three types of drugs used in food-producing animals that may leave residues in human food, such as meat, milk, and eggs. The drugs not only present a problem related to the parent chemicals, but it is also necessary to consider their metabolites, which are produced as a result of the metabolic processes, including bioactivation in the animals, which may possess different toxic properties (Hayes and Borzelleca, 1982).

*Therapeutic drugs,* such as the anthelmintic agents febantel, fenbendazole, and oxfendazole are generally used in individual animals for specific disease and only over short periods. Therefore, they do not pose a widespread health concern. On the other hand, tranquilizing agents such as chlorpromazine and propylpromazine are used shortly before slaughter, and hence, leave residues in the meat. Their use is therefore banned (WHO, 1995).

*Antibiotics* such as benzyl penicillin and oxytetracycline are usually incorporated in the animal feeds to prevent outbreaks of bacterial diseases and to promote growth. The residue levels are generally extremely low and not expected to induce toxic effects. These antibiotics can result in resistance in humans, which is a concern.

*Anabolic agents* are growth-promoting substances and are implanted subcutaneously in a part of the animal that is usually not eaten, such as the ear. Their residue levels in the meat are low enough to be essentially devoid of general toxic effects, except carcinogenicity. A carcinogen may be effective at extremely low-dose levels. Diethylstilbestrol (DES) is no longer used as a growth promoter, because of the discovery that tumors of genital organs had developed in the offspring of mothers who had taken DES in large doses during pregnancy for medical purposes.

The anabolic agents in use may be considered either "endogenous" or "exogenous." The former includes estradiol, progesterone, and testosterone. The latter includes porcine somatotropin and trenbolone acetate. Trenbolone has been shown to be teratogenic and immunotoxic in the avian species (Quinn et al., 2007). The "endogenous" anabolic agents are considered indistinguishable from the endogenous hormones, and the "erogenous" hormones leave very low levels of residues. Acceptable daily intakes (ADI) have been allocated to their residues (WHO, 2000a).

## Food contaminants

There are three main types of food contaminants: mycotoxins, heavy metals, and synthetic chemicals. These contaminate food because of growing or harvesting from contaminated soil or water, improper handling, and accidental release from industrial sources.

## Mycotoxins

*Aflatoxins*, produced by the mold *Aspergillus flavus*, occur in nuts and grains, especially when these commodities are stored in a humid and warm climate. These toxins exist as mixtures of aflatoxins $B_1$, $B_2$, $G_1$, and $G_2$. Among these aflatoxins, $B_1$ is the most potent carcinogen in most species of animals, especially the rat. In one experiment, rats fed on a diet containing 1 ppb of aflatoxin $B_1$ had hyperplastic nodules and carcinoma of the liver (Wogan et al., 1974). Aflatoxins $G_1$ and $M_1$ (a metabolite of $B_1$, occurring in milk) are also carcinogenic, but much less potent. A positive correlation was noted between aflatoxin intake and liver cancer incidence in certain regions of Africa and Thailand (IARC, 1976). Lu (2003) has provided a more extensive review on aflatoxins. As noted in Chapter 3, aflatoxin is bioactivated to aflatoxin-8,9-epoxide, which may covalently bind to DNA, and thus initiate carcinogenesis.

A number of other mycotoxins also occur in foods. Deoxynivalenol occurs commonly in cereal-based foods. Deoxynivalenol was shown to produce gastrointestinal disturbances, immune dysfunction, and anorexia (Pestka and Smolinki, 2005). Ochratoxin A is present in dairy products, chocolate, beer, coffee, wine, poultry, and pork. Ochratoxin A produces Balkan endemic nephropathy as well as cancer (Clark and Snedeker, 2006). Their characteristics are summarized in Table 22.1. Additional information on these and other mycotoxins may be found in two WHO publications (1990, 2000b).

***Table 22.1*** Source, occurrence, and toxicity of certain mycotoxins

| Mycotoxin | Source | Occurrence | Toxic effects |
|---|---|---|---|
| Aflatoxins | *Aspergillus* | Nuts, grains | Liver cancer |
| Ergot | *Claviceps purpurea* | Grains, especially rye | Ergotism (spasm, cramps, dry gangrene) |
| Fumonisin $B_1$ | *Fusarium* | Maize | Esophageal cancer |
| Ochratoxins | *Aspergillus* | Grains | Nephropathy |
| | *Penicillium* | | Cancer |
| Trichothecenes | *Fusarium trichoderma* | Grains | Vomiting, diarrhea, skin inflammation, multiple hemorrhage |
| Zearalenone | *Fusarium* | Grains | Estrogenic effects |

*Source:* WHO, *Environ Health Criteria No. 105*, World Health Organization, Geneva, 1990; WHO, *Environ Health Criteria No. 219*, World Health Organization, Geneva, 2000b.

## *Neurotoxins*

Certain toxins are found in marine animals that are used as food (Table 22.2). The notable ones are saxitoxin, which may be present in clams, and tetradotoxin, which is found in puffer fish, especially in its ovaries. An important and extremely toxic substance is the botulinum toxin. It is produced by the bacteria *C. botulinum* in improperly canned food. The major toxic effects of these toxins are on the nervous system. Descriptions of these effects are provided in Chapter 18. Another toxin (ciguatoxin) is occasionally present in large coastal fish, in certain geographical areas, notably the Caribbean Sea. In addition to the nervous system, it often produces toxic effects on the GI system.

## *Metals*

The toxic properties of a number of metals are described in Chapter 25, but human exposure via food is highlighted in this section. Among the metals that have produced the most concern are mercury, lead, cadmium, and arsenic.

A number of acute and chronic poisoning episodes have resulted from improper application or consumption of alkyl *mercury* compounds used as fungicides to preserve seed grains. Others followed consumption of fish contaminated with methylmercury. The compound can be formed via bioactivation (aided by microorganisms in the mud) of mercury discharged from factories (e.g., in Minamata and Niigata, Japan; Appendix 1.2). On account of the biomagnification factor along the food

***Table* 22.2** Source, occurrence, and toxicity of certain neurotoxins in marine animals

| Toxins | Source | Occurrence | Toxic effects |
|---|---|---|---|
| Botulinum toxin | Clostridium botulinum | Improperly canned food | Impairing ACh release |
| Ciquatoxin | Blue-green algae | Large coastal fishes | Various effects on nervous and GI systems |
| Domoic acid | *Pseudonitzschia multiseries* and *Pseudonitzschia australis* | Mussels, seaweed, and red algae | Memory loss, seizure, and gastroenteritis |
| Saxitoxin | Gonyolax | Clams | Blocking of nerve conduction |
| Tetrodotoxin | Uncertain | Puffer fish | Blocking of nerve conduction |

chain, large carnivorous fish generally contain much higher levels of methylmercury (WHO, 1976; Bayen et al., 2005).

*Lead* has been used as a fuel additive, in lead batteries, paints, and so on. Humans are exposed to this metal via air, water, and food. According to one analysis, daily intakes from these media amount to 15, 20, and 140 μg, respectively (NRC Canada, 1973). One unusual source of lead intake is improperly fired ceramic foodware, which may release large amounts of lead from the glaze, and which has produced a number of poisonings. This fact has prompted the promulgation of limits in the extent of release of lead from various types of foodware (WHO, 1979). The estimated intake of lead from ceramic ware would be in the range of 30–80 μg/day if all the wares in use released this metal to the legal limit (Lu, 1979b). Among certain populations, ceramic foodware still constitutes an important source of lead (Rojas-Lopez et al., 1994).

*Cadmium* is used as a pigment and occurs in the environment, especially through the refining of zinc ores, which contain varying concentrations of cadmium. It enters the food chain through pollution of soil and water. The Itai-Itai disease in Japan has been attributed to chronic exposure to cadmium, through long-term ingestion of contaminated rice. It may also be leached from decorated ceramic foodware.

*Arsenic* contamination is primarily attributed to the smelting and mining industries. It enters the food chain through pollution of soil and water. Arsenic poisoning results in black foot disease (peripheral vascular disorder), hyperkeratotic lesions on the skin leading to cancer, as well as liver cancer (Bernstam and Nriagu, 2000).

*Certain organic compounds*

Among these chemicals are *organochlorine insecticides*, which have been widely used. Their use has been discontinued because of their persistence in the environment. However, they are still present in foods, in trace amounts. Others include *polychlorinated biphenyls* (PCBs), which are used in electrical capacitors and transformers, as plasticizers and heat exchangers, and in paper manufacturing. Through leakage and discharge of waste, they enter the environment. On account of their persistence and biomagnification properties, they enter the food chain. These chemicals have attracted much attention because of the episode of consumption of a batch of rice oil contaminated with PCBs through a leak in a heat exchanger in 1968. Thousands of consumers in Japan were affected (Appendix 1.2). The main sign of toxicity was chloracne, although there were many other symptoms and signs (Chapter 1). Similarly, an inadvertent addition of *polybrominated biphenyls* (PBBs) to cattle feed, in Michigan, resulted in the contamination of a large amount of beef and milk. In addition, some polybrominated flame retardants used in electronics, furniture,

***Table* 22.3** Action levels for certain food contaminants

| Contaminants | Commodity | Action level |
|---|---|---|
| Aflatoxin | Nuts | 20 ppb |
| | Foods and feeds | 20 ppb |
| | Milk[a] | 0.5 ppb |
| Aldrin and dieldrin | Various foods | 0.02–0.3 ppm |
| Cadmium, in leaching solution from ceramic ware | Flatware | 0.5 μg/mL |
| | Small hollowware | 0.5 μg/mL |
| | Large hollowware | 0.25 μg/mL |
| Lead, in leaching solution from ceramic ware | Flatware | 3.0 μg/mL |
| | Small hollowware | 2.0 μg/mL |
| | Large hollowware | 1.0 μg/mL |
| Mercury | Fish, shellfish, crustaceans | 1.0 ppm |
| | Wheat | 1.0 ppm |
| Polychlorinated biphenyls | Red meat (fat basis) | 3 ppm |

*Source:* FDA, Food and Drug Administration, Washington, DC, 2000.

[a] Aflatoxin M1.

and the like, resulted in the contamination of various foods, including fruits, vegetables, and baby food.

The "action levels" for these and other contaminants have been established by the U.S. FDA, to control their levels in food and feed. Some of them are listed in Table 22.3. Poisonous plants are also listed in Table 1.1 in Chapter 1.

## *Appendix 22.1 Major functional groups of direct food additives*

1. Preservatives are added to prolong the shelf life of foods by preventing or inhibiting microbial growth. Examples are benzoic acid, propionic acid, and sorbic acid, their salts, nitrates and nitrites, and sulfur dioxide and related compounds.
2. Antioxidants are added to oils to prevent them from becoming rancid, which is a result of oxidative changes. Some are added to fruits and vegetables to prevent enzymatic browning. The most commonly used ones include butylated hydroxyanisole, butylated hydroxytoluene, various gallates, ascorbic acid and its salts, and α-tocopherol.
3. Emulsifying, stabilizing, and thickening agents are added to improve the homogeneity, stability, and "body" of a variety of food products. These include mono- and diglycerides, sucrose esters of fatty acids, lecithin, salts of various types of phosphates, modified

starches, calcium gluconate, calcium citrate, agar, alginic acid and its salts, various vegetable gums, and cellulose derivatives.
4. Colors are used to enhance the visual appeal of food products. Some of these substances are derived from natural colors, such as carotene, chlorophyll, and cochineal. Others are synthetic, such as allura red, amaranth, azorubine, indigotine, and tartrazine.
5. Flavors and flavor enhancers. The flavors constitute the largest group of food additives. However, they are used, in general, at very low levels in foods. Some are synthetic (mainly esters, aldehydes, and ketones) and others are derived from natural sources (such as oleoresins, plant extracts, and essential oils). Flavor enhancers, such as monosodium glutamate, enhance the flavor of the food to which it is added.
6. Artificial sweeteners have a strong sweet taste, but have little or no caloric value. They are therefore useful for diabetics and for those who wish to enjoy the sweet taste without increasing the caloric intake. The notable ones are the cyclamates, saccharin, and aspartame.
7. Nutrients include vitamins, minerals, and essential amino acids. As noted above, national regulations in most countries, contrary to those of the United States, do not consider these as food additives. However, a food additive used for a technological reason may incidentally have certain nutritional values. For example, riboflavin may be used as a color, but it is also a vitamin.
8. Miscellaneous groups. These include (a) acidity regulators (acids and bases), which are used to adjust the pH of beverages and canned fruits and vegetables; (b) anticaking agents, which are added to salt, sugar, etc., to maintain their free-flowing property; (c) antifoaming agents, which are added to liquids to prevent foaming; (d) flour treatment agents, which are added to flour to improve its baking qualities; (e) glazing agents; (f) propellants; and (g) raising agents.

## References

Andreatta MM, Muñoz SE, Lantieri MJ et al. (2008). Artificial sweetener consumption and urinary tract tumors in Cordoba, Argentina. *Prev Med*. 47, 136–9.

Arnold DL, Moodie CA, Stavric D et al. (1977). Canadian saccharin study. *Science*. 197, 320.

Bayen S, Koroleva E, Lee HK et al. (2005). Persistent organic pollutants and heavy metals in typical seafoods consumed in Singapore. *J Toxicol Environ Health A*. 68, 151–66.

Bernstam L, Nriagu J (2000). Molecular aspects of arsenic stress. *J Toxicol Environ Health B*. 3, 293–322.

Bosetti C, Gallus S, Talamini R et al. (2009). Artificial sweeteners and the risk of gastric, pancreatic, and endometrial cancers in Italy. *Cancer Epidemiol Biomarkers Prev.* 18, 2235–8.
Carr CJ (1987). Food additives: A benefit/risk dilemma. In: Haley TJ, Berndt WO, eds. *Handbook of Toxicology.* Washington, DC: Hemisphere.
Clark HA, Snedeker SM (2006). Ochratoxin A: Its cancer risk and potential for exposure. *J Toxicol Environ Health B.* 9, 265–96.
Classen HG, Marquardt P, Spath M (1968). Sympathomimetic effects of cyclohexylamine. *Arzneimittel Forsch.* 18, 590–4.
FAO/WHO (1994). Food Additives. *Codex Alimentarius, vol. XIV.* Rome: Food Agriculture Organization of the United Nations.
FDA (1982). Toxicological principles for the safety assessment of direct additives and color additives used in food. U.S. Food and Drug Administration. Springfield, VA: National Technical Information Service, PB 83–170696.
FDA (2000). Action levels for poisonous or deleterious substances in human food and animal feed. Washington, DC: Food and Drug Administration.
Hayes JR, Borzelleca JF (1982). Biodisposition of xenobiotics in animals. In: Beitz DC, Hanson R, eds. *Animal Products in Human Nutrition.* New York: Academic Press, 225–59.
Hord NG, Tang Y, Bryan NS (2009). Food sources of nitrates and nitrites: The physiologic context for potential health benefits. *Am J Clin Nutr.* 90, 1–10.
IARC (1976). Evaluation of Carcinogenic Risk of Chemicals to Man, vol. 10. Some Naturally Occurring Substances. Lyon, France: International Agency for Research on Cancer.
IARC (1980). Evaluation of the Carcinogenic Risk of Chemicals to Humans, vol. 22. Some Non-Nutritive Sweetening Agents. Lyon, France: International Agency for Research on Cancer.
Ito N, Fukushima S, Hagiwara A et al. (1983). Carcinogenicity of butylated hydroxyanisole in F344 rats. *J Natl Cancer Inst.* 70, 343–52.
Jinap S, Hajeb P. (2010). Glutamate. Its applications in food and contribution to health. *Appetite.* 55, 1–10.
Juhlin L (1980). Incidence of intolerance to food additives. *Int J Dermatol.* 19, 548–51.
Kenney RA (1986). The Chinese restaurant syndrome: An anecdote revisited. *Food Chem Toxicol.* 24, 351–4.
Kim HS, Kim TS, Shin JH et al. (2004). Neonatal exposure to di(*n*-butyl)phthalate alters male reproductive tract development. *J Toxicol Environ Health A.* 67, 2045–60.
Lu FC (1979a). The safety of food additives: The dynamics of the issue. In: Deichmann WB, ed. *Toxicology and Occupational Medicine.* New York: Elsevier/North Holland.
Lu FC (1979b). Review of Total Intake of Lead from All Sources. WHO: HCS/CER/79.5. Geneva, Switzerland: World Health Organization.
Lu FC (1988). Acceptable daily intake: Inception, evolution and application. *Reg Toxicol Pharmacol.* 8, 45–60.
Lu FC (2003). Assessment of safety/risk vs. public health: Aflatoxins and hepacarcinoma. *Environ Health and Prev Med.* 7, 235–8.
NRC Canada (1973). Lead in the Canadian environment. NRCC No. 13682. Ottawa: National Research Council of Canada.
Olsen P, Bille N, Meyer O (1983). Hepatocellular neoplasms in rats induced by butylated hydroxytoluene (BHT). *Acta Pharmacol Toxicol.* 54, 433–4.

Pestka JJ, Smolinski AT (2005). Deoxynivalenol: Toxicology and potential effects on humans. *J Toxicol Environ Health B*. 8, 39–69.

Price JM, Biava CG, Oser BL et al. (1970). Bladder tumors in rats fed cyclohexylamine or high doses of a mixture of cyclamate and saccharin. *Science*. 167, 1131–2.

Prochaska HJ, DeLong MJ, Talalay P (1985). On the mechanisms of induction of cancer-protective enzymes: A unifying proposal. *Proc Natl Acad Sci USA*. 82, 8232–6.

Quinn MJ, McKernan M, Lavoie ET et al. (2007). Immunotoxicity of trenbolone acetate in Japanese quail. *J Toxicol Environ Health A*. 70, 88–93.

Rojas-Lopez M, Santos-Burgoa C, Rios C et al. (1994). Use of lead-glazed ceramics is the main factor associated to high lead in blood levels in two Mexican rural communities. *J Toxicol Environ Health*. 42, 45–52.

Schaumberg HH, Byck R, Gerstl R et al. (1969). Monosodium glutamate: Its pharmacology and role in the Chinese restaurant syndrome. *Science*. 163, 826.

U.S. Federal Food, Drug, and Cosmetic Act, as Amended (1979). Washington, DC: U.S. Government Printing Office.

WHO (1974). Toxicological Evaluation of Certain Food Additives with a Review of General Principles and of Specifications (17th Report). Tech Rep Ser. 539. Geneva, Switzerland: World Health Organization.

WHO (1976). Mercury. Environmental Health Criteria 1. Geneva, Switzerland: World Health Organization.

WHO (1979). Ceramic Foodware Safety. Report of a Meeting of Experts. HCS/79.7. Geneva, Switzerland: World Health Organization.

WHO (1982). Evaluation of Certain Food Additives and Contaminants (26th Report). Tech Rep Ser. 683. Geneva, Switzerland: World Health Organization.

WHO (1986). Evaluation of Certain Food Additives and Contaminants (29th Report). Tech Rep Ser. 733. Geneva, Switzerland: World Health Organization.

WHO (1989). Evaluation of Certain Food Additives and Contaminants. WHO Food Additives Series 24. Geneva, Switzerland: World Health Organization.

WHO (1990). Selected Mycotoxins: Ochratoxins, Trichothecene, Ergot Environ Health Criteria No. 105. Geneva, Switzerland: World Health Organization.

WHO (1995). Evaluation of Certain Veterinary Drug Residues in Food (38th Report). Tech Rep Ser. 815. Geneva, Switzerland: World Health Organization.

WHO (2000a). Toxicological Evaluation of Certain Veterinary Drug Residues in Food. Food Additives Series No. 43. Geneva, Switzerland: World Health Organization.

WHO (2000b). Fumonisin $B_1$. Environ Health Criteria No. 219. Geneva, Switzerland: World Health Organization.

Wilhite CC, Ball GL, McLellan CJ (2008). Derivation of a bisphenol A oral reference dose and drinking water equivalent concentration. *J Toxicol Environ Health B*. 11, 69–145.

Wogan GN, Paglialunga S, Newberne PM (1974). Carcinogenic effects of low dietary levels of anatoxin B in rats. *Food Cosmet Toxicol*. 12, 681–5.

# *chapter twenty three*

# *Toxicity of pesticides*

***Ramesh C. Gupta***

*Contents*

## Introduction

### Value of pesticides

The word pesticide can be defined as "any substance or mixture of substances intended for preventing, destroying, repelling or mitigating pests (insects, rodents, nematodes, weeds, fungi, etc.)." Among all pests, insects pose a serious threat to human health, since some of them serve as vectors transmitting bacteria, viruses, and parasites (malaria, filariasis, West Nile virus, Zika virus, yellow fever, viral encephalitis, rickettsialpox, typhus, bubonic plague, and others) from animals to humans or from humans to humans. Each year, millions of people become sick and a large number of them die from these deadly diseases. In such scenarios, the use of insecticides is not only important, but also inevitable to prevent and/or combat these vector-borne diseases.

In addition to the protection of human and animal health, insecticides are also used for food protection from production to consumer level. Although most insecticides currently in use are synthetic chemicals, farmers have also used a number of natural substances for centuries. These substances include nicotine from tobacco, pyrethrins from the flowers of *Chrysanthemum cinerariaefolium*, and various compounds of lead, copper, and arsenic.

Besides insects, *weeds* constitute a very important nuisance to the farmer. Before the introduction of herbicides, farmers used to spend much of their time manually removing weeds. More pesticides have also been developed to control other pests, such as *fungi, rodents,* and so forth. The vast array of agricultural uses and chemical categories may be found in a compilation of the 230 pesticides that have been evaluated by the WHO Expert Committee on Pesticide Residues since 1965 (Lu, 1995).

### Adverse effects of pesticides

Adverse effects involve human health and/or the environment. The most dramatic effects on humans are accidental acute poisonings. Several major outbreaks of poisoning with methyl and ethyl mercury compounds, hexachlorobenzene (a fungicide), and methyl and ethyl parathion (an organophosphorus insecticide) have occurred in several parts of the world poisoning thousands of individuals and causing hundreds of deaths. A few examples are listed in Appendix 1.2. Individual cases of acute poisoning have usually resulted from ingestion of large quantities of pesticides accidentally or with suicidal intent.

Occupational exposure to pesticides may involve workers engaged in the production, formulation, and application of pesticides. The pesticides generally enter the body through the respiratory tract and by dermal absorption, but small amounts may also enter the gastrointestinal tract through the use of contaminated hands and utensils; this is the most frequent route of exposure in cases of accidental ingestion of household products by children. This type of poisoning is more likely to happen with pesticides that are acutely toxic. The major public health concern, however, is the ingestion of pesticide residues in foods, as this may involve large populations (especially children) over long periods of time (Infante-Rivard and Weichenthal, 2007; Wigle et al., 2008; Marty, 2015).

In addition to human health hazards, pesticides may have a serious impact on the environment. Apart from large-scale accidental release in the environment, only minimal levels are found in various environmental media. However, the levels are likely to be higher with pesticides that are persistent and/or have a propensity for biomagnification. In the latter case, the concentration of a pesticide increases as it moves through the trophic chain. For example, the bald eagle was nearly extinct because of fragile egg shells, due to the toxic effect of high levels of dichlorodiphenyltrichloroethane (DDT) bioaccumulated through the bird's contaminated food chain. Seafood in Singapore was found to contain excessive amounts of DDT and heptachlor, as a result of biomagnification, putting the population that consumed seafood daily at a significantly higher risk of cancer (Bayen et al., 2005). Such environmental pollution may also affect human health by virtue of contaminated soil and water, which then results in contaminated drinking water and human food production.

## Categories of pesticides

Pesticides are usually classified based on their use and chemistry. The mechanism of action and toxicity of these pesticides are summarized in Table 23.1.

### Insecticides

As noted above, this is the largest group of pesticides and consists of a number of different chemical subgroups.

*Table 23.1* Summary of the mechanism of action and toxic effects of pesticides

| Pesticide | Mechanism of action | Toxic effects | References |
|---|---|---|---|
| | **Insecticides** | | |
| Organophosphates | Irreversible inhibition of AChE at synapses and neuromuscular junction(s) leading to ACh accumulation causing muscarinic and nicotinic ACh receptors | Hyper salivation, lacrimation, urination, diarrhea, tracheobronchial secretion, cyanosis, miosis, hypothermia, muscle tremors, convulsions, seizures, death | Dekundy and Kaminski (2010); Gupta and Milatovic (2010, 2012, 2014); Gupta et al. (2017) |
| Carbamates | Reversible inhibition of AChE at synapses and neuromuscular junction(s) leading to ACh accumulation causing muscarinic and nicotinic ACh receptors | Hyper salivation, lacrimation, urination, diarrhea, tracheobronchial secretion, cyanosis, miosis, hypothermia, muscle tremors, convulsions, seizures, death | Dekundy and Kaminski (2010); Gupta and Milatovic (2010, 2012, 2014); Gupta et al. (2017) |
| Organochlorines | Alter sodium and potassium transport ions across axonal membranes, resulting in negative after potential and prolonged action potential. Interact with $GABA_A$-regulated chloride channels in the brain | Paresthesia of the tongue, lips, and face, apprehension, hyperthermia, tremors, clonic and tonic convulsions, death | Smith (2012); Silva et al (2015); Malik et al. (2017) |
| Neonicotinoids | Bind to nAChRs of the postsynaptic membrane and act as nAChR agonists | Miosis or mydriasis, tremors, convulsions, death | Tomizawa and Casida (2005); Rose (2012); Sheets et al. (2015) |

(*Continued*)

***Table 23.1 (Continued)*** Summary of the mechanism of action and toxic effects of pesticides

| Pesticide | Mechanism of action | Toxic effects | References |
|---|---|---|---|
| Fipronil | Antagonizes $GABA_A$-regulated chloride channels in the brain | Hyperactivity, tremors, convulsions, seizures, death | Anadon and Gupta (2012); Marrs and Dewhurst (2012); Wang et al. (2016) |
| Amitraz | Overstimulation of $\alpha_2$-adrenoreceptors | General CNS depression, impairment of consciousness, respiratory depression, convulsions, disorientation, miosis, vomiting, bradycardia, hypotension, hypothermia, hyper-/hypoglycemia | Gupta (2012a); Gupta and Milatovic (2014); Marrs and Dewhurst (2012) |
| Pyrethrins/Pyrethroids | Interact directly with voltage-gated sodium channels to interfere with the generation and conduction of nerve impulses. This results in repetitive activity in various parts of the brain. | *T syndrome (Type I):* Whole body tremors, incoordination, prostration, tonic-clonic convulsions, death<br>*CS syndrome (Type II):* Hyperactive behavior, profuse salivation, tremors, motor incoordination, death | Ensley (2012); Gammon et al. (2012); Gupta and Milatovic (2014); Malik et al. (2017) |
| Rotenone | Inhibits the oxidation of NADH to $NAD^+$. Also, causes inhibition of mitochondrial respiratory chain complex I and cell death by apoptosis due to excess generation of reactive oxygen species (ROS) | Pharyngitis, nausea, vomiting, gastric pain, clonic convulsions, muscle tremors, lethargy, incontinence, cardio-respiratory failure, death | Li et al. (2003); Gupta (2012); Gupta and Milatovic (2014) |

*(Continued)*

***Table 23.1 (Continued)*** Summary of the mechanism of action and toxic effects of pesticides

| Pesticide | Mechanism of action | Toxic effects | References |
|---|---|---|---|
| Nicotine | Overstimulation of nAChRs in the CNS and PNS | Tremors, convulsions, fasciculations, muscle paralysis, death | Yildiz (2004); Bruin et al. (2010); Rose (2012) |
| | | **Herbicides** | |
| Chlorophenoxy herbicides | Uncouple oxidative phosphorylation, depress ribonuclease synthesis, and increase hepatic peroxisomes | Low mammalian toxicity<br>Death occurs due to ventricular fibrillation | Gupta (2012c, 2014, 2017) |
| Bipyridyls | NADPH depletion as a result of cyclic reduction–oxidation reactions and excess generation of ROS in lungs | Vomiting, abdominal pain, diarrhea, hypotension, dyspnea, death | Gupta (2012c, 2014, 2017) |
| Dinitrophenols | Block oxidative phosphorylation in tissues, resulting in stimulation of metabolism, and impairment of ATP synthesis | Increased respiration rate, tachycardia, hyperthermia, acidosis, anoxia, death | Gupta (2012c, 2014, 2017) |
| Ureas/Thioureas | Mechanism of action not well understood | Low mammalian toxicity, eye and skin irritation | Gupta (2012c, 2014, 2017) |
| Triazines | Induce liver microsomal enzymes | Depression, anorexia, hypothermia, weight loss, gastrointestinal upset, tenseness, weakness, locomotor disturbances | Gupta (2012c, 2014, 2017) |

(Continued)

*Table 23.1 (Continued)* Summary of the mechanism of action and toxic effects of pesticides

| Pesticide | Mechanism of action | Toxic effects | References |
| --- | --- | --- | --- |
| | | **Fungicides** | |
| Halogenated substituted monocyclic aromatic fungicides | Uncoupling of oxidative phosphorylation by targeting $Na^+$/$K^+$-ATPase | Hepatic porphyria, increased respiratory rate, hyperthermia, tremors, convulsions, asphyxial spasms, death | Gupta and Aggarwal (2012), Gupta (2014, 2017) |
| | | **Rodenticides** | |
| Anticoagulants: | Interference of vitamin k synthesis, leading to inhibition of prothrombin formation and capillary damage, resulting in bleeding.<br>Uncoupling of oxidative phosphorylation | Hemorrhage in the cerebral vasculature, pericardial sac, and thorax, convulsions, ataxia, bleeding through all body orifices, death | Murphy (2012); Murphy and Lugo (2015) |
| Nonanticoagulants: Alphanaphthyl thiourea | Stimulates the sympathetic nervous system, thereby causing vasoconstriction and pulmonary edema, anoxia | Excessive pulmonary edema, pleural effusion, emesis, dyspnea, death | Gupta (2012d) |
| Sodium fluoroacetate/ Fluoroacetamide | Inhibit the activity of aconitase, blocking the citric acid cycle | Damage the kidneys, heart, and CNS, death occurs due to cardiac, respiratory, and renal failure | Gupta (2012d) |

(Continued)

*Table 23.1 (Continued)* Summary of the mechanism of action and toxic effects of pesticides

| Pesticide | Mechanism of action | Toxic effects | References |
|---|---|---|---|
| Zinc phosphide | Formation of phosphine following a hydrolytic reaction, causing damage to liver, kidney, and GI tract | Vomiting, anorexia, rapid and deep respiration, terminal hypoxia | Gupta (2012d) |
| Bromethalin | Uncoupling oxidative phosphorylation in mitochondria of the CNS. Decreased $Na^+/K^+$-ATPase activity and ATP levels | Increased intracranial pressure leading to paralysis, convulsions, and death | Gupta (2012d); Gupta and Milatovic (2014) |
| Plant alkaloids: Strychnine | Antagonizes the inhibitory action of glycine in Renshaw cells of the spinal cord and medulla | Rigidity of skeletal muscles, tonic seizures, death due to paralysis of the respiratory muscles | Gupta (2012d); Patocka (2015) |
| Red squill | Scilliroside produces cardiotoxicity similar to that of digitalis | Vomiting, ataxia, hyperesthesia, hypothermia, incoordination, convulsions, death | Gupta (2012d) |

### *Organophosphate insecticides*

Organophosphate (OP) insecticides are esters of phosphoric, phosphonic, or thiophosphoric acid. Examples of some commonly used OP insecticides include chlorpyrifos, diazinon, dichlorvos, fenthion, malathion, and parathion, and their chemical structures are shown in Figure 23.1. Their toxicities vary widely (Table 23.2). For detailed classification, uses, and toxicity see Gupta (2006a).

OPs produce toxicity by inhibiting acetylcholinesterase (AChE) primarily at the synapses and neuromuscular junctions (NMJ), resulting in the accumulation of acetylcholine (ACh) (Pope, 1999). Excess ACh induces a variety of symptoms and clinical signs. The severity of symptoms is more or less correlated with the extent of the inhibition of AChE in blood, but the precise relationship varies depending on the OP compound (Clegg and van Gemert, 1999). Muscarinic ACh receptor (mAChR)-associated effects include hyper salivation, lacrimation, urination, diarrhea, tracheobronchial secretion, vomiting, cyanosis, and miosis. Nicotinic ACh receptor (nAChR) associated effects include muscle tremors, convulsions, and seizures. Evidence suggests that some OPs directly interact with mAChRs and nAChRs. High-dose OP exposure leads to paralysis and death (Gupta and Milatovic, 2012). Figure 23.2 depicts the mechanism of action involved in OP's toxicity. In OP-induced excitotoxicity, *N*-methyl-*D*-aspartate receptor (NMDAR), gamma aminobutyric acid receptor (GABAR), and other neurotransmitter systems are also involved (Dekundy and Kaminski, 2010). Therefore, antidotal treatment includes timely administration of a mAChR blocker, atropine sulfate (0.5 mg/kg; one-third IV and the remainder IM), AChE reactivator pyridine 2-aldoxime methochloride

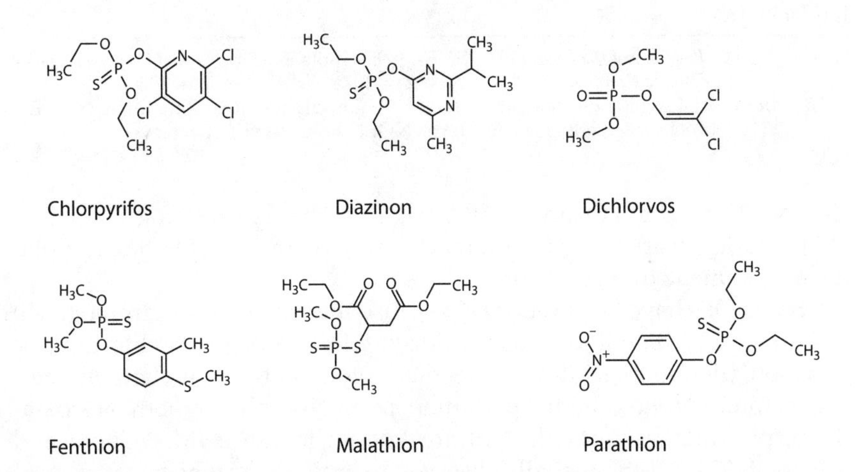


***Figure 23.1*** Commonly used OP pesticides. (Courtesy of Ramesh C. Gupta.)

***Table 23.2*** Toxicological findings and evaluations of certain insecticides

| Pesticide | $LD_{50}$ (mg/kg) | NOAEL (mg/kg) | | | ADI (mg/kg) |
|---|---|---|---|---|---|
| | | Rat | Dog | Human | |
| Azinphosmethyl | 13 | 0.45 | 0.74 | 0.3 | 0.005 |
| Chlorfenvinphos | 15 | 0.05 | 0.05 | | 0.002 |
| Diazinon | 108 | 0.02 | 0.02 | 0.025 | 0.002 |
| Dichlorvos | 80 | | 0.05 (NOEL) | 0.04 | 0.004 |
| Dimethoate | 215 | 0.4 | | 0.2 | 0.02 |
| Disulfoton | 6.8 | 0.06 | 0.03 | 0.01 | 0.0003 |
| Malathion | 1375 | 5.0 | | 0.2 | 0.02 |
| Mevinphos | 6.1 | 0.02 | 0.025 | 0.014 | 0.0015 |
| Parathion | 13 | | | 0.05 | 0.005 |
| Parathion-methyl | 14 | 0.1 | 0.375 | 0.3 | 0.02 |
| Trichlorfon | 630 | 2.5 | 1.25 | | 0.01 |
| Aldicarb | 0.8 | 0.125 | 0.25 | 0.025 | 0.003 |
| Carbaryl | 500~850 | 10 | | 0.06 | 0.01 |
| Propoxur | 83 | 12.5 | 50 | | 0.02 |
| DDT | 113 | 0.05 | | | 0.01 |
| Aldrin/dieldrin | 40 | 0.025 | 0.025 | | 0.0001 |
| Chlordane | 335 | 0.25 | 0.05 | | 0.0005 |
| Endrin | 18 | 0.05 | 0.025 | | 0.002 |
| Heptacholor | 100 | 0.25 | 0.025 | | 0.0001 |
| Lindane | 88 | 1.25 | 1.75 | | 0.008 |
| Methoxychlor | 6000 | 10 | | | 0.1 |
| Imidacloprid | 450 | 5.7 | | | 0.1 |

*Source:* Lu FC, *Reg Toxicol Pharmacol.*, 21, 352–64, 1995; Gupta RC *Toxicology of Organophosphate and Carbamate Compounds*, Academic Press/Elsevier, Amsterdam, 2006b.
*Abbreviations:* ADI, acceptable daily intake; DDT, dichlorodiphenyltrichloroethane; NOAEL, no-observed adverse effect level; NOEL, no-observed effect level.

(2-PAM, 20 mg/kg, IV), and GABAR agonist diazepam (5 mg IV or IM). Other clinically approved AChE reactivating oximes are methoxime, obidoxime, trimedoxime, and HI-6.

Some OPs have been reported to cause intermediate syndrome (IMS) in humans. To date, more than a dozen OPs (bromophos, chlorpyrifos, diazinon, dicrotophos, dimethoate, disulfoton, fenthion, malathion, merfos, methamidophos, methyl parathion, monocrotophos, omethoate, parathion, phosmet, and trichlorfon) are known to cause IMS (Gupta and Milatovic, 2012). IMS is usually observed in individuals who have ingested a massive dose of an OP insecticide either accidentally or intentionally

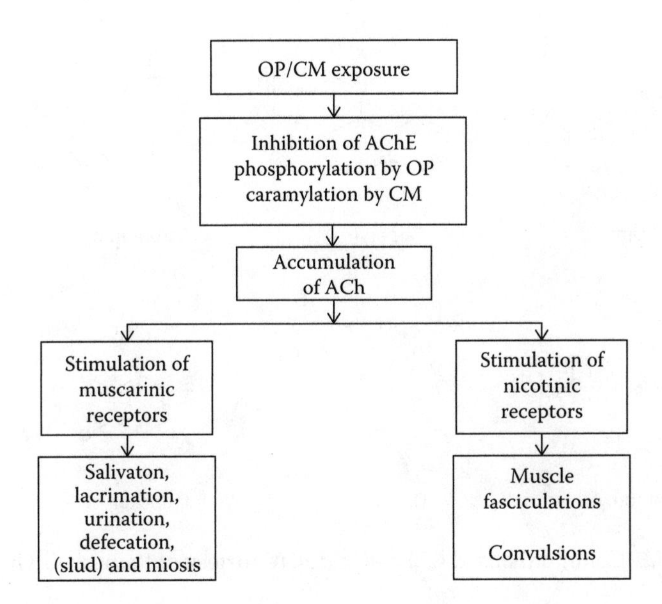


***Figure 23.2*** Mechanisms involved in OP/CM toxicity. (Courtesy of Ramesh C. Gupta.)

in a suicide attempt. IMS is a separate clinical entity from acute toxicity and delayed neuropathy, and is characterized by acute respiratory paresis and muscular weakness, primarily in the facial, neck, and proximal limb muscles, occurring 24–96 hours after exposure. IMS appears to occur due to the interaction of OPs with nAChRs at the motor endplate, oxidative stress, and electrophysiological abnormalities at the NMJ.

Some OPs, such as tri-*o*-cresyl phosphate (TOCP), are known to cause OP-induced delayed polyneuropathy (OPIDPN). Signs and symptoms of this neurodegenerative disorder include tingling of the hands and feet, followed by sensory loss, progressive muscle weakness, and flaccidity of the distal skeletal muscles of the extremities, and ataxia. With higher doses of an OP, symptoms can occur as early as 10 days and, with lower doses symptoms can take as long as 5 weeks to occur. OPIDPN occurs due to inhibition and aging of neuropathy target esterase (NTE) in peripheral nerves.

### *Carbamate insecticides*

Carbamate (CM) insecticides are the esters of methyl or dimethyl carbamic acid. Some commonly used CM insecticides are aldicarb, carbaryl, carbofuran, methomyl, oxamyl, and propoxur, and their chemical structures are shown in Figure 23.3. CMs produce toxicity by reversible inhibition

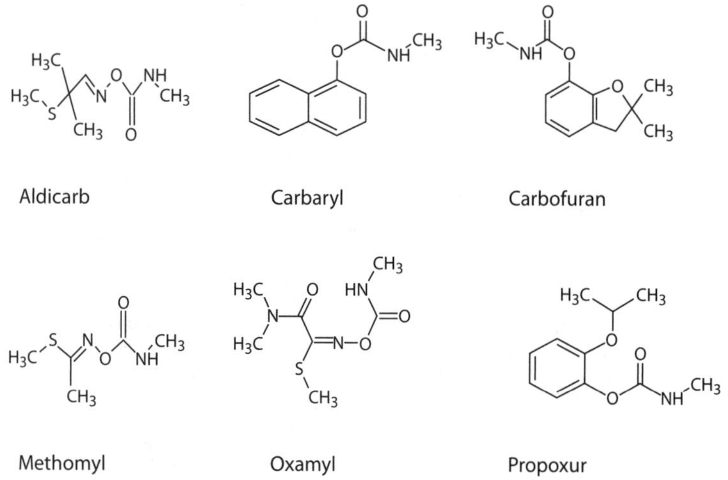

Aldicarb Carbaryl Carbofuran

Methomyl Oxamyl Propoxur

*Figure 23.3* Commonly used CM pesticides. (Courtesy of Ramesh C. Gupta.)

of AChE (Figure 23.2). For this reason, CMs are considered safer than OP insecticides. In mild to moderate poisoning cases, recovery can be anticipated within 1 to 4 hours. Antidotal treatment for CM toxicity rests with atropine sulfate.

### *Organochlorine insecticides*

Organochlorine (OC) insecticides include the chlorinated ethane derivatives, cyclodienes, and hexachlorocyclohexanes. Some of these chemicals (e.g., DDT) were introduced in the 1940s and were widely used in agricultural and public health programs. This was because of their relatively low acute toxicity and their persistence, which reduced the need for repeated applications. However, their persistence in the biological system and the environment has been since recognized as a liability rather than an asset.

Both DDT and methoxychlor are chlorinated ethane derivatives, but methoxychlor is much less toxic and less persistent than DDT. The cyclodiene insecticide endrin is extremely toxic; aldrin and dieldrin are somewhat less toxic; and chlordane, heptachlor, and mirex even less toxic. Lindane is the gamma isomer of hexachlorocyclohexane (HCH), and it is highly toxic, but less cumulative. Consequently, lindane is more widely used than HCH, especially for hair lice in children. OC insecticides are less water soluble than OP or CM insecticides and more environmentally persistent.

OCs alter the transport of sodium and potassium ions across axonal membranes, resulting in increased negative after potential and prolonged action potentials. Consequently, repetitive firing occurs after a single stimulus and spontaneous trains of action potentials. Clinical signs and symptoms appear within 24 hours of exposure. The toxic manifestations with chlorinated ethanes and chlorinated benzenes include paresthesia of the tongue, lips and face, apprehension, tremors, clonic and tonic convulsions, and hyperthermia. With cyclodienes, the signs and symptoms include dizziness, nausea, vomiting, and generalized convulsions. Death may occur within 24 to 72 hours from respiratory failure due to prolonged paralysis of the respiratory muscles. There is no antidotal treatment.

*Neonicotinoids*

Neonicotinoids are a new class of insecticides with widespread use in crop protection and veterinary medicine. Commonly used neonicotinoids are imidacloprid, acetamiprid, clothianidin, dinotefuran, nitenpyram, thiacloprid, and thiamethoxam. These insecticides produce a neurotoxic insecticidal action by binding to nAChRs of the postsynaptic membrane of nerve cells in the CNS and acting as nAChR agonists (Rose, 2012). Neonicotinoids show selective toxicity, that is, lower toxicity in vertebrates compared to insects due to the fact that they have lower affinity for binding to nAChRs in mammals than in insects. In mammals with low dose exposure, the toxic effects include tremors and impaired pupillary function (miosis or mydriasis). At higher doses, death either occurs within 4 hours or recovery takes place within 8 to 24 hours. There is no specific antidote for neonicotinoid toxicity.

*Fipronil*

Fipronil is a member of a new class of insecticides called phenylpyrazoles used in agriculture and veterinary medicine worldwide. Fipronil and its major metabolites (fipronil sulfone and fipronil desulfinyl) produce neurotoxicity by antagonizing $GABA_A$-regulated chloride channels in the brain (Marrs and Dewhurst, 2012). Selective toxicity of fipronil and its metabolites (>500 times in insects over mammals) is due to higher specificity and affinity for receptor binding in insects. Dermal toxicity is low, inhalation toxicity is moderate, and oral toxicity is high. In humans, poisoning is mainly due to accidental ingestion or suicide attempts. The signs and symptoms are hyperactivity including tremors, convulsions, seizures, and death. There is no specific treatment for fipronil toxicity.

*Amitraz*

Amitraz is an amidine insecticide and acaricide used in crop protection and veterinary medicine. Poisoning from amitraz in humans occurs from accidental or intentional ingestion. Amitraz overstimulates $\alpha_2$-adrenoreceptors resulting in general CNS depression, impairment of consciousness, respiratory depression, convulsions, disorientation, miosis, vomiting, bradycardia, hypotension, hypothermia, and hyper-/hypoglycemia (Marrs and Dewhurst, 2012). Onset of symptoms occurs within 1 hour of exposure. Amitraz is of moderate acute toxicity via the oral route, but low acute toxicity via dermal and inhalation exposure. Antidotal treatment includes therapy with $\alpha_2$-adrenoreceptor antagonists (yohimbine and atipamezole).

## *Botanical and other insecticides*

### *Pyrethrins and pyrethroids*

Pyrethrins are insecticidal compounds obtained from the flowers of *Chrysanthemum cinerariaefolium*. There are six compounds that comprise natural pyrethrins (pyrethrin I and II, jasmolin I and II, and cinerin I and II). Synthetic pyrethroids have been developed because natural pyrethrins tend to break down quickly when exposed to air, light, and heat (Ensley, 2012). An enzyme inhibitor, piperonyl butoxide, is often used in combination with pyrethrins/pyrethroids as a synergist. The pyrethroids are divided into two types. Type I pyrethroids lack an alpha cyano substituent. Some common examples of this group are allethrin, kadethrin, permethrin, phenothrin, resmethrin, and tetramethrin. Type II pyrethroids contain an alpha cyano substituent. Some examples of this group are cypermethrin, cyphenothrin, deltamethrin, fenpropanthrin, fenvalerate, and fluvalinate.

Pyrethroids interact directly with voltage-gated sodium channels, thereby interfering with the generation and conduction of nerve impulses. This interference induces pronounced repetitive activity in various parts of the brain. Type I pyrethroids produce tremor ("T") syndrome with symptoms of whole-body tremors, incoordination, prostration, tonic-clonic convulsions, and death. Type II pyrethroids elicit choreoathetosis/salivation ("CS") syndrome with symptoms of hyperactive behavior, profuse salivation, tremors, motor incoordination, and death. Both the central nervous system (CNS) and peripheral nervous system (PNS) are affected by pyrethroids. There is no antidotal treatment for pyrethrin/pyrethroid toxicity.

### *Rotenone*

Rotenone (nicouline) is one of the oldest naturally occurring compounds present in a number of plants (*Derris elliptica, Derris involuta, Lonchocarpus nicou, Lonchocarpus urucu, Lonchocarpus utilis, Mundulea sericea,* and *Tephrosia virginiana*). In general, rotenone is an organic pesticide used in home gardens for insect control, for lice and ticks on pets, and fish eradications as part of water-body management. Rotenone has selective toxicity, as it is highly toxic to insects and fish in comparison to mammalian species. Rotenone converts to highly toxic metabolites in large quantities in insects and fish, while it converts to less toxic metabolites in mammals. Also, rotenone is rapidly absorbed in fish compared to mammalian species. In mammals and fish, it inhibits the oxidation of NADH to $NAD^+$, thereby blocking the oxidation of $NAD^+$ and substrates such as glutamate, alpha-ketoglutarate, and pyruvate. Rotenone causes inhibition of the mitochondrial respiratory chain complex I and cell death by apoptosis due to excess generation of free radicals. With acute exposure, rotenone produces pharyngitis, nausea, vomiting, gastric pain, clonic convulsions, muscle tremors, lethargy, incontinence, and cardiorespiratory failure and death. In experimental animals, it is a neurotoxicant and produces signs similar to Parkinson's disease.

#### *Nicotine*

Nicotine is obtained from the plants *Nicotiana tabacum* and *Nicotiana rustica*. Black Leaf 40® (nicotine sulfate 40%) has been used as an insecticide for more than half a century. Nicotine is known to affect the nervous, cardiovascular, respiratory, endocrine systems, and the gastrointestinal tract. Nicotine is highly toxic to mammals; its pharmacological effects mimic certain effects of ACh and are called "nicotinic effects." Overstimulation of nAChRs at the neuromuscular junction (NMJ) results in tremors, fasciculations, and paralysis of muscles. These effects are blocked by *d*-tubocurarine. Higher dose nicotine exposure often results in death. Nicotine also affects neuroeffector junctions of the parasympathetic system including the iris of the eye, bladder, heart, tear glands, and salivary glands; these effects are blocked by atropine sulfate.

### *Herbicides*

Herbicides, commonly referred to as "weed killers," are chemicals used to destroy unwanted plants. There are several types of herbicides; some retard the growth of weeds by inhibiting photosynthesis, respiration, cell division, or synthesis of protein or lipids, while others act as growth stimulants, disturbing normal growth (Gupta, 2012c). Most human poisoning cases are from accidental exposure to herbicides or suicidal intent.

Chlorophenoxy compounds are exemplified by 2,4-dichlorophenoxyacetic acid (2,4-D) and 2,4,5-trichlorophenoxyacetic acid (2,4,5-T). These compounds act as plant growth hormones and have a relatively low toxicity in mammals. By having an additional chlorine, 2,4,5-T is more toxic than 2,4-D. However, chloracne, the main toxic effect of 2,4,5-T in humans, seems attributable to the contaminant 2,3,7,8-tetrachlorodibenzo-*p*-dioxin

(TCDD or dioxin). There is no specific treatment for chlorophenoxy herbicide poisoning.

Bipyridyl herbicides (paraquat and diquat) are widely used in agriculture and horticulture. Life-threatening pulmonary toxicity occurs from occupational or accidental exposure or suicidal attempts. Lungs accumulate paraquat about ten times more than other tissues, mostly in type I and type II epithelial cells. The mechanism of action of bipyridyls involves cyclic reduction–oxidation reactions that deplete NADPH and generate reactive oxygen species (ROS), which cause cell death by polymerizing unsaturated lipids in cell membranes. Clinical signs include vomiting, abdominal pain, diarrhea, and hypotension, as well as peripheral neuromuscular effects that may persist in surviving victims.

Dinitrophenol herbicides include 2,4-dinitrophenol, 2,4-dinitro-*o*-cresol, and dinoseb. These compounds produce toxicity by blocking oxidative phosphorylation in tissues, which results in stimulation of the metabolism. These compounds also stimulate tissue respiration and impair ATP synthesis. As a result, there is an increase in oxygen demand and an increase in respiration and heart rate, leading to hyperthermia, acidosis, anoxia, and death.

Herbicides of the urea and thiourea group (diuron, flumeturon, isoproturon, linuron, and others) are commonly used in agriculture. These herbicides are of low toxicity and do not pose serious risks to humans; however, they may cause eye and skin irritation.

Common herbicides of the triazine group include atrazine, simazine, prometon, and propazine. These compounds are of low mammalian toxicity and pose no human risk. The clinical signs of toxicity may include depression, anorexia, weight loss, gastrointestinal upset, tenseness, and weakness.

Carbamate herbicides include chloropropham, carbetamide, desmedipham, and asulam; thiocarbamate herbicides include dimepiperate, molinate, eradicane, diallate, thiobencarb, and so forth. These herbicides have low mammalian toxicity and pose little human risk.

### *Fungicides*

Fungicides are agents that are used to prevent or eradicate fungal infections from plants or seeds. In agriculture, they are used to protect tubers, fruits, and vegetables during storage and are applied directly to ornamental plants, trees, field crops, cereals, and turf grasses (Gupta and Aggarwal, 2012).

The inorganic and metallic fungicides include formulations from sulfur, copper, mercury, and potassium. Acute poisoning from sulfur fungicides is very rare and, therefore, does not pose a toxicological threat to mammals (Gupta and Aggarwal, 2012; Gupta and Crissman, 2013). Vineyard sprayers usually develop liver disease after 3–15 years of using fungicidal copper sulfate in a Bordeaux mixture. Mercury compounds such as methyl and ethyl mercury are very effective fungicides and had been widely used to preserve seed grains. However, several tragic accidents involving numerous deaths and permanent neurological damage occurred with their use (Appendix 1.2). In humans, methylmercury disrupts CNS developmental processes in the unborn and infant. These facts have deterred further use of these compounds.

Carbamic acid derivative fungicides include ferbam, thiram, ziram, maneb, mancozeb, metiram, nabam, zineb, and so forth. These compounds have been widely used in agriculture and have relatively low mammalian acute toxicity. However, there is concern about their carcinogenic potential.

Chloroalkylthiodicarboximide fungicides have very low acute and chronic toxicity and include captan, captafol, and folpet. Captan, however, was found to reduce body weight of pups and folpet-induced keratosis of the gastrointestinal tract in rats (FAO, 1990).

Halogenated substituted monocyclic aromatics, such as pentachlorophenol (PCP), have been widely used as wood preservatives. PCP increases metabolic rate through uncoupling of oxidative phosphorylation. It has a low $LD_{50}$, but its technical grade is more toxic, indicating greater toxicity of its contaminants. Pentachloronitrobenzene (PCNB) has been used as a fungicide in treating soil. It is somewhat less acutely toxic than PCP, but may be carcinogenic. Hexachlorobenzene has been used as a seed treatment, but has caused mass poisoning (Appendix 1.2). Other commonly used fungicides in agriculture include benomyl and thiobendazole, which have very low toxicity. Benomyl is known to induce teratogenic effects, such as tetramelia, eye defects, miscarriages, and infants with congenital anomalies.

## *Rodenticides*

Rodenticides are chemical agents that kill rodents and are divided into two categories, anticoagulants and nonanticoagulants. Anticoagulant rodenticides are of two types: (1) coumarin type, such as dicoumarol, warfarin, coumachlor, coumafuryl, coumatetralyl, brodifacoum, and bromadiolone; and (2) indanedione type, such as pindone, diphacinone, and chlorophacinone. The mode of action of these rodenticides is twofold: (1) inhibition of prothrombin formation as a result of interferences with the action of vitamin K in the synthesis of clotting factors (II, VII, IX, and X), and (2) capillary damage resulting in internal bleeding. All mammalian and bird species are susceptible to these compounds, although toxicity varies widely from species to species. In humans, adults are exposed to these compounds because of malicious or suicidal intent, while infants are exposed via accidental ingestion of poisoned baits, and the outcome is usually fatal. Generally, in acute cases, hemorrhage occurs in the cerebral vasculature, pericardial sac, and thorax, and is followed by convulsions and ataxia. In subacute cases, in addition to hematemesis, bleeding occurs through all body orifices. Antidotal treatment includes vitamin $K_1$ (5 mg/kg body wt, IM, SC, or IV) and whole blood transfusion (20 ml/kg body wt, IV).

Of the many thioureas, alphanaphthyl thiourea (ANTU) has the best rodenticidal effect. ANTU stimulates the sympathetic nervous system and causes a significant increase in permeability of the lung capillaries, and consequently, excessive pulmonary edema and pleural effusion. ANTU is extremely toxic to rats, but only moderately toxic to humans.

Sodium fluoroacetate ("Compound 1080") and fluoroacetamide ("Compound 1081") are extremely toxic and their use has been restricted to licensed personnel. In the body, these compounds get converted to toxic metabolites (fluorocitrate) which exert a toxic effect via blockage of the citric acid cycle by inhibiting the activity of aconitase. These compounds cause damage to the kidneys, heart, and CNS, resulting in death.

Zinc phosphide is another rodenticide that has been used for a long time because it is very effective and inexpensive. The toxicity of zinc phosphide is mainly due to phosphine ($PH_3$), which is formed following a hydrolytic reaction in the stomach. The onset of toxicity is fairly rapid, within a few minutes to a few hours. Clinical signs include vomiting, anorexia, rapid and deep respiration, followed by terminal hypoxia.

Bromethalin is a unique, highly potent, single-feeding rodenticide developed in 1985. It was developed specifically as a rodenticide to overcome rodent resistance to certain anticoagulants. Poisoning in humans occurs because of suicidal intent. Bromethalin produces toxicity by uncoupling oxidative phosphorylation in mitochondria of the CNS. Decreased ATP production inhibits the activity of $Na^+/K^+$-ATPase and leads to an accumulation of fluid within myelin lamellae and the cerebroventricular system. The increased intracranial pressure damages axons, inhibiting neural transmission, and leads to paralysis, convulsions, and death within 1–3 days.

Other rodenticides include plant alkaloids, such as strychnine and red squill. Strychnine is obtained from the seeds of *Strychnos nuxvomica* and *S. ignatii*. Strychnine selectively antagonizes the inhibitory action of glycine in Renshaw cells of the spinal cord and medulla. Clinical signs include rigidity of skeletal muscles, tonic seizures, and death due to paralysis of the respiratory muscles. Red squill is a red powder obtained from the dried bulbs of the sea onion (*Urgenia maritima*) having the active principle scilliroside. Clinical signs include convulsions, hyperesthesia, incoordination; death occurs due to cardiac toxicity.

### Fumigants

As the name implies, this group of pesticides includes a number of gases, liquids that readily vaporize, and solids that release gases by chemical reactions. Methyl bromide, chloropicrin, and methyl iodide are broad-spectrum fumigants (Lim, 2015). Other fumigants include dazomet, formadehyde, hydrogen cyanide, iodoform, methyl isocyanate, phosphine, and sulfuryl fluoride. Fumigants are used in buildings, soil, grain, and produce to eradicate pests. Fumigation is a hazardous operation and is conducted by certified operators. These chemicals are hazardous to most forms of life, including humans, and inhalation is the primary route of exposure (Heaps, 2006).

## Toxicological properties of pesticides

### Toxicity on the nervous system

OC insecticides stimulate the nervous system and induce paresthesia, susceptibility to stimulation, irritability, disturbed equilibrium, tremors, and convulsions. The precise mode of action is not known. However, some of these chemicals, such as aldrin, dieldrin, and lindane, induce fasciculation and hyperexcitation at synaptic and neuromuscular junctions (NMJs), resulting in repetitive discharge in central, sensory, and motor neurons. DDT may exert its toxic effect in the nervous system by adversely affecting the action potential in the axon membrane (Narahashi, 1980).

The OP and CM insecticides inhibit AChE. Normally, the neurotransmitter ACh is released at the synapses and NMJs. Once the nerve impulse is transmitted, the released ACh is hydrolyzed to acetic acid and choline by AChE at the active site. Upon exposure to OP and CM insecticides, AChE is inhibited, resulting in an accumulation of ACh. The accumulated ACh in the CNS produces tremors, incoordination, and convulsions. In the autonomic nervous system, AChE inhibition produces diarrhea, involuntary urination, bronchoconstriction, miosis, and so forth. ACh accumulation at the NMJ produces contraction of the muscles, followed by weakness, loss of reflexes, and paralysis. The inhibition of AChE induced by CMs is readily reversible, whereas that by OPs is irreversible. Several OP compounds, including DFP, tri-*o*-cresyl phosphate (TOCP), leptophos, mipafox, and trichlorfon, cause a "delayed neuropathy" by inhibition and aging of neuropathy target esterase (NTE). Pyrethrins and pyrethroids also produce toxicity by adversely affecting the nervous system (Ensley, 2012; Gupta and Milatovic, 2012; Soderlund, 2012).

### *Interactions of pesticides*

The most notable type of interaction is *potentiation* observed between certain OP insecticides. Frawley and coworkers (1957) reported marked potentiation of the toxicity of the *o*-ethyl-*o*-(4-nitrophenyl) phenyl phosphonothioate and malathion. Combinations of a number of OP insecticides have since been tested. Some showed additive effects, others were less than additive, and still others were synergistic. The most pronounced potentiation (about 100-fold increase) was observed between malathion and TOCP. The mechanism of the potentiation was attributed to inhibition of enzymes, such as carboxylesterase and amidases, which are responsible for detoxication of certain OP compounds such as malathion and its more toxic metabolite, malaoxon (Murphy, 1969). For other anticholinesterase pesticide interactions, see Gupta and Milatovic (2010) and for anticholinesterases and metals interaction, see Malik et al (2010).

### *Carcinogenicity*

Generally, OP insecticides are not carcinogenic in adults, with the exception of compounds that contain halogens such as tetrachlorvinphos. These chemicals possess the properties of OC insecticides (see the next paragraph). However, it is worth noting that children are a more susceptible subpopulation (Makri et al., 2004; Rohlman and McCauley, 2010). There is epidemiological evidence of an increased frequency of cancer in children exposed to OP insecticides (Infante-Rivard and Weichenthal, 2007; Wigle et al., 2008). The CM insecticides, per se, are not carcinogenic either. However, carbaryl was shown to form, in the presence of nitrous acid, nitrosocarbaryl, which is known to be carcinogenic. A number of other pesticides are also nitrosatable under extreme conditions and their products are carcinogenic and mutagenic (IARC, 1983). Because of the unrealistic conditions required for such nitrosation to take place, the health concern arising from this type of reaction is questionable.

On the other hand, the OC insecticides tested were all found to induce hepatoma in mice (IARC, 1983). The pesticide that aroused the most controversy has been DDT. It did not produce carcinogenicity in rats, hamsters, and several other mammalian species. Furthermore, epidemiological findings are essentially negative, and so are the short-term mutagenesis tests. For these reasons, the WHO Expert Committee on Pesticide Residues reaffirmed in 1984 the acceptable daily intake (ADI) for DDT and several other OC insecticides. Coulston has provided a comprehensive review and interpretation of toxicological data on DDT (1985). Nevertheless, its use has been restricted or suspended in several nations, based partly on this potential health hazard and partly on its ecological impact. It is worth noting that in certain underdeveloped countries DDT must be applied in order to counteract malaria, West Nile, or Zika, and other diseases by controlling mosquitoes. The only pesticide on which there is some epidemiological evidence of carcinogenicity is hexachlorocyclohexane (Wang et al., 1988).

The fumigants ethylene dibromide and 1,2-dibromo-3-chloropropane were found to produce highly malignant squamous cell carcinoma in the stomach of rats and mice (IARC, 1977). However, their use has not been restricted or suspended because the fumigated foods, upon aeration, contain negligible residue levels.

Amitrole (aminotriazole), a herbicide, produces thyroid tumors through an indirect mechanism (Steinhoff et al., 1983). Thyroid peroxidase normally oxidizes iodine to an oxidized form, which then conjugates with tyrosine to form thyroxine (T4). Amitrole inhibits this enzyme, thus lowering T4 levels. This lowered level, through a biofeedback mechanism, stimulates the pituitary gland to release more thyroid-stimulating hormone (TSH). TSH, in turn, stimulates the thyroid gland to become hyperplastic and eventually forms tumors. Amitrole is a "secondary carcinogen." Similarly, the carbamic acid derivative fungicides (mancozeb, maneb, nabam, and zineb) were also reported to produce thyroid tumors. In general, many endocrine-disrupting chemicals (EDCs) are pesticides and their major toxicities include carcinogenicity, developmental toxicity, mutagenicity, immunotoxicity, and neurotoxicity (Choi et al., 2004; Kitamura et al., 2010; Evans, 2017).

## *Teratogenicity and its effects on reproductive functions*

In the late 1960s, several articles appeared reporting a variety of teratogenic and reproductive effects of carbaryl in dogs (Smalley et al., 1968). Summaries of these reports have been included in a monograph (WHO, 1970). A comprehensive study in rats, given carbaryl in the diet at doses of 100 or 200 mg/kg, showed no effect on various reproductive functions and no teratogenic effects. Some effects were observed in rats given carbaryl by gavage (Weil et al., 1972). The authors attributed the effects in rats to the gavage method of administering the pesticide, and the effects in the dog to its routes of biotransformation of carbaryl since it is different from those in humans and several other species. A cat fetus showed heptadactyly of right and hexadactyly of left forepaw from a cat exposed to dimethoate during day 14–22 of pregnancy (Khera, 1979). Alkylation of nicotinamide adenine dinucleotide ($NAD^+$) coenzyme by OPs seemed to be the major mechanism involved in the induction of teratogenesis (Schoental, 1977). Other proposed mechanisms in OP-induced teratogenesis are altered levels of RNA, glycogen, mucopolysaccharides, and calcium in the developing bone. For the detailed reproductive and developmental effects of OPs and CMs, readers are referred to Gupta et al (2017).

Other pesticides reported as having teratogenic effects include the dithiocarbamate fungicides (Gupta, 2017). Such effects are likely due, at least partly, to their breakdown product ETU (WHO, 1974). In addition, abamectin, dinocap, glyphosate, and procymidone induced cleft palate, defects in the neural tube, renal defects, and hypospadias, respectively (Lu, 1995; Gupta, 2017). An extensive, comprehensive review of pesticides and developmental outcomes including fetal death, intrauterine growth retardation, preterm birth, and birth defects is provided by Weselak et al. (2007). In chicken embryos, the simultaneous administration of 2,4-D herbicide and cadmium or copper produced higher embryo mortality and developmental anomalies than individual administration (Juhász et al., 2006). For detailed reproductive and developmental toxicity of pesticides, readers are referred to Gupta (2017), Malik et al. (2017), and Gupta et al. (2017).

### *Other adverse effects*

Certain renal effects of carbaryl were reported in a group of human volunteers ingesting carbaryl at a daily dose of 0.12 mg/kg for 6 weeks. There was an increase in the ratio of urinary amino acid nitrogen to creatinine, compared with those taking a placebo. This was interpreted as an indication of a decrease in the ability of the proximal convoluted tubules to reabsorb amino acids. This effect was not observed in individuals taking carbaryl at 0.06 mg/kg daily (Wills et al., 1968).

Paraquat produces pulmonary edema, hemorrhage, and fibrosis (Smith and Heath, 1976) following either inhalation or ingestion, but the closely related herbicide diquat does not. Both chemicals are toxic to cultured lung cells. As paraquat is concentrated in the lung and diquat is not, it is evident that the difference between those two herbicides in their pulmonary toxicity is related to the special affinity of paraquat for certain pulmonary cells (alveolar cells). In addition, paraquat produces Parkinson's disease (PD)-like lesions in certain strains of rodents and may increase the risk of developing PD in humans (Berry et al., 2010).

Hypersensitivity reactions to pyrethrum have been reported. The most common form is contact dermatitis (Vial et al., 1996; Bradberry et al., 2005). This type of reaction is not serious in the general population, but may have serious consequences in immunocompromised individuals such as AIDS patients with non-Hodgkin's lymphoma, lupus erythematosus, or rheumatoid arthritis. Asthma has also been reported; however, anaphylactic reactions are rare (Hayes, 1982).

Organochlorine insecticides, such as DDT, chlordecone, and mirex are hepatotoxic, inducing liver enlargement and centrolobular necrosis. They are also inducers of microsomal monooxygenases, thereby affecting the toxicity of other chemicals.

A number of OP, CM, and OC insecticides, the dithiocarbamate fungicides, and herbicides alter various immune functions (Vial et al., 1996). For example, malathion, methyl parathion, carbaryl, DDT, paraquat, and diquat have been shown to depress antibody formation, impair leukocyte phagocytosis, and reduce germinal cells in spleen, thymus, and lymph nodes (Koller, 1979; Street, 1981; Sharma, 2006; Corsini et al., 2013).

## *Bioaccumulation and biomagnification*

Bioaccumulation and biomagnification properties do not necessarily represent adverse biological effects. They are generally associated with substances that are lipophilic and resistant to breakdown. The OC pesticides are generally more persistent in the environment and tend to be stored in the fat depot. However, bioaccumulation is more marked with some chemicals than others. For example, DDT is stored in body fat for a much longer time than methoxychlor. The half-lives of these insecticides in rats are 6–12 months and 12 weeks, respectively.

Persistence of pesticides in the environment may create ecological problems (Carson, 1962). DDT and related chemicals in the environment enhance metabolism of estrogens in birds. In the egg-laying and nestling cycle of certain birds, this disturbance of hormones adversely affects reproduction and survival of the young. There is evidence that the estrogenic actions of DDT are responsible for the development of breast cancer and disorders of female reproductive functions (Roy et al., 1997).

Biomagnification is the result of bioaccumulation in the organism alone or in conjunction with persistence in the environment. For example, DDT is lipophilic and occurs in the fat portion of body fluids, including milk. While a mother's daily intake of DDT may be 0.5 μg/kg, her breastfed baby's daily DDT intake may be 11.2 μg/kg. This magnification results from the fact that DDT is stored in the human body at 10 to 20 times the chronic daily intake level and that the baby consumes, essentially, only milk. Furthermore, the caloric intake per kilogram body weight is higher in babies compared with that of adults. The significance of a greater intake of DDT by babies is not clear because of the relatively short duration of this increased level of intake and the sensitivity of young versus adult (Lu et al., 1965; Makri et al., 2004).

The biomagnification is even more marked in carnivorous animals. DDT and methylmercury can accumulate through a series of plankton, small fish, large fish, and birds, resulting in a magnification of the concentration amounting to several hundred-fold (Woodwell, 1967). The decision to suspend the use of DDT was partly based on its adverse ecological impact, as noted earlier.

## Testing, evaluation, and control

### Categories of data required

Various categories of data are required in the evaluation of pesticides. Basic data required are essentially the same as those listed for food additives (see Chapter 18). However, a number of specific toxicological problems have been encountered with pesticides in the preceding section. Additional studies for certain pesticides include the following:

#### *$LD_{50}$ and short-term toxicity*

Because of the greater acute toxicity of most pesticides, $LD_{50}$ is usually determined more precisely. Furthermore, in view of the fact that certain occupational workers such as manufacturers, formulators, and applicators may be exposed via dermal and respiratory exposure, dermal $LD_{50}$ and $LC_{50}$ by inhalation are generally required. As occupational workers are likely to be exposed for some length of time, the toxicity of repeated exposure through dermal and inhalation routes are generally ascertained (see Chapters 12 and 15).

#### *Delayed neurotoxicity (Peripheral axonopathy)*

Delayed toxicity has been observed with a number of OP insecticides (Wu and Chang, 2010: Gupta and Milatovic, 2012; Gupta and Crissman, 2013). The appropriate test is performed on new chemicals in this group to exclude this potential hazard (see Chapter 17).

#### *Interaction*

Marked interaction exists between certain pairs of OP insecticides. The potential health hazard is assessed using the $LD_{50}$ of the individual chemicals alone and in combination.

### Toxicological evaluation

The assessment of an acceptable daily intake (ADI) involves assessing the database for completeness and relevance, determining a no-observed adverse effect level (NOAEL) in terms of mg/kg body weight, and selecting an appropriate safety factor to extrapolate to an ADI for humans, also in terms of mg/kg body weight. A list of ADIs of the 230 pesticides that have been evaluated by the WHO Expert Committee on Pesticide Residues since 1965, along with the NOAELs, safety factors, and critical effects is included in a review article (Lu, 1995).

While all pesticides are toxic, they vary in nature and magnitude of toxicity. Certain pesticides have an inherent potential for specific toxic effects. The presence of such properties must be assessed by conducting appropriate tests, before determining a NOAEL. The safety factor magnitude depends on a number of factors, as discussed in Chapter 27.

## *Standards*

### *Tolerances*

To protect the health of the consumer, standards are formulated and established in the form of "tolerances" (also known as "maximum residue limits"). Standards provide maximum permitted levels in each food commodity in which the pesticide may leave residues following its use. A pesticide may be used during one or more stages of the preplanting, growth, harvesting, handling, and storage of the food crop.

### *Dietary intakes*

Several procedures are used to ensure that the total intake of each pesticide from its residues in all food commodities does not exceed its ADI. One procedure involves chemical analysis of residue levels in food represented in the "total diet" and calculation of the "dietary intake" of each pesticide by adding the products of residue levels and the per capita consumption of each of these foods. The survey by the U.S. Food and Drug Administration (FDA) showed that the dietary intakes of all pesticides analyzed were considerably lower than the corresponding ADIs (FDA, 1987).

The other procedure, which is much simpler, involves calculating the "potential daily intake" and comparing it with the corresponding ADI. The former potential daily intake is obtained by adding the products of the tolerance levels in each of the foods with the per capita consumption of these foods. Evidently, the potential daily intake represents an overestimation. First, a pesticide is not necessarily used in all the food commodities in which there are tolerances. Furthermore, in a vast majority of cases, the actual residue levels are much lower than the tolerances. Nevertheless, this procedure offers distinct advantages. Apart from a few industrialized countries, figures for dietary intakes of pesticides are not available; for them, the potential daily intakes provide a means of assessing the health hazards to the consumer posed by the dietary intake of pesticides. Overestimation may also compensate for differences in dietary habits in different parts of the world and for variations in levels of pesticide residues in certain foods. According to actual analysis, residue levels may, infrequently, exceed the tolerances (see also Chapter 27).

In addition to assessing the potential hazard of pesticides, dietary intake figures obtained by analysis/calculation are also used in assessing, and possibly in recommending, modification of agricultural use of these chemicals. Where the residue levels appear too high; they may be lowered by a reduction of the rate of application or by an increase in the interval between the last application and harvesting of the food crop.

## *Gulf War syndrome*

Between August 1990 and April 1991, there were over 750,000 military personnel from the United States, Canada, and the United Kingdom who participated in an air, sea, and ground war in the Persian Gulf region. During this war, service personnel were concurrently exposed to certain biological, chemical, and psychological environments. Among some veterans, there was an increased frequency of chronic symptoms including headache, loss of memory, fatigue, muscle and joint pain, ataxia, skin rash, respiratory difficulties, and GI tract disturbances. Potential exposure was to fumes and smoke from the following: military operations, oil-well fires, diesel exhaust, toxic paints, pesticides, fire sand, depleted uranium, chemoprophylactic agents, and multiple immunizations. The variety of symptoms reported by veterans make it unlikely that a single etiological cause was responsible for producing Gulf War illnesses.

It was suggested by news media that chemical interactions among pyridostigmine bromide (PB), permethrin, and *N,N*-diethyl-*m*-toluamide (DEET) might contribute to Gulf War illnesses. This reported mixture served to protect military personnel against insect-borne diseases. Furthermore, PB protected against a potential nerve gas attack. However, heavy use of DEET by 1–5% of the Persian Gulf War veterans (7000–35,000 persons) may be related to the unexpected increase in the number of complaints of some veterans, which included fatigue, joint pain, ataxia, and rash (Institute of Medicine, 1995). Other complaints reported by "heavy users" of DEET were stumbling, weakness, and muscle cramps. The fact that these complaints occurred with excess frequency within this subpopulation can be deemed that exposure to contaminants in the Persian Gulf was responsible for this illness. A comprehensive toxicological assessment of Gulf War veterans has been carried out and some pesticides are described here (Brown, 2006; McCauley, 2006, 2015).

*Pyridostigmine bromide* (PB) is a quaternary ammonium carbamate that has been approved by the FDA as a treatment for myasthenia gravis and the reversal of nondepolarizing neuromuscular blocking agents. PB was used in the Gulf War at a dose of one 30-mg tablet every 8 hours (90 mg/day).

PB was taken for about 2 weeks at the start of the air war in mid-January and again at the start of the ground war in mid-February. The majority of service members in the theater of operations took some PB during these periods. Toxicity from an overdose of PB results from the accumulation of ACh at nicotinic and muscarinic ACh receptors in the peripheral nervous system. The resultant effect is exaggerated cholinergic response, such as muscle fasciculations, cramps, weakness, muscle twitching, respiratory difficulty, tremor, GI tract disturbances, and paralysis (Abou-Donia et al., 1996). Finally, death occurs from asphyxia. It should be clearly noted that a therapeutic oral dose of PB for myasthenia gravis is 200–1400 mg/day, but a much lower dose was taken in the Persian Gulf.

*Permethrin*, a synthetic pyrethroid, has been approved for use as an insecticide by the U.S. Environmental Protection Agency (EPA). This compound has also been used to impregnate army battle-dress uniforms in the field. Formulations for application include a 0.5% aerosol and a 40% solution applied either with a 2-gallon compressed air sprayer or via a passive absorption method in a plastic bag (for uniform impregnation). The impregnation method available to soldiers prior to and during the Gulf War was the aerosol spray can method. The aerosol supply and distribution were limited within the war theater (less than 5% of deployed units had distributional access) (McCain et al., 1997). Permethrin modifies voltage-gated sodium channels to open longer during a depolarizing pulse, evoking repetitive after-discharges by a single stimulus (Gammon et al., 2012; Soderlund, 2012). GABA-gated chloride and calcium channels have also been implicated as additional sites of action. As a result, repetitive nerve action is associated with hyperactivity, tremors, ataxia, convulsions, and eventually, paralysis and death (Bradberry et al., 2005; Morgan et al., 2007; Drago et al., 2014).

*DEET* is an aromatic amide used as a personal insect repellent against mosquitoes, biting flies, and ticks, among other insects. It has been used since 1946 by the U.S. Army and since 1957 by the general population. Approximately 30% of the U.S. population uses DEET as a lotion, stick, or spray at concentrations between 10% and 100% active ingredient. DEET is an EPA-approved insect repellant that is widely used commercially. Several formulations using various concentrations of DEET are available; it is the active ingredient in products such as Deep Woods Off and Cutter Insect Repellent. Formulations prepared for the U.S. Army include 75% DEET in ethanol, 33% in extended duration formulation, and 19% in stick. Entomologists assigned to the Persian Gulf during the conflict indicated a very low usage of personal repellents, including DEET, even at times and in areas where mosquitoes were present and biting. The cool seasonal climatic conditions that prevailed at the time of the war (January and February 1991) resulted in the near absence of biting insects.

Extensive and repeated topical applications of DEET resulted in human poisoning, including two deaths (de Garbino and Laborde, 1983; Roland et al., 1985). Symptoms of poisoning are characterized by tremors, restlessness, slurred speech, seizures, impaired cognitive functions, and coma (Institute of Medicine, 1995). The exact mechanism underlying DEET toxicity is unknown. Pathological findings, following DEET administration, indicate that this compound is a demyelinating agent that produces spongiform myelinopathy, primarily of the cerebellar roof nuclei.

In light of the established safety of PB, it was surprising that approximately half of all military personnel seen in health-care facilities during the Gulf War complained of PB side effects consistent with muscarinic and nicotinic acetylcholine receptors stimulation (Institute of Medicine, 1995). One conclusion reached by the Committee to Review the Health Consequences of Service during the Persian Gulf War was that "studies are needed to resolve uncertainties about whether PB, DEET, and permethrin exert additive effects" (Institute of Medicine, 1995). The Committee also recommended for immediate action that: "appropriate laboratory animal studies of interactions between DEET, PB, and permethrin should be conducted." Regardless of the need for further studies, it is clear that contaminant mixture exposure produced a Gulf War syndrome in humans.

## Acknowledgment

I would like to thank Ms. Michelle A. Lasher for her technical assistance in the preparation of this chapter.

## References

Abou-Donia MB, Wilmarth KR, Jensen KF et al. (1996). Neurotoxicity resulting from coexposure to pyridostigmine bromide, DEET, and permethrin: Implications of Gulf War chemical exposures. *J Toxicol Environ Health*. 48, 35–56.

Anadon A, Gupta RC (2012). Fipronil. In: Gupta RC, ed. *Veterinary Toxicology: Basic and Clinical Principles*. Amsterdam: Academic Press/Elsevier. pp. 604–8.

Bayen S, Koroleva E, Lee HK et al. (2005). Persistent organic pollutants and heavy metals in typical seafoods consumed in Singapore. *J Toxicol Environ Health A*. 68, 151–66.

Berry C, La Vecchia C, Nicotera P (2010). Paraquat and Parkinson's disease. *Cell Death Differ*. 17, 1115–25.

Bradberry SM, Cage SA, Proudfoot AT, Vale JA (2005). Poisoning due to pyrethroids. *Toxicol Rev*. 24(2), 93–106.

Brown M (2006). Toxicological assessments of Gulf War veterans. *Philos Trans R Soc Lond B Biol Sci*. 361, 649–79.

Bruin JE, Gerstein HC, Holloway AC (2010). Long-term consequences of fetal and neonatal nicotine exposure: A critical review. *Toxicol Sci*. 116, 364–74.

Carson R (1962). *Silent Spring.* New York: Houghton Mifflin Company. p. 297.
Choi SM, Yoo SD, Lee BM (2004). Toxicological characteristics of endocrine-disrupting chemicals: Developmental toxicity, carcinogenicity, and mutagenicity. *J Toxicol Environ Health B Crit Rev.* 7, 1–24.
Clegg DJ, van Gemert M (1999). Expert panel report of human studies on chlorpyrifos and/or other organophosphate exposures. *J Toxicol Environ Health B.* 2, 257–79.
Corsini E, Sokooti M, Galli CL, Moretto A, Colosio C (2013). Pesticide induced immunotoxicity in humans: A comprehensive review of the existing evidence. *Toxicology.* 307, 123–35.
Coulston F (1985). Reconsideration of the dilemma of DDT for the establishment of an acceptable daily intake. *Reg Toxicol Pharmacol.* 5, 332–83.
de Garbino JP, Laborde A (1983). Toxicity of an insect repellent: N,N-diethyltoluamide. *Vet Hum Toxicol.* 25, 422–3.
Dekundy A, Kaminski RM (2010). Central mechanisms of seizures and lethality following anticholinesterase pesticides exposure. In: Satoh T, Gupta RC, eds. *Anticholinesterase Pesticides: Metabolism, Neurotoxicity, and Epidemiology.* Hoboken, NJ: John Wiley & Sons. pp. 149–64.
Drago B, Shah NS, Shah SH (2014). Acute permethrin neurotoxicity: Variable presentations, high index of suspicion. *Toxicol Rep.* 1, 1026–8.
Ensley SM (2012). Pyrethrins and pyrethroids. In: Gupta RC, ed. *Veterinary Toxicology: Basic and Clinical Principles.* Amsterdam: Academic Press/Elsevier. pp. 591–5.
Evans TJ (2017). Endocrine disruption. In: Gupta RC, ed. *Reproductive and Developmental Toxicology.* Amsterdam: Academic Press/Elsevier. pp. 1091–110.
FAO (1990). Pesticide Residues in Food—1990. Report of the FAO and WHO Groups of Experts on Pesticide Residues. FAO Plant Production and Protection Paper No. 102. Rome: Food and Agricultural Organization of the United States.
FDA (1987). Residues in Foods. Washington, DC: Food and Drug Administration.
Frawley JP, Fuyat HN, Hagen EC et al. (1957). Marked potentiation in mammalian toxicity from simultaneous administration of two anticholinesterase compounds. *J Pharmacol Exp Ther.* 121, 96–106.
Gammon DW, Chandrasekaran A, Elnaggar SF (2012). Comparative metabolism and toxicology of pyrethroids in mammals. In: Marrs TC, ed. *Mammalian Toxicology of Insecticides.* Cambridge: RSC Publishing. pp. 137–83.
Gupta RC (2006a). Classification and uses of organophosphates and carbamates. In: Gupta RC, ed. *Toxicology of Organophosphate and Carbamate Compounds.* Amsterdam: Academic Press/Elsevier. pp. 5–24.
Gupta PK (2006b). WHO/FAO guidelines for cholinesterase inhibiting pesticide residues in food. In: Gupta RC, ed. *Toxicology of Organophosphate and Carbamate Compounds.* Amsterdam: Academic Press/Elsevier. pp. 643–54.
Gupta RC, Milatovic D (2010). Anticholinesterase pesticides interactions. In: Gupta RC, Satoh T, eds. *Anticholinesterase Pesticides: Metabolism, Neurotoxicity, and Epidemiology.* Hoboken: John Wiley & Sons. pp. 315–27.
Gupta RC (2012a). Amitraz. In: Gupta RC, ed. *Veterinary Toxicology: Basic and Clinical Principles.* Amsterdam: Academic Press/Elsevier. pp. 599–603.
Gupta RC (2012b). Rotenone. In: Gupta RC, ed. *Veterinary Toxicology: Basic and Clinical Principles.* Amsterdam: Academic Press/Elsevier. pp. 620–3.

Gupta PK (2012c). Toxicity of herbicides. In: Gupta RC, ed. *Veterinary Toxicology: Basic and Clinical Principles*. Amsterdam: Academic Press/Elsevier. pp. 631–52.

Gupta RC (2012d). Non-anticoagulant rodenticides. In: Gupta RC, ed. *Veterinary Toxicology: Basic and Clinical Principles*. Amsterdam: Academic Press/Elsevier. pp. 698–711.

Gupta RC, Milatovic D (2012). Toxicity of organophosphates and carbamates. In: Marrs TC, ed. *Mammalian Toxicology of Insecticides*. Cambridge: RSC Publishing. pp. 104–36.

Gupta PK, Aggarwal M (2012). Toxicity of fungicides. In: Gupta RC, ed. *Veterinary Toxicology: Basic and Clinical Principles*. Amsterdam: Academic Press/Elsevier. pp. 653–70.

Gupta RC, Milatovic D (2014). Insecticides. In: Gupta RC, ed. *Biomarkers in Toxicology*. Amsterdam: Academic Press/Elsevier. pp. 389–407.

Gupta PK (2014). Herbicides and fungicides. In: Gupta RC, ed. *Biomarkers in Toxicology*. Amsterdam: Academic Press/Elsevier. pp. 409–31.

Gupta RC, Crissman JW (2013). Agricultural chemicals. In: Haschek WM, Rousseaux CG, Wallig MA, eds. *Haschek and Rousseaux's Handbook of Toxicologic Pathology*, 3rd edition. San Diego: Academic Press/Elsevier. pp. 1349–72.

Gupta PK (2017). Herbicides and fungicides. In: Gupta RC, ed. *Reproductive and Developmental Toxicology*. Amsterdam: Academic Press/Elsevier. pp. 657–79.

Gupta, RC, Miller Mukherjee IR, Doss RB, Malik JK, Milatovic D (2017) Organophosphates and carbamates. In: Gupta RC, ed. *Reproductive and Developmental Toxicology*. Amsterdam: Academic Press/Elsevier. pp. 609–631.

Hayes WJ Jr (1982). *Pesticides Studied in Man*. Baltimore: Williams & Wilkins.

Heaps JW (2006). Insect Management for Food Storage and Processing. AACC Intl. pp. 1–231.

IARC (1977). *Monographs on the Evaluation of Carcinogenic Risk of Chemicals to Man*, vol. 15. Some Fumigants, the Herbicides 2,4-D and 2,4,5-T, Chlorinated Dibenzodioxins and Miscellaneous Industrial Chemicals. Lyon, France: International Agency for Research in Cancer.

IARC (1983). Monographs on the Evaluation of Carcinogenic Risk of Chemicals to Man, vol. 30. Miscellaneous Pesticides. Lyon, France: International Agency for Research in Cancer.

Infante-Rivard C, Weichenthal S (2007). Pesticides and childhood cancer: An update of Zahm and Ward's 1998 review. *J Toxicol Environ Health B*. 10, 81–99.

Institute of Medicine (1995). *Health Consequences of Service during the Persian Gulf War: Initial Findings and Recommendations for Immediate Action*. Washington, DC: National Academy Press.

Juhász E, Szabó R, Keserü M et al. (2006). Teratogenicity testing of a 2,4-D containing herbicide formulation and three heavy metals in chicken embryos. *Commun Agric Appl Biol Sci*. 71, 111–4.

Khera KS (1979). Evaluation of dimethoate (Cygon 4E) for teratogenic activity in the cat. *J Environ Pathol Toxicol*. 2, 1283–8.

Kitamura S, Sugihara K, Fujimoto N, Yamazaki T (2010). Organophosphates as endocrine disruptors. In: Satoh T, Gupta RC, eds. *Anticholinesterase Pesticides: Metabolism, Neurotoxicity, and Epidemiology*. Hoboken, NJ: John Wiley & Sons. pp. 189–202.

Koller LD (1979). Effects of environmental contaminants on the immune system. *Adv Vet Sci Com Med*. 23, 267–95.

Li N, Ragheb K, Lawler G, Sturgis J, Rajwa B et al. (2003). Mitochondrial complex I inhibitor rotenone induces apoptosis through enhancing mitochondrial reactive oxygen species production. *J Biol Chem*. 278, 8516–25.

Lim L (2015). Fumigants: Toxicology and development of acute reference values for methyl bromide, chloropicrin, and methyl iodide. In: Fan AM, Khan EM, Alexeef GV, eds. *Toxicology and Risk Assesment*. Singapore: Pan Stanford Publishing. pp. 369–91.

Lu FC (1995). A review of the acceptable daily intakes of pesticides assessed by WHO. *Reg Toxicol Pharmacol*. 21, 352–64.

Lu FC, Jessup DC, Lavallée A (1965). Toxicity of pesticides to young versus adult rats. *Food Cosmet Toxicol*. 5, 591–6.

Makri A, Goveia M, Balbus J, Parkin R (2004). Children's susceptibility to chemicals: A review by development stage. *J Toxicol Environ Health B*. 7, 417–35.

Malik JK, Telang AG et al. (2010). Interaction of anticholinesterase pesticides with metals. In: Satoh T, Gupta RC, eds. *Anticholinesterase Pesticides: Metabolism, Neurotoxicity, and Epidemiology*. Hoboken, NJ: John Wiley & Sons. pp. 329–39.

Malik JK, Aggarwal M, Kalpana S, Gupta RC (2017). Chlorinated hydrocarbons and pyrethrins/pyrethroids. In: Gupta RC, ed. *Reproductive and Developmental Toxicology*. Amsterdam: Academic Press/Elsevier. pp. 633–55.

Marrs TC, Dewhurst I (2012). Toxicology of some insecticides not discussed elsewhere. In: Marrs TC, ed. *Mammalian Toxicology of Insecticides*. Cambridge: RSC Publishing. pp. 288–301.

Marty MA (2015). Consideration of infants and children in risk assessment. In: Fan AM, Khan EM, Alexeeff GV, eds. *Toxicology and Risk Assessment*. Singapore: Pan Stanford Publishing. pp. 93–133.

McCain WC, Lee R, Johnson MS et al. (1997). Acute oral toxicity study of pyridostigmine bromide, permethrin, and DEET in the laboratory rat. *J Toxicol Environ Health*. 50, 113–24.

McCauley LA (2006). Organophosphates and the Gulf War Syndrome. In: Gupta RC, ed. *Toxicology of Organophosphate and Carbamate Compounds*. Amsterdam: Academic Press/Elsevier. pp. 69–78.

McCauley LA (2015). Epidemiology of chemical warfare agents. In: Gupta RC, ed. *Handbook of Toxicology of Chemical Warfare Agents*. Amsterdam: Academic Press/Elsevier. pp. 47–54.

Morgan MK, Sheldon LS, Croghan CW, Jones PA, Chuang JC, Wilson NK (2007). An observational study of 127 preschool children at their homes and daycare centers in Ohio: Environmental pathways to cis- and trans-permethrin exposure. *Environ Res*. 104, 266–74.

Murphy SD (1969). Mechanisms of pesticide interactions in vertebrates. *Residue Rev*. 25, 201–21.

Murphy MJ (2012). Anticoagulant rodenticides. In: Gupta RC, ed. *Veterinary Toxicology: Basic and Clinical Principles*. Amsterdam: Academic Press/Elsevier. pp. 673–97.

Murphy MJ, Lugo AM (2015). Superwarfarins. In: Gupta RC, ed. *Handbook of Toxicology of Chemical Warfare Agents*. Amsterdam: Academic Press/Elsevier. pp. 223–38.

Narahashi T (1980). Nerve membrane as a target of environmental toxicants. In: Spencer P, Schaumberg HH, eds. *Neurotoxicology*. Baltimore: Williams & Wilkins.

Patocka Y (2015). Strychnine. In: Gupta RC, ed. *Handbook of Toxicology of Chemical Warfare Agents*. Amsterdam: Academic Press/Elsevier. pp. 215–22.

Pope CN (1999). Organophosphorus pesticides: Do they all have the same mechanism of toxicity? *J Toxicol Environ Health B*. 2, 161–81.

Rohlman D, McCauley L (2010). Toxicity of anticholinesterase pesticides in neonates and children. In: Satoh T, Gupta RC, eds. *Anticholinesterase Pesticides: Metabolism, Neurotoxicity, and Epidemiology*. Hoboken, NJ: John Wiley & Sons. pp. 225–36.

Roland EH, Jan JE, Rigg JM (1985). Toxic encephalopathy in a child after brief exposure to insect repellents. *Can Med Assoc J*. 132, 155–6.

Rose PH (2012). Nicotine and neonicotinoids. In: Marrs TC, ed. *Mammalian Toxicology of Insecticides*. Cambridge: RSC Publishing. pp. 184–220.

Roy D, Palangat M, Chen C-W et al. (1997). Biochemical and molecular changes at the cellular level in response to exposure to environmental estrogen-like chemicals. *J Toxicol Environ Health*. 50, 1–29.

Schoental R (1977). Depletion of coenzymes at the site of rapidly growing tissues due to alkylation: The biochemical basis of the teratogenic effects of alkylating agents, including organophosphorus and certain other compounds. *Biochem Soc Trans*. 5, 1016–7.

Sharma RP (2006). Organophosphates, carbamates, and the immune system. In: Gupta RC, ed. *Toxicology of Organophosphate and Carbamate Compounds*. Amsterdam: Academic Press/Elsevier. pp. 495–507.

Sheets LP, Li AA, Minnema DJ, Collier RH, Creek MR et al. (2016). A critical review of neonicotinoid insecticides for developmental neurotoxicity. *Crit Rev Toxicol*. 46, 153–90.

Silva M, Pham N, Lewis C, Iyer S, Kwok E et al. (2015). A comparison of ToxCast test results with *in vivo* and other *in vitro* endpoints for neuro, endocrine, and developmental toxicities: A case study using endosulfan and methidathion. *Birth Def Res*. (Part B) 104, 71–89.

Smalley HE, Curtis JM, Earl FL (1968). Teratogenic action of carbaryl in beagle dogs. *Toxicol Appl Pharmacol*. 13, 392–403.

Smith P, Heath D (1976). Paraquat. *CRC Crit Rev Toxicol*. 4, 411–45.

Smith AG (2012). DDT and other chlorinated insecticides. In: Marrs TC, ed. *Mammalian Toxicology of Insecticides*. Cambridge: RSC Publishing. pp. 37–103.

Soderlund DM (2012). Molecular mechanisms of pyrethroid insecticide neurotoxicity: Recent advances. *Arch Toxicol*. 86, 165–81.

Steinhoff D, Weber H, Mohr U et al. (1983). Evaluation of amitrole (aminotriazole) for potential carcinogenicity in orally dosed rats, mice and golden hamster. *Toxicol Appl Pharmacol*. 69, 161–9.

Street JC (1981). Pesticides and the immune system. In: Sharma RP, ed. *Immunologic Considerations in Toxicology.* Boca Raton, FL: CRC Press. pp. 45–66.
Tomizawa M, Casida JE (2005). Neonicotinoid insecticide toxicology: Mechanisms of selective action. *Ann Rev Pharmacol Toxicol.* 45, 247–68.
Vial T, Nicolas B, Descotes J (1996). Clinical immunotoxicity of pesticides. *J Toxicol Environ Health.* 48, 215–29.
Wang XQ, Gas PY, Lin YZ et al. (1988). Studies on hexachlorocyclohexane and DDT contents in human cerumen and their relationship to cancer mortality. *Biomed Environ Sci.* 1, 138–51.
Wang X, Martinez MA, Wu Q, Martinez-Laranaga MR, Anadon A, Yuan Z (2016). Fipronil insecticide toxicity: Oxidative stress and metabolism. *Crit Rev Toxicol.* In Press. http://dx.doi.org/10.1080/10408444.2016.1223014.
Weil CS, Woodside MD, Carpenter CP et al. (1972). Current status of tests of carbaryl for reproductive and teratogenic effects. *Toxicol Appl Pharmacol.* 21, 390–404.
Weselak M, Arbuckle TE, Foster W (2007). Pesticide exposures and developmental outcomes: the epidemiological evidence. *J Toxicol Environ Health B.* 10, 41–80.
Wigle DT, Arbuckle TE, Turner MC et al. (2008). Epidemiologic evidence of relationships between reproductive and child health outcomes and environmental chemical contaminants. *J Toxicol Environ Health B.* 11, 373–517.
Wills JH, Jameson E, Coulston F (1968). Effects of oral doses of carbaryl on man. *Clin Toxicol.* 1, 265–71.
Woodwell GM (1967). Toxic substances and ecological cycles. *Sci Am.* 216, 24.
World Health Organization (1970). Pesticide Residues in Food. WHO Tech Rep Ser. 458. Geneva, Switzerland: WHO.
World Health Organization (1974). Pesticide Residues in Food. Report of the 1973 Joint FAO/WHO Meeting. Tech Rep Ser. 545. Geneva, Switzerland: WHO.
Wu Y-J, Chang P-A (2010). Molecular toxicology of neuropathy target esterase. In: Satoh T, Gupta RC, eds. *Anticholinesterase Pesticides: Metabolism, Neurotoxicity, and Epidemiology.* Hoboken, NJ: John Wiley & Sons. pp. 109–20.
Yildiz D (2004). Nicotine, its metabolism and an overview of its biological effects. *Toxicon.* 43, 619–32.

# *chapter twenty-four*

# *Nanotoxicology*

***Sang-Hyun Kim and Byung-Mu Lee***

*Contents*



## *Introduction*

Nanotoxicology is the area of toxicology specifically dealing with nanomaterials (NMs) or nanoparticles (NPs). Advances in nanoscience and nanoengineering technology have provided both benefits and risks to human safety as nanoparticles are now being used in many consumer products, such as foods, cosmetics, biosensors, energy, household products, electronic devices, and drug delivery systems and their applications continue to increase rapidly (Zhao and Castranova, 2011). In general, a NP is defined as a particle with a diameter between 1 and 100 nm (ISO, 2008; SCENIHR, 2010), which enters cells either via energy-dependent endocytosis, transmembrane channels, or membrane penetration and may produce adverse effects. Due to rapid increase in nanotoxicological research, a database, NHECD (Nano Health-Environment Commented Database), was developed and is available at: http://www.nhecd-fp7.eu (CORDIS, 2016).

## Types of nanomaterials: Classification

One nanometer (nm) is one billionth of a meter and the term "nanomaterials" refers to any engineered materials of 100 nm or less in at least one direction. Nanomaterials (NMs) are classified as NPs, nanofibers, and nanoplates (ISO, 2008) (Figure 24.1). NMs can be classified as carbon-based NMs, metal-based NMs, dendrimers, and nanocomposites (as summarized below) (Choi and Frangioni, 2010).

1. *Carbon-based nanomaterials*: Carbon nanomaterials (CNMs) exist in several forms, such as hollow spheres, ellipsoids, rings, or tubes. Spherical and ellipsoidal CNMs are called fullerenes, whereas cylindrical CNMs are termed nanotubes. Carbon fullerenes (also termed buckminster fullerenes in full or Bucky balls) are similar to graphite in structure, insoluble, and nonreactive. The most common and smallest fullerene is $C_{60}$. Carbon nanotubes (CNTs) can be further divided into single-walled carbon nanotubes (SWCNTs) and multiwalled nanotubes (MWCNTs). CNMs are used in the electronics industry and for material engineering.
2. *Metal-based nanomaterials*: These include metals (silver, gold), metal oxides (iron oxide, aluminum oxide, cerium oxide, copper oxide, zinc

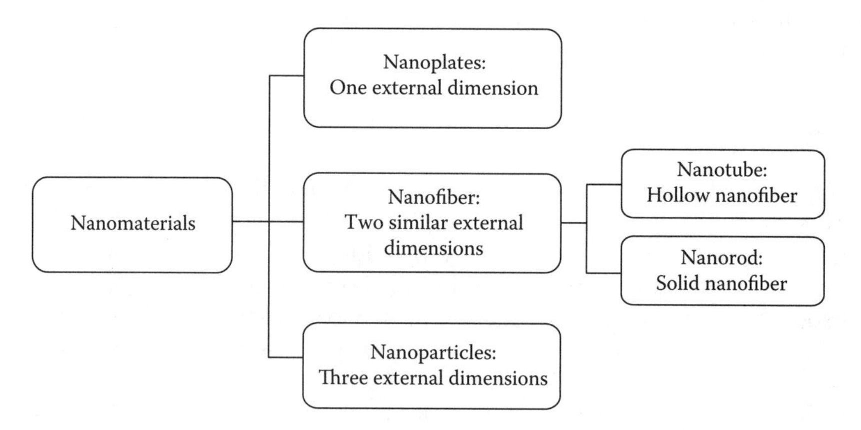


***Figure 24.1*** ISO TS 27687 Categories of nanomaterials: nanoparticles, nanofibers, and nanoplates. (From ISO, *ISO/TS 27687:2008*, 2008.)

oxide, and titanium oxide), and quantum dots (also called nanocrystals, made from ZnSe, ZnS, CdSe, CdTe, PbSe, and PbS compounds). These metal-based NMs are used in consumer products, cosmetics, semiconductors, and in the automobile industry. Of the metal-based NMs, the oxides of zinc and copper are known to be particularly toxic.

3. *Dendrimers*: Dendrimers are hyperbranched materials and nano-sized polymers. Dendrimers are used in nanomedicine for drug delivery and catalysis as well as chemical sensors and reaction vessels.
4. *Nanocomposites*: Nanocomposites are combinations of NPs with other materials or NPs, and are used in auto parts, for drug delivery, in electronics, and in packaging materials to enhance mechanical, thermal, and flame-retardant properties (Hu and Gao, 2010).

Auffan et al. (2009) proposed that for specific "nanoeffects," the particles must be below 30 nm, but particles larger than 30 nm also exhibit NP-like properties.

## *Exposure sources*

Exposure sources are numerous and vary from natural to anthropogenic sources. Humans are exposed to smoke or ash produced by cigarettes, automobile exhaust, combustion, power plants, fires, and volcanoes. Meteorological changes also generate NPs. Aerosols generated by human activities (automobile and industrial exhausts) are estimated to constitute 10% of the total, and the remaining 90% of the airborne aerosols of dust and particulate matter (PM) are generated naturally by volcanic eruptions, forest fires, vegetation, and by sea spray (Taylor, 2002). Humans are exposed to NPs from foods, cosmetics, electronics, medical devices, drugs, and consumer products (e.g., detergents and paper).

## *Physicochemical properties of nanomaterials*

NPs possess various physicochemical properties that depend upon size and chemical composition. As the physicochemical properties of NPs affect both the pharmacological and toxicological effects of NPs in biological systems, information on the physicochemical properties (e.g., size, shape, surface area, surface charge, surface chemistry, solubility, structure, stability, surface porosity, pH, electric properties, light activation, conductivity, agglomeration, magnetic properties, crystal structure, zeta potential, and coatings) is considered important (Johnston et al., 2010).

Physicochemical properties govern the toxicokinetics (e.g., absorption, distribution, metabolism, excretion, and storage) of NPs, toxicodynamics (interactions with biomolecules), and toxicological outcomes. The intratracheal instillation of ultrafine $TiO_2$ particles (20 nm) was found to produce pulmonary inflammation in rats and mice, and its toxicity was found to be correlated with a greater surface area per unit mass (Oberdörster et al., 2000). Further, as the degree of sidewall functionalization of SWCNTs increases, SWCNTs become less cytotoxic to cultured human dermal fibroblasts (HDF) (Sayes et al., 2006). Smaller NPs have substantially greater specific surface areas. NPs produce unique optical effects, because their sizes produce quantum effects. For example, the colors of gold NPs change size dependently from red to black in solution, whereas gold slabs are usually yellow. Further, the melting point of gold NPs of 2.5 nm is ~300°C, whereas that of gold slabs is 1064°C (Buffat and Borel, 1976).

The physicochemical properties of NPs are characterized by using various analytical techniques such as AFM (atomic force microscopy), DLS (dynamic light scattering), DMA (dynamic mechanical analysis), FFF (field flow fractionation), ICP-MS (inductively coupled plasma–mass spectrometry), MALDI-TOF (matrix-assisted laser desorption/ionization time-of-flight mass spectrometry), NMR (nuclear magnetic resonance), SEM (scanning electron microscopy), TEM (transmission electron microscopy), UV/Vis absorption spectroscopy, XPS (x-ray photoelectron spectroscopy), and XRD (x-ray diffraction). The following are examples of the size range of different materials:

- DNA molecules (diameter of 2–12 nm)
- Viruses (typically maximum dimension of 10–100 nm)
- Single red blood cell (diameter of 2500–5000 nm)
- Human hair (thickness of 10,000–50,000 nm)

## *Usage and effects of nanomaterials*

NMs are being used in more than 1800 consumer products from 622 companies in 32 countries and this number is expected to rapidly grow (Vance et al., 2015). It is estimated that consumer products involving nanotechnology applications will reach approximately $75.8 billion by 2020. NPs can be made of many materials, but the specific types of NPs mentioned above are being widely used. $TiO_2$, silicon dioxide, and zinc oxide are the most produced NMs worldwide on a mass basis (Figure 24.2). However, silver NPs are the most popular NMs in the Consumer Products Inventory, present in 24% of products (Keller et al., 2013). NPs are used in the medical and food industries, in cosmetics, electronics, textiles, and in other consumer products such as deodorant, detergent, shampoo, soap, and toothpaste (Zhao and Castranova, 2011) (Table 24.1).

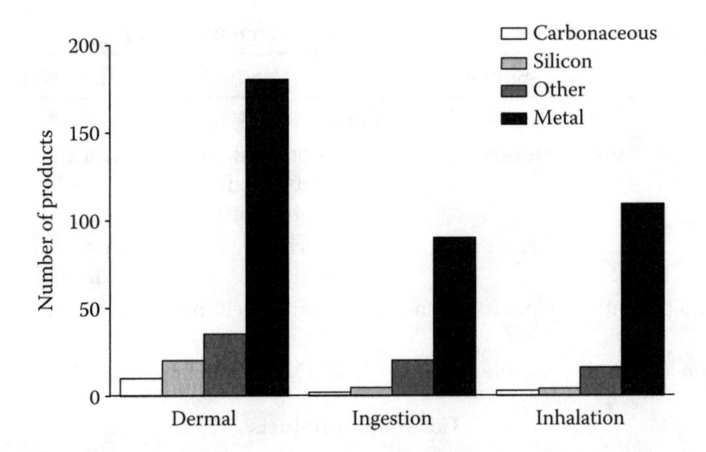


***Figure 24.2*** Potential exposure pathways of nanomaterials from the expected use of consumer products.

Nanomedicine is an emerging area for the development of new drugs, diagnostics, treatments, medical devices, and drug delivery systems (Armstead and Li, 2011). Different types of NPs have also been applied in biomedicine as imaging agents. Liposomes are commonly used NPs for the delivery of drugs or biomolecules such as siRNAs. Silver NPs exhibit effective antibacterial properties against pathogenic bacteria (Gram-negative and Gram-positive), and smaller silver NPs enhance these effects, due to their larger surface area to volume ratios (Panacek et al., 2006).

## *Toxicities of nanomaterials*

The development and application of NMs introduced safety issues, and thus, nanotoxicology emerged as an important part of toxicology and nanoscience. The major concerns relate to the introduction of NMs and nanoproducts without safety evaluations. However, lessons were gleaned, regarding the importance of the toxicology of NPs, from the data reported on asbestos, metal fumes, and smokes, before the era of nanotechnology (Pacurari et al., 2010). The applications of asbestos in building construction produced various lung diseases (e.g., asbestosis and mesothelioma) in exposed workers. In addition, smokes produce various types of diseases such as cancer, respiratory disorders, GI tract diseases, skin diseases, and reproductive diseases. Some key factors such as the physicochemical properties and toxicokinetics/toxicodynamics need to be considered for nanotoxicity (Figure 24.3).

*Table 24.1* List of commercial products containing nanoparticles

| Categories | Subcategories | Products | Exposure route |
|---|---|---|---|
| | | **Food** | |
| Food conservation | Storage | Food containers, baby (milk) bottles, mugs | Dermal/oral |
| | Cleaning | Sterilizing sprays | Inhalation/dermal |
| Food equipment | Cooking utensils | Cutting/chopping boards | Dermal |
| Food consumption | Supplements | AgNPs in water | Oral |
| | | **Consumer products** | |
| Personal care/cosmetics | Skin care/oral hygiene | (Body) cream, beauty soap, etc. | Dermal |
| | | Toothbrushes | Oral |
| | Hair care | Hair brushes, hair masks | Dermal |
| | Cleaning | Elimination sprays | Dermal |
| | Baby care | Pacifiers, teethers | Dermal |
| | Other | Deodorant | Dermal |
| Textile | Clothing | Fabrics/fibers, socks, underwear | Dermal |
| | Other textiles | Sheets, towels, sleeves | Dermal |
| | Toys | Plush toys | Dermal/oral |
| Electronics | Personal care | Hair dryers, shavers | Dermal |
| | Household appliance | Refrigerators, washing machines | Dermal |
| | | Humidifiers | – |
| | Computer hardware | Notebooks, (laser) mouse, keyboards | Dermal |
| | Mobile devices | Mobile phones | Dermal |
| Household products/home improvement | Cleaning | Laundry soap | Dermal |
| | | Detergents, fabric softeners | |
| | Coating | Sprays | Dermal |
| | Others | Pet products, algicide | Dermal |

(*Continued*)

*Table 24.1 (Continued)* List of commercial products containing nanoparticles

| Categories | Subcategories | Products | Exposure route |
|---|---|---|---|
| Filtration, purification, neutralization, sanitization | Filtration | Air filters | Inhalation |
| | Cleaning | Disinfectants/aerosol sprays | Inhalation/dermal |
| | **Medical products** | | |
| Medical instruments | Breathing masks, endotracheal tubes | | Inhalation |
| | Gastrointestinal tube | | Oral |
| | Orthopedic implants | | Intramedullary |
| | Contact lenses | | Ophthalmic |
| | Incontinence materials | | Dermal |
| | Catheters | | Intravascular/urethral/intrathecal/intravesical |
| Others | Sling for reconstructive pelvic surgery | | Intraperitoneal |
| | Surgical masks/textiles | | Inhalation/dermal |
| | Wound dressings | | Dermal |
| | Pharmaceuticals | | Oral/dermal |

Similar safety concerns have been raised regarding CNTs because they possess asbestos-like shapes (Helland et al., 2007). In a 14-week inhalation toxicity study, MWCNTs were found in the lungs of mice, and there was scarring and fibrosis of the lungs, but none of these symptoms were seen in mice exposed to carbon black, which was composed of graphene, the same substance from which nanotubes were made, but in the form of a compact particle (Donaldson and Poland, 2009). Epidemiological studies of fine particles showed that small NMs induced damage in the pulmonary, cardiovascular, and nervous systems (Krug and Wick, 2011). Routes of exposure to NPs were via skin, ingestion, and/or inhalation, and toxic responses could be local or systemic, depending upon physicochemical properties of the NPs concerned.

## *Skin toxicity*

NPs are applied in over 200 commercial skin products such as sunscreens, cosmetics, and personal care products. Nano $TiO_2$ (titanium dioxide, a potent photocatalyst) and nano zinc oxide (ZnO) are utilized as additives in sunscreens to protect the skin from UV radiation. Currently NP

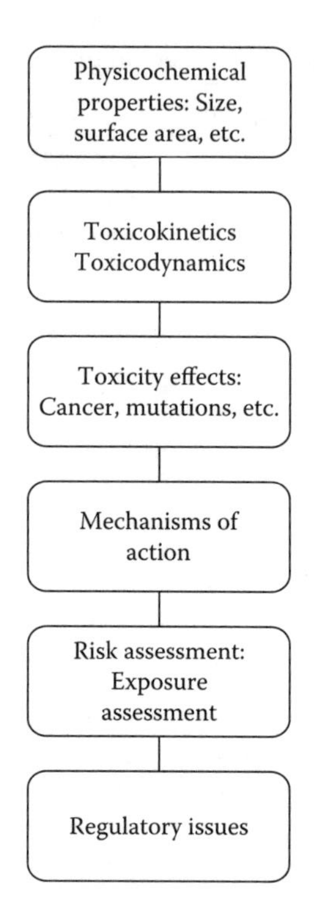


***Figure 24.3*** Consideration of the key toxicological issues posed by nanomaterials.

usages are being examined as treatments for dermatological conditions (Wiesenthal et al., 2011). Wu et al. (2009) reported that $TiO_2$ NPs (4 nm, 60 nm) penetrates the skin of pig ears after treatment for 30 days, and that $TiO_2$ NPs (21 nm) reached the brain in hairless mice after treatment for 60 days. In this investigation, severe pathological changes of the mouse skin and liver were observed, and superoxide dismutase (SOD) activity and malondialdehyde (MDA) levels were significantly changed. Further, it was also reported that typical exposure to SWCNTs produced dermal toxicity, reactive oxygen species (ROS) generation, and inflammation (Shvedova et al., 2003; Murray et al., 2009). Although there are three types of $TiO_2$ (rutile, anatase, and brookite), principally the anatase form has raised concerns over its toxicity.

## *Pulmonary diseases*

NPs initiate pulmonary diseases, such as asthma, cystic fibrosis (CF), and chronic obstructive pulmonary disease (COPD), by altering the mucus rheology in the respiratory tract (Chen et al., 2010). Occupational exposure to NPs (e.g., carbon black, dust, aerosols, fire, and welding fumes) may produce fibrosis, emphysema, bronchitis, pulmonary inflammation, and pulmonary edema. Further, pneumoconiosis might also be associated directly or indirectly with uncharacterized NPs. The underlying mechanisms of NP-induced pulmonary toxicity include generation of oxidative stress, DNA damage, and inflammation leading to fibrosis and pneumoconiosis (Li et al., 2010).

## *Mutations*

Shinohara et al. (2009) reported negative results for the micronucleus (MN) test, after treating ICR mice with fullerene $C_{60}$. SWCNTs were not found to induce MN formation in Chinese hamster lung (CHL) cells, but Totsuka et al. (2009) showed that fullerene $C_{60}$ NPs, depending upon concentration, increased MN frequency in A549 cells. Asakura et al. (2010) reported that MWCNTs significantly increased the rate of polyploidy in CHL/IU cells, as determined by a chromosomal aberration test. In the Ames test, some NPs such as CNTs, fullerenes $C_{60}$, and ZnO were found to be negative. On the other hand, carbon black NPs were reported to induce genotoxicity in the lungs and livers of C57BL/6 mice (Bourdon et al., 2012) and silver NPs were reported to produce DNA damage, chromosomal aberrations, and MN formation (Ahamed et al., 2008; Asharani et al., 2009a,b; Kawata et al., 2009).

## *Cancer*

Various types of NPs have been investigated for tumorigenicity in animals, but the results are contradictory. CNTs may induce granulomas (microscopic nodules) in lungs and skin, and mesothelioma, the type of cancer produced by exposure to asbestos (Poland et al., 2008). MWCNTs (3500 ppm iron content; diameter 100 nm; approximate length 1–5 μm, 25 weeks) induced mesothelioma in the peritoneal cavity of male p53 (+/–) mice (C57BL/6 background), by intraperitoneal injection (Takagi et al., 2008), but another study reported a negative result in male CD1 mice treated intranasally, intratracheally, orally, or intraperitoneally with MWCNTs (approximately 30–50 nm in diameter and 100–300 mm in length) (Carrero-Sanchez et al., 2006). On the other hand, SWCNT was found to be negative for tumor formation in rats and mice (Warheit et al., 2004).

Carbon black was classified as a possible human carcinogen (Group 2B) in 2010, by the International Agency for Research on Cancer (IARC, 2012). Further, inhalation of $TiO_2$ NPs (28 nm) produced lung tumors in female rats (Heinrich et al., 1995), and hydrophilic anatase $TiO_2$ NPs (200 nm) induced a significant incidence of lung tumors (29.5–63.6%) by intratracheal instillation in female rats (Pott and Roller, 2005). In addition, the tumor incidence of chronically inhaled $TiO_2$ NPs was found to correlate better with a specific surface area than with a particle mass.

### *Immunotoxicity*

Interactions between NPs and the immune system produces undesirable immune responses, such as immunostimulation or immunosuppression, which may promote inflammation, autoimmune disorders, and increase susceptibility to infections and cancer (Zolnik et al., 2010). *In vitro* and *in vivo* studies demonstrated that NPs and ultrafine particles induce the production of proinflammatory cytokines, chemokines, and adhesion molecules, which lead to the recruitment of inflammatory cells and disrupt the immune defense (Chang, 2010). NPs can be taken up and processed by dendritic cells in the regional lymph nodes, as well as interact with self-proteins, modify their antigenicities, alter immune responses, and induce autoimmunity (Di Gioacchino et al., 2011). In addition, CoCr NPs enhance cytotoxicity, induce DNA damage and chromosomal aberrations, and possibly stimulate metal hypersensitivity (Gill et al., 2012).

### *Neurotoxicity*

NPs (combustion-derived, manufactured, or engineered) can reach the brain by inhalation and may be associated with neurodegeneration via neuroinflammation, oxidative stress, and alterations of gene expression (Win-Shwe and Fujimaki, 2011). Some NPs cross the blood–brain barrier (BBB) either by passive diffusion or by carrier-mediated endocytosis (Hoet et al., 2004). Another potential route of entry for NPs may be via ionic channels (i.e., $Na^+$, $K^+$, $Ca^{2+}$) present in neuronal cell membranes. The Inhalation of NPs present in PM or ultrafine PM increases cardiopulmonary morbidity and mortality rate (Pope et al., 2004) and may enhance inflammatory processes in the brain via MAP kinase signaling pathways and via translocations of NPs to the central nervous system (Kleinman et al., 2008). In primary rat brain microvessel endothelial cells, silver NPs may interact with the cerebral microvasculature, and induce proinflammatory cascades, inflammation, and neurotoxicity (Trickler et al., 2010). In animal studies, $TiO_2$ NP was shown to produce neurotoxicity due to oxidative stress, inflammation, apoptosis, and genotoxicity (Song et al., 2016). Another potential mechanism of $TiO_2$-mediated nanotoxicity is implicated in epigenetic regulation, which changes gene expression not through genotoxic stress but rather arises during development and cell proliferation (Mizushima and Komatsu, 2011; Stoccoro et al., 2013).

### *Endocrine disruption and reproductive toxicity*

Several reports demonstrated that NPs disrupt the endocrine system. Prenatal exposure of pregnant F344 rats to NP-rich diesel exhaust (NP-DE) suppressed testicular function in male rats after birth (Li et al., 2009). Further, the relative weights of the seminal vesicles and prostate to body weight were decreased as were levels of serum hormones (testosterone, progesterone, corticosterone, and FSH), steroidogenic acute regulatory protein (StAR), and 17-β-hydroxysteroid dehydrogenase mRNA in the testes. NP-DE increased testosterone biosynthesis, StAR, and cytochrome P450 side-chain cleavage (P450scc)-mRNA expressions via growth hormone signaling, which might be the mechanism underlying reproductive toxicity in male rats (Ramdhan et al., 2009). In addition, $TiO_2$ produced reproductive toxicity in zebra fish by reducing the number of zebra fish eggs by 29.5% after 13 weeks of $TiO_2$ exposure (0.1 mg/L) (Wang et al., 2011). *In vitro* and *in vivo* studies demonstrated that NPs may cross the placenta barrier and adversely affect the fetus (Refuerzo et al., 2011; Wick et al., 2011).

## *Mechanisms underlying nanotoxicity*

NMs exert adverse effects such as mutagenicity and carcinogenicity, and these effects are organ specific (e.g., skin, kidney, brain, lung, endocrine system, and immune system) *in vitro* and *in vivo*. Two specific characteristics of NMs are involved: (1) transportation of NMs and the processes of phagocytosis and endocytosis (Beyersmann and Hartwig, 2008; Park et al., 2010), and (2) surface area per unit mass or volume (Oberdörster et al., 2000). Mechanisms underlying nanotoxicity are not fully elucidated, but some of them include free radical generation, inflammation, and mitochondrial perturbation and cell cycle arrest as described further.

### *Free radical generation*

Although the toxic mechanisms attributed to NPs are not clearly understood, it has been proposed that the formation of ROS or free radicals may be associated with nanotoxicity types, including mutagenicity and carcinogenicity (Pacurari et al., 2010). NMs, such as $C_{60}$ fullerenes, CNTs, $TiO_2$, and AgNPs have been reported to produce ROS *in vitro* and *in vivo* (Shvedova et al., 2003; Oberdörster et al., 2005). Free radicals, such as hydroxyl radicals or superoxide anions generated by NPs, attack biomolecules (e.g., lipids, proteins, DNA), produce oxidative damage products (e.g., MDA, carbonyl contents, 8-OHdG), and deplete antioxidant proteins.

ROS generation by NPs has several possible sources: (1) directly from the surfaces of NPs, (2) from Fenton reaction and Fenton-like catalysis associated with metals like Fe, Cu and Ag, and Haber–Weiss cycle reaction, (3) from homeostasis disruption due to effects on respiratory cellular organelles and mitochondria, and (4) due to activations of ROS generating cells, macrophages, and neutrophils (Krug and Wick, 2011). ZnO NPs used in food packaging materials generate ROS to damage the cell wall and cause bacterial death or inhibition of foodborne pathogens (Sirelkhatim et al., 2015).

## Inflammation

NPs with a positive charge may induce inflammation, which is one of the critical responses to NP exposure, leading to the induction of cytokines, interleukins (IL-8, IL-6, IL-2), and TNF-α (Nel et al., 2006). ROS generation may also disturb the immune systems in cells, and oxidative stress or damage produced by the free radicals leads to inflammation, mutations, and cancer. In human lung cells, nano-$SiO_2$ induces inflammation, generating ROS and apoptosis (McCarthy et al., 2012). Oxidative DNA damage, inflammation, and apoptosis were also observed in the lungs of mice treated with $TiO_2$ NPs (Li et al., 2017). Inflammatory responses have been observed in many other toxicity studies of NPs (Shvedova et al., 2003; Murray et al., 2009; Trickler et al., 2010; Song et al., 2016).

### Mitochondrial perturbation and cell cycle arrest

In Ag-NP-induced cytotoxicity and genotoxicity, perturbation of the mitochondrial respiratory chain has led to production of ROS, interruption of ATP synthesis, and production of DNA damage (Asharani et al., 2009b). Subsequently, mitochondrial damage has produced cellular membrane damage, permeability transition pores, interference with energy transfer, and apoptosis and cytotoxicity.

Further, interactions between Ag-NPs and DNA may result in cell cycle arrest in the G(2)/M phase by PKCζ downregulation (Lee et al., 2011). In another *in vitro* study, Ag-NP induced apoptosis was found to be possibly mediated by the mitochondria-dependent jun-N terminal kinase pathway and ROS (Hsin et al., 2008).

## References

Ahamed M, Karns M, Goodson M et al. (2008). DNA damage response to different surface chemistry of silver nanoparticles in mammalian cells. *Toxicol Appl Pharmacol.* 233, 404–10.

Armstead AL, Li B (2011). Nanomedicine as an emerging approach against intracellular pathogens. *Int J Nanomedicine*. 6, 3281–93.

Asakura M, Sasaki T, Sugiyama T et al. (2010). Genotoxicity and cytotoxicity of multi-wall carbon nanotubes in cultured Chinese hamster lung cells in comparison with chrysotile A fibers. *J Occup Health*. 52(3), 155–66.

Asharani PV, Hande MP, Valiyaveettil S (2009a). Anti-proliferative activity of silver nanoparticles. *BMC Cell Biol*. 10, 65.

Asharani PV, Low Kah Mun G, Hande MP et al. (2009b). Cytotoxicity and genotoxicity of silver nanoparticles in human cells. *ACS Nano*. 3, 279–90.

Auffan M, Rose J, Bottero JY et al. (2009). Towards a definition of inorganic nanoparticles from an environmental, health and safety perspective. *Nat Nanotechnol*. 4, 634–41.

Beyersmann D, Hartwig A (2008). Carcinogenic metal compounds: Recent insight into molecular and cellular mechanisms. *Arch Toxicol*. 82, 493–512.

Bourdon JA, Saber AT, Jacobsen NR et al. (2012). Carbon black nanoparticle instillation induces sustained inflammation and genotoxicity in mouse lung and liver. *Part Fibre Toxicol*. 9, 5.

Buffat P, Borel JP (1976). Size effect on the melting temperature of gold particles. *Physical Rev A*. 13, 2287.

Carrero-Sanchez JC, Elias AL, Mancilla R et al. (2006). Biocompatibility and toxicological studies of carbon nanotubes doped with nitrogen. *Nano Lett*. 6, 1609–16.

Chang C (2010). The immune effects of naturally occurring and synthetic nanoparticles. *J Autoimmun*. 34, J234–46.

Chen EY, Wang YC, Chen CS et al. (2010). Functionalized positive nanoparticles reduce mucin swelling and dispersion. *PLoS One*. 5, e15434.

Choi HS, Frangioni JV (2010). Nanoparticles for biomedical imaging: Fundamentals of clinical translation. *Mol Imaging*. 9, 291–310.

CORDIS (Community Research and Development Information System) (2016). Available from: http://cordis.europa.eu/result/rcn/56552_en.html.

Di Gioacchino M, Petrarca C, Lazzarin F et al. (2011). Immunotoxicity of nanoparticles. *Int J Immunopathol Pharmacol*. 24(1 Suppl), 65S–71S.

Donaldson K, Poland CA (2009). Nanotoxicology: New insights into nanotubes. *Nature Nanotechnol*. 4, 708–10.

Gill HS, Grammatopoulos G, Adshead S et al. (2012). Molecular and immune toxicity of CoCr nanoparticles in MoM hip arthroplasty. *Trends Mol Med*. 18, 145–55.

Heinrich U, Fuhst R, Rittinghausen S et al. (1995). Chronic inhalation exposure of Wistar rats and two different strains of mice to diesel engine exhaust, carbon black, and titanium dioxide. *Inhal Toxicol*. 7, 533–56.

Helland A, Wick P, Koehler A et al. (2007). Reviewing the environmental and human health knowledge base of carbon nanotubes. *Environ Health Perspect*. 115, 1125–31.

Hoet PH, Bruske-Hohlfeld I, Salata OV (2004). Nanoparticles–Known and unknown health risks. *J Nanobiotechnol*. 2, 12.

Hsin YH, Chen CF, Huang S et al. (2008). The apoptotic effect of nanosilver is mediated by a ROS- and JNK-dependent mechanism involving the mitochondrial pathway in NIH3T3 cells. *Toxicol Lett*. 179, 130–9.

Hu SH, Gao X (2010). Nanocomposites with spatially separated functionalities for combined imaging and magnetolytic therapy. *J Am Chem Soc.* 132, 7234–7.

IARC (International Agency for Research on Cancer) (2012). IARC Monographs on the Evaluation of Carcinogenic Risks to Humans. Available from: http://monographs.iarc.fr/.

ISO (International Organization for Standardization) (2008). Nanotechnologies-Terminology and definitions for nanoobjects—Nanoparticle, nanofiber and nanoplate. ISO/TS 27687:2008.

Johnston HJ, Hutchison GR, Christensen FM et al. (2010). The biological mechanisms and physicochemical characteristics responsible for driving fullerene toxicity. *Toxicol Sci.* 114, 162–82.

Kawata K, Osawa M, Okabe S (2009). In vitro toxicity of silver nanoparticles at noncytotoxic doses to HepG2 human hepatoma cells. *Environ Sci Technol.* 43, 6046–51.

Keller AA, McFerran S, Lazareva A et al. (2013). Global life cycle releases of engineered nanomaterials. *J Nanopart Res.* 15, 1692.

Kleinman MT, Araujo JA, Nel A et al. (2008). Inhaled ultrafine particulate matter affects CNS inflammatory processes and may act via MAP kinase signaling pathways. *Toxicol Lett.* 178, 127–30.

Krug HF, Wick P (2011). Nanotoxicology: An interdisciplinary challenge. *Angew Chem Int Ed Engl.* 50, 1260–78.

Lee YS, Kim DW, Lee YH et al. (2011). Silver nanoparticles induce apoptosis and G2/M arrest via PKCζ-dependent signaling in A549 lung cells. *Arch Toxicol.* 85, 1529–40.

Li C, Taneda S, Taya K et al. (2009). Effects of in utero exposure to nanoparticle-rich diesel exhaust on testicular function in immature male rats. *Toxicol Lett.* 185, 1–8.

Li JJ, Muralikrishnan S, Ng CT et al. (2010). Nanoparticle-induced pulmonary toxicity. *Exp Biol Med (Maywood).* 235, 1025–33.

Li Y, Yan J, Ding W, Chen Y, Pack LM, Chen T (2017). Genotoxicity and gene expression analyses of liver and lung tissues of mice treated with titanium dioxide nanoparticles. *Mutagenesis.* 32(1), 33–46.

McCarthy J, Inkielewicz-Stepniak I, Corbalan JJ et al. (2012). Mechanisms of toxicity of amorphous silica nanoparticles on human lung submucosal cells in vitro: Protective effects of fisetin. *Chem Res Toxicol.* 25, 2227–35.

Mizushima N, Komatsu M (2011). Autophagy: Renovation of cells and tissues. *Cell.* 147, 728–41.

Murray AR, Kisin E, Leonard SS et al. (2009). Oxidative stress and inflammatory response in dermal toxicity of single-walled carbon nanotubes. *Toxicology.* 257, 161–71.

Nel A, Xia T, Madler L et al. (2006). Toxic potential of materials at the nanolevel. *Science.* 311, 622–7.

Oberdörster G, Finkelstein JN, Johnston C et al. (2000). Acute pulmonary effects of ultra-fine particles in rats and mice. *Res Rep Health Eff Inst.* 96, 5–74.

Oberdörster G, Oberdörster E, Oberdörster J (2005). Nanotoxicology: An emerging discipline evolving from studies of ultrafine particles. *Environ Health Perspect.* 113, 823–39.

Pacurari M, Castranova V, Vallyathan V (2010). Single-and multiwalled carbon nano-tubes versus asbestos: Are the carbon nanotubes a new risk to humans? *J Toxicol Environ health A.* 73, 378–95.

Panacek A, Kvítek L, Prucek R et al. (2006). Silver colloid nanoparticles: Synthesis, characterization, and their antibacterial activity. *J Phys Chem B*. 110, 16248–53.
Park EJ, Yi J, Kim Y et al. (2010). Silver nanoparticles induce cytotoxicity by a trojanhorse type mechanism. *Toxicol In Vitro*. 24, 872–8.
Poland CA, Duffin R, Kinloch I et al. (2008). Carbon nano-tubes introduced into the abdominal cavity of mice show asbestos-like pathogenicity in a pilot study. *Nat Nanotechnol*. 3, 423–8.
Pope CA, Burnett RT, Thurston GD et al. (2004). Cardiovascular mortality and long-term exposure to particulate air pollution: Epidemiological evidence of general pathophysiological pathways of disease. *Circulation*. 109, 71–7.
Pott F, Roller M (2005). Carcinogenicity study with nineteen granular dusts in rats. *Eur J Oncol*. 10, 249.
Ramdhan DH, Ito Y, Yanagiba Y et al. (2009). Nanoparticle-rich diesel exhaust may disrupt testosterone biosynthesis and metabolism via growth hormone. *Toxicol Lett*. 191, 103–8.
Refuerzo JS, Godin B, Bishop K et al. (2011). Size of the nanovectors determines the transplacental passage in pregnancy: Study in rats. *Am J Obstet Gynecol*. 204, 546.e5–546.e9.
Sayes CM, Liang F, Hudson JL et al. (2006). Functionalization density dependence of single-walled carbon nanotubes cytotoxicity in vitro. *Toxicol Lett*. 161, 135–42.
SCENIHR (2010). Scientific committee on emerging and newly identified health risks. Scientific basis for the definition of the term "nanomaterial". Available from: http://ec.europa.eu/health/scientific_committees/emerging/docs/scenihr_o_032.pdf.
Shinohara N, Matsumoto K, Endoh S et al. (2009). In vitro and in vivo genotoxicity tests on fullerene C60 nanoparticles. *Toxicol Lett*. 191, 289–96.
Shvedova AA, Castranova V, Kisin ER et al. (2003). Exposure to carbon nanotubes material: Assessment of nanotube cytotoxicity using human keratinocyte cells. *J Toxicol Environ Health A*. 66, 1909–26.
Sirelkhatim A, Mahmud S, Seeni A et al. (2015). Review on zinc oxide nanoparticles: Antibacterial activity and toxicity mechanism. *Nano-Micro Lett*. 7, 219.
Song B, Zhang Y et al. (2016). Unraveling the neurotoxicity of titanium dioxide nanoparticles: Focusing on molecular mechanisms. *Beilstein J Nanotechnol*. 7, 645–54.
Stoccoro A, Karlsson HL et al. (2013). Epigenetic effects of nano-sized materials. *Toxicology*. 313, 3–14.
Takagi A, Hirose A, Nishimura T et al. (2008). Induction of mesothelioma in p53+/- mouse by intraperitoneal application of multi-wall carbon nanotube. *J Toxicol Sci*. 33, 105–16.
Taylor DA (2002). Dust in the wind. *Environ Health Perspect*. 110, A80–7.
Totsuka Y, Higuchi T, Imai T et al. (2009). Genotoxicity of nano/microparticles in in vitro micronuclei, in vivo comet and mutation assay systems. *Part Fibre Toxicol*. 6, 23.
Trickler WJ, Lantz SM, Murdock RC et al. (2010). Silver nanoparticle induced blood-brain barrier inflammation and increased permeability in primary rat brain microvessel endothelial cells. *Toxicol Sci*. 118,160–70.
Vance ME, Kuiken T, Vejerano EP et al. (2015). Nanotechnology in the real world: Redeveloping the nanomaterial consumer products inventory. *Beilstein J Nanotechnol*. 6, 1769–80.

Wang J, Zhu X, Zhang X et al. (2011). Disruption of zebrafish (Danio rerio) reproduction upon chronic exposure to $TiO_2$ nanoparticles. *Chemosphere*. 83, 461–7.
Warheit DB, Laurence BR, Reed KL et al. (2004). Comparative pulmonary toxicity assessment of single-wall carbon nanotubes in rats. *Toxicol Sci*. 77, 117–25.
Wick P, Malek A, Manser P et al. (2011). Barrier capacity of human placenta for nanosized materials. *Environ Health Perspect*. 118, 432.
Wiesenthal A, Hunter L, Wang S et al. (2011). Nanoparticles: Small and mighty. *Int J Dermatol*. 50, 247–54.
Win-Shwe TT, Fujimaki H (2011). Nanoparticles and neurotoxicity. *Int J Mol Sci*. 12, 6267–80.
Wu J, Liu W, Xue C et al. (2009). Toxicity and penetration of $TiO_2$ nanoparticles in hairless mice and porcine skin after subchronic dermal exposure. *Toxicol Lett*. 191, 1–8.
Zhao J, Castranova V (2011). Toxicology of nanomaterials used in medicine. *J Toxicol Environ Health B*. 14, 593–632.
Zolnik BS, González-Fernández A, Sadrieh N et al. (2010). Nanoparticles and the immune system. *Endocrinology*. 151, 458–65.

# chapter twenty-five

# Toxicity of metals

***Gi-Wook Hwang***

Contents

# *Introduction*

Metals are a unique class of toxicants that occur naturally and persist in nature, but their chemical forms may be changed because of physicochemical, biological, or anthropogenic activities. Their toxicity may be markedly altered as these elements assume different chemical forms. Most metals are of value to humans because of their varied use in industry, agriculture, or medicine. Some are essential elements, required in various biochemical/physiological functions. On the other hand, others may pose health hazards to the public because of their presence in food, water, or air, and to workers engaged in mining, smelting, and a variety of industrial activities.

## *Occurrence*

Most of the metals and "metalloids" occur in nature, dispersed in rocks, ores, soil, water, and air. However, their distribution is grossly uneven. In general, levels of metal sources are relatively low in soil, water, and air. These levels may be increased by geological activities such as degassing that releases, for example, 25,000 to 125,000 tons of mercury (Hg) annually. Anthropogenic activities such as mining of mercury contribute about 10,000 tons a year. It is noteworthy that anthropogenic activities may be more significant in relation to human exposure because they increase the levels of the metals at the site of the human activities.

## *Uses and human exposure*

In ancient times, certain metals such as copper (Cu), iron (Fe), and tin (Sn) were used to make utensils, machinery, and weapons. Mining and smelting were undertaken to supply such demands and these activities increased their environmental levels. In addition, as the ores often contain other metals, such as lead (Pb) and arsenic (As), the levels of these "contaminants" were also elevated.

In later years, a greater variety of metals have found uses in industry, agriculture, and medicine. For example, mercury is used extensively in the chloralkali industry as the cathode in the electrolysis of salt in water to produce chlorine and sodium hydroxide, both of which are important raw materials in the chemical industry. Lead is used in storage batteries and the cable industry. However, the use of various lead compounds as insecticides, fuel additives, and pigments in paints has gradually been discontinued. More recently, the aerospace industry and medico-dental profession require materials that have strength, resistance to corrosion, and nonirritant properties. Alloys of titanium (Ti) and other metals are becoming even more important.

These human activities have increased the extent of exposure not only to occupational workers but also to consumers of these products. In addition, the toxicity of a metal may be significantly altered by changes in its chemical form. For example, inorganic mercury compounds are toxic primarily to kidney, whereas methylmercury (MeHg) is a CNS toxicant.

## Certain common features

Metals exert a wide range of toxicity. Some, for example, lead and mercury, are very toxic; others are almost nontoxic, such as Ti. Nevertheless, there are a number of toxicological features that are shared to some extent by many metals.

### Site of action

#### Enzyme

A major action of toxic metals is inhibition of enzymes. This action usually occurs as a result of the interaction between the metal and the SH group of the enzyme. An enzyme may also be inhibited by a toxic metal through displacement of an essential metal cofactor of the enzyme. For example, lead may displace zinc (Zn) in the zinc-dependent enzyme, δ-aminolevulinic acid dehydratase (ALAD). Another mechanism by which metals interfere with the functions of enzymes is by blocking their synthesis. For example, nickel (Ni) and platinum (Pt) inhibit the δ-aminolevulinic acid synthetase (ALAS), thereby interfering with synthesis of heme, which is an important component of hemoglobin and cytochrome (Maines and Kappas, 1977). The enzymes may be protected from toxic metals by the administration of "chelating agents," such as dimercaprol or British anti-lewisite (BAL) that form stable bonds with metals.

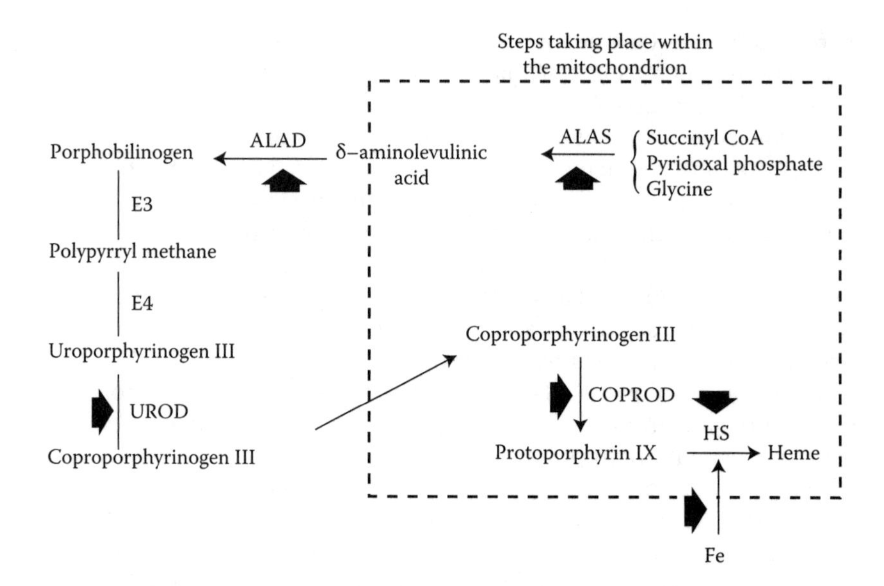


*Figure 25.1* A schematic diagram representing the reactions involved in heme synthesis. Large arrows indicate steps that are inhibited by lead. For further explanation, see the section on lead. *Abbreviations*: ALAD, δ-aminolevulinic acid dehydratase; ALAS, δ-aminolevulinic acid synthetase; COPROD, coproporphyrinogen oxidase; and HS, heme synthetase; UROD, uroporphyrinogen decarboxylase. (From Jaworski JK, National Research Council Canada, 1978.)

Enzymes differ in their susceptibility to metals. Figure 25.1 depicts the synthesis of heme and various enzymes involved, most of which may be inhibited by lead. However, they differ in susceptibility. Inhibition of ALAD occurs at a blood lead level (Bl–Pb) of 10 μg/dl or lower. As a result, δ-aminolevulinic acid will not be processed to become porphobilinogen and thus will be excreted into urine at a Bl–Pb of 40 μg/dl, possibly leading to anemia which occurs at a Bl-Pb level higher than 50 μg/dl (WHO, 1977). However, the lead level at which symptoms appear vary depending upon individual differences.

### *Subcellular organelles*

In general, the adverse effects of metals result from reactions between them and intracellular components. For a metal to exert its toxic effect on a cell, it needs to enter the cell. The entry across the membrane is facilitated if it is lipophilic such as MeHg. When it is bound to a protein, it is absorbed by endocytosis. Passive diffusion is another form of entry of metals such as lead.

After their entry into the cell, metals may affect different organelles. For example, the endoplasmic reticulum contains a variety of enzymes.

These microsomal enzymes are inhibited by many metals, such as cadmium (Cd), cobalt (Co), MeHg, and tin (Sn). Toxic metals also disrupt the structure of the endoplasmic reticulum. The lysosomes are another site of action of metals such as cadmium (as conjugate of metallothionein). Cadmium accumulates in lysosomes of renal proximal tubular cells where this cadmium complex degrades and releases the metal. The cadmium ion inhibits the proteolytic enzymes in the lysosomes and produces cell injury. The mitochondria, because of their high metabolic activity and rapid membrane transport, are also a common target of metals. Metals readily inhibit the respiratory enzymes in these organelles. A number of metals enter the nucleus and may form inclusion bodies. For example, chronic exposure to lead induces inclusion bodies in the nuclei of renal proximal tubular cells. Lead also stimulates DNA, RNA, and protein synthesis. The lead-induced renal adenocarcinoma has been attributed to this mechanism (Goering et al., 1987).

It is therefore evident that the subcellular organelles either enhance or impede the movement of metals across these biological membranes, thereby affecting toxicity. In addition, certain proteins in cytosol, lysosomes, and nuclei may bind with toxic metals such as cadmium, lead, and mercury thereby reducing their availability for adverse effects on sensitive organelles and metabolic sites (Fowler et al., 1984).

## *Factors affecting toxicity*

### *Levels and duration of exposure*

As with other toxicants, the toxic effects of metals are related to the level and duration of exposure. In general, the higher the levels and the longer the duration, the greater are the toxic effects. However, apart from these quantitative differences, changes in the concentrations and duration of exposure may alter the nature of the adverse effects. For example, ingestion of a single, large dose of cadmium induces gastrointestinal tract (GIT) disturbances. Repeated intakes of smaller amounts of cadmium result in renal dysfunction.

### *Chemical form*

A notable example is mercury. Its inorganic compounds are essentially renal toxicants, while MeHg and ethyl mercury compounds are more toxic to the nervous system. The latter type of mercury compound is lipophilic and thus readily crosses the blood–brain barrier. Similarly, tetraethyl lead readily enters the myelin sheath and affects the nervous system. Organic compounds of metals are generally excreted in the bile, while their inorganic compounds are excreted in the urine. Further, the former are biodegradable and the latter are not (Furst, 1987).

### *Metal–protein complexes*

Perhaps as protective mechanisms, various metal–protein complexes are formed in the body. For example, the complexes formed with lead, bismuth, Hg, and Se, are microscopically visible as "inclusion bodies" in the affected cells. Iron may combine with protein to form ferritin, which is water soluble, or hemosiderin, which is not. Cadmium and several other metals (e.g., Zn) combine with metallothionein (MT). MT is low-molecular-weight, cysteine-rich, metal-binding proteins. MT genes are readily induced by various heavy metals, and the metal-regulatory transcription factor-1 (MTF-1) was shown to be essential for basal and heavy metal-induced transcription of MT genes. The induction of MT genes by MTF-1 is mediated by metal response elements (MREs) that are present in multiple copies in the promoter region of these genes (Figure 25.2). For example, the Cd–MT complex is less toxic than $Cd^{2+}$. However, in the renal tubule cells, the Cd–MT complex is degraded by the cysteine protease in lysosomes to release $Cd^{2+}$ and produces toxic effects (Squibb and Fowler, 1984; Min et al., 1992).

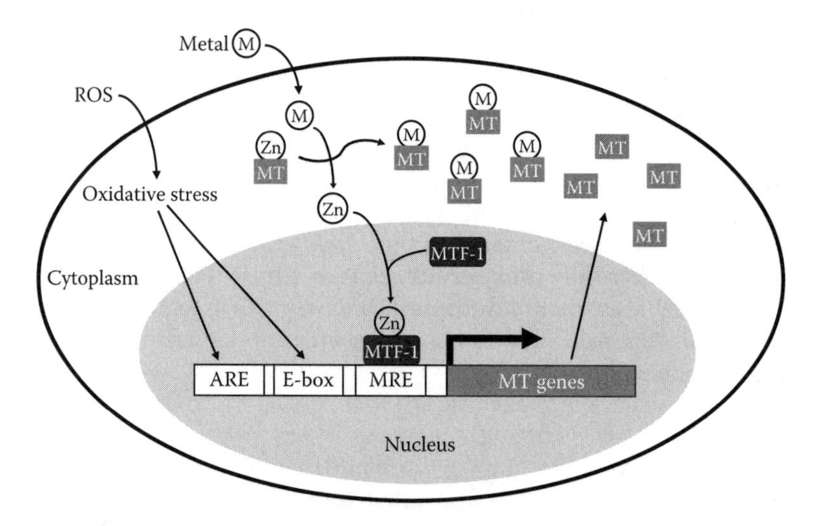


***Figure 25.2*** A model for induction of metallothionein (MT) gene expression by metal. There are many MREs (metal response elements) in the promoter region of MT gene, and the activated MTF-1 by metal induces the MT gene expression through the binding to MRE. Reactive oxygen species (ROS) also induces MT gene expression via the antioxidant response element (ARE) and E-box element (E-box).

#### *Host factors*

As with most other toxicants, young and old animals are in general more susceptible to metals than young adults (Luebke et al., 2006a,b). Young children appear to be especially susceptible to lead because of the generally enhanced sensitivity and greater extent of the GIT absorption. Further, young children have, on a unit body weight basis, a greater intake of food, which is the main source of lead.

Dietary factors such as deficiencies of protein and vitamins C and D enhance the toxicity of lead and cadmium. Certain metals such as lead and mercury cross the placenta, thus affecting the fetus. There is evidence that prenatally exposed children are affected more severely than their mothers: a study found that the median dose that produced ataxia in the mothers was $2.7 \pm 0.18$ mg/kg, whereas that in the prenatally exposed children was $1.23 \pm 0.87$ (Clarkson, 1981). It is worth noting that metals such as lead, cadmium, and mercury bind to albumin and casein, which are subsequently transported to the breast milk and transferred to the lactating infant. The consequences of milk metal exposure remain unknown but accounts for the higher levels seen in these infants (Berlin et al., 2002; Wang and Needham, 2007). As age is a factor in metal-induced toxicity, the lactational component is significant especially for mercury and neuronal effects.

## *Biological indicators/biomarkers*

Exposure to metals can usually be quantitatively assessed. Some of the indicators reveal the extent and approximate time of exposure. Others are early signs of biological effects. The presence and level of the metal in blood and urine are often used as indicators of recent exposure. As the metal compounds are distributed, stored, or excreted, the levels in blood and urine generally diminish.

Many metals are accumulated in hair and nails. Their levels generally bear a relationship with those in blood at the time when the hair and nails are formed. Therefore hair, which grows at a relatively constant rate, has been used to determine the level of past exposures. In the case of black-foot disease, the ingestion of arsenic was correlated with the levels of metal in hair and fingernails and thus reflected a useful biomarker of exposure (Lin et al., 1998). For example, this procedure has been used extensively to ascertain the intake of MeHg among inhabitants in areas where MeHg poisoning was reported. Using different approaches, a fairly reliable conversion factor has been established. Thus, the level of MeHg in hair is about 250 times higher than that in blood, and their relation to the daily intake, after a steady state is reached, is as follows: 0.2 μg/g in blood = 50 μg/g in hair = 3 μg/kg body weight per day (WHO, 1976).

Such biological indicators are also useful in assessing the average blood level of selenium of inhabitants. The level was 3.2 mg/L in areas where there was selenosis and 0.021 mg/L where there was a selenium deficiency syndrome, and in an area where there was neither overexposure nor deficiency, it was 0.095 mg/L (WHO, 1987). Minimal inhibition of ALAD by lead represents a special type of "indicator of exposure" in that this biological effect does not seem to indicate an adverse effect.

## Common toxic effects

### Carcinogenicity

A number of metals were shown to be carcinogenic in humans, animals, or both. As listed in Appendix 8.1, arsenic and its compounds, beryllium (Be), cadmium, certain chromium (Cr) compounds, and Ni and its compounds were categorized as human carcinogens (Group 1) (IARC, 2012). Cisplatin, cobalt metal with tungsten carbide, and lead compounds (inorganic) are probable human carcinogens (Group 2A). Cobalt and cobalt compounds; cobalt metal without tungsten carbide, cobalt sulfate, and other soluble cobalt(II) salts; iron dextran complex; lead; and nickel (metallic and alloys) are possible human carcinogens (Group 2B). Certain other metals may be carcinogenic, but the available information is insufficient to confirm this.

The aforementioned metals, as well as several others, might be carcinogenic through multiple mechanisms of action such as the substitution of $Ni^{2+}$, $Co^{2+}$, or $Cd^{2+}$ for $Zn^{2+}$ in finger loops of transforming proteins (Sunderman and Barber, 1988) and injury to the cytoskeleton by certain metals (Chou, 1989) that affects the fidelity of the polymerase involved in DNA biosynthesis. The carcinogenicity of arsenic involves oxidative stress and induction of the cascade of heat shock proteins (Bernstam and Nriagu, 2000).

### Immune function

Exposure to certain metals may result in the inhibition of immune functions (Sweet and Zelikoff, 2001). Other metals such as beryllium, chromium, nickel, gold, platinum, lead, tributyltin oxide, and zirconium may induce immunotoxicity including hypersensitivity reactions (Lubeke et al., 2006a). The clinical manifestations and mechanism of action of several metals are listed in Table 25.1.

### Nervous system

Because of its susceptibility, the nervous system is a common target for heavy metals. However, even with the same metal, its physicochemical

*Table 25.1* Hypersensitivity reactions to metals

| Metal | Type of reaction[a] | Clinical features | Mechanism of reactions |
|---|---|---|---|
| Platinum, beryllium | I | Asthma, conjunctivitis, urticaria, anaphylaxis | IgE reacts with antigen on mast cell/basophil to release vasoreactive amines |
| Gold, salts of mercury | II | Thrombocytopenia | IgG binds to complement and antigen on cells, resulting in their destruction |
| Mercury vapor, gold | III | Glomerular nephritis, proteinuria | Antigen, antibody, and complement deposit on epithelial surface of glomerular basement |
| Chromium, nickel | IV | Contact dermatitis | Sensitized T cells react with antigen to cause delayed hypersensitivity reaction |
| Beryllium, zirconium | | Granuloma formation | |

[a] For descriptions see the section on "Hypersensitivity and Allergy," Chapter 14.

form often determines the nature of the toxicity. As noted above, metallic mercury vapor and MeHg readily enter the nervous system and induce toxic effects. Inorganic mercury compounds are unlikely to enter the nervous system in significant amounts and thus usually are not neurotoxic. Similarly, the organic compounds of lead are mainly neurotoxic, whereas inorganic lead compounds affect the synthesis of heme first. However, at higher levels of exposure, they may induce encephalopathy. In young children, a moderate level of exposure to these compounds may result in a deficit of mental functions. Other neurotoxic metals include copper, triethyltin, gold, lithium, iron, and manganese. For additional information, see Bondy and Prasad 1988).

## Kidneys

The kidney, as the main excretory organ in the body, is also a common target organ. Cadmium affects the renal proximal tubular cells, producing urinary excretion of small molecule proteins, amino acids, and glucose. In addition, inorganic mercury compounds, lead, chromium, and platinum also induce kidney damage, mainly in the proximal tubules (see Chapter 14).

### Respiratory system

The respiratory system is the primary target organ of most metals following an occupational exposure. There are several types of responses. Many metals induce irritation and inflammation of the respiratory tract; the anatomical structures affected depend upon the metal and the duration of exposure. With acute exposures, hexavalent chromium affects the nasal passage, as the bronchi, and beryllium the lungs. Prolonged exposure may produce fibrosis (Al and Fe), carcinoma (As, Cr, and Ni), or granuloma (Be). The welding fumes or metalloid aerosol may produce various lung diseases including cancer.

## Metals of major toxicological concern

Lead, mercury, arsenic, and cadmium are metals of major health concern because of their impact on large numbers of populations, resulting from environmental pollution, as well as the serious nature of their adverse effects. Several other metals also pose serious toxicological problems.

### Mercury (Hg)

#### General considerations

The elemental form of mercury exists in liquid form at standard conditions of temperature and pressure. It is released from the earth's crust through degassing. It is also present in the environment as inorganic and organic compounds. Elemental mercury may be converted to inorganic compounds by oxidation and revert to elemental mercury by reduction. Inorganic mercury may become organic mercury through the action of certain anaerobic bacteria, and degrade back to inorganic mercury slowly. A variety of anthropogenic activities can raise its levels in the environment. Some of these activities are mining, smelting (to produce metals from their sulfide ores), burning of fossil fuel, and production of steel, cement, and phosphate. Its principal users include the chlor-alkali plants, paper-pulp industry, and electrical equipment manufacturers. Fortunately, these uses have decreased in recent years.

Mercury levels in ambient air are extremely low. The concentrations in water in unpolluted areas are about 0.1 μg/L, but it may reach 80 μg/L near mercury ore deposits. Levels in food, except fish, are low, generally in the range of 5 to 20 μg/kg. Most fish contain higher levels of mercury; the levels in tuna and swordfish usually range from 200 to 1000 μg/kg. In this manner, predators that are larger and located near the top of the food chain have higher quantities of mercury.

*Toxicity*

Because of the massive outbreaks of poisoning from consuming grain treated with mercury fungicide or fish contaminated with MeHg (Appendix 1.2, extensive investigations have been conducted. The populations studied ranged from "normal" subjects to those fatally poisoned. Table 25.2 lists some of these population groups. The "fishermen" were exposed to higher-than-normal levels but showed no signs of poisoning. Those involved in the Niigata episode were exposed to smaller intakes than those in the Iraq episode, and hence the latency in Niigata was generally 2 to 3 years, whereas in Iraq the latency was 2 to 3 months.

These studies revealed that adverse effects are related to the nervous system, which is extremely sensitive to this toxicant and readily susceptible. Paresthesia is usually the earliest symptom. Constricted visual field is pathognomonic. At higher levels of exposure ataxia, dysarthria, deafness, and eventually death occur. Figure 25.3 shows graphically the concentration–response and dose–effect relationships. Pathologically, the major damage is atrophy in the occipital lobe, cerebellar folia, and calcarine cortex. There are also degenerative changes in the axons and myelin sheaths of peripheral nerves.

From these studies it was concluded that MeHg poisoning would be unlikely if the daily intake corresponded to a blood level of 20 μg/dl and a hair level of 50 μg/g (WHO, 1976). Other studies indicated that fetal brain is more susceptible to MeHg than that of adults. This difference is due to the ease of transport across the placenta, preferential uptake by fetal brain, and inhibitory action on cell division and cell migration, both of which are essential for the normal development of the fetal brain (Clarkson, 1991).

*Elemental* mercury *vapor*, for the most part, constitutes a hazard in occupational settings only. Its target organ is also the CNS. The usual symptoms are tremors and mental disturbances. Among workers exposed to mercury vapor the triad of excitability, tremors, and gingivitis are well known (Goldwater, 1972). After continual exposure to a time-weighted

***Table* 25.2** Daily intake of methylmercury by certain populations

| | Daily intake (g) | |
|---|---|---|
| Population | Average | Range |
| "Normal" | – | 1–20 |
| Fisherman | 300 | Up to 1000 |
| Niigata | 1500 | 250–5000 |
| Iraq | 4500 | Up to 12,000 |

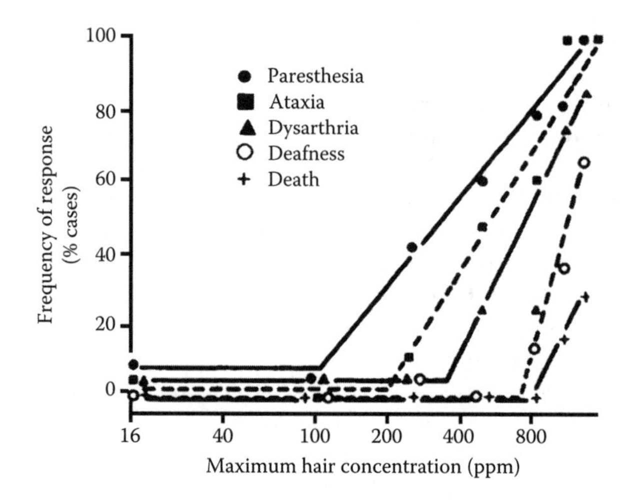


***Figure 25.3*** The frequency of signs and symptoms of methylmercury poisoning in adult victims in Iraq. Plotted according to the estimated maximum hair concentration. Hair samples are not available for all patients and are estimated based on the patient's history of exposure, observed blood levels, blood half-times, and a hair-to-blood concentration ratio of 250 to 1. (From Clarkson, TW, *Environ Health Perspect.*, 75, 59–64, 1987.)

air concentration of 0.05 mg Hg/m$^3$, sensitive workers may exhibit nonspecific (neurasthenic) symptoms, and at a concentration of 0.1–0.2 mg/m$^3$ may display tremors (WHO, 1976).

*Inorganic* mercury *salts* are either monovalent or divalent. The divalent mercuric chloride ($HgCl_2$), the "corrosive sublimate," is corrosive on contact. After ingestion, this metal produces abdominal cramps and bloody diarrhea, with corrosive ulceration, bleeding, and necrosis of the GIT. These effects are followed by renal damage, mainly necrosis and sloughing off of the proximal tubular cells, thereby blocking the tubules and producing oliguria, anuria, and uremia. It may also damage the glomerulus, possibly as a result of a disturbed immune function. The monovalent salt calomel, the mercurous chloride ($Hg_2Cl_2$), is less corrosive and less toxic. However, $Hg_2Cl_2$ may produce the "pink disease," characterized by *dermal* vasodilation, hyperkeratosis, and hypersecretion of the sweat glands. This effect is probably a hypersensitivity reaction, since it is not dose related. Exposure to mercury results in increased susceptibility to infections as evidenced by immunosuppression, and enhanced allergic responses and autoimmune disease as demonstrated by immunostimulation (Sweet and Zelikoff, 2001). Mercury exposure was associated with infertility as attested by luteal insufficiency and menstrual irregularities (Gerhard et al., 1998).

## *Lead (Pb)*

### *General considerations*

Lead is more ubiquitous than most other toxic metals. The environmental levels have been increasing because of lead mining, smelting, refining, and various industrial uses. Generally, lead levels in soil range from 5 to 25 mg/kg; from 1 to 60 μg/L in ground water; somewhat less in natural surface water; and under 1 μg/$m^3$ in air, but may be higher in certain workplaces and areas with heavy motor traffic.

The major industrial uses, such as fuel additives and lead pigments in paints, which contributed greatly to lead levels in the environment, have been gradually phased out. However, its uses in storage batteries and cables have not been significantly reduced. Drinking water may be appreciably contaminated by lead through the use of lead and PVC pipes. Glazed ceramic foodware is another source of lead, as noted in Chapter 20. For most people, the major source of lead intake is food, which contributes generally 100–300 μg/day.

Infants and young children are likely exposed to a greater extent than adults, because of their habit of licking, chewing, or eating foreign objects, such as soil and flakes of old paints from the wall. As the immune system is immature in children, lead produces greater immunotoxic effects in them (Luebke et al., 2006a,b), as manifested by a higher incidence of infections and asthma. In addition, prenatal exposure to lead could be a risk factor to increase blood pressure in females (Zhang et al., 2011).

### *Toxicity*

The *hematopoietic system* is extremely sensitive to the effect of lead. The main component of hemoglobin is heme, which is synthesized from glycine and succinyl coenzyme A, with pyridoxal phosphate as cofactor. After a number of steps, it finally combines with iron to form heme. The initial and final steps take place in the mitochondria, with intermediate steps in the cytoplasm, as shown in Figure 25.1. Among the seven enzymes involved in these steps, five are susceptible for inhibitory effect of lead. ALAD and heme synthetase are the most susceptible, whereas ALAS, uroporphyrinogen decarboxylase, and coproporphyrinogen oxidase are less sensitive to inhibition by lead. Only two of them are not affected, namely, porphobilinogen deaminase and uroporphyrinogen cosynthetase.

Within blood, most of the lead is present in the erythrocytes, leaving only a fraction of less than 1% in the plasma. While clinical anemia is evident only when there is moderate exposure to lead, with a blood level around 50 μg/dl, a number of other effects may be detected at lower levels of exposure. For example, ALAD inhibition becomes perceptible at a Bl–Pb level just over 10 μg/dl and free erythrocyte porphyrins (FEPs) at

20–25 μg/dl. ALAD inhibition, and possibly FEP, may be considered as an indicator of exposure rather than an indicator of toxicity. TI impaired heme synthesis may result in anemia that is hypochromatic and microcytic. The anemia may be due partly to the greater fragility of the erythrocyte membrane (WHO, 1977).

The nervous system is also one of the main targets for lead. After high levels of exposure, with a Bl–Pb level over 80 μg/dl, encephalopathy may occur. There is damage to arterioles and capillaries, resulting in cerebral edema, increased cerebrospinal fluid pressure, neuronal degeneration, and glial proliferation. Clinically, this condition is associated with ataxia, stupor, coma, and convulsions. In children, this clinical syndrome may occur with a Bl–Pb level of 70 μg/dl. At lower levels (40–50 μg/dl), children may exhibit hyperactivity, a decreased attention span, and a lowering of IQ scores (Ernhardt et al., 1981; Schnaas et al., 2006). These subtle manifestations may be a result of impairment of the function of neurotransmitters and calcium ion (Rice and Silbergeld, 1996). Hence, lead perturbs intracellular calcium cycling, altering release ability of organelle stores, such as endoplasmic reticulum and mitochondria. Peripheral neuropathy is characterized by a wrist and foot drop, signs of damage to the motor nerves. Lead produces degeneration of Schwann cells followed by demyelination and possibly axonal degeneration. This syndrome occurs mainly among occupational workers.

Lead generally affects the kidney insidiously, resulting in chronic renal failure after long-term exposure. The proximal tubule is the main target. An early sign of lead toxicity on the kidney is the excretion of the lysosomal enzyme *N*-acetyl-β-D-glucosaminidase (Verschoor et al., 1987). One characteristic of lead poisoning is the presence of lead "inclusion bodies" in the nucleus of tubular cells, which consist of fibrillary lead–protein complexes. In the skeletal system, lead produces osteoporosis and osteomalacia because bones are not only a target organ but also a storage depot for this metal.

#### *Other effects*

The carcinogenicity of lead has been demonstrated in kidneys of rodents, but there is little human data in this respect (IARC, 1980). Lead also adversely affects reproductive functions, mainly through gametotoxicity in both male and female animals, resulting in low sperm counts, decreased sperm motility, sterility, abortion, and neonatal deaths. Young children are likely to be exposed to higher levels of lead, as noted above, and their immature immune system makes them more prone to infections. Further, infants and unborn fetuses are also more sensitive to the toxicity of this metal. Organic lead compounds such as tetraethyl lead and tetramethyl lead are readily absorbed after inhalation and dermal exposures, and rapidly enter the CNS with ensuing encephalopathy. This hazard concerns essentially occupational workers, but not the general public, because the small amounts emitted from automobile exhaust readily degrade.

## *Cadmium (Cd)*

### *General considerations*

Cadmium occurs in nature mainly in lead and zinc ores, and is thus released near mines and smelters of these metals. Cadmium is used as a pigment (such as in ceramics), in electroplating, and making alloys and alkali storage batteries. Cadmium levels in the air are usually in the range of ng/m$^3$, but may amount to several mg/m$^3$ in certain workplaces. The level in water is low (around 1 µg/L) except in contaminated areas. Most foods contain trace amounts of cadmium. Grains and cereal products usually constitute the main source of cadmium. Although meat, poultry, and fish have relatively low levels of cadmium, liver, kidneys, and shellfish have higher levels. The environmental levels are raised by smelting and industrial uses. An additional source is the use of sludge as a food crop fertilizer. Apart from these environmental sources, humans may be exposed to cadmium through cigarette smoking: a pack a day may double the metal intake. Extensively decorated and improperly fired ceramic foodware is another source of cadmium (see Chapter 22). Occupational exposure occurs mainly in smelters.

### *Toxicity*

The acute effects of cadmium exposure result mainly from local irritation. After ingestion, the clinical manifestations are nausea, vomiting, and abdominal pain; after inhalation, the lesions include pulmonary edema and chemical pneumonitis.

Cadmium is excreted slowly with a half-life of about 15–30 years. After chronic exposure, kidney lesions predominate. The primary site of action is the proximal tubules. Damage to these tubules generally occurs when the cadmium level in the kidney reaches 200 µg/g, the "critical concentration." This tubular damage results in their inability to reabsorb small-molecular proteins, the major one of which is $\beta_2$-microglobulin. Other proteins include retinol-binding protein, lysozyme, ribonuclease, and immunoglobulin light chains (Lauwerys et al., 1979). Similarly, aminoaciduria is another result of damage to tubular cells that normally reabsorb the amino acids filtered through the glomeruli. Other related effects are glycosuria and decreased tubular reabsorption of phosphate.

At later stages, there may be hypercalcinuria, which, probably in conjunction with altered bone metabolism, may lead to osteomalacia. However, the association between cadmium and *itai-itai* disease (characterized by chronic renal disease and bone deformity) reported in Toyama, Japan, where the metal levels in rice were high (see Appendix 1.2), has not been firmly established (Nomiyama, 1980).

Effects on the respiratory system result from inhalation exposure. Chronic bronchitis, progressive fibrosis of the lower airway, and rupture of septa between alveoli lead to emphysema. Cadmium exposure was implicated in the exacerbation of pulmonary disorders associated with cigarette smoking (Mannino et al., 2004).

Other effects include hypertension, which may be the result of sodium retention, vasoconstriction, and hyperreninemia. Carcinoma of the prostate has been reported among occupational workers (Kipling and Waterhause, 1967). Cadmium inhibits *N*-acetyltransferase 1 and 2 (NAT1, NAT2), phase II-metabolizing enzymes that play an important role in the metabolism of carcinogenic aromatic amines (Joseph, 2009; Ragunathan et al., 2010). Cadmium also binds to a cysteine-rich metalloprotein, metallothionein (MT)-1 or MT-2, which protect against cadmium-induced toxicities including nephrotoxicity, immunotoxicity, and osteotoxicity (Klaassen et al., 2009).

## Other metals

### Arsenic (As)

Although arsenic is a ubiquitous metalloid, its levels in water and ambient air are generally low. The major source of human exposure is food, which contains somewhat less than 1 mg/kg. However, its level in seafood may reach 5 mg/kg. In certain parts of Taiwan, South America, and Bangladesh, the water perhaps contains hundreds of milligrams of As/L. In these areas, inhabitants may suffer from dermal hyperkeratosis and hyperpigmentation. A more serious condition is gangrene of "lower extremities," called "black foot disease," resulting from peripheral endarteritis (Lin et al., 1998; Chowdhury et al., 2000).

Cancer of the skin and liver is also observed in those areas, as well as among patients who were taking Fowler's solution ($KAsO_2$) as a therapy for leukemia (Bernstam and Nriagu, 2000). Cancer of the lung may occur among workers exposed to arsenic in copper smelters and plants that manufacture arsenic-containing pesticides (Pinto et al., 1978; Enterline et al., 1987; Viren and Silvers, 1994). Evidence is limited for carcinogenesis by arsenic in experimental animal studies, but was found to produce developmental toxicity as evidenced by malformations, growth retardation, and death (Golub et al., 1998). Further, mutagenesis tests have been essentially negative. The mechanism underlying arsenic-mediated carcinogenesis might be associated with epigenetic changes such as modifications of DNA and histone methylation (Marsit et al., 2006; Zhou et al., 2008).

Other effects include toxicity to liver parenchyma, resulting clinically in jaundice in early stages and in cirrhosis and ascites, and carcinoma later. Acutely, large doses of arsenic compounds induce GIT damage with vomiting and bloody diarrhea, muscular cramps, and cardiac abnormality (WHO, 1981). Exposure to excessive amounts of arsenic may interfere with heme formation as evidenced by the increased urinary excretion of porphyrins (Xie et al., 2001).

*Beryllium (Be)*

Beryllium is released into the environment mainly through combustion of fossil fuel and is used in ceramic plants and in making alloys. Beryllium and its alloys have a number of applications in nuclear, space, and other industries. The general population is exposed to beryllium primarily in food and drinking water, with smaller contributions from air and incidental ingestion of dust.

There are no human studies that address the toxicological kinetics of beryllium; however, it has been found in the lungs and urine of non-occupationally exposed individuals. The lung is the primary target of inhalation exposure to beryllium in animals and humans. The major toxic effect is berylliosis, resulting from long-term inhalation exposures. This disease of the lungs is characterized by granulomas, which in time become fibrotic tissues. These lesions reduce the number of alveoli and consequently pulmonary functions.

After dermal contact, beryllium produces hypersensitivity reactions of the skin. The reaction is cell mediated, and therefore delayed (type IV allergy). The soluble compounds of beryllium induce papulovesicular lesions, whereas the insoluble compounds induce granulomatous lesions. Beryllium was shown to be carcinogenic to several species of animals (Kuschner, 1981). Epidemiological data suggest that beryllium is a human carcinogen (IARC, 1994).

*Chromium (Cr)*

Chromium occurs in ores. Mining, smelting, and industrial uses tend to increase its environmental levels. It is used in making stainless steel, various alloys, and pigments. Fossil fuel-powered plants and cement-producing plants are also sources of environmental pollution. However, its levels in air, water, and food are generally low. The major human exposure is occupational.

The toxicity of chromium depends on the oxidation state, hexavalent form $Cr^{6+}$ being more toxic than trivalent form $Cr^{3+}$. $Cr^{3+}$ present in the normal diet is adsorbed by the GIT, while $Cr^{6+}$ is more readily absorbed by both inhalation and oral routes.

Chromium is a human carcinogen, inducing lung cancers among workers exposed to it. The carcinogenicity is generally attributed to the hexavalent form $Cr^{6+}$, which is corrosive and water insoluble. It has been suggested that $Cr^{6+}$, which is more readily taken up by cells, converts to $Cr^{3+}$ intracellularly. The trivalent chromium ion, which is more active biologically, binds to nucleic acid and initiates the carcinogenesis process. The mechanisms underlying $Cr^{6+}$ carcinogenicity are associated with both genotoxic (e.g., Cr-DNA-adducts, crosslinks, strand breaks via oxidative stress) (Zhitkovich, 2005; Jomova and Valko, 2011) and epigenetic events (e.g., histone modification) (Sun et al., 2009). It should be noted that there is no clear evidence to correlate occupational chromium exposure with an increased incidence of cancer in the United Kingdom (Rowbotham et al., 2000). It is worth noting that chromium is present in cigarettes and it was postulated that the rise in cancer incidence in chromium workers was due to the smoking component. The $Cr^{6+}$ is corrosive and produces ulceration of the nasal passages and skin. It also induces hypersensitivity reactions of the skin. Acutely, it induces renal tubular necrosis.

*Nickel (Ni)*

Nickel occurs in ores. Smelting and industrial uses tend to increase its levels in the environment. Its many industrial uses include in the manufacture of storage batteries, electrical contacts and similar devices; electroplating, and as catalysts. It is also emitted from coal gasification.

The absorption of nickel is dependent on its physicochemical form, with water soluble forms being more readily absorbed. The primary target organs for nickel toxicity are the lungs and upper respiratory tract for inhalation exposure and kidneys for oral exposure. Nickel is a human carcinogen among occupational workers. Nasal cancer appears to be the predominant type of neoplasm. Nickel also induces cancer of the lungs, larynx, stomach, and possibly also the kidney. Food and cigarette smoke are the main sources of nickel exposure in the general public. It is one of the most common causative agents of dermal hypersensitivity reactions among the general public. The reactions usually follow contact with nickel-containing metal objects such as coins and jewelry.

## Risk/benefit considerations

The metals discussed in the previous section offer certain benefits because of their industrial and minor medical uses. However, they pose serious toxicological risks either to the population at large or specific occupational workers. On the other hand, there are two groups of metals that are more valuable. One group, the essential metals, is required in certain physiological functions and the other is used for a variety of medical purposes. These three groups of metals are different in their risk/benefit considerations.

## *Toxic metals*

The general population is at risk to these metals mainly through food. Tolerances, or equivalents, are established for various foodstuffs to ensure that the total intake will not exceed the amount that is considered acceptable from a toxicological point of view. However, more targeted action is taken in certain cases. For example, the main source of MeHg is fish. The levels in swordfish range from about 0.5 to 1.2 ppm, and in tuna from 0.2 to 0.5 ppm, whereas those in most other types of fish are 0.1 ppm or lower. The permissible levels for MeHg set by most nations range from 0.4 to 1 ppm. Assuming a daily consumption of fish being 200 g, the intake of MeHg would not exceed 0.2 mg. An intake at this level is considered unlikely to induce MeHg toxicity (WHO, 1976). The safety is provided by the fact that most of the fish samples contain less MeHg than the 1 ppm permitted. The Joint FAO/WHO Expert Committee on Food Additives and Contaminants established a "tolerable intake" of 0.2 mg/week, thus allowing a safety factor of 7, which the Committee considered adequate in this case (WHO, 1972). The rationale was the availability of the exceptionally extensive data obtained from populations exposed to the full gamut of intake levels, ranging from "normal" to questionably poisoned, minimally poisoned, seriously poisoned, and fatally poisoned (Table 25.2), as well as the fact that most of the investigations were thoroughly conducted and properly reported. However, when a pregnant woman is exposed to high concentration of MeHg through seafood intake, it may increase the risk of having a miscarriage, or having a baby with deformities or severe nervous system diseases. Accordingly, the United States issued a national warning in 2001 recommending that pregnant women and infants limit their intake of fish, which was followed by similar warnings from Japan, United Kingdom, Canada, Australia, and Norway. For example, the U.S. EPA and FDA recommend that women who are pregnant or plan to become pregnant within the next 1 or 2 years, as well as young children, avoid eating more than 6 ounces (170 g, one average meal) of fish per week. On the other hand, fish is considered as an important source of nutrients, which should not be discarded for minimal or nonexistent risks. The intake was set on a weekly basis because fish is consumed, in many parts of the world, once a week. Many of the most commonly eaten fish are lower in MeHg. The nutritional value of fish lower in MeHg is especially important during growth and development before birth, in early infancy, and in childhood.

Similarly, targeted action has been taken with respect to cadmium in rice in Japan, where rice is the main source of this contaminant. Permissible levels of release of lead and cadmium from ceramic foodware have been established internationally (WHO, 1979) and in many nations. See also Chapter 22. There are also tolerances set for toxic metals such as arsenic, cadmium, and lead in water and foods for the protection of the consumers' health.

Occupational workers are likely exposed to higher levels of toxic metals in mining, smelting, manufacturing, and similar occupations. The main routes of entry into the body are the skin and respiratory tract. For their protection, threshold limit values of toxicants in air are established. For additional information, see Chapter 26.

### *Essential metals*

Selenium (Se) is a typical element that is toxic at high levels of intake while inducing a deficiency syndrome when the intake is too low. Human overexposure to selenium has been observed in China as well as in few isolated regions in the Americas. The clinical manifestations include hair loss, nail pathology, and tooth decay. In animals overexposure induces more severe ill effects including retarded growth, liver necrosis, enlargement of the spleen and pancreas, anemia, and various disorders of reproductive function.

Deficiency of selenium results in muscular dystrophy in sheep and cattle, exudative diathesis in chicken, and liver necrosis in swine and rats. In rats it may also produce reproductive failures, vascular changes, and cataracts. Selenium is a component of glutathione peroxidase, which is responsible for the destruction of $H_2O_2$ and lipid peroxides. Its function is, therefore, closely related to that of vitamin E, the biological antioxidant. This close relation is reflected in the fact that the minimal intake of selenium in rats is 0.01 mg/kg, but if there is also a vitamin E deficiency, an intake of 0.05 mg/kg will be needed.

It was only in the late 1970s that selenium was recognized as an essential element in humans. In certain regions in China, where selenium levels were low in soil and food, a special type of cardiomyopathy was noted. It was known as *Keshan disease* because it was first observed there. The selenium levels in blood, urine, and hair of the inhabitants were low. As expected, the blood glutathione peroxidase activity was also low. When they were given a sodium selenite supplement, the incidence of this endemic cardiopathy fell sharply. There is also an endemic osteoarthropathy observed in China, known as *Kashin–Beck disease,* and is believed to be due to selenium deficiency; however, the evidence of its etiology is not as strong as that of Keshan disease. Selenium deficiency associated with muscular pain has been reported from New Zealand.

For the general population, selenium exposure is essentially from food, especially cereals. The average daily intake of selenium of inhabitants in areas where there were cases of Keshan disease was about 0.011 mg, whereas in areas where there were cases of selenosis, it was about 5 mg (Yang et al., 1983). It has been estimated that there is about a 100-fold margin between the highest no-toxic effect level and lowest level at which deficiency syndrome is avoided. However, this margin is subject to the influence of various modifying factors. For example, vitamin E deficiency increases toxicity as well as the physiological requirements of selenium, thus effectively reducing the margin. MeHg increases the effect of selenium deficiency, whereas inorganic mercury increases the toxicity of methylated selenium compounds. A hypothetical dose–response (all effects) relationship of selenium is depicted in Figure 4.1 of Chapter 4, which shows that adverse effects are induced when the dose is too low (curve A), whereas other adverse effects are induced when the dose is too high (curve B). Further, because of the great individual variations in susceptibility resulting from host and environmental factors, it is not clear whether there is a dose that can be considered as devoid of deficiency as well as toxic effect on a population basis. Additional details on various aspects of the selenium problem as well as reference citations may be found in a WHO document (WHO, 1987).

Cobalt, copper, and iron are all essential metal elements required in normal development of erythrocytes. Iron is a component of hemoglobin, and copper facilitates the utilization of iron in the synthesis of hemoglobin. Thus a deficiency of either metal results in hypochromatic, microcytic anemia. Cobalt is a component of vitamin $B_{12}$, which is required in the development of erythrocyte. Its deficiency results in pernicious anemia.

Excessive intake of cobalt results in polycythemia, an overproduction of erythrocytes, and cardiomyopathy. Excess copper storage in the body is not a result of overexposure to the metal but rather a genetic disorder (Wilson's disease). Copper accumulates in brain, liver, kidneys, and cornea. Clinical manifestations are thus related to disorders of these organs. Overexposure to iron may result from excessive intake of metal or frequent blood transfusions. The excess iron is deposited as hemosiderin mainly in the liver, causing liver dysfunction. Iron binds to ambient air particles and is believed to be responsible for cardiovascular disturbances and increased morbidity associated with air pollutant exposure. In addition, iron binds to asbestos bodies and is believed to be associated with the observed asbestosis in humans.

Occupational exposure to cobalt induces respiratory irritation and dermal hypersensitivity reactions. Certain iron industry workers have been reported to display pneumoconiosis and an increased lung cancer incidence associated with iron binding to particles and subsequent release. Acute oral poisonings have been noted after consuming improperly canned vegetable juices containing excessive amounts of copper and after taking large doses of iron supplement medications. The clinical manifestations relate mainly to GIT irritations.

Other essential metals include manganese (Mn) and molybdenum (Mo), which are cofactors in a number of enzyme systems such as phosphorylase, xanthine oxidase, and aldehyde oxidase. However, these metals are so plentiful in the human diet that no cases of deficiency syndrome have been reported. These metals have a variety of industrial uses, notably in making high-temperature-resistant steel alloys. Occupational exposure to manganese results in pneumonitis acutely, and encephalopathy chronically. Overexposure to manganese in animals orally induces GIT disturbances followed by fatty degeneration of the liver and kidney.

Zinc is the cofactor in scores of metalloenzymes and is therefore an essential element. Deficiency of zinc thus induces a great variety of effects on the nervous system, hematopoietic system, skin, liver, eye, testis, and so forth. Zinc is readily excreted, and excessive intake by the oral route is thus unlikely to induce toxic effects. Occupational exposure to $Zn_2O_3$ fume leads to *metal fume fever* (Goyer, 1996).

## *Metals used in medicine*

### *Therapeutic agents*

A number of metal compounds have been used in medicine. For example, compounds of mercury have been used as diuretics and vaccines. Because of their toxicity, their uses have been discontinued. Those that are less toxic include compounds of aluminum as antacid, bismuth as astringent, gold for rheumatoid arthritis, lithium for mental depression, platinum complexes as antitumor agents, and thallium as depilatory agents. They may produce toxic effects on the nervous system (e.g., aluminum, bismuth, lithium, and thallium), kidneys (e.g., bismuth, gold, and lithium), skin (e.g., gold and platinum), cardiovascular, and GI systems (e.g., lithium and thallium). Although used as antitumor agents, platinum complexes may induce tumors.

### *Other uses*

Aluminum in hemodialysis for chronic renal failure has resulted in fatal neurological syndrome. The use of barium (Ba) and gallium (Ga) used in conjunction with x-rays, as a radiopaque agent and radioactive tracer has proven to be relatively safe. However, accidental ingestion of soluble barium salts has resulted in serious GIT, muscular, and cardiovascular disturbances. Therapeutic use of radiogallium has resulted in disease conditions related to radioactivity. Of special interest is titanium (Ti) since it is inert and resistant to corrosion, and thus it has been widely used in surgical and dental implants. It is present in trace amounts in a variety of foods of plant origin, and titanium dioxide has been used as a color additive because of its low toxicity.

## References

Berlin CM, Kacew S, Lawrence R et al. (2002). Criteria for chemical selection for programs on human milk surveillance and research for environmental chemicals. *J Toxicol Environ Health A*. 65, 1839–51.

Bernstam L, Nriagu J (2000). Molecular aspects of arsenic stress. *J Toxicol Environ Health B*. 3, 293–322.

Bondy SC, Prasad KN (1988). *Metal Neurotoxicity*. Boca Raton, FL: CRC Press.

Chou IN (1989). Distinct cytoskeletal injuries induced by As, Cd, Co, Cr, and Ni compounds. *Biomed Environ Sci*. 2, 358–65.

Chowdhury UK, Biswas BK, Chowdhury RT (2000). Groundwater arsenic contamination in Bangladesh and West Bengal. *Environ Health Perspect*. 108, 393–7.

Clarkson TW (1981). Dose–response relationships for adult and prenatal exposures to methyl mercury. In: Bery GG, Maillie HD, eds. *Measurements of Risk*. New York: Plenum Press, pp. 111–30.

Clarkson TW (1987). Metal toxicity in the central nervous system. *Environ Health Perspect*. 75, 59–64.

Clarkson TW (1991). Methyl mercury. *Fundam Appl Toxicol*. 16, 20–1.

Enterline PE, Henderson VL, Marsh GM (1987). Exposure to arsenic and respiratory cancer: A reanalysis. *Am J Epidemiol*. 125, 929–38.

Ernhardt CB, Landa B, Schnell NB (1981). Subclinical levels of lead and developmental deficits: A multivariate follow-up reassessment. *Pediatrics*. 67, 911–9.

Fowler BA, Abel J, Elinder CG (1984). Structure, mechanism and toxicity. In: Nriagu J, ed. *Changing Metal Cycles and Human Health*. New York: Springer-Verlag.

Furst A (1987). Relationships of toxicological effects to chemical forms of inorganic compounds. In: Brown SS, Kodama Y, eds. *Toxicology of Metals*. Chichester, UK: Halstead Press.

Gerhard I, Monga B, Waldbrenner A et al. (1998). Heavy metals and infertility. *J Toxicol Environ Health A*. 54, 593–611.

Goering PL, Mistry P, Fowler BA (1987). Mechanism of metal toxicity. In: Haley TJ, Berndt WO, eds. *Handbook of Toxicology*. New York: Hemisphere.

Goldwater LJ (1972). *Mercury: A History of Quicksilver*. Baltimore, MD: York Press.

Golub MS, Macintosh MS, Baumrind N (1998). Developmental and reproductive toxicity of inorganic arsenic: Animal studies and human concerns. *J Toxicol Environ Health B*. 1, 199–241.

Goyer RA (1996). Toxic effects of metals. In: Klaassen CD, ed. *Casarett and Doull's Toxicology*. New York: McGraw-Hill, pp. 691–736.
IARC (1980). Monograph on the Evaluation of the Carcinogenic Risks of Chemicals to Humans. Some Metals and Metallic Compounds, vol. 23. Lyon, France: International Agency for Research on Cancer.
IARC (1994). Monograph on the Evaluation of Risks to Humans. Cadmium, mercury, Benyllium and the Glass Industry, vol. 58. Lyons, France: International Agency for Research on Cancer.
IARC (2012). Monograph on the Evaluation of the Carcinogenic Risks of Chemicals to Humans. Agents Classified by the IARC Monographs, Volumes 1–102. Lyon, France: International Agency for Research on Cancer.
Jaworski JK (1978). *The Effects of Lead in the Canadian Environment*. Ottawa, Canada: National Research Council Canada.
Jomova K, Valko M (2011). Advances in metal-induced oxidative stress and human disease. *Toxicology*. 283, 65–87.
Joseph P (2009). Mechanisms of cadmium carcinogenesis. *Toxicol Appl Pharmacol*. 238, 272–9.
Kipling M, Waterhause J (1967). Cadmium and prostatic carcinoma. *Lancet*. 1, 730–1.
Klaassen CD, Jie L, Bhalchandra DA (2009). Metallothionein protection of cadmium toxicity. *Toxicol Appl Pharmacol*. 238, 215–20.
Kuschner M (1981). The carcinogenicity of beryllium. *Environ Health Perspect*. 40, 101–6.
Lauwerys RR, Roels HA, Poncket JP et al. (1979). Investigations on the lung and kidney function in workers exposed to cadmium. *Environ Health Perspect*. 28, 137–46.
Lin T-H, Huang Y-L, Wang M-Y (1998). Arsenic species in drinking water, hair fingernails and urine of patients with blackfoot disease. *J Toxicol Environ Health A*. 53, 85–93.
Luebke RW, Chen DH, Dietert R et al. (2006a). The comparative immunotoxicity of five selected compounds following developmental or adult exposure. *J Toxicol Environ Health B*. 9, 1–26.
Luebke RW, Chen DH, Dietert R et al. (2006b). Immune system maturity and sensitivity to chemical exposure. *J Toxicol Environ Health A*. 69, 811–25.
Maines MD, Kappas A (1977). Metals as regulators of heme metabolism. *Science*. 198, 1215–21.
Mannino DM, Holguin F, Greves HM et al. (2004). Urinary cadmium levels predict lower lung function in current and former smokers: Data from the Third National Health and Nutrition Examination Survey. *Thorax*. 59, 194–8.
Marsit C, Karagas M, Danaee H et al. (2006). Carcinogen exposure and gene promoter hypermethylation in bladder cancer. *Carcinogenesis*. 27, 112–6.
Min KS, Nakatsubo T, Fujita Y et al. (1992). Degradation of cadmium metallothionein in vitro by lysosomal proteases. *Toxicol Appl Pharmacol*. 113, 299–305.
Nomiyama K (1980). Recent progress and perspectives in cadmium health effects studies. *Sci Total Environ*. 14, 199–232.
Pinto SS, Henderson V, Enterline PE (1978). Mortality experience of arsenic exposed workers. *Arch Environ Health*. 33, 325–31.
Ragunathan N, Dairou J, Sanfins E et al. (2010). Cadmium alters the biotransformation of carcinogenic aromatic amines by arylamine *N*-acetyltransferase xenobiotic-metabolizing enzymes: Molecular, cellular, and in vivo studies. *Environ Health Perspect*. 118, 1685–91.

Rice D, Silbergeld EK (1996). Lead neurotoxicity: Concordance of human and animal research. In: Chang LW, ed. *Toxicology of Metals*. Boca Raton, FL: CRC Press, pp. 659–76.

Rowbotham AL, Levy LS, Shuker LK (2000). Chromium in the environment: An evaluation of exposure of the UK general population and possible adverse health effects. *J Toxicol Environ Health B*. 3, 145–78.

Schnaas L, Rothenberg SJ, Flores MF et al. (2006). Reduced intellectual development in children with prenatal lead exposure. *Environ Health Perspect*. 114, 791–7.

Squibb KS, Fowler BA (1984). Intracellular metabolism of circulating cadmium–metallothionein in the kidney. *Environ Health Perspect*. 54, 31–5.

Sun H, Zhou X, Chen H et al. (2009). Modulation of histone methylation and MLH1 gene silencing by hexavalent chromium. *Toxicol Appl Pharmacol*. 237, 258–66.

Sunderman FW Jr, Barber AM (1988). Fingerloops, oncogenes and metals. *Ann Clin Lab Sci*. 18, 267–88.

Sweet LI, Zelikoff JT (2001). Toxicology and immunotoxicology of mercury: A comparative review in fish and humans. *J Toxicol Environ Health B*. 4, 161–205.

Verschoor M, Wibowo A, Herber R et al. (1987). Influence of occupational low-level lead exposure on renal parameters. *Am J Ind Med*. 12, 341–51.

Viren JR, Silvers A (1994). Unit risk estimates for airborne arsenic exposure: An updated view based on recent data from two copper smelter cohorts. *Reg Toxicol Pharmacol*. 20, 125–38.

Wang RY, Needham LL (2007). Environmental chemicals: From the environment to food, to breast to the infant. *J Toxicol Environ Health B*. 10, 597–609.

WHO (1972). Evaluation of Certain Food Additives and the Contaminants Mercury, Lead and Cadmium. Tech Rep Ser 505. Geneva, Switzerland: World Health Organization.

WHO (1976). Mercury. Environmental Health Criteria 1. Geneva, Swirzerland: World Health Organization.

WHO (1977). Lead. Environmental Health Criteria 3. Geneva, Switzerland: World Health Organization.

WHO (1979). Ceramic Foodware Safety. Document HCS/79.7. Geneva, Switzerland: World Health Organization.

WHO (1981). Arsenic. Environmental Health Criteria 18. Geneva, Switzerland: World Health Organization.

WHO (1987). Selenium. Environmental Health Criteria 58. Geneva, Switzerland: World Health Organization.

Xie Y, Kondo M, Koga H et al. (2001). Urinary porphyrins in patients with endemic chronic arsenic poisoning caused by burning coal in China. *Environ Health Prevent Med*. 5, 180–5.

Yang G, Wang S, Zhou R et al. (1983). Endemic selenium intoxication of humans in China. *Am J Clin Nutr*. 37, 872–81.

Zhang A, Hu H, Sánchez BN et al. (2011). Association between prenatal lead exposure and blood pressure in female offspring. *Environ Health Perspect*. 120, 445–50.

Zhitkovich A (2005). Importance of chromium-DNA adducts in mutagenicity and toxicity of chromium (VI). *Chem Res Toxicol*. 18, 3–11.

Zhou X, Sun H, Ellen T et al. (2008). Arsenite alters global histone H3 methylation. *Carcinogenesis*. 29, 1831–6.

# *chapter twenty-six*

# *Environmental pollutants*

***Sam Kacew and Byung-Mu Lee***

*Contents*

# General remarks

The environment consists of air, water, and soil; the biota is sometimes included as one of the environmental media. Toxic substances may originate from any one medium; however, they are generally transported to other media. Humans are exposed to environmental pollutants from a variety of pathways. Figure 26.1 illustrates the transportation of lead (Pb) to humans, via air, water, food, or dust. The lead that enters humans is returned to the environment via excreta, refuse, dumps, incinerators, and so forth. Many other pollutants also have complex routes of environmental transport and affect humans. A number of more important pollutants are briefly described in this chapter.

# Air pollutants

## Introduction

### Past disasters

Several episodes of severe air pollution affecting the health and lives of large numbers of people have been reported. The notable ones occurred in

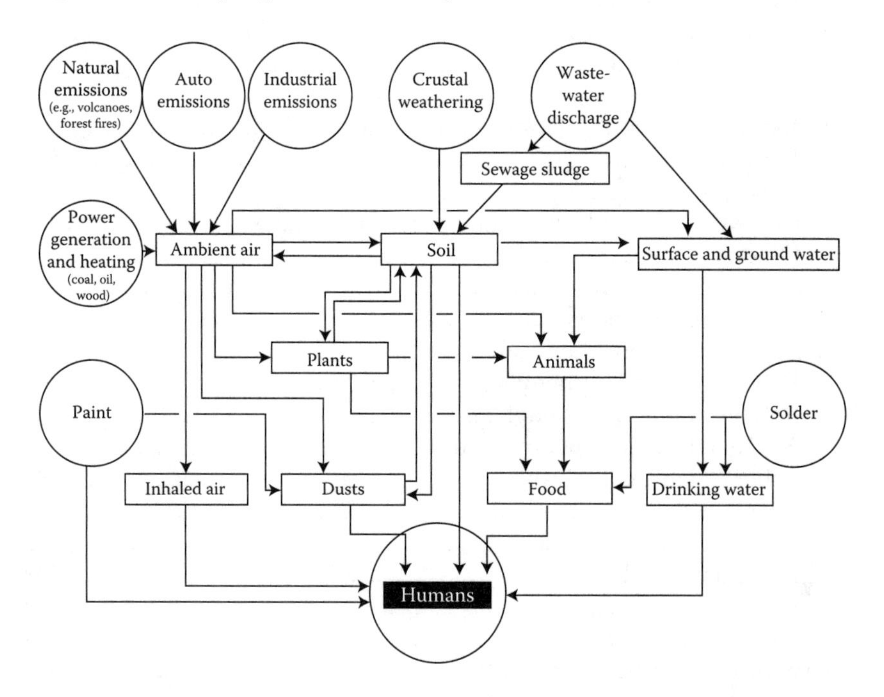


***Figure 26.1*** Environmental pathways of human exposure to lead. (From OECD, *Risk Reduction Monograph No. 1*, Organization for Economic Cooperation, Paris, France, 1993.)

Meusee Valley, Belgium (December 1930); Donora, Pennsylvania (October 1948); London, England (December 1952); Los Angeles, California (August or September 1942, 1952, 1955); and Piscataway, New Jersey (September 1971). These episodes fell into two categories. One type occurred in winters, especially during the night, when domestic burning of coal was an important source of pollution, and the other occurred in summers, during daytime, when photo oxidation of automobile exhaust was the major source of pollutants. In either case, the meteorological conditions, low wind, and high barometric pressure kept the pollutants at ground level. The major effects were related to distress of respiratory and, to a lesser extent, cardiovascular systems. A number of deaths were reported from the air pollution episodes, either directly from the exposure to air pollutants or from strains on preexisting diseases or deficiencies in these systems (Waldbott, 1978). In the case of the London smog in 1952, there was an outbreak of a severe influenza epidemic, which could be attributed to the fraction of elevated mortality for this period (Bell et al., 2004).

### *Current conditions*

As a result of these tragic events, measures have been taken to reduce the extent of air pollution. Nevertheless, health problems still remain, although somewhat abated. For example, Mar et al. (2000) reported that elevated levels of CO and $NO_2$ in Phoenix were associated with increased total nonaccidental mortality, and increased frequency of mortality due to cardiovascular involvement was associated with higher levels of CO, $NO_2$, $SO_2$, and particulate matter (PM). Similar observations in other cities are cited in a review (Krewski et al., 2003; Dominic et al., 2005).

The most important anthropogenic source of ambient air pollutants in many developed nations is automobiles (Krewski and Rainham, 2007). Other sources include combustion (coal, natural gas, fuel oil, incineration of refuse, and wood stoves), metallurgical industry (see Chapter 25), and chemical industry (solvents, chemical intermediates, etc.).

## *Outdoor pollutants*

### *Reducing types of pollutants*

*Composition and sources* The major pollutants are sulfur oxides and suspended PMs. The former includes sulfur dioxide, sulfuric acid, and sulfates; the latter includes finely divided solids and liquids. Particles of 0.1–10 μm in diameter settle slowly, with a velocity of $8 \times 10^{-7}$ m/sec to $3 \times 10^{-3}$ m/sec, while larger particles (1000 μm in diameter) settle at a velocity of 3.9 m/sec (Fuchs, 1964). Thus, particles smaller than 10 μm are suspended in air and are inhalable, as noted in Chapter 2.

The main sources of these pollutants are domestic burning of coal and other fuels for heating, cooking, and industrial combustion to generate energy. Smelting of ores also generates these and other pollutants.

#### *Diverse effects*

$SO_2$ is easily and highly soluble; hence it is readily absorbed in the nose and upper respiratory tract, where it induces irritation. This is followed with thickening of the mucus layer in the trachea and hypertrophy of goblet cells. This irritation produces cough, expectoration, dyspnea, and bronchoconstriction. Respiratory functions are impaired, manifested by a decreased tidal volume, increased pulmonary resistance, and higher respiratory rate. Among exposed individuals, there is a rise in the incidence of respiratory tract infections, which may be attributable in part to an interference of the respiratory tract clearance mechanisms. Under normal conditions, this mechanism is responsible for removing bacteria and other particles from the tract. Aerosols of sulfuric acid formed from $SO_3$ are even more irritating than sulfur dioxide, which forms sulfurous acid (Costa and Amdur, 1996).

The effects of these sulfur pollutants are enhanced by the presence of suspended sulfur dioxide and smoke (suspended particulate matter) and produce deaths, especially among the elderly and those with preexisting diseases of the respiratory tract and heart, as those in Belgium (1930), Pennsylvania (1948), and London (1952).

Even at lower concentrations (e.g., $SO_2 \geq 500\ \mu g/m^3$ and smoke $\geq 500\ \mu g/m^3$), there is likely to be an excess incidence of mortality among the elderly and the chronically sick. When exposure to these pollutants takes place at half of these concentrations, there is likely to be a worsening of existing respiratory disease (WHO, 1979). Willis et al. (2003) reported that an increased risk of mortality attributed to cardiopulmonary complications was correlated with atmospheric $SO_2$ concentrations.

### *Photochemical oxidants*

#### *Composition and sources*

This group of air pollutants consists of nitrogen dioxide ($NO_2$), ozone ($O_3$), and a number of other oxides of nitrogen ($N_2O$, $NO$, $NO_2$, $N_2O_3$, $N_2O_4$, and $N_2O_5$). $N_2O$ is the most abundant among these chemicals, but is generated by anaerobic processes in the soil and surface layer of oceans, and hence is not an important air pollutant, as far as human health is concerned. The last three oxides of nitrogen can be formed from NO and/or $NO_2$. However, their levels are low and they are not known to produce any harmful effects.

NO is the main oxide formed from man-made sources. However, after its discharge from the sources to the atmosphere, it reacts with $O_2$ to form $NO_2$. This reaction is facilitated in the presence of ozone.

Ozone is the most ubiquitous photochemical oxidant. At times, it constitutes as much as 90% of the oxidants in smog. Ozone is also a natural constituent of the upper atmosphere, formed by the photolysis of oxygen. Atmospheric circulation carries some to the lower levels.

The main sources of photochemical oxidants are automobiles and industrial combustion. Domestic heating and power stations also generate significant amounts. Ozone is also produced by a variety of high-voltage electrical equipment. Formaldehyde, which is one of the photochemical oxidants, will be discussed under the section "Indoor Air Pollutants/Sick Building Syndrome."

*Adverse effects*

In contrast to $CO_2$, $NO_2$ is hardly soluble in water. This gas, therefore, passes through the upper respiratory tract to the terminal bronchioles and alveoli, where it forms nitric and nitrous acids. These acids are irritant and corrosive. Acute exposure produces pulmonary edema and congestion and damage ciliated epithelium and type I cells (see Chapter 15), which are then replaced by the less-sensitive nonciliated epithelial cells and cuboidal type II cells. Chronic exposure produces emphysema. Resistance to bacterial and viral infections is decreased (WHO, 1977).

After inhalation exposure, ozone reacts with organic matter in the respiratory tract. Similar to $NO_2$, its main effects are on the epithelial cells of the nasal cavity, terminal bronchioles, and alveoli, affecting the more susceptible ciliated epithelial cells and type I cells. The endothelia surrounding these structures are also damaged, resulting in pulmonary edema. Chronic exposure results in emphysema, atelectasis, focal necrosis, and sometimes bronchopneumonia. In the nasal mucosa, there is destruction of the epithelial lining and release of cytokines, and consequent inflammatory processes develop (Nikasinovic et al., 2003). Resistance to bacterial and viral infection is decreased. Because of the oxidative activity of ozone, vitamin C decreases its toxicity, whereas vitamin E deficiency has the opposite effect (WHO, 1978).

Apart from their toxic effects on the respiratory tract, these air pollutants also produce eye irritation in adults (see Chapter 17). Recently, focus of air pollutants concentrated on neonates, infants, and children (Foos et al., 2008). It is well established that the lung is not mature and full development of architecture and functionality do not occur until age 18. Children have a larger lung surface area per kilogram and under normal circumstances, breathe a greater amount of air. Further, their immune system is still immature. Thus, maternal exposure to air pollutants during pregnancy results in fetal loss, while infant exposure is correlated with a higher frequency of mortality. The effect of air pollutants on children is an increased incidence of cough, bronchitis, and asthma.

## *Indoor air pollutants/"sick building syndrome"*

In recent years, the importance of indoor pollutants has become increasingly appreciated. The more efficient insulation of modern buildings, resulting in inadequate ventilation and in the use of certain insulation materials, has intensified the problem. Some of the more important pollutants and reactions are described in this chapter. Additional details are provided in articles by Karol (1991) and Samet (1993).

### *Formaldehyde*

This organic chemical is a product of photo oxidation of natural and synthetic hydrocarbons. Formaldehyde is more important as a component of urea formaldehyde foam insulation material, which has been widely used in mobile homes and, to a lesser extent, in conventional houses. Because of its volatility and toxicity, it has been a significant indoor air pollutant.

Formaldehyde is water soluble and irritates the eyes, nose, and upper respiratory tract. At higher concentrations, it also affects the bronchioles and alveoli, and induces pulmonary edema and pneumonia. The dose–effect relationship of formaldehyde is listed in Table 26.1. In addition, it has been reported to induce nasal cancers in rodents, while in humans

***Table 26.1*** Acute human health effects of formaldehyde at various concentrations

| Reported effects | Formaldehyde concentration (ppm) |
|---|---|
| None reported | 0.0–0.05 |
| Neurophysiologic effects | 0.05–1.5 |
| Odor threshold | 0.05–1.0 |
| Eye irritation[a] | 0.1–2.0 |
| Upper airway irritation | 0.10–25 |
| Lower airway and pulmonary effects | 5–30 |
| Pulmonary edema, inflammation, pneumonia | 50–100 |
| Death | >100 |

*Source:* NRC, Committee on Aldehydes, *Formaldehyde and Other Aldehydes*. National Academy Press, Washington, DC, 1981.

[a] As measured by the determination of optical chronaxy, electroencephalography, and sensitivity of dark-adapted eyes to light. The low concentration (0.01 ppm) was observed in the presence of other pollutants that may have been acting synergistically.

there is an increased incidence of micronucleated buccal and mucosal cells (Liteplo and Meek, 2003). Some studies reported evidence of genetic defects in humans. In 2004, formaldehyde was upgraded from Group 2A (a probable human carcinogen) to Group 1 (a human carcinogen) by the International Agency for Research on Cancer (IARC). Formaldehyde produces not only nasal cancer, but also common cancers including leukemia (Golden, 2011). Further, formaldehyde was also associated with the increased incidence of asthma in children (McGwin et al., 2010). The modes of action of formaldehyde are related to both genotoxic and epigenetic mechanisms (Rager et al., 2010).

*Asbestos*

Asbestos is a naturally occurring silicate fiber. Because of its heat and electrical insulation properties, it has been widely used in houses, ships, automobiles, and so forth. Workers in certain occupations are the main population at risk. However, the general public may also be exposed to it through the air and, to a lesser extent, the drinking water because it is used as a water filter (Paustenbach et al., 2004).

After inhalation, asbestos enters the alveoli and produces parenchymal asbestosis consisting of fibrosis and asbestos bodies (Vallyathan et al., 1998). Iron bound to asbestos fibers is also believed to be involved in the toxic manifestations observed. It may pierce the alveoli and produce pleural asbestosis. It also produces lung carcinoma, the incidence of which is significantly higher among cigarette smokers (Vallyathan et al., 1998). Mesothelioma is a rare type of malignant tumor, which may originate from the pleural and peritoneal surfaces after inhalation and ingestion, respectively.

Asbestos fibrosis appears to result from its entering the cells (macrophages and lymphocytes), breaking the lysosomal membrane, and releasing hydroxylases. It produces tumors either by carrying carcinogenic hydrocarbons into the body or by acting as a cocarcinogen (Vallyathan et al., 1998).

*CO, $NO_2$, $SO_2$, and suspended particulate matter*

These substances exist indoors as well as outdoors. In fact, this type of indoor air pollution may be more important than that which exists outdoors. This is because people in general spend more time indoors and because domestic heating may involve burning coal or other fuel without adequate ventilation. However, the predominant source of air pollutants arises from vehicular generation (Krewski and Rainham, 2007).

*Others*

Various volatile organic compounds (benzene, toluene, xylene, ethyl benzene, etc.) are present in offices and homes, arising from paints, adhesives, cleaners, cosmetics, furnishings, and printed materials. In addition, there are many types of biological materials such as bacteria, viruses, fungi, fungal spores, and dandruff. These substances may induce allergic reactions. The mixture of pollutants produces a wide range of reactions, which has been termed "sick building syndrome." The common symptoms of this syndrome include irritation of eyes, nose, and throat, headaches, fatigue, and nasal congestion (Samet et al., 1988).

The presence of nanoparticles (NPs) in electronics, various household items, and televisions is ubiquitous. In animals exposed to high concentrations of NPs, via the respiratory route, it is known that these compounds exert adverse effects on lung functions. Although humans are clearly exposed to NP, a direct correlation to adverse effects has not been established. However, considering the fact that NPs are ubiquitous, further investigations are needed to establish the safety of these compounds.

## *Water and soil pollutants*

### *General considerations*

Various pollutants are discharged into environmental media. Those that predominate in the air are described in the preceding section. Others are discharged in wastewater as effluent, or stored in dump sites. Generally these contaminate both the water and soil.

Water and soil contaminants include pesticides and metals, which have been discussed in Chapters 23 and 25. Asbestos is also an important environmental pollutant. Its major health hazard is related to inhalation exposure as outlined in the preceding section. It is also present in water because of various mining, milling, and industrial applications as well as its use in filter pads for wine, beer and so on (Paustenbach et al., 2004).

A great variety of organic chemicals, including some solvents and pesticides, have been detected in water, and most of these are present at extremely low levels. However, some of them are more persistent. In addition, a number of inorganic ions may also present health hazards. Both of these groups are described below. Drugs are released into water from human urine. Hormonal steroids are released into water from livestock and produce endocrine disruption.

### *Synthetic persistent chemicals*

#### *Polychlorinated biphenyls*

Polychlorinated biphenyls (PCBs) are manufactured by the progressive chlorination of biphenyl. Commercial products are mixtures of biphenyl with a different degree of chlorine substitution. These products have a variety of uses in electric insulators, and in the rubber and paper industries as plasticizers. PCBs are stable and hence persistent in the environment with levels in water ranging from 0.5 to 500 ppb, depending upon the extent of contamination. PCBs are lipophilic, and are thus bioaccumulated in aquatic organisms; fish caught from certain lakes contain 520 ppm PCBs. Because of their extreme persistence and toxicity, many nations have suspended or restricted their use. However, they will remain in the environment for a long time.

PCBs, being lipophilic, are stored in adipose tissue and secreted in milk. PCBs are a potent inducer of microsomal enzymes (Hu and Bunce, 1999). As a result, they enhance the metabolism of steroids such as estradiol and androsterone, a fact that may account for some of their effects on reproductive function. Because of this effect on enzymes, they can modify the toxicity of other chemicals and act as carcinogen promoters.

PCBs exert a variety of toxic effects in animals. For example, they induce hepatic adenoma and carcinoma. Among the reproductive functions affected are lengthened estrus cycles and decreased frequency of implanted ova in mice, lowered fertility in mink and Rhesus monkey, and reduced hatchability of eggs in birds. With respect to the immune system, they produce atrophy of lymphoid tissue in chickens and rabbits, and suppress a variety of humoral and cell-mediated immunity functions. The illnesses reported in Japan due to exposure to PCBs were referred to as Yusho disease and in Taiwan as Yu-Cheng disease.

An outbreak of poisoning occurred in Japan in 1968, resulting from a consumption of rice oil contaminated with PCBs, which affected more than 1000 people. The major clinical manifestations were chloracne, hyperkeratosis, and darkening of the skin. Immunosuppression was also noted. Various subjective symptoms were reported, such as numbness of the limbs, coughing, expectoration, general fatigue, and eye discharge. There might have also been an increase of liver and lung cancer rates among the male patients.

#### *Polybrominated biphenyls*

Polybrominated biphenyls (PBBs) are used as flame retardants. They gained notoriety because of a large-scale contamination of cattle feed in Michigan in 1973. The beef was contaminated with PBBs (Weber and Greim, 1997). Polybrominated biphenyls are similar to PCBs in many aspects, such as biotransformation, storage, and effects on reproduction, carcinogenesis, the immune system, and the skin (chloracne). The actions of PBBs on thyroid function and central nervous system disturbances in animals resulted in the banning of some of these chemicals by the European Union and the U.S. Environmental Protection Agency (USEPA).

#### *2,3,7,8-Tetrachlorodibenzo-p-dioxin*

2,3,7,8-Tetrachlorodibenzo-*p*-dioxin (TCDD) attracted wide attention after its accidental release from a factory in Seveso, Italy, in 1976. While its level in water is low, it is important toxicologically because of its extreme potency. Further, TCDD is a contaminant present with other chemicals, notably the herbicide 2,4,5-T, which was extensively used as a defoliant in the Vietnam War. TCDD is extremely toxic, with $LD_{50}$ ranging from 0.0006 to 0.115 mg/kg in different species of animals (NRC, 1977).

TCDD is a potent inducer of microsomal enzymes, by binding to a specific receptor (Hu and Bunce, 1999). TCDD is a potent carcinogen (2 ppb in rats), inducing cancer in a variety of organs such as the liver, the respiratory tract, and the oral cavity (Kociba et al., 1977). At somewhat higher doses, it is hepatotoxic, immunosuppressive, teratogenic, and fetotoxic. In humans, the predominant effect of TCDD is chloracne. In the past, it was not reported to be carcinogenic in humans despite its extremely potent carcinogenicity in rats (Zack and Suskind, 1980). However, epidemiological studies have shown that TCDD produced cancer in humans and was finally classified as a human carcinogen, Group 1 by IARC in 1997 (IARC, 1997; Baan et al., 2009; Warner et al., 2011).

#### *Other organic chemicals*

*Phthalate esters* are extensively used in plastics and are widely distributed in the environment, especially water. Their acute toxicity is low, but di(2-ethylhexyl) phthalate was shown to be carcinogenic and adversely affect reproductive functions in animals (Conference on Phthalates, 1982). *Trihalomethanes* (THMs) are formed through chlorination of water. These chemicals comprise chloroform, bromodichloromethane, dibromochloromethane, and bromoform. They are found in drinking water from less than 0.1–311 ppb. Among them, chloroform had the highest concentration. At high doses, these chemicals are hepatotoxic, produce reproductive and developmental effects, and may be carcinogenic (Teuschler et al., 2004).

### *Inorganic ions*

#### *Nitrates*

The increase of nitrates in soil and water results mainly from intensive application of fertilizers, but also from wastes (excreta) of humans and farm animals. They are converted to nitrites in soil, water, and the gastrointestinal tract through microbial action. Nitrites induce methemoglobinemia, thus reducing the oxygen-carrying capacity of hemoglobin as noted in Chapter 4. Further, they may react with certain amines to form nitrosamines, most of which are carcinogenic (Chapters 8 and 22).

*Phosphates*

These substances arise mainly from fertilizers and detergents and exert low toxicity, but their presence in a body of stagnant water results in excessive growth of algae. The algae reduce the oxygenation of the water, resulting in fish kills. Certain "algae," the cyanobacteria, contain hepatotoxins and neurotoxins (see the respective sections on these toxins).

*Fluoride*

The natural level of fluoride in water varies greatly, depending upon the location. Industrial activities may also raise its level. While fluoride has been added to water to about 1 ppm to reduce dental cavity formation, excessive levels in water (10 ppm) are likely to produce fluorosis. The enamel on the teeth is weakened, resulting in surface pitting. Changes in bones, including osteosclerosis and exostoses, usually affect the spine and produce knee deformity known as *genu valgum*. At lower levels of fluoride intake, chalky-white patches appear on the surface of the dental enamel. These patches are then stained yellow or brown and give rise to the characteristic "mottled" appearance (Dean, 1942).

*Arsenic*

In certain areas of Taiwan, South America, and Bangladesh, high levels of arsenic have been reported to be associated with black foot disease, a peripheral vascular disorder resulting in gangrene. Arsenic also produces skin lesions and possibly visceral cancers, especially in the liver (see Chapter 25).

## Cyanotoxins/eutrophication

Eutrophication occurs in lakes and ponds when there are excessive amounts of phosphorus. In general, this results from runoffs contaminated with fertilizers and detergents. Algae tend to thrive in such waters. Some of the algae produce cyanotoxins. Three groups of cyanotoxins are now recognized: one affects the nervous system, the second termed as cylindrospermopsin inhibits protein synthesis and are cytotoxic, while the third termed as microcystins inhibits protein phosphatases in the liver (Chorus et al., 2000; Zurawell et al., 2005).

*Neurotoxins*

The most important among them is saxitoxin, also known as paralytic shellfish poison. Human exposure to saxitoxin is through consumption of contaminated shellfish. The toxin acts by blocking the conduction of nerve impulse thereby inducing muscle paralysis (see Chapter 18).

*Microcystins*

The other type comprises microcystins and nodulins. These toxins are hepatotoxic to wild and domestic animals (Zurawell et al., 2005). In an epidemiological study in several areas in China, Chorus et al. (2000) found a positive correlation between the use of surface water and high rates of primary liver cancer. Subsequently, Wang and Zhu (1996) showed that an extract of *Microcystis aeruginosa* (a major species of cyanobacteria) promoted cell transformation of Syrian hamster embryo cells which had been exposed to a genotoxic carcinogen. It is thus evident that the extract is a carcinogen promoter. Gilroy et al. (2000) showed that a "health food product," made of blue-green algae, was contaminated with microcystins, as more than 70% of the samples tested contained ≥1 mg/kg.

In 1996 in Caruaru, Brazil, 100 patients suffered acute liver failure from the use of partially treated municipal water for kidney dialysis. More than half of the patients died. The cause of the outbreak has now been attributed to certain cyanotoxins (Chorus et al., 2000). In addition, Li and Han (2012) demonstrated that the reproductive toxicity in male rats might be related to reactive oxygen species generation, and inducing oxidative stress in Sertoli cells, and subsequently leading to apoptosis.

## References

Baan R, Grosse Y, Straif K et al. (2009). A review of human carcinogens—Part F: Chemical agents and related occupations. *Lancet Oncol.* 10, 1143–4.

Bell ML, Davis DL, Fletcher T (2004). A retrospective assessment of mortality from the London smog episode of 1952: The role of influenza and pollution. *Environ Health Perspect.* 112, 6–8.

Chorus I, Falconer IR, Salas HJ et al. (2000). Health risks caused by freshwater cyanobacteria in recreational waters. *J Toxicol Environ Health B.* 3, 323–47.

Conferences on Phthalates (1982). Proceedings of the conference. *Environ Health Perspect.* 45, 11–51.

Costa DL, Amdur MO (1996). Air pollution. In: Klaassen CD, ed. *Casarett and Doull's Toxicology.* New York: McGraw-Hill, pp. 857–82.

Dean HT (1942). The investigation of physiological effects by the epidemiological method. *Am Assoc Adv Sci.* 19, 23–31.

Dominic F, Mcdermott A, Daniels M et al. (2005). Revised analyses of the national morbidity mortality and air pollution study: Mortality among residents of 90 cities. *J Toxicol Environ Health A.* 68, 1071–92.

Foos B, Marty M, Schwartz J et al. (2008). Focusing on children's inhalation dosimetry and health effects for risk assessment: An introduction. *J Toxicol Environ Health A.* 71, 149–65.

Fuchs NA (1964). *The Mechanisms of Aerosol.* Oxford, UK: Pergamon Press, p. 28.

Gilroy DJ, Kauffman KW, Hall RA et al. (2000). Assessing potential health risks from microcystin toxins in blue-green algae dietary supplement. *Environ Health Perspect.* 10, 435–49.

Golden R (2011). Identifying an indoor air exposure limit for formaldehyde considering both irritation and cancer hazards. *Crit Rev Toxicol.* 41, 672–721.

Hu K, Bunce NJ (1999). Metabolism of polychlorinated dibenzo-*p*-dioxins and related dioxin-like compounds. *J Toxicol Environ Health B.* 2, 183–210.

IARC (International Agency for Research on Cancer) (1997). Polychlorinated dibenzo-para-dioxins and polychlorinated dibenzofurans. *IARC Monogr Eval Carcinog Risks Hum.* 69, 33–422.

Karol MH (1991). Allergic reactions to indoor air pollutants. *Environ Health Perspect.* 95, 45–51.

Kociba RJ, Keyes DG, Beyer JE (1977). Results of a two-year chronic toxicity and oncogenicity study of 2,3,7,8-tetrachlorodibenzo-*p*-dioxin in rats. *Toxicol Appl Pharmacol.* 46, 279–303.

Krewski D, Burnett RT, Goldberg MS et al. (2003). Overview of the reanalysis of the Harvard six cities study and American Cancer society of particulate air pollution and mortality. *J Toxicol Environ Health A.* 66, 1507–51.

Krewski D, Rainham D (2007). Ambient air pollution and population health: Overview. *J Toxicol Enviorn Health A.* 70, 275–83.

Li Y, Han X (2012). Microcystin-LR causes cytotoxicity effects in rat testicular Sertoli cells. *Environ Toxicol Pharmacol.* 33, 318–26.

Liteplo RG, Meek ME (2003). Inhaled formaldehyde: Exposure estimation, hazard characterization and exposure response analysis. *J Toxicol Environ Health B.* 6, 85–114.

McGwin G, Lienert J, Kennedy JI (2010). Formaldehyde exposure and asthma in children: A systematic review. *Environ Health Perspect.* 118, 313–7.

Mar TF, Norris GA, Koenig JQ et al. (2000). Associations between air pollution and mortality in Phoenix, 1995–1997. *Environ Health Perspect.* 108, 347–53.

Nikasinovic L, Momas I, Seta N (2003). Nasal, epithelial and inflammatory response to ozone exposure: A review of laboratory-based studies published since 1985. *J Toxicol Environ Health B.* 6, 521–68.

NRC (1977). *Drinking Water and Health.* Washington, DC: National Research Council, National Academy of Sciences.

NRC, Committee on Aldehydes (1981). *Formaldehyde and Other Aldehydes.* Washington, DC: National Academy Press.

OECD (1993). Risk Reduction Monograph No. 1: Lead Background and National Experience with Reducing Risk. Paris, France: Organization for Economic Cooperation.

Paustenbach DJ, Finley BL, Lu ET et al. (2004). Environmental and occupational health hazards associated with the presence of asbestos in brake linings and pads (1900 to present): A state of the art review. *J Toxicol Environ Health B.* 7, 25–80.

Rager JE, Smeester L, Jaspers I et al. (2010). Epigenetic changes induced by air toxics: Formaldehyde exposure alters miRNA expression profiles in human lung cells. *Environ Health Perspect.* 119, 494–500.

Samet JM (1993). Indoor air pollution: A public health perspective. *Indoor Air.* 3, 219–26.

Samet JM, Marbury MC, Spengler JD (1988). Health effects and sources of indoor air pollution. Part II. *Am Rev Respir Dis.* 137, 221–42.

Teuschler LK, Rice GE, Wilkes CR et al. (2004). A feasibility study of cumulative risk assessment methods for drinking water disinfection by-product mixtures. *J Toxicol Environ Health A*. 67, 755–77.

Vallyathan V, Green F, Ducatman B et al. (1998). Roles of epidemiology, pathology, molecular biology and biomarkers in the investigation of occupational lung cancer. *J Toxicol Environ Health B*. 1, 91–116.

Waldbott GK (1978). *Health Effects of Environmental Pollutants*. St. Louis, MO: C.V. Mosby.

Wang HB, Zhu HG (1996). Promoting activity of microcystins extracted from waterbloom in SHE cell transformation assay. *Biomed Environ Sci*. 9, 46–51.

Warner M, Mocarelli P, Samuels S et al. (2011). Dioxin exposure and cancer risk in the Seveso Women's Health Study. *Environ Health Perspect*. 119, 1700–5.

Weber LW, Greim H (1997). The toxicity of brominated and mixed-halogenated dibenzo-*p*-dioxins and dibennzofurans: An overview. *J Toxicol Environ Health*. 50, 195–215.

WHO (1977). Oxides of Nitrogen. Environ Health Criteria 4. Geneva, Switzerland: World Health Organization.

WHO (1978). Photochemical Oxidants. Environ Health Criteria 7. Geneva, Switzerland: World Health Organization.

WHO (1979). Sulfur Oxides and Suspended Particulate Matter. Environ Health Criteria 8. Geneva, Switzerland: World Health Organization.

Willis A, Jerrett M, Burnett RT et al. (2003). The association between sulfate air pollution and mortality at the county scale: An exploration of the impact of scale on a long-term exposure study. *J Toxicol Environ Health A*. 66, 1605–24.

Zack JA, Suskind RR (1980). The mortality experience of workers exposed to tetrachlorodibenzodioxin in a trichlorophenol process accident. *J Occup Med*. 22, 1–114.

Zurawell RW, Chen H, Burke JM et al. (2005). Hepatotoxic cyanobacteria: A review of the biological importance of microcystins in freshwater environments. *J Toxicol Environ Health B*. 8, 1–37.

# *chapter twenty-seven*

# *Occupational toxicology*

***Sam Kacew and Byung-Mu Lee***

*Contents*

## General remarks

As noted in previous chapters, humans are exposed to a variety of substances, by ingestion, inhalation, and dermal contact. Unlike the general population, however, workers are often exposed to higher levels of specific toxicants. Such exposures may clearly result in adverse effects. In fact, as early as 1775, Pott observed that chimney sweeps exposed to soot developed cancer of the scrotum. In 1895, Rehn discovered that bladder tumors occurred among workers in aniline dye factories.

In the late nineteenth century, certain societal changes prompted the development of a variety of new occupations. One of these was the introduction of powerful machinery to facilitate many mining activities. While the machinery increased the output of mining, it also elevated airborne dusts to which miners were exposed.

Another major change was the invention of internal combustion machines, which increased air pollution through their use in motor vehicles. To fuel these vehicles, petroleum was produced in large quantities. In fact, the excess petroleum became an excellent source of new chemicals. These petrochemicals, along with other raw materials, found uses in the production of clothing, furniture, construction material, household, and office commodities, as well as in paints, pesticides, solvents, pharmaceuticals, and so forth. These and other changes in society increased the number of occupational workers as well as the variety of substances they were exposed to.

Workers engaged in the production, processing, or utilization of these substances are thus exposed to some chemical hazard. The severity of the adverse effects, however, depends not only upon the nature of the substance but also on the level and duration of the exposure. Occupational toxicology is thus intended to assess the "permissible" levels of exposure, for a specified duration, to the toxicants encountered in workplaces. For the protection of the workers, the concentrations of the toxicants in the workplaces are to be maintained at or below their corresponding permissible levels. It should be noted that occupational exposure does not occur in a vacuum. A worker can be exposed to more than a single chemical, leading to a mixture of effects. Further, a worker who smokes or drinks, or suffers from a chronic illness such as diabetes or is on a chronic medication regime may be more susceptible than the nonsmoking worker to the same chemical. It needs to be clarified that individuals who spray pesticides are also occupational exposure workers exposed to the outdoors where chemical concentration cannot be determined. However, in the context of this chapter occupational refers to jobs done in an indoor setting.

## *Exposure limits*

Food additives and most medications, if too toxic, can be readily prohibited for use; but occupational toxicants, in general, cannot be eliminated, as the workers who are exposed to these toxicants are dependent on their jobs for an income. To protect the health of occupational workers, permissible ("safe") limits of exposure are assessed.

### *Definitions*

Permissible limits of exposure are present in many countries. In the United States, a yearly booklet listing the threshold limit values (TLVs) is published by the American Conference of Governmental Industrial Hygienists (ACGIH) since 1946 (ACGIH, 2000). The limits refer to airborne concentrations of substances and represent conditions under which "nearly all workers may be repeatedly exposed daily without adverse effects." The list includes solvents, metals and their compounds, pesticides, and others. There are three categories of TLV:

1. TLV-TWA (time-weighted average) refers to the TWA concentration for a normal 8-hour workday and a 40-hour workweek.
2. TLV-STEL (short-term exposure limit) refers to the STEL to which workers may be exposed. It is defined as a 15-minute TWA exposure. This limit is set mostly to avoid irritation and narcosis, but also to avoid chronic or irreversible tissue damage. The short-term exposure is acceptable provided that the TLVTWA is not exceeded.
3. TLV-C refers to the ceiling that should not be exceeded during any part of the working exposure.

These limits are expressed in terms of parts per million (ppm) and/or milligrams per cubic meter (mg/m$^3$). Since 1 mole of an ideal gas at 25°C and 760 mmHg occupies 24.45 L, the following equation can be used to convert the limits: parts of vapor/million parts air (ppm) = C (mg/m$^3$) × 24.45/(molecular weight of the solvents), where the letter "C" denotes a concentration of chemical. For example, 15 mg/m$^3$ of formaldehyde (MW = 30 g/mol) can be converted to 12.225 ppm [= 15 (mg/m$^3$) × 24.45/(30 g/mol)]. The Occupational Safety and Health Administration published a list of "permissible exposure limits" which are essentially similar to the TLV of ACGIH. There are other occupational exposure limits such as the maximum allowable concentration. However, the TLV published by ACGIH have been widely accepted, even outside of the United States.

## *Scientific basis*

The permissible levels of exposure are assessed on the basis of relevant test results in experimental animals as well as in clinical observations and human epidemiological studies.

### *Tests in animals*

These include the various types of tests described in previous chapters. However, with occupational toxicants, the major routes of exposure are the respiratory tract and skin. After inhalation, gases and vapors may exert effects locally, and may also be absorbed. Large particulate matter and liquid droplets (>10 μm) do not enter the respiratory tract but affect the nasal mucosa; very small particles (<0.01 μm) are likely to be exhaled. Those within the range of 0.01–10 μm may be absorbed from the respiratory tract and exert systemic effects and may also induce local effects in the lungs.

Skin is relatively impermeable to most chemicals, but some may be absorbed in sufficient quantities to induce systemic effects. Some toxicants may produce local irritation and hypersensitization.

After absorption, a toxicant is distributed to various parts of the body. Depending upon its nature, a small or large portion of it may be stored. In general, it is excreted as is or after undergoing biotransformation. In general, this process renders the toxicant more water soluble, hence more excretable. However, some chemicals undergo bioactivation, especially in the liver, and become more toxic. For additional information on bioactivation, see Chapter 3.

Although all organs and systems may be adversely affected by occupational toxicants, the most commonly affected targets, apart from the respiratory tract and skin, are the nervous system, liver, and kidneys. In addition, potential adverse effects on the immune system, reproductive function, and fetal development merit special attention.

### *Human data*

To obtain relevant data from humans, a variety of studies may be used. The *case control study* is generally used to unravel the etiology of a specific adverse effect. For example, Cole et al. (1972) observed a higher rate of lower urinary tract cancer among workers engaged in the manufacture of dyestuff, rubber, and leather. This observation provided a basis for further confirmatory studies.

*Epidemiological studies* are more elaborate and usually provide more precise information. Prospective studies are usually carried out to confirm a suspected cause–effect relationship, and/or to provide more precise quantitative data. Retrospective studies involve analysis of clinical data obtained in exposed workers versus a group of unexposed cohort, matched for age, gender, and such lifestyle as smoking and alcohol consumption.

#### *Assessment of permissibility*

With adequate and relevant animal and human data, a "no-observed adverse effect level" (NOAEL) can generally be assessed. The permissible exposure level can be obtained by applying an appropriate "safety factor" to the NOAEL. A detailed description of the procedure used in Europe to assess the permissible levels of exposure to pesticides was described by de Raat et al. (1997). Procedures used in the United States, Canada, Germany, and the Czech Republic are outlined in a WHO document (WHO, 2000).

## *Occupational toxicants*

### *Organic solvents*

Solvents comprise a variety of organic chemicals such as aromatic hydrocarbons (e.g., chloroform and carbon tetrachloride [$CCl_4$]), alcohols, or glycols, and their ethers. These chemicals are used extensively in paints, inks, thinners, adhesives, pharmaceuticals, cosmetics, and so forth. Some solvents are used mainly for dry cleaning clothes and degreasing machinery. Their manufacture and use in industry may pose health hazards to occupational workers. In addition, some of them become components of household products, thereby constituting potential health hazards to the consumer. Their adverse effects are outlined below, and summarized along with their TLV-TWAs in Table 27.1. Chloroform produces toxic effects in the liver, kidneys, central nervous system (CNS), and cardiovascular system (Table 27.1).

#### *General effects*

Most of the solvents exert certain nonspecific effects. These include irritation at the site of contact, and depression of CNS.

### *Irritation*

At room temperature solvents are in liquid form and when they are in contact with the skin, irritation may occur. As these chemicals are volatile, inhalation of their vapors may produce irritation of the nasal epithelium and respiratory tract, and may also produce eye irritation and watering.

***Table 27.1*** Toxic effects and TLV-TWAs of certain organic solvents

| Organic solvents | Toxic effects | TWA (ppm) |
|---|---|---|
| Benzene | Leukemia | 0.5 |
| Carbon disulfide | CNS, neuropathy | 10 |
| Carbon tetrachloride | Liver | 5 |
| Chloroform | CVS, liver, kidneys, CNS | 10 |
| Dioxane | Skin | 20 |
| *n*-hexane | Neuropathy, CNS irritation | 50 |
| Methanol | Neuropathy, vision CNS | 200 |
| Methyl *n*-butyl ketone | Neuropathy | 5 |
| Methylene chloride | CNS, anoxia | 50 |
| Toluene | CNS, skin | 50 |
| Trichloroethylene | CNS, liver | 50 |

*Source:* ACGIH, *Threshold Limit Values for Chemical Substances and Biological Exposure Indices*, Publications Office, American Conference of Governmental Industrial Hygienists, Cincinnati, OH, 2000.

*Abbreviations:* CNS, central nervous system; CVS, central vascular system; TLV, threshold limit value; TWA, time-weighted average.

## *CNS depression*

At sufficiently high levels of exposure, a consistent effect of solvents is CNS depression. The clinical manifestation begins with disorientation, giddiness, and euphoria. The latter effect is responsible for abuse of some of these chemicals. The syndrome may progress to paralysis, unconsciousness, and convulsions. Death may ensue.

The mechanism of action is not clear, but well over half a century ago, Meyer (1937) observed that the narcosis (CNS depression) was related to the solubility of these substances in lipid and was not related to their chemical structure, and hence suggested that narcosis resulted from CNS cell dysfunction following solubilizing of the solvents in the cell membrane.

## *Interaction*

As noted above, most solvents may undergo biotransformation and elevate the activities of cytochrome P-450 isozymes. Since solvents are often present in mixtures, interaction between them may occur. For example, a solvent such as benzene may potentiate the adverse effects of others by enhancing their bioactivation. On the other hand, the toxicity may also be decreased with certain mixtures. For example, toluene may reduce the toxicity of benzene by competitively inhibiting the bioactivation enzyme systems (Andrews et al., 1977). These effects are dependent on normal liver function but become skewed in an alcoholic person. The presence of drugs also affects solvent biotransformation. It is worth noting that there are gender differences and in general men appear to be more susceptible to chemical-induced alterations compared with women.

#### *Specific effects*

Apart from the general effects described earlier, a variety of specific effects may follow exposure to solvents. The diversity of these effects is a result of different reactive metabolites being formed. Some of the specific effects are described next.

### *Liver*

As noted in Chapter 12, ethanol is a common cause of fatty liver and liver cirrhosis. These effects likely result from the direct toxicity of ethanol and nutritional deficiency commonly present among alcoholics. Various chlorinated hydrocarbons may produce liver damage. These include fatty liver as well as liver necrosis, cirrhosis, and cancer. The liver lesions are induced by reactive metabolites of these solvents. For example, the likely metabolite of carbon tetrachloride is trichloromethyl radical, that of chloroform is phosgene, and those of halogenated aromatic hydrocarbons such as bromobenzene are their epoxides (Reid and Krishna, 1973). However, the recurrent cytotoxicity and chronic tissue regeneration may be the cause of carcinogenicity.

### *Kidneys*

As noted in Chapter 13, certain chlorinated hydrocarbons such as chloroform and carbon tetrachloride are nephrotoxic in addition to being hepatotoxic. At lower levels of exposure, renal effects are related to tubular functions, such as glycosuria, amino aciduria, and polyuria. At higher levels, there may be cell death along with elevated BUN and anuria. In humans, $CCl_4$ affects mainly the kidneys when the route of exposure is inhalation, whereas the liver is the major target organ when the chemical is ingested. Ethylene glycol is nephrotoxic because of its direct cytotoxicity as well as the blocking of proximal tubules with formation of crystals of its metabolite, calcium oxalate. Trichloroethylene, a solvent used as a degreasing agent, was shown to produce damage to the proximal tubules as well as nephrocarcinogenicity.

### *Nervous system*

Apart from their effects on CNS, as noted above, aliphatic hydrocarbons and certain ketones such as *n*-hexane and methyl *n*-butyl ketone also affect the peripheral nervous system. The clinical manifestation of this polyneuropathy begins with numbness and paresthesia, as well as motor weakness of both hands and feet. These effects then involve both arms and legs. Pathologically, it is characterized by distal axonopathy (Chapter 18). The reactive metabolite of these two solvents is 2,5-hexanedione (Krasavage et al., 1980). Perchloroethylene (tetrachloroethylene) present in dry cleaning fluids was found to produce central nervous system disturbances.

### Hematopoietic system

Benzene is an outstanding example of a solvent affecting this system. It depresses bone marrow in animals and humans, thereby decreasing the circulating erythrocytes, leukocytes, and thrombocytes. Leukemia has been reported in humans exposed to benzene (Snyder, 2000).

### Carcinogenesis

As noted above, a number of chlorinated hydrocarbons are known to produce liver tumors. Benzene is carcinogenic in animals and produces leukemia in humans. In addition, dioxane is also a liver carcinogen and produces nasopharyngeal cancers (Andrews and Snyder, 1996).

Diethylene glycol induced bladder tumors in rats fed with large doses of the solvent. In all the tumor-bearing rats, there were bladder stones that were composed of calcium oxalate, a metabolite of this chemical (Fitzhugh and Nelson, 1946). This solvent has thus been considered a secondary carcinogen (Chapter 8). Chloroform (Group 2B, a possible human carcinogen) was reported to induce renal tumors only in male rats and mice (Meek et al., 2002) but appears to have a limited evidence for humans. Trichlorethylene (Group 2A, a probable human carcinogen) was found to induce renal tumors that are relevant for humans, whereas perchloroethylene (Group 2A, a probable human carcinogen) was shown to be a weak renal carcinogen.

### Other effects

*Testicular degeneration* and *cardiovascular abnormalities* have been observed in animals exposed to ethylene glycol monoethyl ether. Methanol may damage the *retina* through its metabolite and affect mainly the part that is responsible for central vision. Methylene chloride produces CNS depression and irritation to the eye and skin. However, it also induces *carboxy hemoglobinemia*, because CO is formed in the biotransformation (WHO, 1984). Chloroform may induce *cardiac arrhythmias*, probably as a result of sensitization of the myocardium to epinephrine. This is one of the reasons why chloroform has been discontinued as a general anesthetic.

It should be noted that certain solvents are practically nontoxic. For example, propylene glycol possesses low toxicities, with $LD_{50}$ values of 32 and 18 ml/kg in rats and rabbits, respectively, and rats fed on this solvent at 1.8 ml/kg for 2 years showed no adverse effects. This chemical has thus been used as a food additive.

## *Metals*

Metals are mined, smelted, refined, and processed for a great variety of uses. Workers are therefore exposed to metals and their compounds in many ways through their occupations. The target organs and the nature of toxicity depend upon the metal and its chemical form. For example, elemental mercury vapor produces excitability, tremors, and gingivitis. On the other hand, the divalent mercuric chloride is corrosive on contact, whereas the monovalent mercurous chloride produces dermal vasodilatation, hyperkeratosis, and hypersecretion of the sweat gland.

Table 27.2 lists the main toxic effects and/or target organs as well as the TLV-TWAs of a number of toxic metals.

***Table* 27.2** Toxic effects and TLV-TWAs of toxic metals

| Metals | Toxic effects | TWA ($mg/m^3$) |
|---|---|---|
| Arsenic | Cancer (lung, skin) | 0.01 |
| Beryllium | Cancer (lung), berylliosis | 0.002 |
| Cadmium | Cancer (lung, prostate), kidney lesions | 0.01 |
| *Metal fume fever* | | |
| Cr, metal, and Cr III | Skin, irritation | 0.5 |
| Cr VI, soluble | Cancer, liver, kidneys | 0.05 |
| Cr VI, insoluble | | 0.01 |
| Lead | CNS, GI, blood, kidneys, reproduction | 0.05 |
| *Mercury* | | |
| Alkyl | CNS | 0.01 |
| Aryl | CNS, neuropathy, eye, kidneys | 0.1 |
| Inorganic and elemental | CNS, neuropathy, eye | 0.025 |
| Nickel, elements | Skin | 1.5 |
| Soluble compounds | CNS, skin | 0.1 |
| Insoluble compounds | Cancer (lung) | 0.2 |

*Source:* ACGIH, *Threshold Limit Values for Chemical Substances and Biological Exposure Indices*, Publications Office, American Conference of Governmental Industrial Hygienists, Cincinnati, OH, 2000.

*Abbreviations:* CNS, central nervous system; Cr, chromium; TLV, threshold limit value; TWA, time-weighted average.

*Pesticides*

Pesticides are widely used in agriculture and public health programs to control vector-borne diseases. There are several types of pesticides, that is, insecticides, herbicides, fungicides, rodenticides, and fumigants.

The organochlorine insecticides include aldrin, chlordane, DDT, lindane, and methoxychlor. Their major adverse effects are on the CNS and liver. The organophosphorus insecticides, such as azinphos-methyl (guthion), diazinon, malathion, methyl parathion, and parathion, inhibit acetylcholinesterase (AChE). The inhibition of AChE in the central, peripheral, and autonomic nervous systems produces a variety of adverse effects, as described in Chapter 23. Carbaryl, a carbamate insecticide, also inhibits AChE, but its effects are short lived.

The herbicides, 2,4-D and diquat, irritate the skin. Paraquat is stored in the lungs, hence it produces lung edema. The TLV-TWA for this chemical is lower. The fungicide thiram produces skin irritation and may disturb reproductive function. The fumigant metam sodium produces allergic dermatitis and exacerbates asthma. The irritant effects are attributed to account for the observed neurotoxicity (Pruett et al., 2001).

***Table 27.3*** Toxic effects and TLV-TWAs of certain pesticides

| Pesticides | Toxic effects | TWA (mg/m$^3$) |
|---|---|---|
| Aldrin | Liver | 0.25 |
| Azinphos-methyl | AChE inhibition | 0.2 |
| Carbaryl | AChE inhibition | 0.5 |
| Chlordane | CNS, liver lesion | 0.5 |
| 2,4-D | Skin irritation | 10 |
| DDT | CNS, liver lesion | 1 |
| Diazinon | AChE inhibition | 0.1 |
| Diquat | Irritation of eye, skin | 0.5 |
| Lindane | CNS, liver lesion | 0.5 |
| Malathion | AChE inhibition | 10 |
| Methoxychlor | CNS, liver lesion | 10 |
| Methyl parathion | AChE inhibition | 0.2 |
| Paraquat | Lung edema, kidneys, liver | 0.5 |
| Parathion | AChE inhibition | 0.1 |
| Thiram | Skin irritation, reproduction | 1 |

*Source:* ACGIH, *Threshold Limit Values for Chemical Substances and Biological Exposure Indices*, Publications Office, American Conference of Governmental Industrial Hygienists, Cincinnati, OH, 2000.

*Abbreviations:* AChE, acetylcholinesterase; CNS, central nervous system; Cr, chromium; DDT, dichloro-diphenyl-trichloroethane; TLV, threshold limit value; TWA, time-weighted average.

Table 27.3 lists the main toxic effects and/or target organs as well as the TLV-TWA of the above-mentioned pesticides. Additional details on their toxicity are provided in Chapter 23. Their acute toxicity in humans is listed in Appendix 27.1.

## *Miscellaneous toxicants*

### *Particulate matter*

As noted above, particulate matter (PM) of sizes in the range of 0.01 to 10 μm ($PM_{0.01}$ to $PM_{10}$) are readily inhaled and exert adverse effects. A notable example is asbestos. It is widely used to provide thermal and acoustic insulation as well as fire protection, but produces pulmonary fibrosis (asbestosis), and cancers of the bronchus and mesotheliomas of the pleura and peritoneum (Vallyathan et al., 1998). Its TLV-TWA is "1 fiber/$cm^3$" (ACGIH, 2000).

Other common PM include coal dust, kaolin, silica, and talc. All these substances may induce pulmonary fibrosis (Vallyathan et al., 1998). Coke oven emissions initiate tracheobronchial cancers (Vallyathan et al., 1998). Tobacco smoking enhances the toxic effects of PM, such as asbestos (see Chapter 5) and cement dust (Table 27.4). Particulate matter is a complex mixture of different sizes, shapes, types, and chemical compositions (Donaldson et al., 2005). Exposure to PM produced from combustion induced oxidative damage to DNA and lipids (Møller and Loft, 2010) and was associated with cardiovascular and pulmonary diseases (Salvi and Barnes, 2009).

### *Gases*

A number of gases, such as CO, $CO_2$, $NO_2$, $O_3$, and $SO_2$, are encountered in certain occupational settings. However, these also occur in the general environment, as described in Chapter 26.

### *Plastics*

There are many types of plastics. They are polymerized monomers, with molecular weights generally in the range of 10,000–1,000,000 Da, hence

***Table 27.4*** Prevalence of respiratory symptoms in cement workers

| Cement dust exposure | Smoking history | Prevalence of respiratory symptoms (%) | Ratio |
|---|---|---|---|
| – | – | 1.6 | 1 |
| – | + | 3.3 | 2 |
| + | – | 9.0 | 5.6 |
| + | + | 11.7 | 7.3 |

*Source:* Lu, PL and Gu, XQ, *Biomed Environ Sci.*, 2, 17–23, 1989.

are inert and nontoxic. However, some monomers are toxic. For example, vinyl chloride was reported to induce hepatic malignant tumors (angiosarcomas) among exposed workers (Creech and Johnson, 1974). Vinyl chloride may also produce cancer in the lung, skin, and lymphatic and hematopoietic tissues (WHO, 1999). Acrylamide, unlike other monomers, is readily absorbed through the skin and may induce peripheral neurotoxicity. After absorption it releases cyanide and induces CNS toxicity (Drew, 1993).

Among the additives, the catalyst benzoyl peroxide was found to promote cancer on mouse skin initiated by genotoxic carcinogen (Slaga et al., 1981). Phthalates, used as plasticizers, produce proliferation of peroxisomes, thereby acting as nongenotoxic carcinogens (Rao and Reddy, 1987).

Toluene diisocyanate is used in the manufacture of flexible polyurethane foams, surface coatings, fibers, sealants, and adhesives. It is a potent irritant to the eyes, skin, and especially respiratory system, producing allergic asthma (Wilder et al., 2011). There is an immunologic component in this syndrome with an increased immunoglobulin E (Karol et al., 1994).

## *Occupational monitoring*

To ensure that the specified permissible exposure limits are complied with, both the workplace and some workers are monitored.

### *Workplace monitoring*

In general, using appropriate instruments, the air is monitored for concentrations of airborne pollutants. These include gases, vapors, dusts (total, inhalable, and respirable), fibers, liquid droplets, and smokes. For details see Gray (1993).

### *Biological monitoring*

Workers exposed to the same workplace environment may not be equally affected by, or even equally exposed to, the toxicants. This is due to differences in age, gender, body build, diet, medication, disease state, and so forth. In addition, there are differences in work intensity and duration, temperature, humidity, coexposure to other chemicals, and so forth. (ACGIH, 2000). ACGIH has, therefore, published a number of biological exposure indices, values used for guidance to assess biological monitoring results. Human samples frequently used for biological monitoring include urine, blood, hair, feces, nails, expired air and human tissues. The most commonly used methods involve monitoring of the exposure to the toxicants or their biological effects.

*Effects*

Inhibition of AChE in whole blood or plasma is a reliable, sensitive indicator of exposure to organophosphorus insecticides such as parathion and methyl parathion and the carbamates such as carbaryl.

Zinc protoporphyrin is a sensitive indicator of a minimal effect of lead. Carboxy hemoglobin is an indicator of the effect of CO.

*Exposure*

The levels of lead and mercury in blood are good indicators of the extent of exposure to these metals. The level of mercury in urine is also useful. As the volume of urine varies greatly from day to day and between different individuals, the level of mercury in urine is expressed in terms of microns per gram of creatinine, because a fairly constant amount of creatinine is excreted daily. The extent of exposure to benzene and carbon disulfide is also determined in urine and expressed in terms of microns per gram of creatinine.

Another type of monitoring measures the biochemical reaction products, such as mercapturic acids (*N*-acetyl-l-cysteine *S*-conjugates) in wine. This procedure has shown to be useful in monitoring benzene, acrolein, acrylamide, acrylonitrile, trichloroethane, and so forth (DeRooij et al., 1998).

## *Appendix 27.1 Acute pesticide toxicity, general signs, and symptoms in humans*

| Pesticide | Symptoms and signs |
|---|---|
| *Insecticides*<br>Organophosphates, carbamates | *Mild*: Headache, dizziness, perspiration, lacrimation, salivation, blurred vision, tightness in chest, twitching of muscles in eyelids, lips, tongue, face |
| | *Moderate*: Abdominal cramps, nausea, vomiting, diarrhea, bronchial hypersecretions, bradycardia or tachycardia, muscle (skeletal) spasms, tremors, general weakness |
| | *Severe*: Pinpoint pupils, profuse sweating, urinary and/or fecal incontinence, mental confusion, pulmonary edema, respiratory difficulty, cyanosis, progressive cardiac and respiratory failure, and unconsciousness leading to coma |
| Organochlorines | *Mild*: Systemically, toxic action is confined to the central nervous system with stimulation resulting in dizziness, nausea, vomiting, headache, and disorientation |

(*Continued*)

| Pesticide | Symptoms and signs |
| --- | --- |
| | *Moderate to severe*: Hyperexcitability, apprehension, weakness of skeletal muscles, incoordination, tremors, seizures, coma, and respiratory failure (progressive clinical findings related to severity of poisoning) |
| Pyrethroids | Generally of low toxicity but can cause irritation of oral and nasal mucosa. Some agents cause dermal tingling, stinging, or burning sensation followed by numbness (paresthesia). Facial contamination results in lacrimation, pain, photophobia, congestion, and edema of eyelids and conjunctiva |
| | Ingestion of large amounts may cause salivation, epigastric pain, nausea, vomiting, headache, dizziness, fatigue, coarse muscular twitching in limbs, convulsive seizures, loss of consciousness |
| *Herbicides* Bipyridyls | Irritation of nose and throat, hemorrhage, eye irritation with conjunctivitis and corneal stripping, skin irritation, and dermatitis |
| | Ingestion results in initial signs of ulceration of tongue, throat, and esophagus; sternal and abdominal pain; general muscular pain; vomiting; and diarrhea. After 48–72 hours, signs of renal and hepatic damage (oliguria, jaundice), respiratory difficulty (cough, dyspnea, tachypnea, pulmonary edema), and progressive respiratory failure |
| Phenoxy acids<br>Urea<br>Triazines<br>Chloroaliphatics<br>Aryl carbamates | Generally of low toxicity but, during handling, may cause irritation of eye, nose, throat, and skin. Ingestion may cause gastroenteritis, nausea, vomiting, diarrhea. Respiratory symptoms include burning sensation, cough, and chest pain. Muscle weakness and muscle twitching may be encountered, and central nervous system signs include dizziness, weakness, anorexia, and lethargy |
| *Fungicides* | |
| Dithiocarbamates<br>Phenolics<br>Chlorobenzenes<br>Benzimidazoles<br>Thiophanate | Generally of low toxicity but local contamination of skin may cause itching, rash, and dermatitis. Ingestion of large amounts may cause nausea, vomiting, diarrhea, and muscle weakness. The dithiocarbomates exert a disulfiram-like effect in the presence of alcohol, causing flushing, sweating, dyspnea, hyperpnea, chest pains, and hypotension |

(*Continued*)

| Pesticide | Symptoms and signs |
|---|---|
| *Rodenticides* | |
| Fluorinated agents<br>Zinc phosphide<br>Strychnine<br>α-Naphthyl thiourea<br>Anticoagulants | Accidental rodenticide poisoning is difficult to achieve because agents are packaged as baits attractive only to the pest. When ingested, these agents may cause nausea, vomiting, intestinal cramps, diarrhea, excitation, abnormal cardiac rhythms, muscle spasms, and seizures. The anticoagulants require laboratory assessment of coagulation status and treatment with vitamin $K_1$ |

*Source:* Ecobichon, DJ, *Occupational Hazards of Pesticide Exposure*, Taylor & Francis, Philadelphia, 1999.

# References


ACGIH (2000). *Threshold Limit Values for Chemical Substances and Biological Exposure Indices*. Cincinnati, OH: Publications Office, American Conference of Governmental Industrial Hygienists.

Andrews LS, Lee EW, Witmer CM et al. (1977). Effect of toluene on metabolism, disposition, and hematopoietic toxicity of (3H) benzene. *Biochem Pharmacol.* 26, 293–300.

Andrews LS, Snyder R (1996). Toxic effects of solvents and vapors. In: Klaassen CD, ed. *Casarett and Doull's Toxicology*. New York: McGraw-Hill.

Cole P, Hoover R, Friedell GH (1972). Occupation and cancer of the lower urinary tract. *Cancer.* 29, 1250.

Creech JL, Johnson MN (1974). Angiosarcoma of the liver in the manufacture of PVC. *J Occup Med.* 16, 150–1.

de Raat WK, Stevenson H, Hakhert BC et al. (1997). Toxicological risk assessment of worker exposure to pesticides: Some general principles. *Reg Toxicol Pharmacol.* 25, 204–10.

DeRooij BM, Commandeur JNM, Vermeulen NPE (1998). Mercapturic acids as biomarkers of exposure to electrophilic chemicals: Applications to environmental and industrial chemicals. *Biomarkers.* 3, 239–303.

Donaldson K, Tran L, Jimenez LA et al. (2005). Combustion-derived nanoparticles: A review of their toxicology following inhalation exposure. *Part Fibre Toxicol.* 2, 1–14.

Drew R (1993). Toxicity of plastics. In: Stacey NH, ed. *Occupational Toxicology*. London and Bristol, PA: Taylor & Francis.

Ecobichon DJ (1999). *Occupational Hazards of Pesticide Exposure*. Philadelphia, PA: Taylor & Francis.

Fitzhugh OG, Nelson AA (1946). Comparison of the chronic toxicity of triethylene glycol with that of diethylene glycol. *J Ind Hyg Toxicol.* 28, 40–3.

Gray C (1993). Occupational hygiene-interface with toxicology. In: Stacey NH, ed. *Occupational Toxicology*. London and Bristol, PA: Taylor & Francis, pp. 269–93.

Karol MH, Tollerud DJ, Campbell TP et al. (1994). Predictive value of airways hyper-responsiveness and circulating IgE for identifying types of responses to tolerance diisocyanate inhalation challenge. *Am J Respir Cont Care Med.* 143, 611–5.

Krasavage WJ, O'Donoghue JL, DiVincenzo GD et al. (1980). The relative neurotoxicity of methyl *n*-butyl ketone, n-hexane and their metabolites. *Toxicol Appl Pharmacol.* 52, 433–41.

Lu PL, Gu XQ (1989). New challenges for occupational health services facing economic reform in China. *Biomed Environ Sci.* 2, 17–23.

Meek ME, Beauchamp R, Long G et al. (2002). Chloroform: Exposure estimation, hazard characterization and exposure–response analysis. *J Toxicol Environ Health B.* 5, 283–334.

Meyer KH (1937). Contributions to the theory of narcosis. *Faraday Soc Transl.* 33, 1062–4.

Møller P, Loft S (2010). Oxidative damage to DNA and lipids as biomarkers of exposure to air pollution. *Environ Health Perspect.* 118, 1126–36.

Pruett SB, Myers LP, Keil DE (2001). Toxicology of metam sodium. *J Toxicol Environ Health B.* 4, 207–22.

Rao MS, Reddy JK (1987). Peroxisome proliferators and cancer: Mechanisms and implications. *Carcinogenesis.* 8, 631–6.

Reid WD, Krishna G (1973). Centrolobular hepatic necrosis related to covalent binding of metabolites of halogenated aromatic hydrocarbons. *Exp Med Pathol.* 18, 80–99.

Salvi SS, Barnes PJ (2009). Chronic obstructive pulmonary disease in nonsmokers. *Lancet.* 374, 733–43.

Slaga TW, Klein-Szanto AJP, Triplett LL et al. (1981). Skin promoting activity of benzoyl peroxide, a widely used free radical generating compound. *Science.* 213, 1023–5.

Snyder R (2000). Overview of the toxicology of benzene. *J Toxicol Environ Health A.* 61, 339–46.

Vallyathan V, Green F, Ducatman B et al. (1998). Roles of epidemiology, pathology, molecular biology and biomarkers in the investigation of occupational lung cancer. *J Toxicol Environ Health B.* 1, 91–116.

WHO (1984). Methylene chloride. Environ Health Criteria 32. Geneva, Switzerland: World Health Organization.

WHO (1999). Vinyl chloride. Environ Health Criteria 215. Geneva, Switzerland: World Health Organization.

WHO (2000). Human exposure assessment. Environ Health Criteria 214. Geneva, Switzerland: World Health Organization.

Wilder LC, Langley RL, Middleton DC et al. (2011). Communities near toluene diisocyanate sources: An investigation of exposure and health. *J Expo Sci Environ Epidemiol.* 21, 587–94.

# *chapter twenty-eight*

# *Exogenous agents and childhood exposure*

***Sam Kacew***

*Contents*



## *Introduction*

It should be noted that, unlike the case of drugs, a child is not normally administered a chemical that has no direct therapeutic potential. However, exposure of children to environmental chemicals can occur due to the presence of toxicants in food, water, and air via the oral and inhalation routes. In addition, the presence of chemicals in air or water can also result in contact with the skin, that is, the dermal route. Therefore, it is worth noting that a fetus can be exposed to chemicals via the mother (placental route) or an infant can be exposed when nursing (lactational route) but the consequences are not observed until the child develops; that is, the occurrence of adverse effects is delayed. It needs to be kept in mind that data obtained for chemical exposure in adults is not always applicable to children. The infant needs to be regarded as a distinct organism. A lack of appreciation of this fact may result in serious harm and potentially lead to death. Hence, it is essential to understand that the pharmacokinetic principles applied in pediatric toxicology are based upon knowledge obtained from drug therapy studies in adults.

### *Pharmacokinetics*

The pharmacokinetic principles applied in pediatric chemical exposure are, in general, similar to those utilized for adults. However, data obtained from adult studies are not necessarily applicable to observations in infants or young children based upon distinct differences between a mature adult organ versus that of a developing child, as described hereafter.

A number of important characteristics exist that distinguish infants from adult with respect to chemical exposure. Although the examples described arise from drug therapy, the basic principles are similar for environmental contaminant exposure. The reactions of infants to cardiac glycosides and anticonvulsants are examples of adverse effects attributed to altered drug absorption. In the case of oral ingestion by the child of contaminants such as lead in soil, the distribution of the metal may be similar to that of the adult's, but the susceptibility to neurological alterations is higher in the younger population as the central nervous system is not fully developed in the child.

In the infant, absorption from the gastrointestinal tract of an orally administered drug differ from that in adults. In both adults and infants, the rate and extent of drug absorption depend on the degree of ionization, which is influenced by pH. Within the first 24 hours of life, gastric acidity increases rapidly, and this is followed by an elevation in alkalinity over the next 4–6 weeks. These conditions result in drugs existing in the infant gastrointestinal tract in states of ionization different than might be observed in adults. With respect to metals such as arsenic or chromium, it is the ionic species that is critical for an effect. Therefore, the role of gastric ionization in the absorption of metals and species released into the circulation needs to be considered. Other factors that modify gastrointestinal drug absorption in the young infant, as summarized by Roberts (1986), include an irregular neonatal peristalsis, a greater gastrointestinal tract surface to body ratio, and enhanced β-glucuronidase activity in the intestinal tract. The significance of the β-glucuronidase is that it releases drug-bound glucuronide to the free form and thus increases drug bioavailability.

Differences exist in distribution of drugs in the organs between newborns and adults. In the newborn, a higher percentage of body weight is composed of water, therefore extracellular water space is proportionally larger. To initiate a receptor response, the distribution of chemicals needs to occur predominately in the extracellular space; as a result the concentration of a substance reaching the receptor sites is higher in neonates. Further, the ability of newborns to bind chemicals in plasma is significantly lower than in adults. This again suggests that neonates might be expected to be more susceptible to the effects of compounds. Differences also exist with respect to drug-metabolizing enzymes, such as the cytochrome P450 system. It has been clearly demonstrated that the chemical inactivation rate is generally slower in newborns. In addition, the ability of neonates to eliminate substances via the kidneys, the major excretion pathway, is significantly limited by the state of development of these organs. Consideration of these factors indicates that the susceptibility and responsiveness of newborns to chemical exposure are different from those of adults.

Differences also exist with respect to cytochrome P450 system enzymes. It has been clearly demonstrated that chemical inactivation rate is generally slower in newborns. However, one cannot generalize regarding the cytochrome P450 system metabolizing capacity in newborns since there is a marked variability among infants, and this capacity is highly dependent on the substance being examined. Further, certain metabolic pathways exist uniquely in the neonate. Although drug metabolism is a means of chemical inactivation, it is also a process utilized to form an active component. In an effort to effectively remove the unwanted consequences of chemical exposure, this factor needs to be considered in light of the fact that hepatic cytochrome P450 system enzyme capacity is age related.

As mentioned before, the ability of the neonate to eliminate chemicals via the kidneys, the major excretion pathway, is significantly limited by their state of development. It is well established that the half-life of several antibiotics is prolonged in neonates due to a decreased glomerular filtration rate. However, the glomerular filtration rate reaches the level seen in adults by 5 months of age. In addition, renal tubular secretory capacity increases during the first few months to attain adult values at 7 months of age. Consequently, an agent eliminated via the secretory renal pathway would have a three times greater half-life in an infant. As an example, the clearance of phenytoin and phenobarbital was rapid in the first week or two of age, yet theophylline and caffeine clearance remained low until the age of 6 weeks. The knowledge of clearance rates is essential in the evaluation of initial as well as subsequent effects of chemicals and metals on children.

The discussion relating to drug absorption from the gastrointestinal tract is also pertinent to the absorption of environmental contaminants.

As previously discussed, significant quantities of a chemical may be transferred to an infant by ingestion of mother's milk. Young children past the age of suckling are prone to accidental poisoning from ingestion of household chemicals and toxic plants.

The lung is not mature at birth, and development of its full architecture and functionality does not occur until about 18 years of age. During early childhood, the bronchial tree is still developing. For example, the number of alveoli in the human lung increases from 24 million at birth to 257 million at the age of 4, and the lung epithelium is not fully developed. Children also have a larger lung surface area per kilogram of body weight than adults, and under normal breathing, they breathe a greater amount of air per kilogram of body weight than adults, with the highest levels in the youngest children. This process of early growth and development, whose outcome is important for the future health of the child, suggests that there is a critical exposure time where air pollution may have persistent effects on respiratory health.

At the same time the child's lung is developing, the child's immune system, immature at birth, is also beginning to develop. Much attention in asthma research has focused on immune development and factors that influence the development of TH-2 (humoral immunity dominant) versus TH-1 (cellular immunity dominant) phenotypes. Significant industrial pollution and photochemical smog have the potential for producing adverse effects in both adults and infants. Respiratory irritation, edema, and hyperplasia can occur in the most severe cases. A concentration-dependent immunologic response can also occur as a result of exposure to certain chemicals. Because the lung cells of neonates are not well developed, there is an increased potential for significant damage.

## *Chemicals and the older child*

Within the context of this chapter, the final stage constitutes the older child, where patterns of chemical disposition are far less important than dose calculation based on normal growth. As the child grows, the pathways of chemical biotransformation and metabolism are similar to those in the adult. In addition, the total body water distribution, albeit on a smaller scale, is similar in the child and adult. Despite these recognized similarities, there are examples of drugs (exogenous chemicals) that behave differently and uniquely in the child. Barbiturates produce CNS stimulation in the child as opposed to sedation in the adult. Further, cationic amphiphilic drugs, such as gentamicin and chlorphentermine, are more toxic to the adult than the newborn. In a study of 1327 children attending outpatient clinics, the incidence of adverse drug reactions was 0.75%. The nature of these adverse reactions was slight, occurred predominantly in females, and was associated with polypharmacy. As in the case of the neonate, polypharmacy is believed to play an important role in the initiation of adverse drug reactions.

There are other problems associated with therapy, the major component being compliance. At this stage of development, the physician is still reliant on an adult, who at the best of times may not be consistent. Ultimately, the onus is on the physician to adequately inform the responsible individual of the necessity for compliance and the consequences resulting from failure to adhere.

In the case of contaminants, it is well-established that children are more susceptible to lead and mercury, possibly attributable to differences in distribution as the blood–brain barrier is not fully developed, enabling the metals to enter the central nervous system more readily. The issue of compliance is not applicable to environmental contaminants as exposure is inadvertent but can be controlled by changing residence or moving to a nonindustrialized area.

## *Summary*

The neonate and infant are unique organisms, and their responsiveness to drugs and environmental chemicals cannot simply be predicted from known effects in adults. The consequences of maternal drug or chemical exposure during infancy can take years to manifest themselves; therefore women who believe they are pregnant should take caution.

The following sections of this chapter are devoted to a discussion of specific chemicals encountered during gestation and early life, which have potential subsequent effects on the development to adulthood.

### *Bisphenol A*

Bisphenol A (BPA, 4-hydroxy-phenyl propane) is a high-production-volume chemical that is widely used in the production of polycarbonate plastics and epoxy resins. These materials are present in a wide variety of consumer products, including food containers, baby feeding bottles, storage containers, food cans, and tanks for drinking water or the food industry. As a result of dietary intake and other sources, there is a widespread exposure of the general population to BPA. Concern has been raised regarding the potential impact of BPA exposure, particularly on children's health (Kasper-Sonnenberg et al., 2012). Bisphenol A displays weak estrogenic activity, which may exert a low impact on the endocrine system. Based on the known toxicokinetics of BPA in humans, low concentrations of free BPA in human blood are detected as a result of rapid biotransformation and excretion. Only unconjugated "free" BPA is presumed to act as endocrine-disrupting agent. Hence, the actual circulating active amount of BPA is very small and the effects at this concentration are not significant. At present the effects of BPA on childhood development and health outcomes remain to be determined. However, in order to err on the side of caution, the use of BPA in nursing baby bottles has been banned from use in several countries, nevertheless, it should be noted that no apparent reports of adverse effects on the endocrine system have been recorded in children.

## *Mercury*

Table 28.1 summarized the consequences of childhood exposure to various chemicals. Human exposure to methylmercury (MeHg) presents a high health risk due to metal-induced neurotoxicity, teratogenicity, nephrotoxicity, cardiotoxicity, and immunotoxicity. Developmental neurotoxicity is widely recognized and considered the most sensitive endpoint in humans as it results in widespread deranged cytoarchitecture of the brain. The sensitivity of the developing brain, during pregnancy and early childhood, to the impact of neurotoxic substances is higher compared to the adult brain's sensitivity. Indeed, evidence demonstrated the vulnerability of young children to mercury (Hg) exposure. Studies showed that early exposure to low-level MeHg produced higher risks of neurodevelopmental delays. However, there are still unresolved issues regarding the benefits of fish consumption and the negative effects of accompanying pollutants. Fish is an excellent source of high-quality protein and is one of the best sources of long-chain omega-3 fatty acids, docosahexaenoic acid, (DHA) and eicosapentaenoic acid (EPA), which are important for brain and eye development and for protection of the cardiovascular system. An

***Table 28.1*** Examples of reported infant responses due to chemical exposure

| Class/chemical | Consequences |
|---|---|
| Metals | |
| Arsenic | Ultrastructural changes in liver, peripheral vascular disease, skin lesions |
| Lead | Neurotoxicity, ototoxicity |
| Methylmercury | Altered neurodevelopment |
| Chlorinated compounds | |
| Hexachlorobenzene | |
| Polychlorinated biphenyls | Skin rash, diarrhea, vomiting, neurotoxicity, death |
| Dioxin | hypotonia, lethargy, chloracne, alopecia |
| Tetrachloroethylene | Obstructive jaundice |

increasing number of studies also provided evidence for the nutritional benefits of selenium (Se), also commonly found in fish. In addition to the benefits of selenium as an antioxidant and for disease prevention, this element has been examined with respect to its ability to counteract the adverse effects of mercury. Other important fish nutrients are iodine, magnesium, iron, copper, and vitamins D and B12, which the body requires for diverse functions such as growth, repair, and normal functioning. When considering the risk assessment and prevention of human exposure to MeHg, care needs to be taken as a risk communicator not to remove fish from the diet, since the regular consumption of fish (two to three times per week) is recommended because of its high nutritional value.

Globally, dietary studies identified fish as the primary source of MeHg intake for the average population. The Portuguese are the greatest consumers of fish in Europe, with 57 kg fish/year/inhabitant, and the third greatest worldwide. Infants and children, due to their higher food consumption rates per body weight, are expected to have an increased relative risk and are therefore considered a susceptible group (Nunes et al., 2014). Fish is a natural and abundant food resource in the Amazon, consumed in large quantities by riverine populations as the main source of nutritional subsistence (Carneiro et al., 2014). In this high fish-consumption environment, a toddler's exposure to MeHg in fish may occur during pregnancy and through breast milk. In addition to that, in countries using thimerosal-containing vaccines (TCV) in pregnant mothers and young children, a substantial part of organic mercury exposure may also occur during the first 6 months through ethylmercury (EtHg) in TCV. Mercury exposure is of particular concern during the neonatal period when consumption of breast milk and a more concentrated TCV schedule result in higher exposure to both forms of mercury (EtHg and MeHg). This exposure is even higher, on a body weight basis, than that of older infants and children. The estimated Hg exposure from TCV, as a bolus dose of EtHg at 2 months, is 80% of the total mercury ingested as small daily doses in breast milk, thus increasing the risk of higher impact by cumulative (chronic and acute) exposure to both forms of organic mercury.

Thimerosal during pregnancy may also affect experimental animals, and administration of EtHg, at levels reflecting those in TCV given to infants, produced untoward effects on neurodevelopment in animals. However, data on neurodevelopmental effects, due to exposure to EtHg administered in vaccines, are conflicting in population studies conducted in developed countries or are not sufficiently extensive in Third World countries. In an accidental mass poisoning in Iraq, children exposed while in the womb to food contaminated with organic mercury (which included both MeHg and EtHg) showed neurodevelopment effects measured by criteria such as the age at which the child first walked, the age at which the child first talked, and by a score derived from neurologic examinations. Research into mercury exposure and neurodevelopment has mainly focused on a single mercury species—most often MeHg. While there are population studies that examined the effects of low-dose MeHg on neurobehavior, few of these addressed EtHg exposure. Neurodevelopment outcomes in relation to TCV EtHg are not consistent but may be summarized as: (a) there is ambiguity in some studies reporting neurodevelopment outcomes that seem to depend on confounding variables; (b) the risk of neurotoxicity due to low doses of Thimerosal is plausible at least for susceptible infants; and (c) there is a need to address these issues in less developed countries still using TCV in pregnant mothers, newborns, and young children suggesting significant, albeit weak, interactions between TCV EtHg exposure and untoward neurological outcomes where possible interactions were noted.

Presently, traditional food items are consumed less by riverine populations in western Amazonia due to the transitioning socioeconomic situation there. The consumption of fish is less prominent among migrant populations with different dietary preferences and also among former riverine families that have found new sources of income from modern economic activities. The proportion of the total dietary protein that comes from fish has been replaced by other sources. This does not seem to impact anthropometric growth in children of former subsistence-living communities or in newly formed tin ore mining settlements. When evaluating the interactions of nutrients and mercury exposure, one needs to consider the complex nature of the nutrient components of fish and the types of exposure to different organic mercury forms, such as persistent (fish MeHg) and episodic or acute (EtHg in TCV), or both (Dorea et al., 2014). Studies that compared the toxicity of MeHg and EtHg found that both forms of organic mercury are toxic, both *in vitro* and *in vivo,* to several systems (immune, neurologic, and renal); and that both these compounds are comparably toxic.

There is increasing evidence of widespread mercury exposure among children who live near gold mining operations. Indigenous people in the rain forests of Latin American and in other locations, where elemental mercury is used in the gold extraction process, are at high risk for mercury intoxication as residues from this activity are released into the environment. The developing nervous system of children is particularly sensitive to mercury exposure, which may induce neurological damage even in small doses by targeting the lipid-rich neurons of the central nervous system. Children living near rainforest gold mines who were found to suffer from mercury intoxication are generally exposed to MeHg from the consumption of contaminated fish and other foods. Exposure to the neurotoxicant MeHg may induce severe neurological impairment in children. Aquatic microorganisms in river sediments, where indigenous people fish, convert inorganic mercury deposits through methylation into MeHg, which bioaccumulates in several smaller species before concentrating in the eaten species. Exposure to mercury from aquatic sources may also impair the immune response in humans. A second source of MeHg intoxication in children is that of food contaminated by mercury-based fungicides. Lipid-soluble MeHg compounds may cross the blood–brain barrier, where MeHg acts as a potent neurotoxicant.

In addition to MeHg poisoning, exposure to elemental mercury (Hg°), can be from inhalation of mercury vapors. This occurs during the burning of metallic mercury amalgams used to separate gold particles from soil and alluvial sediment, and has become a more common route of intoxication among gold miners and their families. Mercury vapors diffuse through the capillaries of the alveolar sacs, permeate the blood–brain barrier, and accumulate in the brain. Acute and chronic exposure to both MeHg and Hg° vapors has been reported to induce a variety of neurological symptoms and disorders, including mercurial erethism, headache, dysarthria, malaise, loss of memory, blurred vision, tremors, paresthesia, hearing and visual impairment, cognitive deficits, neurobehavioral disorders, and cerebral palsy.

The indigenous Andean Saraguro "Amer-Indians" of Ecuador form a major part of the formal and informal (gold-panning) labor force in the remote Andean gold mining settlement of Namibia. The Saraguro and others make extensive use of mercury amalgam burning to separate gold particulates from soil. Case history interviews with Saraguro and non-Saraguro (Mestizo) gold miners and their families in Namibia revealed that both groups engage in this gold-extraction process within the close confines of their homes and in their yards, and that both groups consume fish from the local rivers where mercury residues are released. Their children also participate directly and are thus exposed to the mercury burning process, as well as infants carried on their mothers' backs. However, no known risk assessment study has been conducted among these children. Such a study would represent a first step in evaluating the effects of persistent chemicals on the health of the indigenous children, and in identifying other toxicological agents in the study area.

## *Lead*

It has been well established that pediatric lead (Pb) exposure impairs the developing brain of children and damages other vital organs, such as the kidneys. Lead exposure adversely affects neuronal development in the prenatal and postnatal developing brain, inhibits neurotransmitter storage and release at synapses, and impedes mitochondrial and glial cell function. Neurosensory impairment is ostensibly related to damage of the inner ear receptors and, as reported by some investigators, auditory brainstem neurons can be affected by lead exposure, even at low blood lead (PbB) levels; however, this effect has not always been noted. A range of neurocognitive and behavioral deficits are associated with lead exposure, including intellectual disabilities, learning disabilities, and behavioral disorders in children. Lead exposure has also been linked to specific deficits in visual-motor integration, short-term auditory memory, attention span, and visual-spatial perception.

The main intake route of lead is by ingestion, but environmental exposure by ambient air and soil is also highly correlated to the internal lead burden in children. Therefore, lead concentrations in ambient air and soil are regulated as precautionary measures. The contribution of lead in ambient air and soil to the internal metal burden has been estimated by several groups in epidemiological studies (Nancano et al., 2014). During the last decades, lead in ambient air has decreased considerably, but the relative contribution of soil ingestion to the internal metal burden presumably increased, at least for children, because lead concentration in soil has remained nearly constant. Most cases of pediatric lead poisoning during child development arises from exposure to lead dust and ingestion of lead contaminated materials through pica. Chronic lead poisoning is generally a feature of occupational exposure, which is typically observed in adults. However, some children in developing countries displayed chronic lead poisoning from residing in environments highly contaminated from occupational activities, such as from automobile garages and shops (batteries and radiators), or lead glazing of ceramics. Children in some communities in Ecuador, South America, demonstrated chrome lead poisoning from occupational exposure to the lead-glazing of ceramic roof tiles and other marketable ceramic objects. In cases of pediatric lead poisoning exceeding the Centers for Disease Control and Prevention (CDC) III classification, and in cases where blood lead (PbB) level do not decline, despite environmental abatement and nutritional supplementation, chelation therapy is the recommended treatment. The traditional chelation therapy has consisted of using dimercaprol or British anti Lewisite (BAL), ethylenediamine tetraacetic acid (EDTA), or the oral chelating agents D-penicillamine and mesa-2, 3-dimercaptosuccinic acid (DMSA), which were found to reduce the lead body burden in children. However, in order for chelation therapy to be effective, exposure to the source of lead must be discontinued. In a milieu with widespread environmental lead contamination from continuous occupational lead use, reintoxication of treated patients can occur. This leads to a chronic and persistent intoxication difficult to manage medically, which may result in irreversible neurological, neurocognitive, and renal impairment.

A population of children with chronic lead poisoning from persistent exposure to environmental and occupational sources from a lead–glazing village industry has been examined (Counter et al., 2009, 2015). Some of the children in this area were found to have extreme plumbism, exhibiting elevated PbB levels over a period of years, even after chelation therapy and family counseling. These children also had elevated zinc protoporphyrin (ZPP) levels, substantiating the presence of chronic lead intoxication. However, it was surprising to find that many of the children did not exhibit the expected neurological and intellectual impairments that are generally reported in such extreme cases of plumbism. In fact, most of the children displayed normal adaptive community behaviors, such as age-appropriate daily living skills, age-appropriate socialization skills, and age appropriate communication skills. Although many of these children were reported by their teachers to have some learning difficulties, the majority of them attend regular classes.

Lead (Pb) exposure has been associated with adverse neurocognitive and neurobehavioral outcomes in children as well as auditory neurosensory impairments. A number of recent review articles on the developmental consequences of lead exposure by, among others, the American Academy of Pediatrics concluded that exposure induces hearing impairment or subclinical auditory sensory deficits. However, these studies on auditory sensory function have shown mixed results. Some studies have reported an association between lead exposure and cochlear (inner ear) hearing impairment in both children and adults, leading some investigators to suggest that lead-induced hearing loss in children may contribute to the neurodevelopmental learning disabilities that are associated with pediatric lead exposure. Other studies found no unequivocal association between lead exposure and sensory hearing loss or any change in auditory sensitivity. Children living in highly lead-contaminated environments in rural Andean villages of Ecuador displayed extremely elevated PbB levels, but the results showed no statistical association between PbB levels and auditory sensory function. These disparate findings suggest that lead exposure is not invariably associated with hearing impairment, and that behavioral auditory sensitivity measures may not be a reliable marker of lead toxicity.

A more direct and objective technique for examining inner ear integrity involves the physiologic measurement of otoacoustic emissions, a non-invasive procedure that is routinely used to screen infants' hearing, part of universal newborn hearing screening programs (Buchanan et al., 2011). Otoacoustic emissions refer to sounds generated by the active mechano-electric transduction processes of intact cochlear sensory cells, the outer hair cells of the inner ear. These low-intensity-level sounds are transmitted in a retrograde manner from the inner ear to the ear canal, where they are recorded in a noninvasive manner via a miniature microphone placed at the entrance to the ear canal. The outer hair cells are quite susceptible to acoustic trauma or certain toxic agents resulting in a reduction or absence of otoacoustic emission. Otoacoustic emissions were found to be diminished in individuals treated with ototoxic medications, such as aminoglycoside antibiotics or cisplatin, even before changes in behavioral auditory thresholds became apparent. Thus, if lead exposure exerts an adverse effect on the inner ear, otoacoustic emissions may be a more sensitive index of auditory sensory impairment than behavioral pure-tone thresholds, which were used in most previous studies. Nevertheless, a preliminary otoacoustic emissions study on 14 lead-exposed children found no unequivocal associations of lead exposure with hearing impairment, even though the study group was found to have abnormally elevated lead levels, which contrasts with some earlier reports.

## *Air pollution and children's health*

The adverse health effects attributed to air pollution exposure have become an area of increasing focus in the last 30 years. A growing body of evidence has demonstrated that there are serious health consequences to community air pollution, and that these consequences are not spread equally among the population (Slezakova et al., 2015). Relative to adults, children spend a greater portion of their days outside and at greater exertion levels, both of which may increase exposure to pollution from traffic, power plants, and other combustion sources, which are generally higher outdoors. For ozone, in particular, exposure is generally outdoors (as ozone disappears quickly indoors) and during the afternoon on sunny days. Children's exposure to air pollution is of special concern since their immune system and lungs are not fully developed, raising the possibility of different responses than those seen in adults.

The following provides a brief overview of up to date findings from epidemiological studies on the association of air pollution with a number of children's health outcomes important for risk assessments. This topic has been reviewed from different perspectives (Madureira et al., 2015). While most of these studies do not compare children and adult risks, the findings remain important because they reinforce the fact that the health of children is adversely affected by air pollution.

### *Air pollution health effects observed in children*

#### *Infant mortality*

Studies have reported that air pollution is associated with infant mortality. In considering air pollution and death, one is inevitably reminded of

***Table 28.2*** Ambient air pollutants and infant/child responses

| Ambient air pollutant | Consequences | Reference |
|---|---|---|
| Particulate matter (traffic emissions) | Infant mortality | Anderson, 1999<br>Woodruff et al., 2006<br>Bobak and Leon, 1992 |
| Particulate matter | Chronic cough and bronchitis | Dockery et al., 1996<br>Mar et al., 2004 |
| Particulate matter, ozone, nitrogen dioxide, sulfur oxides | Asthma | Mar et al., 2004<br>Kim et al., 2004<br>Gent et al., 2004 |
| Ozone | Decreased lung function, wheeze | Gauderman et al., 2004<br>Kunzil et al., 1997 |

the great air pollution episode of December 1952 in London. A low-level thermal inversion that trapped coal smoke in the Thames valley, coupled with a stationary front that dropped wind speed to zero, resulted in a rapid buildup of pollution to extremely high levels. Approximately 4000 excess deaths occurred in London during that week, and elevated death rates continued for weeks afterwards, indicating that there were delayed as well as early-onset effects. While most of the deaths were in adults, infant mortality doubled during that period. This episode is important because it implies causality. Several investigators found that incidence of infant deaths in the United States and levels of $PM_{10}$ in the air was associated with higher infant death rates at ages 2–12 months (the first month after birth was excluded as likely to reflect complications of pregnancy and delivery). This excess risk seemed to result principally from respiratory illnesses, although sudden infant death syndrome deaths were also elevated. Across towns in the Czech Republic, there was a marked cross-sectional association between air pollution and infant mortality rates. A significant association was seen between infant death rates and particle (TSP-10) and $SO_2$ concentration. Another population-based case control study demonstrated significant associations between infant mortality from respiratory causes, and total TSP and $SO_2$. Other studies examined day-to-day changes in air pollution and day-to-day changes in infant deaths and reported that infant death from respiratory disease was associated with air pollution, particularly from traffic. Ambient air pollutants and infant or children's adverse outcomes are summarized in Table 28.2.

*Respiratory effects: Chronic cough and bronchitis*

Chronic bronchitis and chest illness in children were associated with exposure to particulate air pollution. Subsequent studies confirmed the association of particulate exposure with higher rates of chronic cough and bronchitis symptoms in children. A similar large study ($n = 4470$) comparing school children in 10 communities in Switzerland reported an adjusted odds ratio for bronchitis of 2.88 for $PM_{10}$ exposure between the most and least polluted community. The largest study examined 13,369 children in 24 communities in the United States and Canada. Again, particulate air pollution was associated with bronchitis episodes across these communities. Chronic cough in children was also associated with air pollution in a number of studies. A recent study looking at eastern Germany, where there has been a reduction in pollution since the reunification of Germany, showed that this decrease was correlated with a fall in rates of chronic cough and bronchitis symptoms in a cohort of children. This demonstrates not merely an association, but that an intervention produces improvements in health. A similar result was found in Switzerland.

*Respiratory effects: Asthma*

Air pollution, including particulate matter, ozone, $NO_2$, and sulfur oxides, has long been known to exacerbate asthma, including increasing symptoms, causing the need for bronchodilator medication, decreasing lung function, and increasing emergency visits due to attacks. Several studies suggested that air pollution, particularly traffic-related pollution, was associated with development of asthma and atopy (Greenberg et al., 2016; Madureira et al., 2016). In eight small rural communities, a strong association between asthma prevalence and $NO_2$ levels was found, with odds ratios reaching 5.81 when contrasting the highest and lowest exposures. In 317 children in three German communities, $NO_2$ measurements outside each child's home were significant predictors of hay fever, symptoms of allergic rhinitis, wheezing, and sensitization against pollen, house dust mites or cats, while indoor $NO_2$ was not, indicating that outdoor $NO_2$ functioned as a surrogate for other traffic-related pollutants. In the Netherlands, residence on a high-traffic street was associated with more than a two fold rise in the risk of wheezing after control for confounders. Similar results were seen in other studies of traffic-related pollution. Overall, diesel exhaust was shown to be a potent adjuvant for atopic sensitization, and also seems the most important traffic indicator for prediction of asthma and atopy.

*Respiratory effects: Lung development*

Finally, there is increasing evidence that air pollution negatively impacts lung growth. Chronic ozone exposure during childhood was associated with decreased lung function and increased risk of wheeze and chronic respiratory symptoms in college freshmen. Results from the chronic exposure to air pollutants including $NO_2$, acid vapors, $PM_{2.5}$, and elemental carbon during childhood decreases lung function growth, producing significant decrements at age 18 years, and that this reduction may be permanent with adverse implications for long-term respiratory health as adults.

## Ontogeny of lung structure and function, breathing patterns, and implications for dose and deposition

As discussed in the previous section, epidemiological evidence of childhood susceptibility is substantial, and more importantly, epidemiological studies suggest children may be more susceptible than adults to lower respiratory tract effects of inhaled particulate matter. Clearly, adverse effects on developmental processes, such as lung function growth, occur only in children and not in adults. While children may be especially predisposed to adverse effects from airborne particulates, they may also receive an increased dose of particles to their lungs compared to adults.

At least three factors may contribute to enhanced lung deposition in children versus adults:

1. *Lesser nasal contribution to breathing at rest and during exercise in children*
2. *Less efficient uptake of particles in the nasal airways of children*
3. *Greater efficiency of particle deposition within the lower respiratory tract of children*

The nose is a more effective filter than the mouth for preventing penetration of particles to the lower respiratory tract. Thus, the route of breathing, oral versus nasal, is an important determinant of particulate dose to the lung. The efficiency of the nose itself for filtering particles is dependent on the anatomy of the nasal passage, which changes with age. Lung growth and changes in breathing patterns with age (from child to adult) may affect the fractional deposition of inhaled particles in the lower respiratory tract. Further, among children, there are several risk factors that may contribute to enhanced pulmonary deposition of inhaled particles, including race, obesity, and presence of allergic rhinitis or asthma.

Very large (>5 μm aerodynamic diameter) and very small (<0.01 μm) particles are deposited efficiently in the nose by inertial impaction and diffusion, respectively, during nasal breathing. The ability of the nose to filter particulate matter (as well as soluble or reactive gases) serves as a protective mechanism against toxicity to the lower respiratory tract. Thus, the pattern of breathing (nose or mouth) due to different activities is a critical factor in determining the location and amount of deposition of inhaled particles in the respiratory tract.

Only a few studies attempted to measure oronasal breathing in children as compared to adults. In both cases, only a limited number of children were studied. It was found that children (age 7–16, $n = 10$) displayed more variability than adults with respect to their oronasal pattern of breathing with exercise. However, it was not possible to predict the pattern of partitioning of ventilation during exercise based on age, gender, or nasal airway resistance. Further, in a limited number of children (age 8–16, $n = 10$), children tended to display more oral breathing both at rest and during exercise than the adults. The highest oral fractions were also found in the youngest children. None of the studies was able to show a relationship between nasal resistance and relative contribution of nasal breathing in these children. Further, a recent study in adults found that nasal ventilation during exercise varied as a function of both race and gender. African Americans possessed a greater nasal contribution to breathing during exercise than Caucasians. At similar exercise efforts (i.e., normalized as % maximum work capacity) females also had a greater nasal contribution to breathing during exercise than males. Whether these race and gender effects occur in children as well has not been investigated. While a number of investigators measured the oronasal pattern of ventilation in adults, few addressed this parameter in children. Additionally, those that have done so, in either adults or children, did not fully characterize *nasal anatomy/physiology* in their study subjects, such that the mechanisms/determinants of oronasal breathing during exercise are not fully understood.

*Breathing rates* are also an area that would benefit from further experimental data, as models are only as useful as the data that goes into them. Limited data are available to verify the current models for breathing rates. A recent development called a "life shirt" was identified as a tool; it is worn for 24 hours to measure not only breathing rate (or minute ventilation), but also the tidal volumes and breathing frequencies associated with those rates throughout the entire day. An alternative method for validating breathing rates has been evaluated by the California EPA. This validation exercise (OEHHA, 2000, Appendix K) examined data from energy expenditure studies using doubly labeled water to determine how much oxygen subjects consumed. From these data it was possible to determine the quantity of air the individual subjects inhaled over a few weeks. Such data may be compared to estimates of inhalation rates obtained through other approaches.

A concern was raised about focusing on breathing rate when other kinetic parameters, such as metabolism and blood flow, may be important factors. Current assessment methods involve PBPK models (when available), and these models take into account more factors than breathing rate; moreover, breathing rate may be applied as a variable parameter in the exposure assessment. Quantitative allowances are made for variability due to age (insofar as suitable age-dependent parameter values can be identified) and for issues of internal dosimetry. Under the California Air Toxics Hot Spots Program, the air pollution control districts in California have a number of emissions sources for which public health impacts are assessed via emissions inventories and subsequent health risk assessments. The reporting is somewhat similar to the U.S. EPA Toxic Release Inventory (TRI) but with lower reporting triggers (lb/yr) and a more comprehensive accounting for small facilities. Facilities are ranked based on a prioritization procedure, and for high priority facilities, a risk assessment is completed using the guidelines already described briefly in the fourth section. Other issues identified for further examination included the risk assessment of nanoparticles on children's health, the effects of in utero exposures, and the mode of breathing (nasal versus mouth breathing). A broad concern is that, generally, the application of available knowledge in current risk assessment practice sometimes lags behind and particularly for children's health risk assessments, thus updating needs to become more routine.

## Conclusions

The scientific evidence presented above is an introduction that helps to illustrate the scientific basis of evidence concerning children's exposure to air pollutants. The following sums up its main points:

i. Available epidemiological evidence indicates adverse health effects in children from exposure to current levels of ambient air pollution.
ii. A review of the ontogeny of lung structure and function, breathing patterns, and the resulting implications for dose and deposition reveals age-related differences that increase risk for children.
iii. New methods for the estimation of inhalation rates illustrate variability with age, which is greater than was previously estimated.
iv. Reviewing the current risk assessment methods illustrates how children are taken into account, as well as areas where additional analysis may be warranted to adequately characterize their risk.

## References

Anderson RH (1999). Health effects of air pollution episodes. In: Holgate ST, Samet JM, Koren HS, Maynard RL, eds. *Air Pollution and Health*. Academic Press, San Diego, CA: pp. 461–84.

Bobak M, Leon DA (1992). Air pollution and infant mortality in the Czech Republic, 1986–88. *Lancet*. 340, 1010–4.

Buchanan LH, Counter SA, Ortega F (2011). Environmental lead exposure and otoacoustic emissions in Andean children. *J Toxicol Environ Health A*. 74, 1280–93.

Carneiro MFH, Grotto D, Barbosa F Jr (2014). Inorganic and methylmercury levels in plasma are differentially associated with age, gender, and oxidative stress markers in a population exposed to mercury through fish consumption. *J Toxicol Environ Health A*. 77, 69–79.

Counter SA, Buchanan L, Ortega F (2009). Neurocognitive screening of lead-exposed Andean adolescents and young adults. *J Toxicol Environ Health A*. 72, 625–32.

Counter SA, Buchanan L, Ortega F (2015). Blood lead levels in Andean infants and young children in Ecuador: An international comparison. *J Toxicol Environ Health A*. 78, 778–88.

Dockery DW, Cunningham J, Damokosh AI, Neas LM, Spengler JD, Koutrakis P, Ware JH et al. (1996). *Environ Health Persp*. 105, 500–5.

Dorea JG, Marquesm RC, Abreu L (2014). Milestone achievement and neurodevelopment of rural Amazonian toddlers (12 to 24 months) with different methylmercury and ethylmercury exposure. *J Toxicol Environ Health A*. 77, 1–13.

Gauderman WJ, Avol E, Gilliland CF et al. (2004). The effect of air pollution on lung development from 10 to 18 years of age. *N Engl J Med*. 351, 1057–67.

Gent JF, Triche EW, Holford TR et al. (2003). Association of low-level ozone and fine particles with respiratory symptoms in children. *J Am Med Assoc*. 290, 1859–67.

Greenberg N, Carel RS, Derazne E et al. (2016). Different effects of long-term exposures to $SO_2$ and $NO_2$ air pollutants on asthma severity in young adults. *J Toxicol Environ Health A*. 79, 342–51.

Kasper-Sonnenberg M, Wittsiepe J, Koch HM et al. (2012). Determination of bisphenol A in urine from mother–child pairs—Results from the Duisburg birth cohort study, Germany. *J Toxicol Environ Health A*. 75, 429–37.

Kim KJ, Smorodinsky S, Lipsett M et al. (2004). Traffic-related air pollution near busy roads: The East Bay Children's Respiratory Health Study. *Am J Respir Crit Care Med*. 170, 64–70.

Kunzil N, Lurmann F, Segal M, Ngo L, Balmes J, Tager IB (1997). Association between lifetime ambient ozone exposure and pulmonary function in college freshman—Results of a pilot study. *Environ Res*. 72, 8–23.

Madureira J, Paciencia I, Ramos E et al. (2015). Children's health and indoor air quality in primary schools and homes in Portugal—Study design. *J Toxicol Environ Health A*. 78, 915–30.

Madureira J, Paciencia I, Cavaleoro-Rufo J, Fernandes EO (2016). Indoor air risk factors for schoolchildren's health in Portugese homes: Results from a case-control survey. *J Toxicol Environ Health A*. 79, 938–53.

Mar T, Larson TV, Stier RA, Claiborn C, Koenig JQ (2004). An analysis of the association between respiratory symptoms in subjects with asthma and daily pollution in Spokane, Washington. *Inhal Toxicol*. 16, 809–15.

Nacano LR, de Freitas R, Barbosa F Jr (2014). Evaluation of seasonal dietary exposure to arsenic, cadmium and lead in school children through the analysis of meals served by public schools of Ribeiro Preto, Brazil. *J Toxicol Environ Health A*. 77, 367–74.

Nunes E, Cavaco A, Carvalho C (2014). Children's health risk and benefits of fish consumption: Risk indices based on a diet diary follow-up of two weeks. *J Toxicol Environ Health A*. 77, 103–14.

OEEHA (2000). Adequacy of California Ambient Air Quality Standards: Children's Environmental Health Protection.

Roberts, RJ (1986). Developmental aspects in clinical pharmacology. In: Spector R, ed. The Scientific Basis of Clinical Pharmacology. Boston, Littele, Brown pp. 153–170.

Slezakova K, Texeira C, Morais S, Pereira MC (2015). Children's indoor exposures to ultra(fine) particles in an urban area: A comparison between school and home environments. *J Toxicol Environ Health A*. 78, 886–96.

Woodruff TJ, Parker JD, Schoendorf KC (2006). Fine particulate matter (PM 2.5) air pollution and selected causes of postnatal infant mortality in California. *Environ Health Persp*. 114, 786–90.

# *chapter twenty-nine*

# *Clinical toxicology*

***Byung-Mu Lee***

*Contents*



## *Introduction*

*Clinical toxicity* refers to adverse effects of toxic agents produced in humans whereas preclinical toxicity is in animals. Clinical toxicology focuses not only on human adverse effects but also on mechanism of action, detoxification or management for a variety of toxic substances such as metals, pesticides, radiation, animal and plant toxins, food additives, environmental contaminants, industrial chemicals, cosmetic ingredients, and pharmaceutical agents (i.e., drugs). In this chapter, the toxicological profile for pharmaceutical agents is covered because other compounds are described in previous chapters. The ten drugs responsible for the most deaths in the United States induced 43,981 and 47,055 fatalities in 2013 and 2014, respectively (NIDA, 2016; Warner et al., 2016; Xu et al., 2016). The top 10 drug overdose deaths in 2014 are due to (1) heroin 10,863, (2) cocaine 5856, (3) oxycodone 5417, (4) alprazolam 4217, (5) fentanyl 4200, (6) morphine 4022, (7) methamphetamine 3728, (8) methadone 3495, (9) hydrocodone 3274, and (10) diazepam 1729.

The FD&C Act defines drugs, in part, by their intended use, as *"articles intended for use in the diagnosis, cure, mitigation, treatment, or prevention of disease" and "articles (other than food) intended to affect the structure or any function of the body of man or other animals"* [FD&C Act, sec. 201(g)(1)] (FDA, 2016). *Pharmaceutical agents* required by law to be prescribed to patients are called prescription drugs. However, over the years there have been an escalating number of products available to treat various ailments for which a written prescription is not necessary. This latter group of compounds is termed over-the-counter (OTC) or nonprescription drugs. OTC drugs are believed to be relatively safe and effective in the view of the general public simply because regulatory agencies allow these drugs to be sold without medical advice. It is the popular belief that if a drug needs to be prescribed then it must be regulated, as there are inherent adverse effects. However, the public does not know that many of these OTC products have not undergone extensive clinical testing and may not be safe. Although it may be laudable to treat serious illnesses and make available the compounds that are prescribed and required for these purposes, one must question the trend toward easy access of an uneducated public to more OTC drugs that are self-administered and have not undergone proper testing.

It is safe to assume with respect to OTC drugs that the public:

i. Is generally overwhelmed and confused by the wide array of products available
ii. Probably uses those that are most heavily advertised
iii. Uses these drugs inadvertently and inappropriately in some cases
iv. May be subjected to adverse effects (Kacew, 1999)

A paradox exists with respect to public awareness and drug use. An increased awareness of adverse drug effects has led to a decrease in the use of prescription drugs during pregnancy (De Jongvan den Berg et al., 1992, 1993). However, because of the perception that OTC drugs are safe, there was a disproportionate rise in the quantity of OTC self-administered medications such as laxatives, nonsteroidal anti-inflammatory drugs (NSAIDs), cold remedies, and vitamins. From an epidemiological point of view, the population most at risk for adverse effects from OTC drugs are children, resulting from the absence of safety caps, attractive packages, and administration of overdoses by parents. It is worthwhile to note that Kacew (1992, 1997) clearly demonstrated that pharmacokinetics and pharmacodynamics are different between children and adults, with differences associated to variation in the responsiveness to drugs. Thus, prediction of therapeutic effectiveness based on adult data may lead to grave consequences in children (Kogan et al., 1994; Smith and Kogan, 1997).

## Over-the-counter medicines and toxicities

In 1989, the American public spent approximately $10 billion on an estimated 300,000 OTC products to medicate themselves for self-diagnosed ailments ranging from acne to warts, colds, headaches, upset stomach, or constipation (Koda-Kimble, 1992). These 300,000 products represent approximately 700 active ingredients in various forms and combinations.

It is thus apparent that many are no more than "me too" products advertised to the public in ways that suggest that there are significant differences between them. The American public spent almost $2 billion per year on cough and cold remedies (Rosendahl, 1998). There are more than 800 OTC preparations for the common cold (Lowenstein and Parrino, 1987), over 100 for treatment of diarrhea (Dukes, 1990), over 200 different systemic analgesic products, almost all of which contain aspirin, acetaminophen, salicylamide, phenacetin, ibuprofen, or a combination of these agents as primary ingredients (Leist and Banwell, 1974). OTC drugs can be made different from one another in the following ways:

i. Addition of questionable ingredients such as caffeine or antihistamines
ii. Creation of an identity by brand names chosen to suggest a specific use of strength ("feminine pain," "arthritis," "maximum," "extra")
iii. Indication of their special dosage form (enteric-coated tablets, liquids, sustained-release products, powder, seltzers, etc.)

Hence, the consumer could utilize a product without the realization that an analgesic agent was being ingested (Kacew, 1994).

In 2015, the OTC category in the United States is about $40 billion in size and grew by about 2.8% during 2014 (IRI, 2015). The top five categories within OTC contribute about 72% of total OTC sales: respiratory ($7.7B), analgesics ($4.7B), oral care ($4.2B), gastrointestinal ($4.2B), and eye care ($1.7B) (CHPA, 2016). In addition, it is estimated that to alleviate symptoms of diseases, 8 in 10 consumers use OTC medicines without seeing a health-care professional.

### Excipients and OTC usage

OTC preparations also contain excipients and/or inactive ingredients such as dyes, sweeteners, flavorings, or preservatives. The so-called "hidden ingredients" in OTC products may on their own initiate adverse effects or potentiate the actions of the active components (Golightly et al., 1998; Kumar et al., 1993). The findings that excipients produce adverse effects, including skin disorders, gastrointestinal upset, and cardiovascular abnormalities, clearly indicate that OTC drugs should not be used merely due to the improper perception of safety from adverse effects.

The enormity and severity of OTC drug usage in our society has received little, if any, attention. In addition to the economics, it has been estimated that 70% of illnesses, predominantly in the adult population, are treated with OTC agents (Knapp and Knapp, 1972; Conn, 1991; Chrischelles et al., 1992). However, of greater concern is the fact that 48–63% of children, a population known to be far more susceptible to drug-induced adverse effects (Lock and Kacew, 1988; Kacew, 1997) received OTC drugs during a 2-week period (Dunnell and Cartwright, 1972; Kovar, 1994) and that approximately 40% of these children received at least two preparations (Kogan et al., 1994; Smith and Kogan, 1997). Due to serious adverse events and infant deaths associated with OTC cough and cold remedies, there are suggestions that the OTC drugs should not be given to infants and very young children (Rimsza and Newberry, 2008; Vassilev et al., 2010).

## *Nonsteroidal anti-inflammatory drugs*

Nonsteroidal anti-inflammatory drugs (NSAIDs) are the most commonly medicated drugs available by OTC or prescription. In the United States, more than 100 million NSAID prescriptions are written annually, excluding OTC NSAIDs and aspirin (Laine, 2001). NSAIDs are used to alleviate fever, inflammation, and pain associated with headaches, toothache, arthritis, menstrual cramps, colds, sports injuries, and many other illnesses. Adverse reactions of NSAIDs are produced in various organs such as the gastrointestinal (GI) tract, liver, kidney, brain, skin, heart, and lung. It is estimated that GI toxicity related to NSAID use causes more than 100,000 hospitalizations and more than 16,000 deaths per year in the United States, mostly as a consequence of upper GI tract bleeding (Singh, 1998; Wolf, 1999). To minimize GI toxicity (bleeding and ulcer) due to medication of NSAIDs, GI risk factors (caffeine-containing drinks, smoking, alcohol, irritating diet, stress, steroids, high and chronic intake of NSAIDs, and concomitant intake of multiple NSAIDs) should be avoided (Dhikav et al., 2003). The adverse effects of some NSAIDs (aspirin, acetaminophen, ibuprofen) are described below (Table 29.1).

### *Aspirin*

Aspirin (acetylsalicylic acid, ASA) is one of the most commonly used NSAIDs. However, the use of ASA has declined significantly as it has been replaced with acetaminophen because of a typical adverse effect, observed in children taking ASA, called "*Reye syndrome,*" a rare, acute, and sometimes fatal encephalopathy (Arrowsmith et al., 1987; Casteels-Van Daele et al., 2000). A case of fetal death was reported in a 17-year-old, 37-week-pregnant girl who had ingested aspirin daily for 1 month (Palatnick and Tenenbein,

***Table 29.1*** Adverse effects for some NSAIDs

| NSAIDs | Adverse effects | Reference |
|---|---|---|
| APAP | • Hepatotoxicity, nephrotoxicity<br>• GI toxicity, pacreatic toxicity (pancreatitis)<br>• CNS stimulation and then depression<br>• Hematotoxicity (pancytopenia) | McGill et al., 2012; Jóźwiak-Bebenista and Nowak, 2014; Mohammad et al., 2014 |
| Aspirin | • Hypersensitivity, hemolysis<br>• GI ulceration, nephrotoxicity | Krause et al., 1992; Ymer et al., 2015 |
| Celecoxib | • Cardiovascular toxicity (myocardial infarction, heart failure) | Chau-In et al., 2012; Gong et al., 2012 |
| Diclofenac | • GI toxicity including bleeding<br>• Anorexia<br>• Skin reactions (dryness, rash, pruritus) | Zimmerman et al., 1995; Rostom et al., 2005; Gan, 2010; Nair & Taylor-Gjevre, 2010; Peterson et al., 2010; TGA, 2014 |
| Ibuprofen | • Nephrotoxicity, hematemesis<br>• Peptic ulcer, heart failure<br>• GI bleeding, rash, tinnitus<br>• Optical neuritis | Tsokos and Schmoldt, 2001; Yang et al., 2008; Bushra and Aslam, 2010; Peterson et al., 2010 |
| Ketoprofen | • Bronchospasm, peptic ulceration<br>• Renal insufficiency<br>• Hepatotoxicity, GI toxicity | Green, 2001; Lees et al., 2004; Junot et al., 2008; Mustonen, 2012 |
| Nafroxen | • Myocardial infarctions and strokes<br>• Renal dysfunction, Hepatotoxicity<br>• Hypertension, ulceration | Duggan et al., 2010; NAVC, 2012; Bhala et al., 2013 |
| Piroxicam | • Hepatotoxicity<br>• GI toxicity | JFC, 2013; LiverTox, 2016 Stephen et al., 1982 |
| Rofecoxib | • Cardiotoxicity, hepatotoxicity<br>• GI toxicity | Langman et al., 1999; Loewen, 2002; LiverTox, 2016 |

1998). Autopsy of the fetus revealed petechiae of the lungs, heart, thymus, and kidneys. Aspirin is not contraindicated for treatment of headaches during pregnancy (Underhill, 1994), but it is stressed that aspirin and other NSAID products should be avoided during the third trimester (Bonati et al., 1990; Koren et al., 1998). It is of interest that ingestion of aspirin during the first 20 weeks of gestation does not significantly affect IQ at 4 years of age (Klebanoff and Berendes, 1988). These confusing messages are relayed to the public with the recommendation that even though aspirin can be taken safely during pregnancy, paracetamol has been recommended as the drug of choice. The mechanism underlying ASA-induced hemolytic anemia is related to glucose-6-phosphate-dehydrogenase (G-6-PD) inhibition by salicylate and gentisate (2,5-dihydroxybenzoic acid, an ASA metabolite) (Shahidi and Westring, 1970). Such an inhibition would further curtail NADPH regeneration, rendering the cells more vulnerable to oxidants. In principle, aspirin detoxification strategies aim to

1. *Decrease absorption of drugs*—Activated charcoal, emetics, and gastric lavage
2. *Enhance excretion*—Ion trapping (alkalinize urine), forced diuresis, hemodialysis
3. *Administer antidote*—No specific antidote, but correct any fluid for rehydration, electrolyte or metabolic imbalance
4. *Take supportive measures I*—Ion trapping (alkalinize urine), forced diuresis, hemodialysis if necessary
5. *Take supportive measures II*—Mechanical ventilation, blood pressure support, seizure medications

#### *Acetaminophen*

Since the declining use of ASA, poisoning cases with APAP have exceeded those of other NSAIDs due to increased use of acetaminophen (*N*-acetyl-para-aminophenol, APAP, paracetamol). APAP toxicity was recorded as the single most common cause of liver failure in the United States and United Kingdom, and associated with nearly 500 fatalities per year (Davern et al., 2006). APAP in humans produces various adverse effects such as hepatotoxicity, nephrotoxicity, cardiotoxicity, esophageal toxicity, pancreatic toxicity, hematotoxicity, and muscular toxicity. APAP is metabolized by CYP2E1 and CYP3A to the reactive intermediate NAPQI (*N*-acetyl-*p*-benzoquinone imine), which binds to mitochondrial proteins and leads to mitochondrial oxidative stress, hepatocyte necrosis, and liver failure. Overdose of APAP is associated with GSH depletion and free radical generation (McGill et al., 2012; Jóźwiak-Bebenista and Nowak, 2014; Mohammad et al., 2014). For ibuprofen, a NSAID considered relatively safe, the mechanism of acute toxicity is related to (1) decreased production of intrarenal prostaglandin (PG), (2) reduced renal blood flow, and (3) diminished glomerular filtration rate (GFR).

### *Estrogens*

It is worthwhile noting that during pregnancy, both mother and fetus are equally exposed to a chemical, but the risk of fetal toxicity far exceeds that of the mother or neonate (Kacew, 1997, 1999). Hence, the presumption of safety for the mother cannot be applied with certainty to the fetus. The hair cream Le Kair contains estrogens (Koda-Kimble, 1992) and presumably, if used appropriately does not produce toxicity. However, there have been reports that the use of estrogenic cosmetics resulted in gynecomastia in the child (Kacew, 1999). Although a correlation between estrogenic OTC products and fetal toxicity has not been examined, it is known that estrogens are teratogenic (Lock and Kacew, 1988; Safe, 1998). It should be noted that various foods are estrogenic (Safe, 1998) and thus the combination of certain foods and OTC products may potentially affect fetal development. This latter scenario is further compounded, as there are numerous environmental estrogenic contaminants to which a pregnant mother is inadvertently exposed on a daily basis (Shore et al., 1993). Since estrogens are lipophilic and accumulate in tissue fat, the potential for fetal exposure to excess estrogens is dependent on diet and environment. These compounds can certainly convert a relatively safe OTC into a toxic agent. Adverse effects for estrogen, testosterone, and corticosteroids are summarized in Table 29.2.

***Table 29.2*** Adverse effects for corticosteroids, estrogens, and testosterone

| Name | Adverse effects | Reference |
|---|---|---|
| Corticosteroids | • Osteoporosis, susceptibility to infection<br>• Cataract, glaucoma, weight gain, ischemia<br>• Na+ retention (edema, hypertension, heart failure)<br>• Moon face, loss of skin collagen<br>• Hyperglycemia, immunosupression<br>• Peptic ulcer, gastritis, ulcerative colitis | Korte, 2001; Donihi et al., 2006; Canalis, 2007; Aulakh and Singh, 2008; Ong et al., 2008; Hasselgren et al., 2010 |
| Estrogens (E2) | • Breast cancer, endometrial cancer<br>• Hypertension, hyperlipidemia<br>• Increase in HDL and decrease in LDL and cholesterol<br>• Myelotoxicity | Crane and Harris, 1978; Gapstur et al., 1999; Sontas et al., 2009; Soltysik and Czekaj, 2013 |
| Testosterone (T) | • Cardiovascular disease, prostate cancer<br>• Increase in Hb levels and serum erythropoietin, leading to erythrocytosis | Calof et al., 2005; Coviello et al., 2008; Corona et al., 2011; Grech et al., 2014 |

*Abbreviations:* DHT, dihydrotestosterone; Hb, hemoglobin.

## *Adverse consequences from medication*

As a general rule, all drugs, including OTC preparations, should be avoided whenever possible. High-risk subpopulations have been identified, including children and the elderly. Of even greater risk is the use of OTC during pregnancy where the fetus is the target (Hays and Pagliaro, 1987; Karboski, 1992) (Table 29.3). Although it is falsely perceived that OTC preparations are virtually without any adverse fetal consequences, the reverse may be the case.

Apart from the intrinsic toxicity of drugs, adverse effects and fatality may occur due to medication errors by health-care professionals (prescriber, pharmacist, nurse):

1. Prescription of wrong drugs or dosage
2. Illegible prescription, illegible handwriting
3. Inappropriate use of decimal points, use of abbreviations
4. Confusion with similar sounding drug names
5. Insufficient pharmacological knowledge of health professionals
6. Dispensing wrong drugs or dosage

***Table 29.3*** Over-the-counter preparations: Their adverse effects in susceptible populations

| Populations | OTC preparation | Adverse effects |
|---|---|---|
| Pregnant women | Aspirin | Fetal death with internal hemorrhage |
| | Cimetidine | Liver toxicity |
| | Imidazolines | Mental depression, hypertension, miosis |
| | Vitamin A | Spontaneous abortion, hydrocephalus, cardiac anomalies |
| | Vitamin D | Mental retardation, hemorrhage |
| | Vitamin K | Liver dysfunction |
| Infants | Loperamide | Paralytic ileus, persistent drowsiness |
| Geriatric patients | Saline laxatives | Hypotonia, CNS, and respiratory depression |
| | Bulk laxatives | Cramping, nausea, fluid loss, electrolyte imbalance |
| General | Hyperglycemic drugs and aspirin | Aggravation of diabetes |
| | Multivitamin preparation + iron | Interference of iron absorption |
| | Cimetidine + tea | Cimetidine interferes with metabolism of theophylline |

The medication errors can be reduced or are preventable by using computerized entire medication systems, automated dispensing systems, and barcode technology (van den Bemt et al., 2000). Further, all professionals (pharmacists, physicians, and nurses) involved in the medication process should have a good pharmacological knowledge and be trained for the use of the error-free system of medication (Krähenbühl-Melcher et al., 2007).

## *Fetal exposure to drugs during pregnancy*

As a result of pressure from the pharmaceutical industry, a number of prescribed drugs have been switched to OTC status (Fletcher et al., 1995). Although the effects of the antidiarrheal agent loperamide on fetal outcome have not been established, administration of this drug to infants produced paralytic ileus and persistent drowsiness in 20% of the cases (Motala et al., 1990). The recent inclusion of the antiulcerogenic histamine blocker, cimetidine, in the OTC list is a further example of a drug with potential effects on the fetus and easy public accessibility. The finding that cimetidine concentrations in neonatal plasma exceeded those in the mother's suggested that there was a substantial uptake by the fetus (Somogi and Gugler, 1983). The fact that cimetidine is known to inhibit hepatic microsomal enzymes and is reported to produce fetal liver toxicity when used in late pregnancy (Glode et al., 1980) indicates that self-administration of this drug for reflux esophagitis during pregnancy could have adverse consequences. This could be of particular concern if a pregnant epileptic mother with impaired liver function was to ingest cimetidine; plasma concentrations of anticonvulsants would be increased, with adverse consequences for the fetus. In patients who are taking tricyclic antidepressants for depression, cimetidine potentiates the actions of the antidepressant resulting in cardiovascular abnormalities, hallucinations, vomiting, and hypotension. In the elderly, cimetidine causes confusion, which could have dire consequences, as this population tends to be more forgetful.

A number of current OTC products are associated with adverse consequences. The industry has applied pressure to make certain drugs more accessible and, because of a presumed history of safety and the public perception that self-administered therapies will hasten recovery, even more compounds will be transferred from prescription to nonprescription status (Splinter et al., 1997). Consequently, a larger assortment of OTC drugs will be available to the pregnant mother and the geriatric population. Indeed, Rubin et al. (1993) reported that OTC preparations were used 1.5 times more often than prescription drugs during pregnancy; this figure is presumably underestimated because they failed to include vitamins in their study. It is disturbing to note that approximately 50% of products taken during pregnancy are OTC medications (Rayburn et al., 1982). With aging, there is also an increased use of drugs.

Clearly, some pregnant women are self-medicating themselves during a period of fetal vulnerability. Although it is stressed that pregnant women should not drink alcoholic beverages or smoke cigarettes, these activities still occur during pregnancy. Indeed, a study showed that the maternal characteristics associated with increased OTC medication use were Caucasian, smoking more than 20 cigarettes per day, and drinking alcohol (Buitendijk and Bracken, 1991). Hence, it is likely that despite warnings, pregnant women use OTC medications, the choice of which is expanding. An example of this problem arises with the use of imidazolines as topical vasoconstrictors for nasal decongestion. These compounds are used for sinusitis, colds, and allergic rhinitis, and are known to produce CNS depression, bradycardia, hypotension, and miosis (Liebelt and Shannon, 1993). There is a lack of clinical data regarding the use of these compounds in high-risk subpopulations, yet the potential for adverse effects is quite serious as these drugs produce vasoconstriction.

The misconception that frequent bowel movements are essential has resulted in the misuse of cathartics among some women, especially geriatric populations. Saline cathartic magnesium sulfate induces hypotonia, CNS, and respiratory depression. Bulk-forming laxatives produce cramping and nausea, and result in fluid loss and electrolyte imbalance. In patients with congestive heart failure, this type of OTC product is contraindicated.

### *Vitamins and minerals*

Ingestion of a proper diet is sufficient to provide the necessary requirement for vitamins and iron. However, the erroneous belief that vitamin supplements provide extra energy and create a feeling of "well-being" has resulted in the ingestion of quantities of vitamins vastly in excess of the recommended dietary allowance. This widespread nutritional self-medication promoted through effective massive advertising can have dire consequences in susceptible populations.

*Vitamin A* in the fetus is associated with spontaneous abortion, hydrocephalus, and cardiac anomalies, while in the adult there are menstrual irregularities, exophthalmos, and skin hyperpigmentation. With *vitamin D*, hypercalcemia occurs in the adult and is manifested by anorexia, fatigue, kidney dysfunction, and aortic stenosis. In the fetus, hypervitaminosis D results in elfin facies, mental retardation, and aortic stenosis. Liver dysfunction, jaundice, and hemorrhage occur as a result of excessive *vitamin K* intake. Excessive *iron* intake results in vomiting, cyanosis, and circulatory collapse. In the fetus, there are congenital anomalies and GIT

**Table 29.4** Adverse effects for some antibiotics

| Antibiotics | Adverse effects | References |
|---|---|---|
| Amoxicillin | • GI toxicity, nephrotoxicity<br>• Hematotoxicity<br>• Hypersensitivity (allergy) | Burke and Cunha, 2001; Lewis, 2013; Anderson, 2016 |
| Ampicillin | • GI toxicity, nephrotoxicity<br>• Hematotoxicity | Burke and Cunha, 2001; Lewis, 2013; Anderson, 2016 |
| Cephazolin | • GI toxicity, nephrotoxicity<br>• Hematotoxicity<br>• Neurotoxicity | Schwankhaus et al., 1985; Burke and Cunha, 2001; Lewis, 2013; Anderson, 2016 |
| Chloramphenicol | • Hematologic toxicity<br>• Anemia, pancytopenia | Burke and Cunha, 2001; Lewis, 2013 |
| Gentamycin | • Nephrotoxicity<br>• Neurotoxicity<br>• Ototoxicity | Burke and Cunha, 2001; Grill and Maganti, 2011; Lewis, 2013; Anderson, 2016 |
| Isoniazid | • Hematotoxicity<br>• Hepatic toxicity<br>• Peripheral neuropathy | Banerjee et al., 1994; Bruke and Cunha, 2001; Lewis, 2013; Anderson, 2016 |
| Neomycin | • Nephrotoxicity<br>• Neurotoxicity, ototoxicity | Burke and Cunha, 2001; Lewis, 2013; Anderson, 2016 |
| Pipemidic acid | • Cartilage toxicity insomnia,<br>• Photosensitivity | Linseman et al., 1995; Lewis, 2013; Anderson, 2016 |
| Rifampicin | • Hepatotoxicity, hemolytic anemia<br>• Pulmonary toxicity,<br>• Peripheral neuropathy | Burke and Cunha, 2001; Lewis, 2013; Anderson, 2016 |
| Sulfadiazine | • Hematotoxicity<br>• Photosensitivity, anorexia | Burke and Cunha, 2001; Lewis, 2013; Anderson, 2016 |
| Tetracycline | • Hepatic toxicity, neurotoxicity<br>• Discolored nails and teeth | Burke and Cunha, 2001; Lewis, 2013; Anderson, 2016 |
| Vancomycin | • Hematotoxicity, phlebitis<br>• Red man syndrome (flushing, hypotension, itching) | Burke and Cunha, 2001; Lewis, 2013; Anderson, 2016 |

upset. This reiterates the fact that essential nutritional OTC in excess is not safe. The use of OTC mixtures of vitamins and minerals is not effective in abolishing iron deficiency anemia and this practice should be discouraged. Although there is an increased demand for iron in pregnancy, the prophylactic use of iron to correct any deficiency should be carried out with caution.

An issue that still remains to be considered is the interaction between two OTC preparations or between a prescribed medication and an OTC preparation. In a situation where a mother is being treated for a peptic ulcer with cimetidine, it is conceivable that there is simultaneous consumption of large quantities of tea (theophylline). Cimetidine, by preventing the metabolism of theophylline, results in increased theophylline concentrations and potentially a higher risk of toxicity. Aspirin displaces oral hypoglycemic agents from protein-binding sites, which can lead to severe manifestations in diabetes. Another example is the ingestion of iron to correct iron-deficiency anemia. If the mother is ingesting iron plus a multivitamin preparation, the latter preparation interferes with iron absorption. Consequently, less iron is available and the hematological response is impaired. The omnipresence of OTC preparations and concerted advertising may be a fact of life; however, increased awareness of the dangers associated with the use of self-medication must be stressed (Table 29.3).

### *Antibiotics*

Adverse effects of some antibiotics are briefly summarized in Table 29.4. Although adverse effects produced by antibiotics are different, GI toxicity (abdominal pain, nausea, vomiting, gastritis, etc.), hepatotoxicity, nephrotoxicity, hematotoxicity, and neurotoxicity are commonly observed.

## References

Anderson L (2016). Common Side Effects, Allergies and Reactions to Antibiotics. Available at: https://www.drugs.com/article/antibiotic-sideeffects-allergies-reactions.html.

Arrowsmith JB, Kennedy DL, Kuritsky JN, Faich GA (1987). National patterns of aspirin use and Reye syndrome reporting, United States, 1980 to 1985. *Pediatrics.* 79, 858–63.

Aulakh R, Singh S (2008). Strategies for minimizing corticosteroid toxicity: A review. *Indian J Pediatr.* 75(10), 1067–73.

Banerjee A, Dubnau E et al. (1994). inhA, a gene encoding a target for isoniazid and ethionamide in Mycobacterium tuberculosis. *Science.* 1994; 263(5144), 227–30.

Bhal N et al. (2013). Vascular and upper gastrointestinal effects of non-steroidal anti-inflammatory drugs: Meta-analyses of individual participant data from randomised trials. *Lancet.* 382(9894), 769–79.

Bonati M, Bortolus R, Machetti F et al. (1990). Drug use in pregnancy: An overview of epidemiological (drug utilization) studies. *Eur J Clin Pharmacol.* 38, 325–8.

Buitendijk S, Bracken MB (1991). Medication in early pregnancy: Prevalence of use and relationship to maternal characteristics. *Am J Obstet Gynecol.* 165, 33–40.

Burke A, Cunha MD (2001). Antibiotic side effects. *Med Clin North Am.* 85(1), 149–85.

Bushra R, Aslam N (2010). An overview of clinical pharmacology of Ibuprofen. *Oman Med J.* 25(3), 155–66.

Calof O, Singh A, Lee M, Kenny A et al. (2005). Adverse events associated with testosterone replacement in middle-aged and older men: A meta-analysis of randomized, placebo-controlled trials. *J Gerontol.* 60, 1451–7.

Canalis E, Mazziotti G, Giustina A, Bilezikian JP (2007). Glucocorticoid-induced osteoporosis: Pathophysiology and therapy. *Osteoporos Int.* 18, 1319–28.

Casteels-Van Daele M, Van Geet C, Wouters C, Eggermont E (2000). Reye syndrome revisited: A descriptive term covering a group of heterogeneous disorders. *Eur J Pediatr.* 159, 641–8.

Chau-In W et al. (2012). Analgesic effects of celecoxib following total abdominal hysterectomy. *Clin Trials.* 2, 3.

CHPA (Consumer Healthcare Products Association) (2016). Statistics on OTC Use. Available at: http://www.chpa.org/MarketStats.aspx.

Chrischelles EA, Foley DJ, Wallace RB et al. (1992). Use of medications by persons 65 and over; data from the established populations for epidemiologic studies of the elderly. *J Gerontol.* 47, M137–44.

Conn VS (1991). Older adults: Factors that predict the use of over-the-counter medication. *J Adv Nurs.* 16, 1190–6.

Corona G, Rastrelli G, Vignozzi L et al. (2011). Testosterone, cardiovascular disease and the metabolic syndrome. *Best Pract Res Clin Endocrinol Metab.* 25, 337–53.

Coviello A et al. (2008). Effects of graded doses of testosterone on erythropoiesis in healthy young and older men. *J Clin Endocrinol Metab.* 93, 914–9.

Crane MG, Harris JJ (1978). Estrogens and hypertension: Effect of discontinuing estrogens on blood pressure, exchangeable sodium, and the renin-aldosterone system. *Am J Med Sci.* 276, 33–55.

Davern TJ, James LP, Hinson JA et al. (2006). Measurement of serum acetaminophen-protein adducts in patients with acute liver failure: Acute liver failure study group. *Gastroenterology.* 130, 687–94.

De Jong-van den Berg LTW, Van Den Berg PB, Haaijer-Ruskamp FM et al. (1992). Handling of risk-bearing drugs during pregnancy: Do we choose less risky alternatives? *Pharm Weekbl Sci.* 14, 38–45.

De Jong-van den Berg LTW, Waardenburg CM, Haaijer-Ruskamp FM et al. (1993). Drug use in pregnancy: A comparative appraisal of data collecting methods. *Eur J Clin Pharmacol.* 45, 9–14.

Dhikav V, Singh S, Pande S et al. (2003). Non-steroidal drug-induced gastrointestinal toxicity: Mechanisms and management. *J Ind Acad Clin Med.* 4, 315–22.

Donihi AC et al. (2006). Prevalence and predictors of corticosteroid-related hyperglycemia in hospitalized patients. *Endocr Pract.* 12 (4), 358–62.

Duggan et al. (2010). Molecular basis for cyclooxygenase inhibition by the nonsteroidal anti-inflammatory drug naproxen. *J Biol Chem.* 285(45), 34950–9.

Dukes GE (1990). Over-the-counter antidiarrheal medications used for the self-treatment of acute non-specific diarrhea. *Am J Med.* 88, 24S–6S.

Dunnell K, Cartwright A, eds. (1972). *Medicine Takers, Prescribers and Hoarders.* New York: Routledge and Kegan Paul.

FDA (U.S. Food and Drug Administration) (2016). Is It a Cosmetic, a Drug, or Both? (Or Is It Soap?) Available at: http://www.fda.gov/Cosmetics/GuidanceRegulation/LawsRegulations/ucm074201.htm.

Fletcher P, Stephen R, Du Pont H (1995). Benefit/risk considerations with respect to OTC descheduling of loperamide. *Arzeimittelforschung* 45, 608–13.

Gan TJ (2010). Diclofenac: An update on its mechanism of action and safety profile. *Curr Med Res Opin.* 26(7), 1715–31.

Gapstur SM, Morrow M, and Sellers TA (1999). Hormone replacement therapy and risk of breast cancer with a favorable histology: Results of the Iowa women's health study. *JAMA.* 281, 2091–7.

Glode G, Saccar CL, Pereira GR (1980). Cimetidine in pregnancy and apparent transient liver impairment in the newborn. *Am J Dis Child.* 134, 87–8.

Golightly LK, Smolinske SS, Bennett ML et al. (1998). Pharmaceutical excipients: Adverse effects associated with "inactive" ingredients in drug products (Part II). *Concepts Toxicol Rev.* 3, 209–40.

Gong L (2013). Celecoxib pathways: Pharmacokinetics and pharmacodynamics. *Pharmacogenet Genomics.* 22(4), 310–8.

Grech A, Breck J, Heidelbaugh J (2014). Adverse effects of testosterone replacement therapy: An update on the evidence and controversy. *Ther Adv Drug Saf.* 5, 190–200.

Green GA (2001). Understanding NSAIDs: From aspirin to COX-2. *Clin Cornerstone Sport Med.* 3, 50–9.

Grill MF, Maganti RK (2011). Neurotoxic effects associated with antibiotic use: Management considerations. *Br J Clin Pharmacol.* 72(3), 381–93.

Hasselgren PO et al. (2010). Corticosteroids and muscle wasting role of transcription factors, nuclear cofactors, and hyperacetylation. *Curr Opin Clin Nutr Metab Care.* 13(4), 423–8.

Hays DP, Pagliaro LA (1987). Human teratogens. In: Pagliaro LA, Pagliaro AM, eds. *Problems in Pediatric Drug Therapy.* Hamilton, IL: Drug Intelligence Publications, pp. 51–191.

IRI (Information Resources, Inc.) (2016). Available at: https://www.iriworldwide.com/.

JFC (Joint Formulary Committee) (2013). British national formulary (BNF) (65 ed.). London, UK: Pharmaceutical Press, p. 665, pp. 673–4.

Jóźwiak-Bebenista M, Nowak JZ (2014). Paracetamol: Mechanism of action, applications and safety concern. *Acta Pol Pharm.* 71(1), 11–23.

Junot S et al. (2008). Renal effect of meloxicam versus ketoprofen in anaesthetized pseudo-normovolaemic piglets. *CJPP.* 86, 55–63.

Kacew S (1992). General principles in pharmacology and toxicology applicable to children. In: Guzelian PS, Henry CJ, Olin SS, eds. *Similarities and Differences Between Children and Adults.* Washington, DC: ILSI Press.

Kacew S (1994). Fetal consequences and risks attributed to the use of over-the-counter (OTC) preparations during pregnancy. *Int J Clin Pharmacol Ther.* 32, 335–43.

Kacew S (1997). General principles in pediatric pharmacology and toxicology. In: Kacew S, Lambert GH, eds. *Environmental Toxicology and Pharmacology of Human Development*. Washington, DC: Taylor & Francis.

Kacew S (1999). Effect of over-the-counter drugs on the unborn child. *Pediatr Drugs*. 1, 75–80.

Karboski JA (1992). Medication selection for pregnant women. *Drug Ther.* 22, 53–61.

Klebanoff MA, Berendes HW (1988). Aspirin exposure during the first 20 weeks of gestation and IQ at four years of age. *Teratology*. 37, 249–55.

Knapp DA, Knapp DE (1972). Decision-making and self-medication between medication and preliminary findings. *Am J Hosp Pharm*. 29, 1004–12.

Koda-Kimble MA (1992). Therapeutic and toxic potential of over-the-counter agents. In: Katzung BG, ed. *Basic and Clinical Pharmacology*. Norwalk, CT: Appleton and Lange.

Kogan MD, Pappas G, Yu SM et al. (1994). Over-the-counter medication use among pre-school aged children in the United States. *J Am Med Assoc*. 272, 1025–30.

Koren G, Pastuszak A, Ito S (1998). Drugs in pregnancy. *N Engl J Med*. 338, 1128–37.

Korte SM (2001). Corticosteroids in relation to fear, anxiety and psychopathology. *Neurosci Biobehav Rev*. 25(2), 117–42.

Kovar MG (1994). Use of medications and vitamin-mineral supplements by children and youths. *Public Health Rep*. 100, 470–3.

Krähenbühl-Melcher A, Schlienger R, Lampert M et al. (2007). Drug-related problems in hospitals: A review of the recent literature. *Drug Saf.* 30(5), 379–407.

Krause DS et al. (1992). Acute aspirin overdose: Mechanisms of toxicity. *Ther Drug Monit*. 14(6), 441–51.

Kumar A, Rawlings RD, Bearman DC (1993). The mystery ingredients: Sweeteners, flavorings, dyes, and preservatives in analgesic/antipyretic, antihistamine/decongestant, liquid theophylline preparations. *Pediatrics*. 91, 927–33.

Laine L (2001). Approaches to nonsteroidal anti-inflammatory drug use in the high-risk patient. *Gastroenterology*. 120, 594–606.

Langman et al. (1999). Adverse upper gastrointestinal effects of rofecoxib compared with NSAIDs. *JAMA*. 282(20), 1929–33.

Lees P (2004). Pharmacodynamics and pharmacokinetics of nonsteroidal anti-inflammatory drugs in species of veterinary interest. *J Vet Pharmacol The*. 27, 479–90.

Leist ER, Banwell JG (1974). Products containing aspirin. *N Engl J Med*. 291, 710–12.

Lewis K (2013). Platforms for antibiotic discovery. *Nat Rev Drug Discov*. 12(5), 371–87.

Liebelt EL, Shannon M (1993). Small doses, big problems: A selected review of highly toxic common medications. *Pediatr Emerg Care*. 9, 292–7.

Linseman DA, Hampton LA, Branstetter DG (1995). Quinolone-induced arthropathy in the neonatal mouse. Morphological analysis of articular lesions produced by pipemidic acid and ciprofloxacin. *Fundam Appl Toxicol*. 28(1), 59–64.

LiverTox (2016). Clinical and Research Information on Drug-Induced Liver Injury. NLM (U.S. National Library of Medicine). Available at: https://livertox.nlm.nih.gov//Piroxicam.htm, https://livertox.nlm.nih.gov//Rofecoxib.htm.

Lock S, Kacew S (1988). General principles in pediatric pharmacology and toxicology. In: Kacew S, Lock S, eds. *Toxicologic and Pharmacologic Principles in Pediatrics*. Washington, DC: Hemisphere Publishing, pp. 1–15.

Loewen PS (2002). Review of the selective COX-2 inhibitors celecoxib and rofecoxib: Focus on clinical aspects. *CJEM*. 4(4), 268–75.
Lowenstein SR, Parrino TA (1987). Management of common cold. *Adv Intern Med*. 32, 207–34.
McGill MR (2012). The mechanism underlying acetaminophen-induced hepatotoxicity in humans and mice involves mitochondrial damage and nuclear DNA fragmentation. *J Clin Invest*. 122(4), 1574–83.
Mohammad S et al. (2014). The effect of intravenous paracetamol on postoperative pain after lumbar discectomy. *Asian Spine J*. 8(4), 400–4.
Motala C, Hill ID, Mann MD et al. (1990). Effect of loperamide on stool output and duration of acute infectious diarrhea in infants. *J Pediatr*. 117, 467–71.
Mustonen K (2012). Pharmacology of ketoprofen administered orally to pigs: An experimental and clinical study. Department of Equine and Small Animal Medicine University of Helsinki, Finland.
Nair B, Taylor-Gjevre R, (2010). A review of topical diclofenac use in musculoskeletal disease. *Pharmaceuticals (Basel)*. 11; 3(6), 1892–908.
NIDA (National Institute on Drug Abuse) (2016). Overdose Death Rates. Available at: https://www.drugabuse.gov/related-topics/trends-statistics/overdose-death-rates.
Ong SL, Zhang Y, Whitworth JA (2008). Reactive oxygen species and glucocorticoid-induced hypertension. *Clin Exp Pharmacol Physiol*. 35, 477–82.
Palatnick W, Tenenbein M (1998). Aspirin poisoning during pregnancy: Increased fetal sensitivity. *Am J Perinatol*. 15, 39–41.
Peterson K et al. (2010). Drug Class Review: Nonsteroidal Antiinflammatory Drugs (NSAIDs): Final Update 4 Report [Internet]. Portland (OR): Oregon Health & Science University; 2010.
Rayburn W, Wible-Kaut J, Bledsoe P (1982). Changing trends in drug use during pregnancy. *J Reprod Med*. 27, 569–75.
Rimsza ME, Newberry S (2008). Unexpected infant deaths associated with use of cough and cold medications. *Pediatr*. 122, 318–22.
Rosendahl I (1998). Expense of physician care spurs OTC, self-care market. *Drug Top*. 132, 62–3.
Rostom A et al. (2005). Nonsteroidal anti-inflammatory drugs and hepatic toxicity: A systematic review of randomized controlled trials in arthritis patients. *Clin Gastroenterol Hepatol*. 3, 489–98.
Rubin JP, Ferencz C, Loffredo C (1993). Use of prescription and nonprescription drugs in pregnancy. *J Clin Epidemiol*. 46, 581–9.
Safe S (1998). Dietary estrogens: An overview (abstract). *J Toxicol Sci*. 42, 352.
Schwankhaus JD, Masucci EF, Kurtzke JF (1985). Cefazolin-induced encephalopathy in a uremic patient. *Ann Neurol*. 17, 211.
Shahidi NT, Westring DW (1970). Acetylsalicylic acid-induced hemolysis and its mechanism. *J Clin Invest*. 49, 1334–40.
Shore LS, Gurevitz M, Shemesh M (1993). Estrogen, an environmental pollutant. *Bull Environ Contam Toxicol*. 51, 361–6.
Singh G (1998). Recent considerations in nonsteroidal anti-inflammatory drug gastropathy. *Am J Med*. 105, 31S–38S.
Smith MBH, Kogan MD (1997). Over-the-counter medication use and toxicity in children. In: Kacew S, Lambert GH, eds. *Environmental Toxicology and Pharmacology of Human Development*. Washington, DC: Taylor & Francis.

Soltysik K, Czekaj P (2013). Membrane estrogen receptors—Is it an alternative way of estrogen action? *J Physiol Pharmacol.* 64(2), 129–42.
Somogi A, Gugler R (1983). Clinical pharmacokinetics of cimetidine. *Clin Pharmacokinet.* 8, 463–95.
Sontas HB, Dokuzeylu B, Turna O et al. (2009). Estrogen-induced myelotoxicity in dogs: A review. *CVJ.* 50(10), 1054.
Splinter M, Sagraves R, Nightengale B et al. (1997). Prenatal use of medications by women giving birth at a university hospital. *South Med J.* 90, 498–502.
Stephen LD et al. (1982). Pharmacology, clinical efficacy, and adverse effects of piroxicam, a new nonsteroidal anti-inflammatory agent. *Pharmacotherapy.* 2, 80–9.
TGA (Therapeutic Goods Administration) (2014). Therapeutic Goods Administration. Version 2.1, October.
Tsokos M, Schmoldt A (2001). Contribution of nonsteroidal anti-inflammatory drugs to death associated with peptic ulcer disease: A prospective toxicological analysis of autopsy blood samples. *Arch Patholg Lab Med.* 125(12), 1572–4.
Underhill R (1994). OTC products (correspondence). *Pharm J.* 253, 112.
van den Bemt PM, Egberts TC, de Jong-van den Berg LT et al. (2000). Drug-related problems in hospitalised patients. *Drug Saf.* 22(4), 321–33.
Vassilev ZP, Kabadi S, Villa R (2010). Safety and efficacy of over-the-counter cough and cold medicines for use in children. *Expert Opin Drug Saf.* 9, 233–42.
Warner M, Trinidad JP, Bastian BA (2016). National Vital Statistics Reports. Drugs Most Frequently Involved in Drug Overdose Deaths: United States, 2010–2014. 65:10.
Wolfe MM, Lichtenstein D, Singh G (1999). Gastrointestinal toxicity of nonsteroidal anti-inflammatory drugs. *N Engl J Med.* 340(24), 1888–99.
Xu J, Sherry L, Murphy BS et al. (2016). National Vital Statistics Reports. Deaths: Final Data for 2013. CDC (Centers for Disease Control and Prevention). 64(2). Available at: https://www.cdc.gov/nchs/data/nvsr/nvsr64/nvsr64_02.pdf.
Yang ZF et al. (2008). Possible arrhythmiogenic mechanism produced by ibuprofen. *Acta Pharmacol Sin.* 29(4), 421–9.
Ymer HM et al. (2015). New insights into the mechanisms of action of aspirin and its use in the prevention and treatment of arterial and venous thromboembolism. *Ther Clin Risk Manag.* 11, 1449–56.
Zimmerman J et al. (1995). Upper gastrointestinal hemorrhage associated with cutaneous application of diclofenac gel. *Am J Gastroenterol.* 90(11), 2032–4.

# chapter thirty

# Risk assessment and regulatory toxicology

**Seok Kwon and Byung-Mu Lee**

Contents

## Introduction

As described in Chapter 1, one of the most important goals of toxicology is to protect humans and ecosystems from hazardous substances. Toxic substances such as biological agents (e.g., microorganisms), chemicals, and physical agents (e.g., radiation, temperature, sound) differ greatly in the nature and potency of their toxicity. Because human exposure to these agents (individual or mixture) is not always avoidable, risk assessments need to be carried out to determine the allowable safe level of exposure under which no risk is likely to occur. Comprehensive reviews evaluating the procedure and methodology of risk assessments are available (Paustenbach, 2000; Song et al., 2013). In principle, the critical point for the safety and risk assessment of chemicals is the protection of human and ecosystem health, and therefore conservative approaches or options need to be considered because of gaps in our toxicological knowledge. However, when undue caution or emotional factors are incorporated into the process, chemicals of great value may be willfully ignored under public pressure and society may be burdened with unnecessary economic costs resulting from pollution prevention measures and environmental cleanups. Therefore, the most important function of toxicology is to establish the scientific basis for regulating the use (and disposal) of chemicals without undue human health hazards or undue cost based on risk assessment.

## Principles of risk assessment and regulation

In order to regulate hazardous substances to protect human health, national or international regulatory agencies have to rely on risk assessment results. Therefore, the principles and methodologies for risk assessment are important and need to be prepared scientifically using toxicological data and human exposure. Depending upon the toxicological endpoints of chemicals or physical agents, three different types of risk assessment methods can be applied to carcinogens, noncarcinogens, and skin sensitizers.

In the United States, the first Federal Food and Drugs Act (FFDA) was enacted in 1906: *For preventing the manufacture, sale, or transportation of adulterated or misbranded or poisonous or deleterious foods, drugs, medicines, and liquors, and for regulating traffic therein, and for other purposes.* Similar action was taken in several other countries. At that time, health hazards were based essentially on *qualitative* assessment; the mere presence of a toxic substance in food was considered adulteration and "adulterated" food was banned outright.

To permit the judicious use of food additives, Lehman and Fitzhugh (1954) of the U.S. Food and Drug Administration initiated a *quantitative* assessment by the use of a "100-fold margin of safety" approach. This assessment of food additives stipulated that "the chemical additive should not occur in the total human diet in a quantity greater than 1/100 of the amount that is the maximum safe dosage in long-term animal experiments."

Although this margin of 100 seemed reasonable for food additives, it could not be applied to other chemicals, such as contaminants and pesticide residues, whose levels in food are not readily controllable. In 1961, the Joint Food and Agricultural Organization/World Health Organization (FAO/WHO) Expert Committee on Food Additives (JECFA) therefore coined the term *acceptable daily intake* (ADI). Later that year, this term was adopted by the Joint FAO/WHO Meeting on Pesticide Residues.

In 1977, the U.S. National Research Council (NRC) extended the concept to the assessment of contaminants in water, and the Environmental Protection Agency (EPA) extended it to pollutants in air, with a slight variation in terminology.

In carcinogenic chemicals the Delaney Amendment of 1958 to the Federal Food, Drug, and Cosmetic Act stipulates *"any chemical that has been shown to be carcinogenic in man or animal shall not be used as a food additive."* For other chemicals such as veterinary drugs, the concept of "negligible residues" was introduced to regulate carcinogenic chemicals. As will be seen in subsequent sections, these measures were no panacea. Mathematical models were then devised to estimate doses that could be considered as "virtually safe" (Mantel and Bryan, 1961).

NRC (1983) divided the management of risk assessment into the following steps:

1. *Hazard identification*: Scrutinizing all relevant toxicological and related data to identify the hazard associated with a chemical.
2. *Dose–response assessment*: Determining the relationship between the magnitude of exposure and probability of adverse health effects.
3. *Exposure assessment*: Determining the extent of human exposure either by environmental monitoring (e.g., air, water, food, soil, consumer products) or biological monitoring.
4. *Risk characterization*: Estimating the nature and magnitude of human risk, and the uncertainty of the estimate. Basically, the risk estimation can be obtained by the function of *Potential Human Hazard and Human Exposure. Risk = Hazard × Exposure (Dose).*

The terminology used for risk assessment was published by WHO (2004) and EPA (2006, 2012) as summarized in Appendix 30.1.

## Thresholds and risk assessment approaches

There are threshold doses below which chemicals do not elicit adverse effects for a majority of these agents. These chemicals are noncarcinogenic agents and there are a variety of reasons for which thresholds exist. The chemical in question may not reach the site of action because of its limited absorption and distribution or prompt elimination. Metabolic detoxification often plays an important role. Further, repair and regeneration of affected cells and excess functional capacity may overcome/compensate any minor, temporary effects.

The "safety" of such chemicals can be estimated by using the "ADI" approach, which involves identification of the most sensitive, yet *appropriate,* indicator of adverse effect and the application of a suitable safety factor to the no-observed adverse effect level (NOAEL) to compensate for potential differences between animals and humans, and between the relatively small number of test subjects and a large human population which is more heterogeneous.

Genotoxic carcinogens, on the other hand, probably have no threshold doses. The rational is that a cancer cell can be induced by a single change in the cellular genetic material, and the cancer cell has the capacity of self-replicating. Therefore, theoretically, a single molecule of such a chemical can induce cancer. In the absence of threshold doses, it is not possible to identify a NOAEL, thus rendering the ADI approach impracticable. Mathematical models have been designed to estimate, from the dose–response relationship and a variety of assumptions, a *"virtually safe dose* (VSD)" exposure to which an extremely small risk, say $10^{-6}$ (1 extra cancer death per in 1 million people exposed) results.

## Regulatory safe limits (ADI, RfD) for risk assessment

### Definition and application

The term ADI was coined by the JECFA in 1961 (WHO, 1962a) and adopted by the Joint FAO/WHO Meeting of Experts on Pesticide Residues (WHO, 1962b). This term has been used at all subsequent meetings of these two international expert bodies in their toxicological evaluation, and reevaluation, of large numbers of food additives and pesticides that leave residues in food. The term has also been adopted by a number of other bodies in the toxicological evaluation of chemicals in food, water, and so on as a basis for setting standards, for example, the U.S. EPA (Cotruvos, 1988). The term tolerable daily intake (TDI) is similar to ADI by definition and also applied for contaminants and other chemicals used unintentionally.

ADI is defined as *"the daily intake of a chemical which, during an entire lifetime, appears to be without appreciable risk on the basis of all the known facts at the time."* It is expressed in milligrams of the chemical per kilogram of body weight (mg/kg). It is worth noting that the ADI is qualified by the expressions "appear to be" and "on the basis of all the known facts at the time." This caution is in keeping with the fact that it is not possible to be absolutely certain regarding the safety of a chemical and that ADI may be altered in light of new toxicological data.

Toxicological evaluations of food additives and pesticides, in terms of ADIs by these international expert bodies, have been employed by the regulatory agencies in many countries as an important consideration in the formulation of national regulations. ADIs have also been utilized collectively by national authorities in the framework of the Codex Alimentarius Commission. The Commission is an intergovernmental body with more than 150 countries as its members. Its principal function is to elaborate international food standards for the protection of the health of the consumer and facilitate international food trade. These food standards contain provisions for food additives that are accepted by the Commission only when ADIs have been allocated by the Expert Committee on Food Additives. The latter goal is achieved through the removal of "noneconomic" trade barriers based on unjustified claims of health hazards alleged to be associated with certain additives or pesticides.

There are a number of variations of the terminology. For instance, in dealing with food contaminants, the JECFA in 1972 coined the term *"provisional tolerable weekly intake* (PTWI)." The procedure used in arriving at such intakes is identical to that for ADIs. The JECFA Committee, however, felt that unlike food additives, which serves certain useful purposes, contaminants do not. Therefore they are not acceptable but merely "tolerable." Further, the intakes were expressed in terms of "weekly" because the contaminants dealt then (mercury, lead, and cadmium) were cumulative, and vary (especially mercury) in the *daily* intake, but less so on a *weekly* basis.

Another variation is used by U.S. EPA, which assesses *"Reference Doses* (RfDs)" instead of ADIs, by using essentially the same procedure, except that the safety factor is called *"uncertainty factor* (UF)." It might be noted that the term ADI is widely used on an international level as well as by regulatory agencies in many nations, including the U.S. FDA.

For noncarcinogenic compounds, risk assessment can be carried out as follows:

*Hazard index* (HI) = Chronic daily dose/safe limit (e.g., ADI, RfD, or TDI)

when the HI value is greater than 1, human exposure to a specified chemical is considered not safe. A HI of less than 1 suggests an exposure lower than the safety limit of the chemicals and the risk expected from the specified chemical is assumed not to be of concern (Bang et al., 2012).

## *Procedures for estimating ADIs*

The steps involved in estimating ADIs are discussed in detail.

### *Collection of adequate relevant data*

As noted in previous chapters, chemicals produce different toxicities. Consequently, a great variety of toxicity studies need to be carried out (see Chapter 20). Further, pharmacokinetic studies facilitate the assessment of the effects on humans from findings obtained in experimental animals. In addition, data need to be obtained from *relevant* studies. For example, findings of epithelial hyperplasia in the forestomach of rats given an irritant fumigant by gavage have little, if any, bearing on the possible adverse effects on humans consuming food that has been fumigated by the fumigant (Lu and Coulston, 1996).

The assessment of certain chemicals required less data for establishing their ADIs. Examples are food additives obtained from edible animals, plants, and microbes. The extent of testing and the reasons thereof have been described by WHO (1987).

### *No-observed adverse effect level (NOAEL)*

This is the maximal dose level that has not induced any sign of toxicity (adverse effect) in the most susceptible but appropriate species of animals tested, and using the most sensitive indicator of toxicity. As a rule, this level is selected from a long-term study. However, certain signs of toxicity such as cataracts, delayed neurotoxicity, and effects on reproduction are demonstrable in short-term studies. The NOAEL is not necessarily an absolutely no-effect level; rather it is a "no-observed adverse effect level," because the use of a more sensitive indicator of toxicity or a more susceptible animal species may reveal a lower NOAEL. Hence these chemicals are reassessed whenever significant new toxicological data become available. In addition, an effect might well be demonstrable if a sufficiently large number of animals were used in the tests. However, using experimental data and mathematical extrapolation, Lu (1985) and Lu and Seilken (1991) showed that increasing the number of animals would only reduce the NOAEL slightly. It should also be noted that part of the safety factor is intended to compensate for the limited sample number used in most tests.

On the other hand, certain effects are generally considered as physiological, adaptive, or otherwise "nontoxic." These effects are therefore excluded in establishing the NOAEL. For example, liver enlargement may result from stimulation in the activity of hepatic mixed-function oxidases and de novo protein synthesis in the smooth endoplasmic reticulum. A decrease of body weight may follow reduced food consumption, which in turn may be a result of unpalatability of the feed due to the chemical. The U.S. EPA has designated that a change in body weight greater than 10% denotes a relevant adverse manifestation that needs to be considered in the risk assessment. Feeding large amounts of inert substances such as mannitol and cellulose derivatives may produce diarrhea and malnutrition. However, before disregarding these effects in evaluating the toxicity of a chemical, care needs to be taken to ensure that these are not manifestations of toxicity.

NOAEL has been traditionally used for the estimation of ADI, RfD, or TDI, but the NOAEL approach cannot provide information regarding the shape of dose–response curves, and is strictly dependent upon dose selection, dose interval, and sample size. Therefore, a benchmark dose (BMD) model was alternatively introduced and BMD software programs are now available (Davis et al., 2011). In general, the BMD and BMD 95% lower confidence limit were higher than the NOAEL, but lower than the lowest-observed-adverse-effect level (Izadi et al., 2012).

### *Safety factors*

Safety is defined as the likelihood that a substance does not produce toxic response at given situations or exposure. Safety factor (SF) (also known as UF) is a composite (reductive) factor by which an observed or estimated NOAEL is divided to arrive at a criterion or standard that is considered safe or without appreciable risk. To extrapolate from the NOAEL in animals to an acceptable intake in humans, a safety factor of at least 100 is generally used (10 for individual variation in humans, 10 for the differences between humans and animals on the basis of a chronic study). This was originally proposed by Lehman and Fitzhugh (1954). This factor is intended to allow for differences in sensitivity of the animal species and humans, to allow for wide variations in susceptibility among the human population, and enable the fact that the number of animals tested is small compared to the size of the human population that may be exposed (WHO, 1958, 1974a; Food Safety Council, 1973).

Although the factor 100 is often used, the WHO expert committees have used figures that ranged from 10 to 2000. The size of the safety factor is determined according to the nature of the toxicity, the period of treatment (acute, subacute, chronic), and quality of data. Therefore, additional modifying factors (MFs) from 3 to 10 are multiplied by SF 100 to attain the final value of the safety factor (i.e., the final SF = MF × SF 100). In addition, a larger figure is used to compensate for slight deficiencies in toxicity data, such as relatively small numbers of animals on test. On the other hand, minimal, reversible, and inconsequential effects such as slight inhibition of acetylcholinesterase by an organophosphorus pesticide may justify the use of a smaller safety factor. In addition, available human data may warrant the use of a smaller figure, for example 10, since they obviate the need for interspecies extrapolation.

Biochemical data relating to absorption, distribution, metabolism (detoxication and bioactivation) and excretion (ADME) of the toxicant in various species of animals and in humans are often useful in determining the size of the safety factor. These and other bases for altering the safety factor are elaborated in two WHO documents (WHO, 1987, 1990). The reasons for the use of different safety factors, by WHO in the evaluation/reevaluation of the 230 pesticides in the past three decades, are noted and explained in a review by Lu (1995).

Some toxicologists prefer the use of individual uncertainty (safety) factors in extrapolating from a NOAEL to the corresponding oral RfD. These usually include a factor of 10 for intraspecies differences, a 10 for interspecies differences, a 10 for NOAEL derived from short-term toxicity studies, and so forth. (Dourson and Stara, 1983).

## *Exposure assessment*

The ADI is used as a yardstick to check the acceptability of the proposed uses. This is done by comparing the ADI with the "potential daily intake" (PDI). PDI is the sum of the products of the amounts of the food (calculated on the basis of the average per capita consumption) and permitted use levels of additives in them.

1PDI = $(F_1 \times L_1) + (F_2 \times L_2) + (F_3 \times L_3)$ ...where $F_1$, $F_2$, $F_3$,... are per capita consumption of food commodities and $L_1$, $L_2$, $L_3$,... are use levels of food additives, or maximum residue levels of pesticide residues or other contaminants.

If the PDI exceeds the ADI, the use levels may be lowered or some of the uses may be deleted. The Commission follows the same procedure in accepting the maximum limits for pesticide residues in food. The utilization of "PDI" and other estimated intakes by WHO in assessing the acceptability of food additives and pesticides is provided in some detail in a document WHO (1989) and summarized by Lu and Seilken (1991).

#### *Margins of safety for risk assessment*

The ADI approach is not designed to provide quantitative information on the risks involved with intakes higher than the ADI. This is because of the wide "gray area" between NOAEL and ADI. However, the margin of safety (MOS) between the estimated intake and ADI is sometimes used to indicate the degree of confidence in the safety at a specified intake. In general, the MOS needs to be greater than 100 to ensure human safety on the basis of SF 100 (10 for human variation and 10 for the difference between humans and animals), and lower values are considered unsafe for humans.

However, the acceptable criteria for MOS (= NOAEL/human exposure dose) may be dependent upon the quality of NOAEL values, whether data are obtained from a 3-month repeated toxicity test in animals (MOS = 100), are from a general human study (MOS = 10), or a susceptible human study such as a pregnant women study (MOS = 1). The MOS approach has been used for risk assessment of consumer products including cosmetics (Choi and Lee, 2015).

## *Mathematical models/risk assessment*

As discussed in Chapter 8, there are genotoxic and nongenotoxic carcinogens. It is generally agreed that there are probably no thresholds for genotoxic carcinogens. In view of the theoretical absence of threshold doses and absence of a reliable procedure to determine a threshold for a carcinogen for an entire population, estimating the levels of risk has been considered to be more appropriate.

### *Estimation of risks*

#### *Definition*

Risk has been defined as the expected frequency of undesirable effects arising from exposure to a pollutant or the probability that a substance might produce harm in humans under the specified condition. It may be expressed in absolute terms as the risk due to exposure to a specific pollutant. It may also be expressed as a relative risk, which is the ratio of the risk among the exposed population to that among the unexposed (WHO, 1978).

The term was first adopted by the International Commission on Radiological Protection (ICRP, 1966) in evaluating the health hazards related to ionizing radiation. The use of this term stems from the realization that often a clear-cut "safe" or "unsafe" decision cannot be made.

*Criteria for virtually safe doses*

Estimation of risks involves development of suitable dose–response data and extrapolation from observed dose–response relationship to expected responses at doses occurring at actual exposure situations. A number of mathematical models were proposed for this purpose. Such models are also used to estimate the dose that is expected to be associated with a specific level of risk.

Mantel and Bryan (1961) first introduced the concept of virtual safety. The term was defined as a probability of carcinogenicity of less than 1/100 million ($10^{-8}$) at a statistical assurance level of 99%. The U.S. FDA, however, found that the doses associated with such a low risk level were too small to be enforceable in most actual situations and thus adopted a risk level of $10^{-6}$ (FDA, 1977). These levels of risk are so low that the doses associated with them are referred to as VSDs.

*Human risks expected from man-made or natural activities*

In order to place the risk levels in perspective, risks associated with certain commonplace activities and natural occurrences are sometimes cited. Table 30.1 includes a number of estimates of such risks. The risks in Table 30.1, apart from lightning, are considerably greater than $10^{-6}$. Estimates of risks associated with other common activities and occupations have been compiled by others, for example, Wilson (1980).

The acceptability of a risk depends upon, apart from its magnitude, the nature of the activity. In general, risks associated with voluntary, pleasurable, and/or beneficial activities, such as smoking and driving, are more acceptable to the individual. On the other hand, risks associated with activities that are perceived as having no benefit and those that are not controllable by the individual tend to be rejected, such as food colors suspected of being carcinogenic.

***Table 30.1*** Estimated risks for certain activities and natural occurrences

| Activity | Risk[a] |
|---|---|
| Smoking (10 cigarettes/day) | 1/400 |
| All accidents | 1/2000 |
| Driving (16,000 km/yr) | 1/5000 |
| All traffic accidents | 1/8000 |
| Work in industry | 1/30,000 |
| Natural disasters | 1/50,000 |
| Being struck by lightning | 1/1,000,000 |

*Source:* Courtesy of the Controller of Her Majesty's Stationery Office, London.

[a] Risk is expressed as probability of death of an individual for a year of exposure and is given in round figures.

## *Models for estimating risks/virtually safe doses*

A number of mathematical models have been developed for the purpose of estimating the risks. In general, they involve extrapolating from the observed dose response to either of the following:

1. The risks at a specific exposure level.
2. The "risk-specific dose" is the dose associated with a specified risk. When the specified risk is low enough, for example, $10^{-5}$ or $10^{-6}$, the dose associated with it is generally known as the VSD.

### *Probability models*

As noted above, Mantel and Bryan (1961) first introduced the concept of virtual safety and developed a model based on the assumption that the responses (tumor formation) will be the same as most other quantal (all-or-none) toxicological responses, namely, normally distributed among the subjects.

This S-shaped dose–response curve can be straightened, as described in Chapter 6, by plotting the points on a *probit* basis. Variations of this probit model include *logit* and *Weibull*. These are also known as "tolerance models," as they are based on the probability of individuals in a population whose tolerances to the carcinogen will be exceeded.

### *Mechanistic models*

Several other models have been designed based on presumed mechanisms of action of carcinogenesis. The *one-hit* model assumes that a critical hit in a cell by a carcinogen may induce a cancer through initiation, promotion, and progression. On the other hand, the *multihit* model assumes that several hits are required for a response to occur. The *multistage* model is built on the assumption that induction of a carcinogenic response follows random biological events, the time rate of occurrence of each event being in linear proportion to the dose rate.

The conservativeness of these models is achieved through the use of upper confidence limits to responses on the risk estimated, shallow slopes, or the lower confidence limits on the VSD estimated. Figure 30.1 shows the observed responses, the upper confidence limit, and the linear interpolation.

Several U.S. regulatory agencies, including the EPA (1986), use the linearized multistage model (Anderson, 1986). With this model, it is presumed that no threshold dose exists, a multistage process (i.e., initiation, promotion, and progression) is involved in chemical carcinogenesis, and the time rate of occurrence of each event is linearly proportional to the dose.

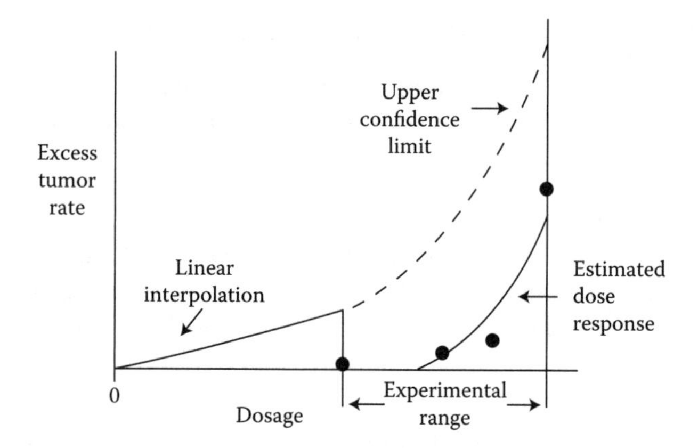


***Figure 30.1*** Linear extrapolation showing the observed responses, the upper confidence limit of the response at the lowest experimental dose, and the linear interpolation. (From Gaylor, DW, Kodell, RL, *J Environ Pathol Toxicol.*, 4, 305–12, 1980.)

Based on a set of aflatoxin $B_1$ carcinogenesis data, low-dose extrapolation was conducted with various models. The marked difference among these is clearly visible in Figure 30.2. The one-hit and multistage models yielded the most conservative estimates, whereas the probit model yielded the least conservative figure. According to the calculations of

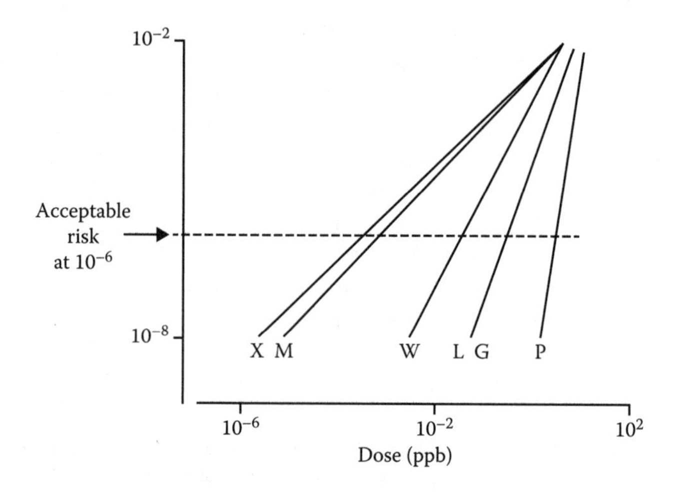


***Figure 30.2*** The low dose–response relationships based on a set of aflatoxin $b_1$ data, using different models: X, one-hit; M, multistage; W, Weibull; L, logit; G, multihit; and P, probit models. (From Krewski, D, Van Ryzin, J, *Statistical and Related Topics*, Elsevier/North Holland, New York, 1981.)

the Food Safety Council (1980), the VSDs at a risk of $10^{-6}$ are $3.4 \times 10^{-5}$ ppb (one-hit), $7.9 \times 10^{-4}$ (multistage), $4.0 \times 10^{-2}$ (Weibull), 0.28 (multihit), and 2.5 (probit).

In addition, *physiologically based pharmacokinetic (PBPK)* modeling was developed to utilize toxicokinetic (TK) differences between test animals and humans. For example, the target concentration of dichloromethane was about 150-fold higher in mice than in humans; these data provided a lower, probably more realistic estimate of the risk of this toxicant (Andersen et al., 1987). For additional examples, see Andersen and Krishnan (1994) and Dallas et al. (1995). A modified version, the *biologically based pharmacodynamic* model, also incorporates data on the interaction of the toxicant with tissues and response of the tissues (Conolly and Andersen, 1991). Although such modeling has certain advantages, it involves complex mathematical equations and the fact that the physiological parameters regarding various species and strains, disease states, and the like are often ill defined.

### *Other variations*

The *time-to-response,* instead of the response itself, has also been proposed for use in the mathematical models (Chand and Hoel, 1974; Sielken, 1981). The importance of this approach has been pointed out by the SOT ED01 Task Force (1981). *Background responses,* that is, those occurring also among the unexposed, are often observed. They can also be incorporated into mathematical models (Hoel, 1980).

The response of an organism to a toxicant is related to dose and duration of exposure. It is also affected by *competing risks.* Kalbfleisch et al. (1983) proposed mathematical models that take these three factors into account.

Since many carcinogens require bioactivation, the importance of incorporating *metabolic data* in evaluating their risks is obvious. For example, vinyl chloride is carcinogenic after bioactivation. Gehring et al. (1978) showed that the tumor incidence in rats exposed to various concentrations of this chemical was proportional to the metabolized amount rather than the exposure concentration (Table 30.2).

## *Cancer risk assessment*

Risk assessment is conducted by estimating the risk associated with a toxicant at an ascertained level of exposure, using an appropriate mathematical model described earlier. Where the risk level is low, for example, $10^{-6}$ or lower, the exposure might be considered acceptable. However, where the risk is higher, various *risk management* decisions may have to be taken. The options consist of lowering the exposure level, shortening the exposure duration, suspending the manufacture/use of chemicals, and others.

***Table 30.2*** Correlation between exposure concentration of vinyl chloride (VC), metabolism, and induction of hepatic angiosarcoma in rats

| Exposure concentration (ppm of VC) | VC/L of Air (μg) | VC metabolized (μg) | Percentage liver angiosarcoma |
|---|---|---|---|
| 50 | 128 | 739 | 2 |
| 250 | 640 | 2435 | 7 |
| 500 | 1280 | 3413 | 12 |
| 2500 | 6400 | 5030 | 22 |
| 6000 | 15,360 | 5003 | 22 |
| 10,000 | 25,600 | 5521 | 15 |

*Source:* Gehring, PJ et al., *Toxicol Appl Pharmacol.*, 44, 581–91, 1978.

For a carcinogenic agent (A), cancer risk can be estimated from the slope factor [$q_1^*$, $(\text{mg/kg-day})^{-1}$] of each carcinogen or carcinogenic potency factor (CPF) multiplied by a lifetime average daily dose (LADD, mg/kg/day) of the carcinogen as follows:

$$\text{Cancer risk} = \text{Slope factor } (q_1^*) \times \text{LADD}$$

## Other procedures

### Noncarcinogenic chemicals

Not all chemicals require the whole gamut of described toxicological testing for estimating ADIs. For example, for chemicals to which humans are not likely to be exposed to an appreciable extent, such as indirect food additives and certain pesticides, a *toxicologically insignificant amount* may be estimated on the basis of toxicological data that include at least 90-day feeding studies in two species of mammals and by the use of a larger safety factor (generally 1000) (NAS, 1965). The U.S. FDA and the U.S. EPA have adopted variations of this principle administratively.

Further, a *decision to reject a chemical* may be made on more limited data, especially in the course of developing new chemicals. Such data include extreme acute toxicity, positive response in short-term mutagenesis tests, or undesirable features in biochemical studies or short-term feeding studies in animals.

As discussed in the next section, most, if not all, of the nongenotoxic carcinogens are assessed by the ADI approach. Risk assessment protocols for various types of toxic agents such as noncarcinogens, carcinogens, nonsensitizers, and sensitizers are summarized in Table 30.3.

***Table 30.3*** A summary of risk assessment protocols for various types of toxic agents

| Types of agents | Critical information | Exposure data | Risk assessment | Criteria for human safety |
|---|---|---|---|---|
| Non-carcinogen | Safe limits (ADI, RfD, TDI) | CDI[a] | HI= CDI/ ADI | HI < 1 |
| Carcinogen | Slope factor ($q_1^*$) | LADD | Cancer risk = ($q_1^*$) × LADD | Risk < $1 \times 10^{-6}$ for consumers |
| Non-sensitizer (skin application) | NOAEL[b] or LOAEL | SED | MOS = NOAEL/SED | MOS ≥ 100[c] |
| Sensitizer | AEL (=NESIL/SAF) | CEL | AEL/CEL | AEL ≥ CEL |

*Note:* All abbreviations are summarized at Appendix 30.1.

[a] CDI: Chronic daily intake from all sources and routes (aggregate exposure).

[b] NOAEL: Assuming that NOAEL or LOAEL values obtained from at least a 3-month repeated toxicity test in animals.

[c] Criteria for MOS value may be varied depending upon the quality of NOAEL. If NOAEL is obtained from general human study or susceptible human study (e.g., pregnant women), the criteria for MOS will be 10 or 1.

## *Carcinogenic chemicals*

### *Chemicals with questionable data*

The Joint FAO/WHO Expert Committee on Food Additives during its second meeting (WHO, 1958) recommended that "no proved carcinogen should be considered suitable for use as a food additive in any amount." This principle has been followed at subsequent meetings of the Committee and at the Joint FAO/WHO Meetings on Pesticide Residues in not allocating ADIs to affirmed carcinogens by IARC. *Temporary or conditional ADIs,* however, have been estimated for chemicals with equivocal carcinogenicity data, such as nitrites and amitrole. On the other hand, *discontinuation* of the use of chemicals without essential functions has been recommended. The basis for the decisions on these and other such chemicals has been reviewed and summarized by Lu (1979). The principle of considering both the soundness of the carcinogenesis data and usefulness of the chemical is consistent with the policies of many national regulatory agencies (Somers, 1986).

### *Secondary and nongenotoxic carcinogens*

The concept of *secondary carcinogens,* which induce tumors only after certain noncarcinogenic effects, has been accepted by many toxicologists. For example, a WHO scientific group (WHO, 1974b) indicated that urinary bladder cancers in rats treated with Myrj 45 (polyoxyethylene monostearate) were induced by the bladder calculi rather than by the chemical directly and that a no-observed-effect level can therefore be established. A variety of other types of nongenotoxic carcinogens were discussed in Chapter 8. Many investigators suggested that the predominant mechanism whereby a chemical elicits a carcinogenic response needed to be considered in extrapolating lab data to humans (Reitz et al., 1990).

### *Risk assessment for nonsensitizers and sensitizers*

A risk assessment procedure for nonsensitizing ingredients in cosmetics requires information as to NOAEL of a chemical, skin absorption, and systemic exposure dose (SED) to estimate MOS (= NOAEL/SED). SED can be estimated as follows (SCCS, 2012):

$$SED\ (\text{mg/kg bw/day}) = A\ (\text{mg/kg bw/day}) \times C(\%)/100 \times DAp(\%)/100$$

$A$ (mg/kg bw/day) = Estimated daily exposure to a cosmetic product per kg body weight, based upon the amount applied and the frequency of application: See the calculated relative daily exposure levels for different cosmetic product types

$C$ (%) = the Concentration of the substance under study in the finished cosmetic product on the application site

$DAp$ (%) = Dermal Absorption expressed as a percentage of the test dose assumed to be applied in real life conditions

For quantitative risk assessment (QRA) of skin sensitizing agents, risk is acceptable if the acceptable exposure level (AEL) is equal to or larger than the consumer exposure level (CEL), that is AEL> CEL. If the CEL exceeds the AEL (AEL< CEL), the risk is not acceptable and reevaluation of the risk management is required. AEL (μg/cm$^2$) (= NESIL (μg/cm$^2$)/SAF) is derived from no expected sensitization induction level (NESIL) divided by sensitization assessment factors (SAFs), uncertainties associated with inter-individual variation (age, gender, genetics, etc.) (UF = 10) matrix differences (presence of irritants, penetration enhancer) (factors of 1–3 or 10) and use considerations (e.g., site of contact, barrier function, occlusion) (factors of 1–3 or 10) (RIFM, 2006; Api et al., 2008). This guideline was specifically developed for fragrance ingredients in cosmetics.

NESIL can be derived from animal and human data. From human studies, NOEL (no observed effect level) may be obtained from a Human Repeat Insult Patch Test (HRIPT) on at least 100 healthy volunteers or a Human Maximization Test (HMT, earlier precursors to the HRIPT such as the Modified Draize Test) to get NESIL.

NESIL value is also obtained from the EC3 value (%, the dose estimated to produce a three-fold increase in local lymph node proliferative activity from murine local lymph node assay [LLNA]) that can be used as a measure of relative potency (ECETOC, 2000). From the equation described below, an NESIL value can be obtained.

$$\text{Log (NESIL } (\mu g/cm^2)) = 1.16 \times (\text{Log EC3 } (\mu g/cm^2)) - 0.64 \text{ (Safford, 2008)}$$

## *Threshold of toxicological concern*

The Threshold of Toxicological Concern (TTC) approach is a tool that estimates a human exposure value below which no adverse health effects associated with a chemical of concern is expected to occur (Munro et al., 1999; Kroes et al., 2004). This TTC approach has been proposed to determine a conservative estimate of a chronic exposure to a chemical that is protective for both cancer and noncancer endpoints when sufficient chemical-specific safety information cannot be obtained (Munro et al., 1991; Kroes et al., 2000). This approach utilizes existing safety data on many hundreds of chemicals that are binned into different potency groups to establish exposure limits that are then considered to be protective for any chemical that is assigned to each bin. It is based on the concept that the chemical structure correlates with its potential toxicity, and structural features can be employed to categorize chemicals to different groups of chemicals of toxicological concern. The TTC values for no adverse effects have been established based on the analysis of the distribution of toxicity data, derived from various safety databases, using conservative assumptions on the potential toxicity of untested chemicals:

1. 0.15 μg/day (0.0025 μg/kg/day) for chemicals with a structural alert for genotoxicity
2. 18 μg/day (0.3 μg/kg/day) for organophosphates and carbamates
3. 90 μg/day (1.5 μg/kg/day), 540 μg/day (9 μg/kg/day), and 1800 μg/day (30 μg/kg/day) for Cramer Classes I, II, and III, respectively

Kroes at al. (2004) developed a decision tree which can be utilized to systematically assign a TTC value to a chemical of concern (Table 30.4). The decision tree considers first chemical structural characteristics associated with potential genotoxicity and carcinogenicity, and then potential systemic toxicity. Understanding of the chemical structure along with consumer exposure to a chemical of concern enables one to assess a chemical with limited safety information.

The application of the TTC approach as a pragmatic risk assessment tool has been well-established and accepted by several regulatory agencies

*Table 30.4* Tiered TTC limits

| TTC tier | TTC exposure limit in µg/day | TTC exposure limit in µg/kg/day* |
|---|---|---|
| Chemical with structural alerts or positive genotoxicity | 0.15 | 0.0025 |
| FDA threshold of regulation | 1.5 | 0.025 |
| Organophosphates/carbamates | 18 | 0.3 |
| Cramer class III (most toxic) | 90 | 1.5 |
| Cramer class II (intermediate) | 540 | 9 |
| Cramer class I (least toxic) | 1800 | 30 |

*Source:* Kroes, R et al., *Food Chem Toxicol.*, 42, 65–83, 2004.
**Assume body weight of 60 kg.*

(EFSA SC, 2012; SCCS, 2016; EFSA/WHO, 2016). There are still ongoing activities to expand the applicability domain of the TTC approach.

## *International activities in risk assessment*

### *Chemicals in food*

The World Health Organization and the Food and Agricultural Organization of the United Nations (FAO) have jointly established the Joint FAO/WHO Expert on Food Additives and Contaminants (JECFA) and the Joint FAO/WHO Meeting on Pesticide Residues (JMPR). JECFA deals with food additives, contaminants, and residues of veterinary drugs, and JMPR deals with residues of pesticides.

The principles of evaluation followed by these two expert bodies, culminating in the assessment of ADIs, are described in detail in two WHO documents (WHO, 1987, 1990). In this article, Lu emphasized two factors contributing to the wide acceptance of the ADIs assessed by JECFA and JMPR. First, there existed a close collaboration between these expert bodies and research scientists in academia, government, and industry. Second, the ADIs assessed by these expert bodies were used as a basis in the elaboration of international food standards, the Codex Alimentarius.

*Bisphenol A* (BPA), known as an endocrine-disrupting chemical (EDC), has been used for manufacturing a variety of industrial products and consumer products including baby bottles. However, the use of BPA in plastic food contact materials (FCMs) has been banned due to public issues on the potential adverse effects of BPA on reproductive, developmental, neurological, and endocrine toxicities. Denmark, in May 2010, banned the use of BPA in infant feeding bottles and all FCMs of foods particularly intended for children between 0 to 3 years of age (EU, 2011). Other European Union (EU) Member States including Sweden, France, Belgium, and Austria followed the ban on use of BPA in baby bottles, pacifiers, and soothers (EU, 2012). Further, BPA is listed as entry 1 176 in the Annex II list of substances prohibited in cosmetic products (EC, 2009). Since then, a ban on the use of BPA has been extended to other countries globally.

Canada is the first country that prohibited BPA in polycarbonate (PC) baby bottles on March 31, 2010. In the United States, the FDA has banned the use of BPA-based PC resins in baby bottles and spill-proof cups (sippy cups) since July 12, 2012 and a number of states in the United States also joined the ban on BPA. South America, Ecuador, Brazil, and the Republic of Argentina banned BPA in baby bottles between October 2011 and April 3, 2012.

In Asia, South Korea has banned the use of BPA in infant feeding bottles (including bottle nipples) since March 1, 2011, and China has banned BPA since June 1, 2011.

## *Other chemicals*

The WHO in conjunction with the United Nations Environment Program (UNEP), and the International Labor Organization (UNEP), have compiled, evaluated, and published more than 240 documents in the "Environmental Health Criteria" series. In general, they deal with subjects such as the identity, sources of human exposure, environmental transport, environmental levels, human exposure, kinetics, metabolism in animals and humans, effects on lab animals and *in vitro* systems, effects on humans, and evaluation of human health risks. These are critical reviews and summaries of the literature on these topics, including citations and references. These documents are thus a good source of toxicological and related topics on the environmental and occupational toxicants.

## *Websites for risk assessment*

There are useful websites available for researchers and the public on risk assessment and regulation: Integrated Risk Information System IRIS, https://www.epa.gov/iris), National Institute for Public Health (RIVM, http://www.rivm.nl/en), TOXNET (https://toxnet.nlm.nih.gov/newtoxnet/iter.htm), National Industrial Chemicals Notification and Assessment Scheme (NICNAS, http://www.nicnas.gov.au), Online interactive Risk Assessment (OiRA, https://osha.europa.eu/en/tools-and-publications/oira), Scientific Committee on Consumer Safety (SCCS, http://ec.europa.eu/health/scientific_committees/consumer_safety_en), and so forth.

# *Appendix 30.1 Terminology used in risk assessment*

| Term | Definition |
|---|---|
| Acceptable daily intake (ADI) | Estimated maximum amount of an agent, expressed on a body mass basis, to which individuals in a (sub) population may be exposed daily over their lifetimes without appreciable health risk. |
| Benchmark dose (BMD) | A dose that produces a predetermined change in response rate of an adverse effect (called the benchmark response or BMR) compared to background. |
| Biomarker | Indicator of changes or events in biological systems. Biological markers of exposure refer to cellular, biochemical, analytical, or molecular measures that are obtained from biological media such as tissues, cells, or fluids and are indicative of exposure to an agent. |
| Cancer potency Factor (or slope factor) | A value that expresses the incremental increased risk of cancer incidence from a lifetime exposure to a substance per unit dose. |
| Exposure scenario | A combination of facts, assumptions, and inferences that define a discrete situation where potential exposures may occur. These may include the source, the exposed population, the time frame of exposure, microenvironment(s), and activities. Scenarios are often created to aid exposure assessors in estimating exposure. |
| Extra risk | A measure of the proportional increase in risk of an adverse effect adjusted for the background incidence of the same effect. In other words, the ratio between the increased risk above background for a dose (d) divided by the proportion of the population not responding to the background risk. Extra risk is calculated as follows: $[P(d)-P(0)]/[1-P(0)]$, where P(d) is the probability of response risk at a dose d and P(0) is the probability of response at zero dose (i.e., background risk). |
| Extrapolation | Process of inferring an unknown from something that is known. (e.g., extrapolate from animal data to humans, from high dose effect to low dose effect, route-to-route extrapolation species extrapolation). |
| Hazard | Inherent property of an agent or situation having the potential to cause adverse effects when an organism, system, or (sub)population is exposed to that agent. |
| Interpolation | The process of determining a value within two known values in a sequence of values. |

*(Continued)*

| Term | Definition |
|---|---|
| Margin of safety (MOS) | Ratio of the NOAEL for the critical effect to the theoretical, predicted, or estimated exposure dose or concentration. |
| Margin of exposure (MOE) | Ratio of a dose that produces a specified effect, e.g., a benchmark dose, to an expected human dose. Alternatively, the LED10 or other point of departure divided by the actual or projected environmental exposure of interest. MOS is often interchangeably used as MOE. |
| Maximum likelihood estimate (MLE) | Estimate of a population parameter (under a specified model for sampling error), found by maximizing the likelihood function that is most likely to have produced the sample observations. |
| Point of departure (POD) | The dose-response point that marks the starting point for low-dose extrapolation. The POD may be a NOAEL/LOAEL, but ideally is established from BMD modeling of the experimental data, and generally corresponds to a selected estimated low-level of response (e.g., 1 to 10% incidence for a quantal effect). Depending on the mode of action and other available data, some form of extrapolation below the POD may be employed for estimating low-dose risk or the POD may be divided by a series of uncertainty factors to arrive at a reference dose (RfD). |
| Probability | The chance of a particular outcome or event occurring. Probability takes on values between 0 and 1 with 0 indicating that the event never occurs and 1 indicating that the event always occurs. |
| Reference dose (RfD) | An estimate of the daily exposure dose that is likely to be without deleterious effect even if continued exposure occurs over a lifetime. |
| Risk | The probability of an adverse effect in an organism, system, or (sub)population caused under specified circumstances by exposure to an agent; typically expressed on a scale of 0 to 1. |
| Risk analysis | A process for controlling situations where an organism, system, or (sub)population could be exposed to a hazard. The risk analysis process consists of three components: Risk assessment, risk management, and risk communication. |

(*Continued*)

| Term | Definition |
|---|---|
| Risk assessment | A process intended to calculate or estimate the risk to a given target organism, system, or (sub)population, including the identification of attendant uncertainties, following exposure to a particular agent, taking into account the inherent characteristics of the agent of concern as well as the characteristics of the specific target system. |
| Risk communication | Interactive exchange of information about (health or environmental) risks among risk assessors, managers, news media, interested groups, and the general public. |
| Risk management | Decision-making process involving considerations of political, social, economic, and technical factors with relevant risk assessment information relating to a hazard so as to develop, analyze, and compare regulatory and non-regulatory options and to select and implement appropriate regulatory response to that hazard. Risk management comprises three elements: Risk evaluation; emission and exposure control; and risk monitoring. |
| Safety | Practical certainty that adverse effects will not result from exposure to an agent under defined circumstances. It is the reciprocal of risk. |
| Safety factor (SF) | Composite (reductive) factor by which an observed or estimated NOAEL is divided to arrive at a criterion or standard that is considered safe or without appreciable risk. Uncertainty factor. |
| Stressor | Any entity, stimulus, or condition that can modulate normal functions of the organism or induce an adverse response (e.g., agent, lack of food, drought). |
| Threshold | Dose or exposure concentration of an agent below which a stated effect is not observed or expected to occur. |
| Tolerable daily intake (TDI) | Analogous to acceptable daily intake. |
| Toxicity | Inherent property of an agent to cause an adverse biological effect. |
| Uncertainty factor (UF) | Reductive factor by which an observed or estimated NOAEL is divided to arrive at a criterion or standard that is considered safe or without appreciable risk. |
| Validation | Process by which the reliability and relevance of a particular approach, method, process, or assessment is established for a defined purpose. |

*Source:* WHO, *IPCS Risk Assessment Terminology*, 2004; EPA, *A Framework for Assessing Health Risks of Environmental Exposures to Children*, 2006; EPA, *Benchmark Dose Technical Guidance*, 2012.

## *Further reading*

Crump KS (1984). A new method for determining allowable daily intakes. *Fundam Appl Toxicol.* 4, 854–71.

Dourson ML, Lu FC (1995). Safety/risk assessment of chemicals by different groups. *Biomed Environ Sci.* 8, 1–13.

EPA (1989). Biological Data for Pharmacokinetic Modeling and Risk Assessment. EPA/600/3–90/019, Washington, DC

FDA (1971). Food and Drug Administration Advisory Committee on Protocols for Safety Evaluation: Panel on carcinogenesis report on cancer testing in the safety evaluation of food additives and pesticides. *Toxicol Appl Pharmacol.* 20, 419–38.

Hart RW, Fishbein L (1985). Interspecies extrapolation of drug and genetic toxicity data. In: Clayson DB, Krewski D, Munro I, eds. *Toxicological Risk Assessment, vol. I.* Boca Raton, FL: CRC Press.

Munro IC (1988). Risk assessment of carcinogens: Present status and future direction. *Biomed Environ Sci.* 1, 51–8.

National Academy of Sciences (NAS) (1984). Toxicity Testing: Strategies to Determine Needs and Priorities. Washington, DC: National Academy of Sciences.

Ramsey JC, Gehring PJ (1980). Application of pharmacokinetic principles in practice. *Fed Proc.* 39, 60–5.

WHO (1957). General Principles Governing the Use of Food Additives. First Report of the Joint FAO/WHO Expert Committee on Food Additives. WHO Tech Rep Ser No. 129.

## *References*

Andersen ME, Clewell HJ, Gargas ML et al. (1987). Physiologically based pharmacokinetics and risk assessment process for methylene chloride. *Toxicol Appl Pharmacol.* 87, 185–205.

Andersen ME, Krishnan K (1994). Physiologically based pharmacokinetics and cancer risk assessment. *Environ Health Perspect.* 102(Suppl. 1), 103–8.

Anderson P (1986). Ninth Symposium on Statistics and the Environment. Washington, DC: National Academy of Sciences.

Api AM, Basketter DA, Cadby PA, Cano MF, Ellis G, Gerberick GF, Griem P et al. (2008). Dermal sensitization quantitative risk assessment (QRA) for fragrance ingredients. *Regul Toxicol Pharmacol.* 52(1), 3–23.

Bang DY, Kyung M, Kim MJ, Jung BY, Cho MC, Choi SM, Kim YW et al. (2012). Human risk assessment of endocrine-disrupting chemicals derived from plastic food containers. *Compr Rev Food Sci Food Safety.* 11(5), 453–70.

Chand N, Hoel W (1974). A comparison of models for determining safe levels of environmental agents. In: Proschan F, Serfling RJ, eds. *Reliability and Biometry.* Philadelphia, PA: SIAM, p. 681.

Choi SM, Lee BM (2015). Safety and risk assessment of ceramide 3 in cosmetic products. *Food Chem Toxicol.* 84, 8–17.

Conolly RB, Andersen ME (1991). Biologically based pharmacodynamic models: Tools for toxicological research and risk assessment. *Ann Rev Pharmacol Toxicol.* 31, 503–23.

Cotruvos JA (1988). Drinking water standards and risk assessment. *Regul Toxicol Pharmacol.* 8, 288–99.
Dallas CE, Chen XM, Muraledhara S et al. (1995). Physiologically based pharmacokinetic model useful in prediction of the influence of species, dose, and exposure route on perchloroethylene pharmacokinetics. *J Toxicol Environ Health.* 44, 301–17.
Davis JA, Gift JS, Zhao QJ (2011). Introduction to benchmark dose methods and U.S. EPA's benchmark dose software (BMDS) version 2.1.1. *Toxicol Appl Pharmacol.* 254, 181–91.
Dourson ML, Stara JF (1983). Regulatory history and experimental support of uncertainty (safety) factors. *Regul Toxicol Pharmacol.* 3, 224–38.
European Commission (EC) (2009). Regulation (EC) No 1223/2009 of the European Parliament and of the Council of 30 November 2009 on cosmetic products, OJ L 342, 22.12.2009, pp. 59–209.
ECETOC (2000). ECETOC Monograph 29: Skin Sensitisation Testing for the Purpose of Hazard Indentification and Risk Assessment.
EFSA SC (2012). Scientific opinion on exploring options for providing advice about possible human health risks based on the concept of Threshold of Toxicological Concern (TTC). *EFSA J.* 10, 2750.
EFSA/WHO (2016). Review of the Threshold of Toxicological Concern (TTC) approach and development of new TTC decision tree. EFSA Supporting publication 2016: EN–1006.
EPA (1986). Guides for carcinogenic risk assessment. *Fed Regul.* 51, 33992–4003.
EPA (2006). A Framework for Assessing Health Risks of Environmental Exposures to Children. EPA/600/R-05/093F September 2006. Available at: https://cfpub.epa.gov/ncea/risk/recordisplay.cfm?deid=158363.
EPA (2012). Benchmark Dose Technical Guidance. EPA/100/R-12/001 June 2012. Available at: https://www.epa.gov/sites/production/files/2015-01/documents/benchmark_dose_guidance.pdf.
EU (European Commission) (2011). Commission Regulation (EU) No 10/2011 of 14 January 2011 on plastic materials and articles intended to come into contact with food. OJ L 12, 15.1.2011, pp. 1–89.
EU (European Commission) (2012). Regulation No 1442/2012 of 24 December 2012 aiming at banning the manufacture, import, export and commercialization of all forms of food packaging containing bisphenol A. OJ of the French Republic (OJFR), 26.12.2012, text 2 of 154.
FDA (1977). Chemical compounds in food-producing animals: Criteria and procedures for evaluating assays for carcinogenic residues in edible products of animals. *Fed Regul.* 42(35), 10412–37.
Food Safety Council (1973). Proposed system for food safety assessment. *Food Cosmet Toxicol.* 16, 1–136.
Food Safety Council (1980). Proposed system for food safety assessment. *Food Cosmet Toxicol.* 16(Suppl. 2), 160.
Gaylor DW, Kodell RL (1980). Linear interpolation algorithm for low dose risk assessment of toxic substances. *J Environ Pathol Toxicol.* 4, 305–12.
Gehring PJ, Watanabe PC, Park CN (1978). Resolution of dose–response toxicity for chemicals requiring metabolic activation: Example vinyl chloride. *Toxicol Appl Pharmacol.* 44, 581–91.

Hoel DG (1980). Incorporation of background in dose–response models. *Fed Proc.* 39, 73–5.
ICRP (1966). Recommendations of the International Commission on Radiological Protection. ICRP Publication No. 9. Oxford: Pergamon Press.
Izadi H, Grundy JE, Bose R (2012). Evaluation of the benchmark dose for point of departure determination for a variety of chemical classes in applied regulatory settings. *Risk Anal.* 32, 830–5.
Kalbfleisch JD, Krewski D, van Ryzin J (1983). Dose–response models for time to response toxicity data. *Can J Stat.* 11, 25–49.
Krewski D, Van Ryzin J (1981). Dose–response models for quantal response toxicity data. In: Csorgo M, Dawson D, Rao JNK, Shilah E, eds. *Statistical and Related Topics.* New York: Elsevier/North Holland.
Kroes R, Galli C, Munro I, Schilter B, Tran L, Walker R, Würtzen G (2000). Threshold of toxicological concern for chemical substances present in the diet: A practical tool for assessing the need for toxicity testing. *Food Chem Toxicol.* 38, 255–312.
Kroes R, Renwick AG, Cheeseman M, Kleiner J, Mangelsdorf I, Piersma A, Schilter B et al., (2004). Structure-based thresholds of toxicological concern (TTC): Guidance for application to substances present at low levels in the diet. *Food Chem Toxicol.* 42, 65–83.
Lehman AJ, Fitzhugh OG (1954). 100-Fold margin of safety. *Q Bull Assoc Food Drug Officials US.* 18, 33–5.
Lu FC (1979). The safety of food additives. The dynamics of the issue. In: Deichman WB, ed. *Toxicology and Occupational Medicine.* New York: Elsevier/North-Holland.
Lu FC (1985). Safety assessment of chemicals with thresholded effects. *Regul Toxicol Pharmacol.* 5, 460–4.
Lu FC (1995). A review of the acceptable daily intakes of pesticides assessed by WHO. *Regul Toxicol Pharmacol.* 21, 352–64.
Lu FC, Coulston F (1996). A safety assessment based on irrelevant data. *Ecotoxicol Environ Saf.* 33, 100–1.
Lu FC, Seilken RL (1991). Assessment of safety/risk of chemicals: Inception and evolution of the ADI and dose–response modeling procedures. *Toxicol Lett.* 59, 5–40.
Mantel N, Bryan WR (1961). "Safety" testing of carcinogenic agents. *J Natl Cancer Inst.* 27, 455–70.
Munro IC, Kennepohl E, Kroes R (1999). A procedure for the safety evaluation of flavouring substances. Joint FAO/WHO Expert Committee on Food Additives. *Food Chem Toxicol.* 37, 207–32.
National Academy of Sciences (NAS) (1965). Report on "No Residue" and "Zero Tolerance." Washington, DC: National Academy of Sciences.
NRC (National Research Council) (1977). Drinking Water and Health, vol. 1. Washington, DC: National Academy of Sciences.
NRC (National Research Council). (1983). Risk Assessment in the Federal Government: Managing the Process. Washington, DC: National Academy Press.
Paustenbach DJ (2000). The practice of exposure assessment: A state-of-the-art review. *J Toxicol Environ Health Part B.* 3, 179–291.
Reitz RH, Mendrala AL, Corley R et al. (1990). Estimating the risk of liver cancer associated with human exposure to chloroform. *Toxicol Appl Pharmacol.* 105, 443–59.

RIFM (The Research Institute for Fragrance Materials). (2006). Dermal Sensitization Quantitative Risk Assessment (QRA) for Fragrance Ingredients. Available at: www.ifraorg.org/view_document.aspx?docId=22180.
Safford RJ (2008). The Dermal Sensitisation Threshold—A TTC approach for allergic contact dermatitis. *Regul Toxicol Pharmacol.* 51(2), 195–200.
SCCS (Scientific Committee on Consumer Safety) (2012). The SCCS notes of guidance for the testing of cosmetic ingredients and their safety evaluation (8th revision).
SCCS (Scientific Committee on Consumer Safety) (2016). The SCCS notes of guidance for the testing of cosmetic ingredients and their safety evaluation (9th revision).
Sielken RL Jr (1981). Re-examination of the ED01 study: Risk assessment using time. *Fundam Appl Toxicol.* 1, 88–123.
Somers E (1986). The weight of evidence: Regulatory toxicology in Canada. *Regul Toxicol Pharmacol.* 6, 391–8.
Song JB, Ahn IY, Cho KT, Kim YJ, Kim HS, Lee BM (2013). Development and application of risk management system in Korea for consumer products to comply with global harmonization. *J Toxicol Environ Health Part B.* 16(1), 1–16.
SOT ED01 Task Force (1981). Re-examination of the ED01 Study. *Fundam Appl Toxicol.* 1, 26–128.
WHO (1958). Procedures for the Testing of Intentional Food Additives to Establish Their Safety in Use. Second Report. WHO Tech Rep Ser No. 144.
WHO (1962a). Evaluation of the Toxicity of a Number of Antimicrobials and Antioxidants. Sixth Report. WHO Tech Rep Ser No. 228.
WHO (1962b). Principles Governing Consumer Safety in Relation to Pesticide Residues. Report of a Joint FAO/WHO Meeting on Pesticide Residues. WHO Tech Rep Ser No. 240.
WHO (1974a). Toxicological Evaluation of Certain Food Additives with a Review of General Principles and of Specifications. Seventeenth Report. WHO Tech Rep Ser No. 539.
WHO (1974b). Assessment of the Carcinogenicity and Mutagenicity of Chemicals. Report of a WHO Scientific Group. WHO Tech Rep Ser No. 546.
WHO (1978). Principles and Methods for Evaluating the Toxicity of Chemicals. Environ Health Criteria 6. Geneva, Switzerland: World Health Organization.
WHO (1987). Principles for the Safety Assessment of Food Additives and Contaminants in Food. Environ Health Criteria No. 70.
WHO (1989). Guidelines for Predicting Dietary Intakes of Pesticide Residues. Geneva, Switzerland: World Health Organization.
WHO (1990). Principles for the Toxicological Assessment of Pesticide Residues in Food. Environ Health Criteria 104.
WHO (2004). IPCS Risk Assessment Terminology. Available at: http://www.inchem.org/documents/harmproj/harmproj/harmproj1.pdf.
Wilson R (1980). Risk-benefit analysis for toxic chemicals. *Ecotoxicol Environ Safety.* 4, 370–83.

# Chemical Index

## A

*B*

*D*

## N



## O

## W



## X



## Y



## Z

# Subject Index

## A

## D

## *I*



## *J*



## *K*

## N



## O

## *P*

## S



## T